Geriatrics, Lifestyle Medicine and Healthy Aging

Geriatrics, Lifestyle Medicine and Healthy Aging: A Practical Guide is a book for those interested in promoting healthy aging through lifestyle approaches. The book is divided into three sections covering various aspects of lifestyle medicine for older individuals including general concepts of lifestyle medicine practices; lifestyle "pillars" as applied to older adults; and a broad range of target conditions of importance to older adults, and how a lifestyle medicine approach may impact them. Readers gain an understanding of how lifestyle medicine and geriatrics can work together to provide a holistic approach that fosters healthy aging throughout life.

Features

- Research-supported analysis of the relevance of lifestyle medicine in geriatric populations
- Evidence-based discussion of conditions that impact quality of life in older adults, including sarcopenia, incontinence, bone health, polypharmacy and falls, and how lifestyle medicine can prevent and treat such conditions
- Edited by a leading expert in the fields of healthy aging and lifestyle medicine in older adults

As part of the *Lifestyle Medicine* series edited by Dr. James M. Rippe, this book is useful to geriatric medicine clinicians who would like to increase the tools in their practice of caring for older adults; lifestyle medicine clinicians who want to understand how to effectively use lifestyle pillars to care for older adults; and anyone who is interested in their own, or a loved one's, healthy aging.

LIFESTYLE MEDICINE

Series Editor

James M. Rippe
Professor of Medicine, University of Massachusetts Medical School

Led by James M. Rippe, MD, founder of the Rippe Lifestyle Institute, this series is directed to a broad range of researchers and professionals consisting of topical books with clinical applications in nutrition and health, physical activity, obesity management, and applicable subjects in lifestyle medicine.

Manual of Lifestyle Medicine
James M. Rippe

Obesity Prevention and Treatment
A Practical Guide
James M. Rippe and John P. Foreyt

Improving Women's Health across the Lifespan
Michelle Tollefson, Nancy Eriksen, and Neha Pathak

Lifestyle Nursing
Gia Merlo and Kathy Berra

Integrating Lifestyle Medicine in Cardiovascular Health and Disease Prevention
James M. Rippe

Integrating Lifestyle Medicine for Prediabetes, Type 2 Diabetes, and Cardiometabolic Disease
Michael Via and Jeffrey Mechanick

Empowering Behavior Change in Patients
Practical Strategies for the Healthcare Professional
Beth Frates and Mark Faries

Lifestyle Psychiatry
Through the Lens of Behavioral Medicine
Gia Merlo and Christopher P. Fagundes

Lifestyle Nutrition
Eating for Good Health by Lowering the Risk of Chronic Diseases
James M. Rippe

Lifestyle Medicine and the Primary Care Provider
A Practical Guide to Enabling Whole Person Care
Ron Stout, Daniel Reichert, and Rebecca Kelly

Geriatrics, Lifestyle Medicine and Healthy Aging
A Practical Guide
Susan M. Friedman

For more information, please visit: www.routledge.com/Lifestyle-Medicine/book-series/CRCLM

Geriatrics, Lifestyle Medicine and Healthy Aging

A Practical Guide

Edited by
Susan M. Friedman, MD, MPH
Founding Director, Highland Hospital
Lifestyle Medicine
Professor of Medicine
University of Rochester School of
Medicine and Dentistry

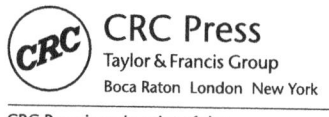

CRC Press
Taylor & Francis Group
Boca Raton London New York

CRC Press is an imprint of the
Taylor & Francis Group, an **informa** business

Designed cover image: Shutterstock

First edition published 2026
by CRC Press
2385 NW Executive Center Drive, Suite 320, Boca Raton, FL 33431

and by CRC Press
4 Park Square, Milton Park, Abingdon, Oxon, OX14 4RN

CRC Press is an imprint of Taylor & Francis Group, LLC

© 2026 Taylor & Francis Group, LLC

This book contains information obtained from authentic and highly regarded sources. While all reasonable efforts have been made to publish reliable data and information, neither the author[s] nor the publisher can accept any legal responsibility or liability for any errors or omissions that may be made. The publishers wish to make clear that any views or opinions expressed in this book by individual editors, authors or contributors are personal to them and do not necessarily reflect the views/opinions of the publishers. The information or guidance contained in this book is intended for use by medical, scientific or health-care professionals and is provided strictly as a supplement to the medical or other professional's own judgement, their knowledge of the patient's medical history, relevant manufacturer's instructions and the appropriate best practice guidelines. Because of the rapid advances in medical science, any information or advice on dosages, procedures or diagnoses should be independently verified. The reader is strongly urged to consult the relevant national drug formulary and the drug companies' and device or material manufacturers' printed instructions, and their websites, before administering or utilizing any of the drugs, devices or materials mentioned in this book. This book does not indicate whether a particular treatment is appropriate or suitable for a particular individual. Ultimately it is the sole responsibility of the medical professional to make his or her own professional judgements, so as to advise and treat patients appropriately. The authors and publishers have also attempted to trace the copyright holders of all material reproduced in this publication and apologize to copyright holders if permission to publish in this form has not been obtained. If any copyright material has not been acknowledged please write and let us know so we may rectify in any future reprint.

Except as permitted under U.S. Copyright Law, no part of this book may be reprinted, reproduced, transmitted, or utilized in any form by any electronic, mechanical, or other means, now known or hereafter invented, including photocopying, microfilming, and recording, or in any information storage or retrieval system, without written permission from the publishers.

For permission to photocopy or use material electronically from this work, access www.copyright.com or contact the Copyright Clearance Center, Inc. (CCC), 222 Rosewood Drive, Danvers, MA 01923, 978-750-8400. For works that are not available on CCC please contact mpkbookspermissions@tandf.co.uk

Trademark notice: Product or corporate names may be trademarks or registered trademarks and are used only for identification and explanation without intent to infringe.

ISBN: 9781032638539 (hbk)
ISBN: 9781032632889 (pbk)
ISBN: 9781032638560 (ebk)

DOI: 10.1201/9781032638560

Typeset in Times
by Deanta Global Publishing Services, Chennai, India

In loving memory of my mother – my role model for aging with grace, purpose, love and dignity. Her influence helped shape both the content of and the approach to this book.

And with enormous gratitude to my husband – my rock and my steadying influence – who always encourages me to take things one step at a time, and to keep moving forward.

Contents

Preface x
Acknowledgments xii
Editor xiii
Contributors xiv

SECTION 1 General Principles

Chapter 1 The Rationale for Lifestyle Medicine in Geriatrics 3
Kamal Wagle and Susan M. Friedman

Chapter 2 Promoting Healthy Aging: A Lifecycle Approach 17
Susan M. Friedman

Chapter 3 The Reality of Aging 33
Rebecca Masutani and Rosanne Leipzig

Chapter 4 Confronting Ageism with Language and Lifestyle Medicine 45
Kaitlin Kyi

Chapter 5 Climate Change, Lifestyle Medicine and Older Adults 52
Matthew Nelson and Jennifer Muniak

Chapter 6 Lifestyle Medicine in a Geriatric Primary Care Practice 71
Kamal Wagle

SECTION 2 Lifestyle Medicine Pillars as Applied to Older Adults

Chapter 7 Why Exercise? Sedentarism, Physical Activity and Exercise among Older Adults 89
Jorge C. Mora and Willy Marcos Valencia

Chapter 8	Physical Activity and Exercise Recommendations among Older Adults	104
	Jorge C. Mora, and Edgar Ramos Vieira	
Chapter 9	Nutrition Care for the Older Adult	117
	Melissa Bernstein and Alison Reyes	
Chapter 10	Malnutrition in Older Adults: A Lifestyle Medicine Approach	133
	Susan M. Friedman, Melissa Bernstein and Alison Reyes	
Chapter 11	Sleep and Older Adults	149
	Brian House	
Chapter 12	Social Connection: An Essential Lifestyle Pillar for Older Adults	162
	Susan M. Friedman	
Chapter 13	Stress and Its Impact on Older Adults	177
	Meredith Troutman-Jordan and Boyd H. Davis	
Chapter 14	Toxins and Older Adults	191
	Kaku Kuroda	

SECTION 3 Target Issues

Chapter 15	Sarcopenia	209
	Aruna Nathan	
Chapter 16	Navigating the Landscape of Dementia and Elevating Brain Health in Later Life	229
	Ecler Ercole Jaqua, Mai-Linh N. Tran and Monica Gupta	
Chapter 17	Depression	248
	Fiona Yan-Yee Ho and Vincent Wing-Hei Wong	

Contents

Chapter 18 Urinary Incontinence in Older Adults: A Lifestyle Medicine Approach 264

Cristina H. Davis, Dawn Woods, Kamal Wagle and Kelly Freeman

Chapter 19 Resilience 282

Halina Kusz and Ali Ahmad

Chapter 20 Palliative Care in Older Adults: A Lifestyle Medicine Approach 302

Tiffany Jackson and Cristina H. Davis

Chapter 21 Polypharmacy and Deprescribing 320

Fatoumata Jallow, Patti A. Parker and Kathryn M. Daniel

Chapter 22 Caregiver Health 328

Paul Mulhausen

Chapter 23 Reducing Fall Risk with Lifestyle Changes 342

Crystal Arrendell

Chapter 24 Obesity in Older Adults: Lifestyle Medicine Perspective 353

Shenbagam Dewar and John A. Batsis

Chapter 25 Osteoporosis and Bone Health 367

Jatupol Kositsawat, Faryal Mirza and Patrick P. Coll

Chapter 26 A Lifestyle Medicine Approach to Constipation 379

Aarti Oza Bedi, Susan Spell and Deborah Chielli

Index 403

Preface

The field of lifestyle medicine has grown exponentially over the last few decades. This has been driven in part by a recognition by both practitioners and patients that the current system is not adequately addressing the need for the prevention and management of chronic disease. We are witnessing the earlier onset of chronic illness and a system that was built on a framework of acute illness, poorly prepared to address the overwhelming preponderance of chronic disease. Because insurance incentives are not aligned to help guide patients to make and sustain meaningful changes, these efforts are often done outside of standardized medicine, without oversight to ensure evidence-based approaches. For many, there is a perception that lifestyle medicine is focused on prevention when its real power is in managing and reversing the impact of chronic disease through addressing root causes.

Geriatrics, which has been recognized by the ABIM since 1988 as a specialty, focuses on the care of older adults. Older adults bear the brunt of chronic illness, with nearly 95% of people over the age of 65 experiencing at least one chronic condition, and nearly 80% having two or more. Older adults understand the impact of chronic disease and want to maintain function and quality of life for as long as possible. Geriatricians have expertise in eliciting goals of care, understanding and addressing complexity and working with a patient's care network to assure the best outcomes according to a patient's values and priorities.

Geriatrics shares a common set of goals and values with lifestyle medicine. Both fields are evidence-based, and both acknowledge the importance of systems in assuring optimal outcomes. Both provide patient-centered care, guided by the patient's wishes, with the goal of preserving function and optimizing quality of life.

The two fields have skills and approaches that can inform and complement each other. Because Geriatrics works predominantly with patients with established chronic disease, the issues relevant to the treatment of patients with chronic illness and multimorbidity can inform lifestyle medicine. Geriatricians understand heterogeneity – heterogeneity of goals, strengths, resources, levels of physical function and cognition. On the other hand, lifestyle medicine provides an opportunity to treat the root causes of disease, thereby facilitating outcomes that are important in Geriatrics, such as reducing polypharmacy and preventing or reducing frailty.

Geriatrics, Lifestyle Medicine and Healthy Aging: A Practical Guide provides a cohesive resource of evidence-based information about lifestyle medicine in the older adult, written by experts in both geriatric medicine and lifestyle medicine. By bringing the two fields together, this book provides material that helps practitioners in both disciplines to improve care for their patients. For the lifestyle medicine clinician, it provides overall and condition-specific information to facilitate working with older adults. For the geriatrician, it provides an additional "arrow in the quiver" for helping patients improve function and quality of life by reducing the burden of multimorbidity.

Preface

This book covers a variety of important topics in providing lifestyle medicine to older adults, in three sections. The first section discusses general concepts that are important to the application of lifestyle medicine to older adults. The introductory chapter presents the rationale for lifestyle medicine in Geriatrics. The second describes healthy aging as a lifecycle event, reviewing the origins and progression of chronic disease. The third chapter in this section discusses the realities of aging, and the fourth addresses ageism, its impact, and ways to address it. The next chapter addresses climate change as a lifestyle issue, and how it will impact older adults and opportunities for healthy aging. The final chapter of the initial section presents a framework for incorporating lifestyle medicine principles into a Geriatrics primary care practice.

The second section discusses the lifestyle "pillars" that have been identified by the American College of Lifestyle Medicine (exercise, nutrition, sleep, social connection, stress management and toxin avoidance) as applied to older adults. Each chapter presents epidemiologic considerations in older adults, and then discusses issues specific to older adults in addressing these lifestyle pillars.

The final section provides a review of issues that are of importance in Geriatrics, and how a lifestyle medicine approach can impact these target conditions. Target conditions for discussion include sarcopenia; dementia and brain health; depression; urinary incontinence; resilience; palliative care; polypharmacy and deprescribing; caregiver health; falls; obesity; osteoporosis and bone health; and constipation.

As our older adult population continues to grow, it is essential that we develop systems that enable individuals to live their best lives at every stage of life. This requires thinking about healthy aging throughout the lifecycle, and provides opportunities over many decades to improve health and well-being in old age. The fields of lifestyle medicine and geriatric medicine have substantial overlap, as well as complementary approaches, that can help to foster this outcome. I hope that this book will help to inform providers from multiple disciplines in a way that helps us all to age well.

Susan M. Friedman, MD, MPH
Rochester, New York

Acknowledgments

Numerous individuals have made significant contributions to every phase of the writing, editing and production of this textbook, and for that, I am sincerely grateful.

First and foremost, I would like to thank and acknowledge the outstanding work of each chapter author of the book. Their expertise in the fields of geriatric medicine and lifestyle medicine has led to an evidence-based book that provides clinically useful information in providing care to older patients.

Many thanks to Dr. James Rippe, whose foresight in developing this series provided this opportunity, and whose guidance and encouragement throughout this process have been invaluable.

Thanks to the editorial staff at Taylor & Francis/CRC Press: Randy Brehm, Senior Editor, who has been an early champion of lifestyle medicine books; and Tom Connelly, Editorial Assistant in the Life Sciences, who handled many of the details of the book prior to publication. Thanks also to Pradiksha Dharsini, who served as Project Manager for the book.

Editor

Susan M. Friedman has been a practicing geriatrician for over 30 years, and has spent more than a decade focusing on fostering healthy aging, incorporating geriatrics and lifestyle medicine into her clinical work, teaching, program development, research and advocacy. She obtained her undergraduate, MD and MPH degrees from Northwestern University, Chicago, Illinois, and completed a General Internal Medicine residency and Geriatrics Fellowship in the Johns Hopkins University system, based at Hopkins Bayview Hospital, Baltimore, Maryland. She was on faculty at Johns Hopkins for five years before moving to the University of Rochester, Rochester, New York, in 2000.

Dr. Friedman is a Professor of Medicine at the University of Rochester School of Medicine and Dentistry, in the Division of Geriatrics. She is the Medical Director of the university's lifestyle medicine program based at Highland Hospital. She has authored more than 50 peer-reviewed papers, which have been cited more than 3000 times, and was the lead author of the American Geriatrics Society's White Paper on Healthy Aging.

Contributors

Ali Ahmad, MD, DABIM
Department of Medicine
McMaster University
Western University
Ontario, Canada

Crystal Arrendell, MD
Department of Medicine
Johns Hopkins University
Baltimore, Maryland

John A. Batsis, MD
Department of Nutrition
University of North Carolina
Chapel Hill, North Carolina

Aarti Oza Bedi, MD, FASGE, DipABLM
Ann Arbor, Michigan

Melissa Bernstein, PhD, RDN, LD, FAND, DipACLM, FACLM
Department of Nutrition
Rosalind Franklin University of Medicine and Science
Chicago, Illinois

Deborah Chielli, MSN, AGNP, DipACLM
Passan School of Nursing
Wilkes University
Wilkes-Barre, Pennsylvania

Patrick P. Coll, MD, AGSF, CMD
Center on Aging
UConn Health
Farmington, Connecticut

Kathryn M. Daniel, PhD, APRN, AGPCNP-BC, GS-C, AGSF, FAAN
(Deceased)
University of Texas at Arlington
College of Nursing and Health Innovation
Arlington, Texas

Boyd Davis, PhD
University of North Carolina at Charlotte
Charlotte, North Carolina

Cristina H. Davis, MSN, APRN, AGPCNP-BC, ACHPN, DipACLM
Four Seasons Palliative Care and Buncombe County Employee Health
Asheville, North Carolina

Shenbagam Dewar, MD
Department of Internal Medicine
University of Michigan Medical School
Ann Arbor, Michigan

Kelly Freeman, MSN, AGPCNP-BC, DipACLM
American College of Lifestyle Medicine
Chesterfield, Missouri

Monica Gupta, DO
Family Medicine Department
Hoag Medical Group
Costa Mesa, California

Fiona Yan-Yee Ho, PhD
Department of Psychology
The Chinese University of Hong Kong
Hong Kong

Contributors

Brian House, MD, MPH
Department of Medicine
University of Rochester School of
 Medicine and Dentistry
Rochester, New York

Tiffany Jackson, DNP, NP-C, ACHPN
School of Nursing
University of North Carolina at
 Charlotte
Charlotte, North Carolina

Fatoumata Jallow, PhD, RN, APRN,
 FNP-C
University of Texas at Arlington
College of Nursing and Health
 Innovation
Arlington, Texas

Ecler Ercole Jaqua, MD, MBA,
 FAAFP, AGSF, FACLM, DipABOM,
 AAHIVS
Family Medicine Department
Loma Linda University School of
 Medicine
Loma Linda, California

Jatupol Kositsawat, MD, DMSc, MPH
Center on Aging
UConn Health
Farmington, Connecticut

Kaku Kuroda, MD, CAS
Department of Medicine
University of Rochester School of
 Medicine and Dentistry
Rochester, New York

Halina Kusz, MD, FACP, AGSF,
 DipABLM
Department of Medicine
Michigan State University
East Lansing, Michigan

Kaitlin Kyi, MD
Department of Medicine
University of Michigan
Ann Arbor, Michigan

Rosanne Leipzig, MD, PhD
Brookdale Department of Geriatrics
 and Palliative Medicine
Icahn School of Medicine at Mount
 Sinai
Mount Sinai, New York

Rebecca Masutani, MD
Brookdale Department of Geriatrics
 and Palliative Medicine
Icahn School of Medicine at Mount
 Sinai
Mount Sinai, New York

Faryal Mirza, MD, FACE, FACP
Department of Medicine
UConn Health
Farmington, Connecticut

Jorge C. Mora, MD, MPH
Department of Internal Medicine
Herbert Wertheim FIU College of
 Medicine
Westchester, Florida

Paul Mulhausen, MD, MHS, FACP,
 AGSF
Department of Internal Medicine
University of Iowa Carver College of
 Medicine
Iowa City, Iowa

Jen Muniak, MD
Department of Medicine
University of Rochester School of
 Medicine and Dentistry
Rochester, New York

Aruna Nathan, MD, DipABLM
Absolute Care LLC
Columbia, Maryland

Matthew Nelson, MD
Department of Medicine
University of Rochester School of Medicine and Dentistry
Rochester, New York

Patti A. Parker, PhD, RN, ANP, GNP, BC, GS-C
Department of Graduate Nursing
University of Texas at Arlington
College of Nursing and Health Innovation
Arlington, Texas

Alison Reyes, MS, RDN, LDN, IFNCP
Sodexo Health Care Services
West Newbury, MA

Susan Spell, MSN, FNP-BC, DipACLM
Vital Transformations LLC
University of Florida St. Johns Care Connect, Mobile Outreach Clinic
St. Johns, Florida

Mai-Linh N. Tran, MD, FAAFP, DipABLM, DipABOM, AAHIVS
Family Medicine Department
Loma Linda University School of Medicine
Loma Linda, California

Meredith Troutman-Jordan, PhD, RN, PMHCNS-BC, FGSA
School of Nursing
College of Health and Human Services
University of North Carolina at Charlotte
Charlotte, North Carolina

Willy Marcos Valencia, MD, MSc
Cleveland Clinic
Department of Endocrinology, Diabetes & Metabolism and Center for Geriatric Medicine
Cleveland, Ohio

Edgar Ramos Vieira, PhD, MSc PT, BSc PT
Nicole Wertheim College of Nursing and Health Sciences
Westchester, Florida

Kamal Wagle, MD, MPH, CMD, DipABLM, AGSF
Department of Family Medicine
Hackensack Meridian School of Medicine
Hackensack, New Jersey

Vincent Wing-Hei Wong, PhD
Department of Psychology
The Chinese University of Hong Kong
Hong Kong

Dawn Woods, PharmD, DipACLM
Birmingham, Alabama

Section 1

General Principles

1 The Rationale for Lifestyle Medicine in Geriatrics

Kamal Wagle and Susan M. Friedman

HISTORY OF LIFESTYLE MEDICINE AND GERIATRICS

Physicians and healers from ancient times have highlighted lifestyle as a foundation for good health. In modern times, the fields of basic science, public health, clinical care and clinical research recognize lifestyle factors as root causes of diseases. The term "lifestyle medicine" was first coined over five decades ago.[1] In recent years, there has been a movement in two major components of lifestyle medicine: Exercise as Medicine[2] and Food as Medicine.[3] Other lifestyle factors are also emphasized in various guidelines: stress management, avoidance of risky substances, restorative sleep and social connection. The American College of Lifestyle Medicine (ACLM) was founded in 2004 and is composed of individuals from multiple and diverse disciplines under one umbrella. It was founded with a vision of lifestyle medicine being "the foundation of health and all health care," and with a mission of "advancing evidence-based lifestyle medicine to treat, reverse and prevent non-communicable, chronic diseases."[4] Lifestyle medicine encompasses a holistic view of all these six important lifestyle factors otherwise known as lifestyle pillars and their assessment is also referred to as lifestyle vital signs[5] (see Table 1.1).

"Geriatrics," on the other hand, was first coined in 1914 by Ignatz Leo Nascher.[6] The term was derived from the word "geronto" which referred to a counsel of men over 60 years of age in Athens.[6] Marjory Warren (1897–1960) laid much of the groundwork for the field, through 27 articles in geriatrics, and introduced rehabilitation programs and a discussion on the positive attributes of aging.[6,7] The inclusion of geriatrics in research, scholarly activities, and policy created momentum in the field of geriatrics. The American Geriatrics Society was founded in 1942, and its mission is "to improve the health, independence and quality of life of all older adults." Some of the key components of the vision include person-centered care, a team-based approach, promoting the health and safety of older adults, and advocacy.[8]

TABLE 1.1
Lifestyle Pillars

🍎	Healthy diet
🏃	Physical exercise
🧠	Stress management
☠️	Avoidance of risky substances
🛏️	Restorative sleep
👥	Social connections

PHYSIOLOGICAL CHANGES IN AGING

Understanding changes in the human body and its physiological systems is key to understanding geriatrics practice. It is probably one of the most important concepts that health care team members should consider while making assessments and plans for every patient. Every aspect of cellular metabolism is known to be affected by the aging process.[9] Aging is a systemic process with physiological changes that occur in every organ and body system.[10] Changes in cellular metabolism lead to physiological changes, and understanding these fundamental changes is important to appreciate the approach to caring for the older adult population.[11] However, every individual's aging is also a unique journey; there are multiple facets influencing the complexities of aging, adding heterogeneity to the aging process.

A strength of the human body is its physiologic reserve, which will let us maintain our physiology despite external stressors such as infections, dehydration, changes in daily routine, etc. This phenomenon is called "homeostasis." Due to cellular and systemic changes with aging, physiologic reserve gradually declines, leading to impairment of homeostasis, otherwise known as "homeostenosis."[12] Lifestyle factors can help preserve physiologic reserve and delay homeostenosis by delaying or preventing the onset of chronic diseases.[13,14] Shortening of telomere length is recognized as a hallmark of aging and a pilot study has indicated that comprehensive lifestyle intervention increased relative telomere length, further underscoring its relationship with healthy aging.[15]

TRENDS IN GERIATRICS

LIFESTYLE TRENDS

Diet is the leading cause of mortality and disability-adjusted life years in the United States.[16] Studies of national surveys indicate that diet quality among older US adults is getting poorer over time.[17] For example, from 2001 to 2018, the mean consumption of whole grains, fruits and vegetables decreased, whereas the mean consumption of sugar-sweetened beverages, sodium and processed meat increased.[17] Sedentary behavior is correlated with poor health outcomes.[18] A systematic review on the prevalence of sedentary behaviors in older adults found that 60% of older adults sit for more than 4 hours a day and 65% of older adults sit in front of a screen for more than 3 hours a day.[19] This clearly represents an opportunity to intervene to create a healthier community. National surveys indicate that adherence to physical activity guidelines in older adults has modestly improved over time but continues to remain low (27.3% for the National Health and Nutrition Examination Survey [NHANES], 35.8% for the National Health Interview Survey [NHIS] and 44.3% for the Behavioral Risk Factor Surveillance System [BRFSS]), further illustrating a significant public health opportunity for intervention.[20] A recent report showed less than 15% of older adults meeting the criteria for aerobic and muscle-strengthening activity recommendation from Physical Activity Guidelines for Americans.[21]

Social isolation has always been a health concern for older adults even pre-COVID. Social isolation and loneliness have been recognized as risk factors for mortality.[22] The National Health and Aging Trends Study report in 2020 suggested that 24% of older adults in the community were socially isolated.[23]

The American Psychological Association (APA) defines psychosocial stressors as those factors in one's life that lead to an increase in the level of stress and that may contribute to overall health and behavior.[24] Some reasons for the psychosocial stressors in an aging population are high levels of loneliness, reduction in the subjective sense of social status, increase in financial burden, reduction in social bonding and increased prevalence of chronic diseases. Psychosocial stressors are known to independently increase frailty in older adults.[25] A study by Almeida et al, revealed that compared to prior decades, American adults, in general, have higher levels of stress.[26] Their study showed that the greatest increase is among the middle-aged group, many of whom are entering older adulthood; it will be interesting to follow the trends as those who are currently middle-aged become older adults. This highlights the need for targeted interventions to cope with psychosocial stressors as we age. A more complete discussion of these lifestyle pillars – their trends, and relevance to the health of older adults – can be found in the second section of this book.

CHRONIC DISEASE TRENDS

As per the National Center for Health Statistics National Health Interview Survey, 13.2% of older adults reported diabetes in 1997, with an increase to 21.5% in 2018. In this 21-year time period (1997 to 2018), the prevalence of other chronic diseases among older adults changed as follows: cancer, 19.4% to 25.8%; COPD, 10.6% to 13.7%; asthma, 7.6% to 11.7%; stroke, 7.8% to 8.9%; hypertension, 46.7% to 57%; and heart disease, 31.6% to 29.1%.[27] Of note, the prevalence of heart disease is reported to be stable among 18–54 year olds and among those who are 75 and over; and has been decreasing for individuals who are 55–74.[28] This is speculated to be due to improved interventions in cardiovascular diseases and their risk factors.

Obesity rates among older adults increased from 22% in 1988–1994 to 40% in 2015–2018.[27] The prevalence of older adults with two or more chronic comorbidities increased from 60.8% to 63.7% from 2010 to 2018.[29] Overall, more older adults now have multimorbidity, and the prevalence of chronic diseases has increased as well.[30] A multi-state population study projects a significant increase in the prevalence of older adults with chronic diseases and multiple chronic diseases in the next three decades.[31]

Longevity

The population is aging globally, and for the first time in 2018, older adults outnumbered children 5 years or younger in 2018.[32] In the United States, older adults are expected to outnumber children in 2034.[33] Life expectancy for the US population decreased from 2019 to 2021, going from 78.5 in 2019 to 77 in 2020, and 76.4 in 2021.[34] In 2022, life expectancy in the United States increased to 77.5 years, but it is still lower than it was in 2019. Although the dip in 2020 was secondary to COVID, the trend also illustrates the overall state of public health in the United States, and the gap between the United States and comparable countries is increasing.[32]

CLINICAL EVALUATION OF OLDER ADULTS AND GERIATRICS PRINCIPLES OF CARE

Geriatric Syndromes

Older adults' health problems are often affected by multiple factors and their management plans are multifaceted. "Geriatric syndromes" are complex problems with multiple contributing factors, leading to various clinical symptoms and signs and needing a multi-pronged approach for management.[35,36] Examples include: impaired gait, falls, incontinence, depression, forgetfulness, weight loss, failure to thrive and frailty. A systematic literature review concluded that multiple geriatric syndromes share some common risk factors such as advanced age, cognition, function and mobility.[36] Other than age, these risk factors can be reduced through lifestyle medicine pillars.

COMPREHENSIVE GERIATRIC ASSESSMENT (CGA)

CGA is a framework that provides a comprehensive and holistic assessment of an older adult. How a patient gets up, walks, uses the bathroom, dresses, eats and manages their personal hygiene are the basic functions, otherwise known as activities of daily living, or ADLs. The ability to prepare meals, go from one place to another, pay bills, use devices such as cell phones, manage health concerns and keep appointments are other important facets of function, known as instrumental activities of daily living, or IADLs. CGA includes evaluation of ADLs and IADLs; cognition; home safety; mobility; falls screening; screening for geriatric syndromes; assessment of vision and hearing; advance care planning; and evaluation of family and social support. Patients can undergo CGA in every setting from community-dwelling older adults to those in hospitals or senior care facilities, and are evaluated by a multidisciplinary team.[37] CGA is an approach to evaluating an older adult that leads to an understanding of their functional strengths and limitations and guides the approach to improving their quality of life.[38] CGA is a proactive and holistic approach to evaluating older adults and has been shown to improve the care of older adults.

GERIATRICS 5MS ASSESSMENT

The core competencies of the CGA have been packaged by US and Canadian geriatric societies as the Geriatric 5Ms: Mind, Mobility, Medications, Multicomplexity and Matters Most.[39,40] An assessment of the 5Ms can also guide a health care team to decide which areas of the assessment needs more in-depth focus. The Geriatric 5M concept is a simple way of communicating what CGA offers.[38-40] _Mind_ includes assessment of mood and cognition, and uncovers problems such as depression, anxiety, cognitive impairment and delirium. _Medication_ includes assessment of high-risk medications for older adults, medication interactions, supplements and over-the-counter medicines a patient is taking and polypharmacy. _Mobility_ includes assessment of function, gait and fracture risk, as well as fall prevention. _Multicomplexity_ includes assessment of recent hospitalizations, transitions of care, social support and complex multimorbidities of the older adult that cumulatively influence well-being. And the fifth M, what _Matters most_, encompasses older adults' core goals and care preferences, which are assessed by doing advance care planning, assessment of core values (a "what-matters" discussion) and understanding what provides meaning and purpose in their life. Table 1.2 shows these 5Ms of geriatrics and what is assessed in each of the Ms.[40,41]

TABLE 1.2
5Ms of Geriatrics

5Ms of Geriatrics	What Do We Assess?
Mind	Mentation, cognition
Mobility	Gait, balance, falls
Medications	Polypharmacy, high-risk medication usage
Multi-complexity	Multimorbidity and their overall effects on health, complexity of living conditions and social factors that influence health
Matters most	Eliciting each individual's health outcome goals and care preferences

Geriatrics 5M assessment nudges health care teams to focus on patient priorities, maximize functional abilities, address geriatric syndromes, initiate interventions to help address multiple health problems/geriatric syndromes and optimize social and behavioral health; thereby setting the stage for further evaluation.

HEALTHY AGING: MODELS AND FRAMEWORKS

Successful Aging

Rowe and Kahn developed a construct for successful aging which they proposed as a state where all three conditions are met: a) avoiding diseases and disability related to disease; b) maintaining high cognitive and physical function; and c) staying highly engaged in life.[42] This construct may help in nudging older adults to stay engaged in life, to continue to do physical activities and pursue hobbies that can help them maintain physical and cognitive function, and can encourage them in health promotion and staying on top of chronic disease management.

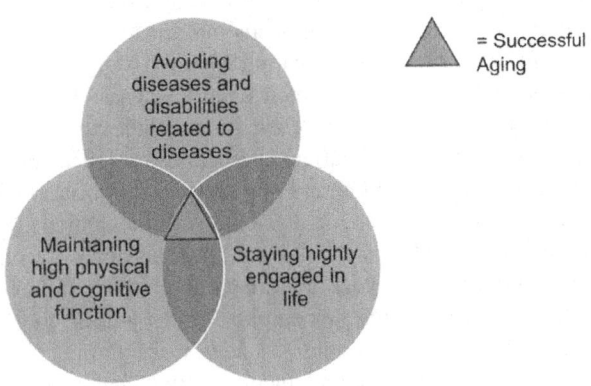

FIGURE 1.1 Successful aging as per the Rowe and Khan model.

Compression of Morbidity

Chronic diseases are the leading cause of disability.[43] With modern medicine, life expectancy increased over time, but we are also seeing an increase in the population living with chronic diseases[28] and disabilities.[44] Compression of morbidity is a term suggesting a reduction in years of life spent with chronic conditions.[45] One goal of healthy aging is the compression of morbidity, with a delay in the onset of diseases and disabilities and an increase in the years of a healthy lifespan. From an epidemiological metrics point of view, a health-adjusted life expectancy (HALE) and disability-adjusted life years (DALYs) can provide some data in understanding

The Rationale for Lifestyle Medicine in Geriatrics

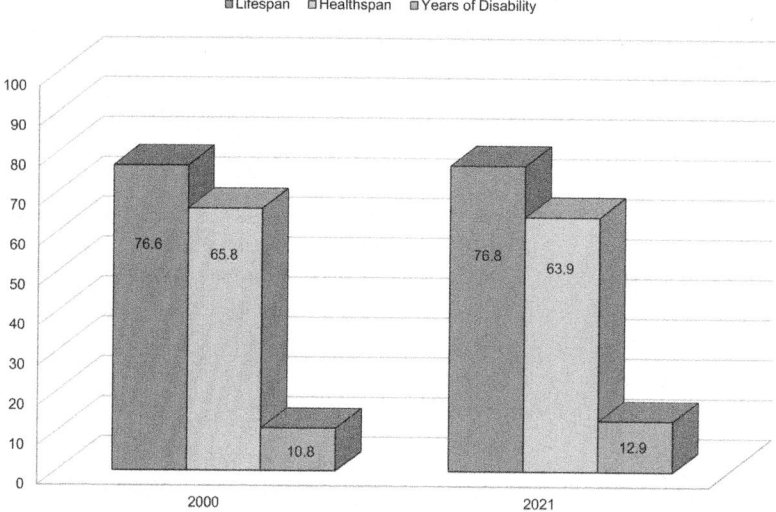

FIGURE 1.2 Total lifespan and healthspan in the United States in 2000 and 2021.

the compression of morbidity and healthy lifespan of a country. HALE is a measure of the number of years a person lived in good health, whereas DALYs are the years of life lost in disability and due to premature death. HALE can be looked at as a "healthspan" of an individual's life, whereas lifespan would include both HALE and years spent with disability. In the United States, HALE decreased from 65.8 years in 2000 to 63.9 years in 2021.[46] Years spent with a disability increased during that time, from 10.8 to 12.9 years. The goal of healthy aging is to increase lifespan and healthspan while decreasing the time spent with a disability.

GLIDEPATHS

The population of older adults is heterogeneous in terms of their overall health, life expectancy, functional independence, and frailty. Addressing clinical concerns has to consider this heterogeneity while being mindful of patient preferences and goals of care and engaging them in shared decision-making.[47] In general, older adults may fit into these four categories in terms of their overall health: (a) robust – with a life expectancy of 5 or more years and functional independence; (b) frail – with a life expectancy of less than 5 years and significant dependence in functional status; (c) moderate dementia with or without functional impairment and life expectancy of 2 to 10 years; and (d) near end-of-life older adult with less than 2 years of life expectancy.[47,48] Consideration of these categories may help frame discussions and clinical decision-making.

TABLE 1.3
Clinical Glidepath for Older Adults

Categories in Terms of Overall Health	Description
Robust	Life expectancy of 5 years and functional independence
Frail	Life expectancy of less than 5 years and significant dependence on functional status
Moderately demented	Life expectancy from 3 to 10 years
End of life	Life expectancy less than 2 years

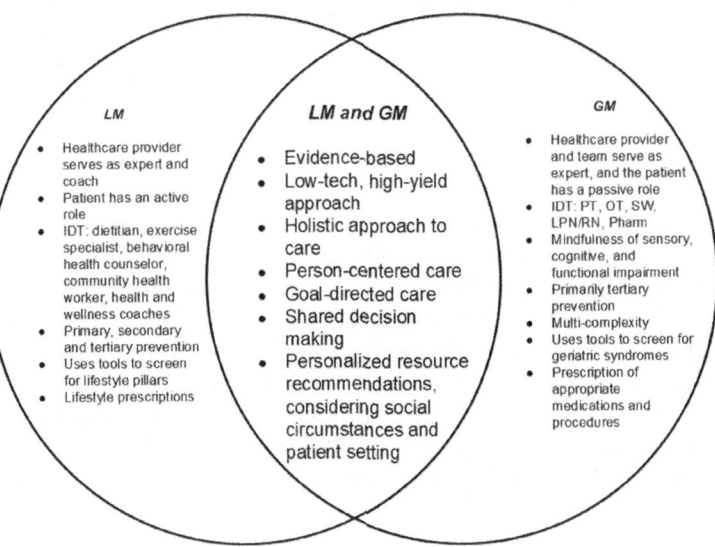

FIGURE 1.3 Venn diagram illustrating common attributes of lifestyle medicine and geriatric medicine. (LM = lifestyle medicine, GM = geriatric medicine, IDT = interdisciplinary team, PT = physical therapy, OT = occupational therapy, SW = social worker, LPN/RN = licensed practical nurse, registered nurse, Pharm= pharmacist.)

INTER-RELATIONSHIP OF LIFESTYLE MEDICINE AND GERIATRICS

Geriatrics and lifestyle medicine have significant commonalities in both their approaches and goals, but also have distinct differences (Figure 1.3).

The relationship between the geriatrician and patient is different from that of the lifestyle medicine physician and patient. In the former, the physician is viewed as the "expert," and gives recommendations that are then discussed by the patient and their caregivers. In lifestyle medicine, the physician has a dual role that includes the educational component of the "expert" role, but also incorporates the role of the coach. The patient has an active role in carrying out mutually agreed-upon steps and behavior changes.

The Rationale for Lifestyle Medicine in Geriatrics

Both geriatrics and lifestyle medicine use an interdisciplinary team, but the makeup of the core members differs. In lifestyle medicine, the core team may include a dietician, an exercise specialist, a behavioral health counselor, a community health worker and health and wellness coaches.[49] In geriatrics, interdisciplinary core team members include physical and occupational therapists, a social worker, a nurse and may include a pharmacist in some settings.[50]

The focus of lifestyle medicine is on all levels of prevention: primary, secondary and tertiary; but the focus of geriatric medicine is primarily on tertiary prevention. In lifestyle medicine, the team assesses lifestyle pillars, whereas in geriatric medicine, the team does a comprehensive assessment of function including sensory assessment (hearing and vision) along with screening for geriatric syndromes. In lifestyle medicine, lifestyle prescriptions are prescribed, whereas in geriatric medicine there is judicious and appropriate prescription of medications and procedures. Both specialties are evidence-based; despite the emphasis on tertiary prevention in geriatric medicine, both specialties also address all three levels of prevention. Both specialties are low-tech and high-yield approaches and have holistic approaches to care. Both specialties are person-centered and incorporate an understanding of social determinants of health while employing shared decision-making for interventions.

HOW THE PILLARS OF LIFESTYLE MEDICINE IMPACT OUTCOMES IMPORTANT IN GERIATRICS

Lifestyle medicine pillars provide a common approach to preventing and treating chronic conditions and geriatric syndromes. Figure 1.4 depicts lifestyle medicine pillars as a foundation of older adults' health and hence the 5M approach to their

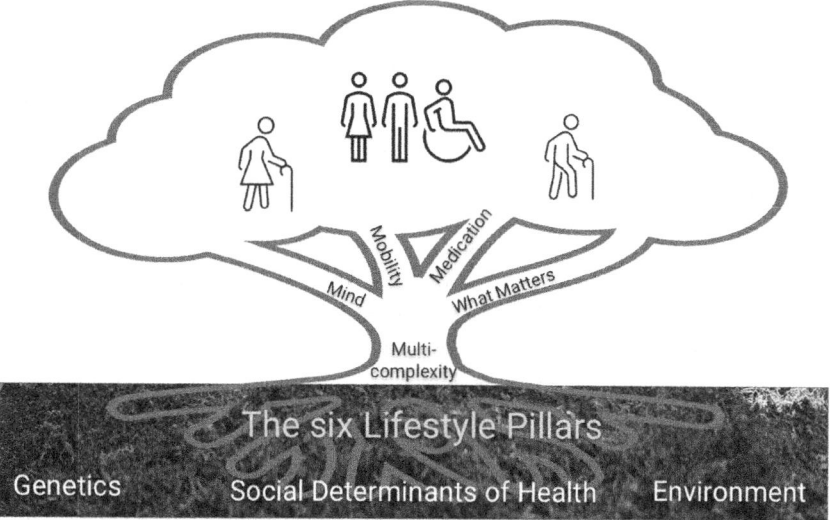

FIGURE 1.4 The six pillars of lifestyle support the 5Ms of geriatrics with the goal of patient-centered and holistic care.

assessment and care. It is never too early and never too late to optimize one's lifestyle to prevent and stabilize chronic diseases. A healthy lifestyle in older adults has been established as an approach to increase healthspan and reduce years with disability.[51] Incidence of geriatric syndromes such as depression and dementia are shown to be reduced by lifestyle modifications[52,53] and a healthy lifestyle reduces polypharmacy.[54] A healthy lifestyle is also helpful to prevent other geriatric syndromes such as falls and osteoporosis.[55] Subsequent chapters will discuss the connection between lifestyle and various disorders and syndromes in more detail. As depicted in Figure 1.4, the treatment of the patient results from addressing both lifestyle pillars and the 5Ms of geriatrics. The approach in lifestyle medicine is personalized by considering the patient outcomes as the goal, based on what matters to them; this fosters the geriatric medicine approach of patient-centeredness.

HOW THE PRINCIPLES OF GERIATRICS IMPACT OUTCOMES IN LIFESTYLE MEDICINE

Geriatrics focuses on function and well-being, which are probably the core and fundamental health outcomes for an individual. Using the goal of improving function and assessing and addressing patient goals can help to motivate them to make lifestyle changes. For example, a patient may want to improve their mobility so as to be able to play with their grandchildren, and so the lifestyle pillar of physical activity becomes important.

A comprehensive geriatric assessment uncovers geriatric syndromes including sensory health such as hearing and vision. Uncovering these concerns and addressing them can pave the path to improving communication for discussing lifestyle medicine interventions.

Similarly, understanding geriatric syndromes can help prioritize lifestyle interventions that are of most importance to the patient. Reducing polypharmacy is often a priority for older adults, and understanding this priority helps tailor lifestyle medicine approaches and motivate patients. An example would be limiting salt intake to reduce hypertension, and eating more fiber to address constipation, thereby reducing pill load for the patient. The geriatrics approach includes addressing a dyad of a patient and caregiver or a family partner who is closely supporting the older adult. Lifestyle interventions can be more effective when the older adult–caregiver dyad is considered and their support is incorporated into care planning that considers a person's frailty level or where the person is in the Glidepath framework discussed above. It should be noted that social determinants of health, functional status, life expectancy and 5M assessment of older adults guide what lifestyle interventions would be most valuable for the older adult.

CONCLUSIONS

Older adulthood is a vulnerable stage of life due to physiological changes, the prevalence of chronic diseases and changing environments and support systems. Geriatric medicine provides principles of geriatrics assessments and a comprehensive approach to addressing complex health problems of older adults. Lifestyle pillars serve as shared root causes for complex health problems and with the lens of lifestyle medicine, one can positively influence a person's whole health. Both of these specialties go hand-in-hand in improving the health of older adults and each of these specialties can influence the other, leading to improved outcomes for older adults. Older adults are the "canary in the coalmine," so if systems are improved for older adults, it is likely to provide better outcomes for all.

CLINICAL APPLICATIONS

- Ample studies provide evidence supporting the notion that it is never too early or too late to optimize lifestyle factors, to impact the quality of life of older adults and to make progress in healthy aging.
- Strengthening one's lifestyle pillars can lead to prevention, reduction, or delay in the onset of geriatric syndromes.
- Lifestyle interventions are first-line approaches for not only prevention but also for the treatment of multiple morbidities of older adults.

REFERENCES

1. Yeh BI, Kong ID. The advent of lifestyle medicine. *J Lifestyle Med*. 2013 Mar;3(1):1-8. Epub 2013 Mar 31. PMID: 26064831; PMCID: PMC4390753.
2. Tipton CM. The history of "exercise is medicine" in ancient civilizations. *Adv Physiol Educ*. 2014;38(2):109–117. doi:10.1152/advan.00136.2013.
3. Bleich SN, Dupuis R, Seligman HK. Food is medicine movement–key actions inside and outside the government. *JAMA Health Forum*. 2023;4(8). doi:10.1001/jamahealthforum.2023.3149.
4. American College of Lifestyle Medicine. About us. *ACLM*. Published online 2024. https://lifestylemedicine.org/about-us/.
5. Grega ML, Shalz JT, Rosenfeld RM. American College of Lifestyle Medicine expert consensus statement: lifestyle medicine for optimal outcomes in primary care. *Am J Lifestyle Med*. 2024;18(2):269–293. doi:10.1177/15598276231202970.
6. Morley JE. A brief history of geriatrics. *J Gerontol Ser A*. 2004;59(11):1132–1152. doi:10.1093/gerona/59.11.1132.
7. Dr MDA. Marjory Warren and the origin of British geriatrics. *J Am Geriatr Soc*. 1984;32:253–258.
8. Published online 2024. www.americangeriatrics.org.
9. Catic A. Cellular metabolism and aging. *Prog Mol Biol Transl Sci*. 2018;155:85–107. doi:10.1016/bs.pmbts.2017.12.003.
10. Boss GR, Seegmiller JE. Age-related physiological changes and their clinical significance. *West J Med*. 1981 Dec;135(6):434-40. PMID: 7336713; PMCID: PMC1273316.
11. Taffet GE. Physiology of aging. In: Wasserman MR, Bakerjian D, Linnebur S, Brangman S, Cesari M, Rosen S, eds. *Geriatric Medicine*. Springer; 2023. doi:10.1007/978-3-030-01782-8_103-1.

12. Kuchel GA. Systems physiology of aging and selected disorders of homeostasis. In: Halter JB, Ouslander JG, Studenski S, et al., eds. *Hazzards Geriatric Medicine and Gerontology.* 8th ed. McGraw-Hill; 2022.
13. Kreouzi M, Theodorakis N, Zones CCLLFB. Lifestyle medicine pillars and beyond: an update on the contributions of behavior and genetics to wellbeing and longevity. *Am J Lifestyle Med.* 2022. doi:10.1177/15598276221118494.
14. Song S, Stern Y, Gu Y. Modifiable lifestyle factors and cognitive reserve: a systematic review of current evidence. *Ageing Res Rev.* 2022. doi:10.1016/j.arr.2021.101551.
15. Ornish D, Lin J, Chan JM, et al. Effect of comprehensive lifestyle changes on telomerase activity and telomere length in men with biopsy-proven low-risk prostate cancer: 5-year follow-up of a descriptive pilot study. *Lancet Oncol.* 2013;14(11):1112–1120. doi:10.1016/S1470-2045(13)70366-8.
16. Murray CJ. The state of us health, 1990–2010: burden of diseases, injuries, and risk factors. *JAMA.* 2013;310(6):591–608. doi:10.1001/jama.2013.13805.
17. Long T, Zhang K, Chen Y, Wu C. Trends in diet quality among older us adults from 2001 to 2018. *JAMA Netw Open.* 2022;5(3):e221880. doi:10.1001/jamanetworkopen.2022.1880.
18. Dogra S, Stathokostas L. Sedentary behavior and physical activity are independent predictors of successful aging in middle-aged and older adults. *J Aging Res.* 2012;2012(190654). doi:10.1155/2012/190654.
19. Harvey JA, Chastin SF, Skelton DA. Prevalence of sedentary behavior in older adults: a systematic review. *Int J Environ Res Public Health.* 2013 Dec 2. doi:10.3390/ijerph10126645.
20. Keadle SK, McKinnon R, Graubard BI, Troiano RP. Prevalence and trends in physical activity among older adults in the United States: a comparison across three national surveys. *Prev Med.* 2016. doi:10.1016/j.ypmed.2016.05.009.
21. U.S. Department of Health and Human Services. *Physical Activity Guidelines for Americans Midcourse Report: Implementation Strategies for Older Adults.* 2023.
22. Holt-Lunstad J, Smith TB, Baker M, Harris T, Stephenson D. Loneliness and social isolation as risk factors for mortality: a meta-analytic review. *Perspect Psychol Sci.* 2015. doi:10.1177/1745691614568352.
23. Donovan NJ, Blazer D. Social isolation and loneliness in older adults: review and commentary of a national academies report. *Am J Geriatr Psychiatry.* 2020. doi:10.1016/j.jagp.2020.08.005.
24. https:/dictionary.apa.org/ (accessed 11/10/2024)
25. Shakya S, Silva SG, McConnell ES, McLaughlin SJ, MP C Jr. Psychosocial stressors associated with frailty in community-dwelling older adults in the United States. *J Am Geriatr Soc.* 2024. doi:10.1111/jgs.18821.
26. Almeida DM, Charles ST, Mogle J, et al. Charting adult development through (historically changing) daily stress processes. *Am Psychol.* 2020. doi:10.1037/amp0000597.
27. Aging-Related Statistics FIF. *Older Americans 2020: Key Indicators of Well-Being.* U.S. Government Printing Office; 2020.
28. https://www.cdc.gov/nchs/hus/topics/heart-disease-prevalence.htm#ref2
29. Ward BW, Schiller JS, Goodman RA. Multiple chronic conditions among US adults: a 2012 update. *Prev Chronic Dis.* 2014. doi:10.5888/pcd11.130389.
30. Boersma P, Black LI, Ward BW. Prevalence of multiple chronic conditions among US adults, 2018. *Prev Chronic Dis.* 2020;17(200130). doi:10.5888/pcd17.200130.
31. Ansah JP, Chiu CT. Projecting the chronic disease burden among the adult population in the United States using a multi-state population model. *Front Public Health.* 2023 Jan 13. doi:10.3389/fpubh.2022.1082183.

32. https://www.healthsystemtracker.org/chart-collection/u-s-life-expectancy-compare-countries/#Life%20expectancy%20at%20birth,%20in%20years,%201980-2022
33. Vespa J, Medina L, Armstrong DM. *Demographic Turning Points for the United States: Population Projections for 2020 to 2060.* Current Population Reports, P25–1144, U.S. Census Bureau; 2020.
34. Xu JQ, Murphy SL, Kochanek KD, Arias E. Mortality in the United States, 2021. *NCHS Data Brief.* 2022(456). doi:10.15620/cdc:122516.
35. Flacker JM. What is a geriatric syndrome anyway? *J Am Geriatr Soc.* 2003. doi:10.1046/j.1532-5415.2003.51174.x.
36. Inouye SK, Studenski S, Tinetti ME, Kuchel GA. Geriatric syndromes: clinical, research, and policy implications of a core geriatric concept. *J Am Geriatr Soc.* 2007. doi:10.1111/j.1532-5415.2007.01156.x.
37. Stuck AE, Siu AL, Wieland GD, Adams J, Rubenstein LZ. Comprehensive geriatric assessment: a meta-analysis of controlled trials. *Lancet.* 1993 Oct 23. doi:10.1016/0140-6736(93)92884-v.
38. Watanabe Y, Yamada Y, Yoshida T, Yokoyama K, Miyake M, Yamagata E. Comprehensive geriatric intervention in community-dwelling older adults: a cluster-randomized controlled trial. *J Cachexia Sarcopenia Muscle.* 2020;11(1):26–37.
39. Tinetti M, Huang A, Molnar F. The geriatrics 5M's: a new way of communicating what we do. *J Am Geriatr Soc.* 2017. doi:10.1111/jgs.14979.
40. Molnar F, Frank CC. Optimizing geriatric care with the geriatric 5Ms. *Can Fam Physician.* 2019 Jan;65(1):39. PMID: 30674512; PMCID: PMC6347324.
41. Tinetti M, Huang A, Molnar F. The geriatrics 5M's: a new way of communicating what we do. *J Am Geriatr Soc.* 2017;65(9):2115. doi:10.1111/jgs.14979
42. Rowe JW, Kahn RL. Successful aging. *Gerontologist.* 1997;37(4):433–440. doi:10.1093/geront/37.4.433.
43. About Chronic Diseases. Accessed December 13, 2024. https://www.cdc.gov/chronic-disease/about/index.html
44. Annual Statistical Report on the Social Security Disability Insurance Program. Published online 2021. Accessed December 13, 2024. https://www.ssa.gov/policy/docs/statcomps/di_asr/2021/sect01.html.
45. Fries JF, Bruce B, Chakravarty E. Compression of morbidity 1980–2011: a focused review of paradigms and progress. *J Aging Res.* 2011;2011(261702). doi:10.4061/2011/261702.
46. HALE Country Table–Sort Highest. Datadot. Accessed November 10, 2024. https://data.who.int/dashboards/global-progress/hale.
47. Flaherty JH, Morley JE, Murphy DJ, Wasserman MR. The development of outpatient clinical glidepaths. *J Am Geriatr Soc.* Published online 2002. doi:10.1046/j.1532-5415.2002.50521.x.
48. Gillick M. *Choosing Medical Care in Old Age: What Kind, How Much, When to Stop,* 1st ed. Harvard University Press; 1994.
49. Lacagnina S, Moore M, Mitchell S. The lifestyle medicine team: health care that delivers value. *Am J Lifestyle Med.* 2018 Aug 22. doi:10.1177/1559827618792493.
50. Welsh TJ, Gordon AL, Gladman JR. Comprehensive geriatric assessment – a guide for the non-specialist. *Int J Clin Pract.* 2014;68(3):290–293. doi:10.1111/ijcp.12313.
51. Jacob ME, Yee LM, Diehr PH, et al. Can a healthy lifestyle compress the disabled period in older adults? *J Am Geriatr Soc.* 2016. doi:10.1111/jgs.14314.
52. Wallensten J, Ljunggren G, Nager A, et al. Stress, depression, and risk of dementia – a cohort study in the total population between 18 and 65 years old in Region Stockholm. *Alzheimers Res Ther.* 2023 Oct 2. doi:10.1186/s13195-023-01308-4.

53. Raichlen DA, Aslan DH, Sayre MK, et al. Sedentary behavior and incident dementia among older adults. *JAMA*. 2023 Sept 2. doi:10.1001/jama.2023.15231.
54. Koren MJ, Kelly NA, Lau JD. Association of healthy lifestyle and incident polypharmacy. *Am J Med*. 2024;137(5):433–441. doi:10.1016/j.amjmed.2023.12.028.
55. Sports Medicine AC, WJ CZ, DN P. American College of Sports Medicine position stand. Exercise and physical activity for older adults. *Med Sci Sports Exerc*. 2009;41(7):1510–1530. doi:10.1249/MSS.0b013e3181a0c95c.

2 Promoting Healthy Aging
A Lifecycle Approach

Susan M. Friedman

INTRODUCTION

Aging is a process that starts at the beginning of life and continues throughout the lifecycle. Similarly, healthy aging – the process of maximizing health as one ages – can also be promoted at every stage of life. As a result, it is never too early, and almost never too late, to promote healthy aging. However, different approaches may be more impactful at different stages of life. This chapter defines health and its drivers and provides examples of common chronic illnesses and the opportunities over the lifecycle for prevention and remission.

WHAT IS HEALTHY AGING?

In its Constitution, adopted at the International Health Conference in 1946, the World Health Organization defined health broadly as "a state of complete physical, mental and social well-being and not merely the absence of disease or infirmity."[1] It further noted that this principle was "basic to the happiness, harmonious relations, and security of all peoples." This holistic view of health dovetails well with what older adults identify as elements important to healthy or successful aging, noting positive aspects of thriving, such as enjoying meaningful relationships, having the physical and cognitive function needed to meet one's goals and remain independent, remaining engaged and having a sense of perspective and purpose.[2]

In their groundbreaking MacArthur study on successful aging, Jack Rowe and Robert Kahn defined a three-component model. This model included avoiding chronic illness, maintaining high physical and cognitive function and remaining engaged with life.[3] They defined the co-occurrence of these three elements as "successful aging," and pointed out that the aging experience was malleable, so that successful aging could be promoted or thwarted based on health behaviors and life circumstances.

The American Geriatrics Society's White Paper on healthy aging, recognizing the heterogeneity of the older adult population, and with a goal of encouraging *all* older adults to embrace healthy aging, used the National Prevention, Health Promotion and Public Health Council strategy[4] to incorporate primary, secondary and tertiary prevention to promote health in five domains.[5] These five domains built upon the Rowe and Kahn model, including promoting health, preventing injury and managing chronic conditions; optimizing cognitive health; optimizing physical health; optimizing mental health; and facilitating social engagement.

HEALTHY AGING AND CHRONIC DISEASE

Chronic illnesses are defined as "conditions that last one year or more and require ongoing medical attention or limit activities of daily living or both."[6] They are the leading causes of death and disability in the United States,[6] with seven out of ten deaths attributable to chronic disease.[7] In recent years, the leading causes of death have been heart disease, cancer, accidents, stroke, chronic lower respiratory diseases, Alzheimer's disease and diabetes.[8] Chronic disease is also expensive, accounting for about 75% of aggregate health care spending and 96% of Medicare spending.[7]

The prevalence of chronic disease in the United States is high and rising over time, and also increases with age.[7] About one in four older adults has one chronic disease, with almost two-thirds having two or more.[9] The prevalence of multiple chronic conditions is rising in adults aged 45–64, as well as in adults over the age of 65, which will impact healthy aging in future generations.[10]

Chronic disease is the major cause of physical disability.[11] Chronic disease can result from a sentinel event, such as a hip fracture or stroke, as risk builds over time and crosses a threshold, or from slowly progressive diseases, such as heart disease or arthritis.[11] In addition to its impact on disability, chronic disease affects other realms that are of central importance to older adults. For example, the presence of chronic illness increases the risk of social isolation and loneliness.[12]

SOCIAL DETERMINANTS OF HEALTH

Because the risk of chronic disease accrues over the lifecycle, early life events and lifestyle over time impact the onset and progression of chronic illness. There is a growing awareness within the medical community of the impact of social determinants of health (Table 2.1). In 2007, Schroeder noted that the combination of social circumstances and behaviors accounted for more than half of premature deaths in the United States and that social determinants contribute to health behaviors.[13] He further stated that "since all the actionable determinants of health... disproportionately affect the poor, strategies to improve national health rankings must focus on this population." Strategies to address health care disparities among marginalized groups, whether due to socioeconomic status, race and ethnicity, sexual orientation and gender, cognitive or functional impairment or others, is a critical component in optimizing health across the lifecycle for all.

Experiences in childhood can impact health throughout the lifecycle, adversely affecting health and well-being into old age. Adverse childhood experiences (ACEs) are potentially traumatic events that include issues of abuse, neglect and household challenges. It has been estimated that nearly half of US children have experienced at least one ACE, and the CDC has reported that one in six adults have experienced four or more ACEs as children.[14] Examples include emotional, physical or

TABLE 2.1
Social Determinants of Health

Realm	Examples
Economic stability	Income, job benefits, job opportunities, socioeconomic status, cost of living, employment, food security, housing stability
Education	School quality, access to information (e.g., digital technology), health literacy, high school graduation, college access
Health care access	Insurance/health care coverage, access to primary care
Neighborhood	Safety, transportation, built environment
Social connection	Proximity of family and friends; quality of relationships
Racism	Discrimination, weathering, structural violence
Environment	Air and water pollution, toxin exposure
Access to nutritious food and physical activity	Food deserts, access to safe spaces for exercise and physical activity
Language	Access to health information, literacy, potential for isolation
Culture	Health behaviors, approach to aging

sexual abuse; separation from a parent or guardian due to death, divorce or incarceration; witnessing domestic violence; growing up in a household with substance abuse or mental health problems; housing instability; bullying; and racism. There is significant racial disparity in the prevalence of ACEs, with 63.7% of Black children, 40.9% of White children and 25% of Asian children exposed to ACEs. Women, racial and ethnic minorities, members of the LGBTQ+ community, individuals with low income or unemployment and those with less than a high school education are the groups most likely to have experienced ACEs in the United States. ACEs lead to a higher risk of many of our most common chronic diseases, such as diabetes, obesity, cancer and heart disease.[15]

In recognition of the impact that these upstream factors have on health, Healthy People – the longest-running health promotion and disease prevention initiative in the United States – is focusing on social determinants of health as one of its five overarching goals for the Healthy People 2030 initiative. The Healthy People program identifies public health priorities, and provides 10-year, measurable public health objectives. In focusing on social determinants of health, the aim is to "create social, physical, and economic environments that promote attaining the full potential for health and well-being for all."[16]

LIFESTYLE CHANGES OVER TIME

Health habits start early in life and are shaped by family, community and life circumstances. These, in turn, influence healthy behaviors into adulthood.[17] Habits such as diet and exercise start in childhood, whereas others, such as smoking, alcohol and drug use, often start in adolescence and early adulthood.[18]

Due to both structure (e.g., schools) and high energy levels, children often have a significant amount of physical activity, although in the digital age, this may be changing. Unhealthy eating habits such as processed food can be affected by peers and dietary choices at home. Habits such as regular exercise and a healthy diet are often solidified in early adulthood, as individuals become more health conscious. In middle age, the combined stresses and time commitments of work and family responsibilities may take a toll, with negative impacts on exercise, diet, sleep and other health behaviors. As chronic illnesses emerge in later adulthood, people may become more attuned to the impact of lifestyle as they work to manage these conditions.[18]

Health habits can and often do change throughout the lifecycle. The primary source of influence that others exert transitions from parents during childhood, to peers and friends as adolescents and young adults, to spouses or partners in midlife. In later life, family may again exert more influence on health habits. Life transitions, such as marriage, childbirth, changes in career and retirement, can lead to changes in health behaviors.

MOTIVATION

Levels of motivation and reasons for choosing healthy behaviors may change throughout the lifecycle. Younger and older adults are most likely to be motivated to take care of themselves, with those in middle age being less motivated.[19] The source of motivation changes over time as well. Younger adults may be more focused on appearance and overall well-being, whereas people in middle age may be more concerned about aging well, avoiding or addressing health diagnoses or maintaining energy. Older adults, in turn, may be driven by the goal of maintaining independence and quality of life.

The onset of chronic illness can both act as a motivator for lifestyle change and may also provide barriers to change. If the illness is seen as serious and the benefit of making changes is clear, health behaviors might be expected to improve. Improvements in fitness and well-being, or reduction in medication, may incentivize an individual to continue a new health habit. However, if the chronic illness impairs function, this may be a barrier to changing habits. In a nationally representative study of adults aged 50 to 85 who were newly diagnosed with heart disease, diabetes, cancer, stroke or lung disease, most did not change their smoking, alcohol or exercise habits, although this varied according to specific disease and health behavior. Every new diagnosis was associated with a significant reduction in smoking, with a 40% relative reduction in smoking (from 25% to 15%) among those with heart disease, as well as a reduction in number of cigarettes smoked among those who continued to smoke. However, there were no increases in the percentage of people who reported exercising at least three times weekly. Among those diagnosed with cancer, stroke or lung disease, there was an increase in the percentage of people who became non-drinkers or drank infrequently.[20] On the other hand, in an online survey of a younger cohort (median age 41), 68% of those who had a chronic illness had made lifestyle changes after a diagnosis.[21] Changes were often made to maintain the ability to work or to care for children or parents, with maintaining health ranking third in the surveyed group.

Throughout life, motivation can be enhanced by fostering the three components of self-determination theory, namely, autonomy, competence and relatedness. Autonomy is the sense that one has a choice over their behavior, and that the behavior supports their goals and values. Competence denotes having a sense of mastery and effectiveness. Relatedness refers to feeling connected and having a sense of belonging.[22]

LIFESTYLE AS A COMMON PATHWAY TO ADDRESSING CHRONIC DISEASE

There is growing evidence that lifestyle and health behaviors play a key role in promoting health and addressing chronic disease.[23] The American College of Lifestyle Medicine recognizes six pillars as significant contributors to health and longevity: a whole food plant-predominant eating pattern; regular physical activity; restorative sleep; stress management; avoiding risky substances; and positive social connections.[24]

A Lifestyle Medicine Research Summit, convening in 2019 to review the connections between lifestyle pillars and health outcomes, articulated three pathways by which lifestyle impacts chronic disease, namely, alterations in microbiome; epigenetic changes; and cellular stress and injury[25] (adapted in Figure 2.1). The human microbiome – the collection of approximately 100 trillion microorganisms that live in and on the body, and predominantly in the gut – can be impacted by multiple pillars, potentially causing dysbiosis, which can change the permeability of the GI tract, leading to an inflammatory cascade. Intensive lifestyle modification has been shown to modulate gene expression, demonstrating that there is an interplay between genetics and lifestyle that can alter the timing and intensity of expression.[26] Observational studies from monozygotic twins with dissimilar lifestyles support these findings.[27] Lifestyle pillars may cause oxidative stress and generate free radicals, damaging

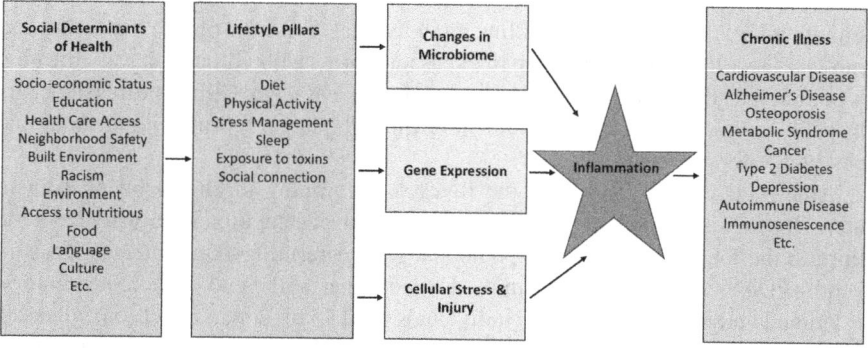

FIGURE 2.1 Framework for the impact of social determinants of health and lifestyle pillars on chronic disease outcomes. (Adapted from Vodovotz et al.[25] and Furman et al.[28])

cells and impairing tissue function. As discussed above, the social determinants of health impact lifestyle, which in turn impacts these three processes.

The three processes each contribute to a state of systemic chronic inflammation. Where acute inflammation is critical for survival in the setting of infection or injury, low-grade systemic chronic inflammation, interacting with genetic predisposition, can lead to many of our most common chronic conditions, including metabolic syndrome, type 2 diabetes, cardiovascular disease, cancer, depression, sarcopenia and neurodegenerative diseases.[28] A healthy lifestyle positively impacts these three processes, thereby reducing systemic chronic inflammation, which in turn reduces the risk of chronic illness.

COMMON CHRONIC ILLNESSES AND LIFETIME OPPORTUNITIES FOR PREVENTION AND REMISSION

Since chronic diseases develop over time, there are opportunities across the lifecycle for prevention and treatment, utilizing the pillars of lifestyle. This section will illustrate some of these opportunities, focusing on three common chronic illnesses and conditions that are associated with significant morbidity in older adults, namely, coronary artery disease, dementia, and osteoporosis and hip fracture.

Coronary Artery Disease

Since the early 20th century, heart disease has been the leading cause of mortality in the United States[29] and currently accounts for about one in five deaths. Coronary artery disease is the most common type of heart disease, leading to more than half of heart disease deaths.[30]

Atherosclerosis is the process that underlies coronary artery disease, leading to arterial wall thickening and plaque development. Progression results from a combination of endothelial damage, lipid deposition, necrosis, inflammatory cell infiltration, fibrosis and calcification.[29] Lesions evolve from adaptive intimal thickening to fatty streaks, as a result of lipid deposits primarily within foam cells in the intima. Atheromas form, with a lipid core covered by a thin fibrous cap that results from smooth muscle cell migration, putting an individual at risk for plaque instability and rupture. Over time, the fibrous cap thickens and forms a fibroatheroma. Calcification is common as the lesion progresses, and increases with age. Clinical disease occurs through narrowing of the vessel lumen, or through plaque rupture and thrombi that obstruct flow.

Atherosclerosis accrues over the lifecycle, beginning in childhood or even in utero. It progresses in all artery sites with age, with acceleration in severity from the third to the fourth decade.[31] The pathobiological determinants of atherosclerosis in youth (PDAY) study, conducted in the United States at the end of the 20th century, examined autopsies of over 3,000 individuals aged 15 to 34 without chronic disease, most of whom had died as a result of trauma. It found that all US teenagers had fatty streaks in some portion of their arterial system. The extent of the lesions increased steadily from age 15 to 34. Obesity was a risk factor for developing vascular lesions, and smoking and hypertension had the greatest impact on developing advanced plaques, with a six-fold and four-fold increase in incidence, respectively. Further, 10% of the individuals autopsied had advanced atherosclerosis and 80% of those individuals were smokers.[32] Wissler et al. concluded from this study that there were multiple opportunities for prevention in childhood and young adulthood, including smoking prevention, monitoring of cholesterol, prevention and treatment of obesity and control of hypertension and hyperglycemia.[33] A study by Lawrence et al. showed that young adults who were inactive and had a poor diet and poor sleep had increased cardiovascular risk.[34]

Among individuals with established coronary artery disease, two lifestyle approaches have been shown to lead to the regression of atherosclerosis. In a randomized, controlled trial led by Dr. Dean Ornish, 48 participants with one-, two- or three-vessel coronary artery disease were assigned to an intensive lifestyle intervention vs usual care. The lifestyle intervention involved eating a low-fat vegetarian diet, smoking cessation, training in stress management, group support and moderate aerobic exercise.[35] The diet contained approximately 10% of calories from fat, and consisted of fruits, vegetables, grains, legumes and soybean products without calorie restriction, and no animal products except egg white and a cup per day of non-fat milk or yogurt. Stress management techniques included stretching, breathing techniques, meditation, progressive relaxation and imagery, and participants were asked to practice techniques for at least 1 hour per day. Participants were instructed to exercise within a target heart rate for 3 hours or more per week. Social support was provided through twice-weekly group discussions.

Individuals in the intervention group reported a 91% reduction in the frequency of angina, where those in the control had a 165% increase in anginal frequency. Participants underwent cardiac catheterization at the beginning of the study and one year later. Average stenosis of lesions regressed in the intervention group, and progressed in the control group, with a dose-response relationship to outcomes.[35] Repeat catheterization at 5 years showed further regression of lesions in the intervention group, suggesting that the longer that these health behaviors are sustained, the greater the improvement.[36]

Dr. Caldwell Esselstyn led a cohort study of 198 individuals with cardiovascular disease to investigate the impact of a low-fat whole food plant-based diet on clinical outcomes after an average of 3.7 years. The average age of participants was 62.9 years of age, and 91% were men. The intervention was a diet of whole grains, legumes, lentils, vegetables and fruit, with a multivitamin and vitamin B12 supplements, as well as ground flax seed. Oils, processed foods containing oil, fish, meat, poultry, dairy, avocado, nuts and excess salt, as well as sugary foods and caffeine, were excluded.[37] Eighty-nine percent of participants were adherent, and 11% were non-adherent. Of the participants who were adherent to the eating pattern, 81% had improvement – 59% had symptom reduction and 22% had reversal. Eight percent were stable and 10% had further events. By comparison, of the participants who were nonadherent, none had improvement, 38% were stable and 62% had further events.

These interventions and their outcomes suggest that a higher intensity of lifestyle intervention may be indicated as atherosclerosis advances. Ornish notes that "small changes in lifestyle may slow the progression of atherosclerosis, whereas substantial changes… may be required to halt or reverse coronary atherosclerosis."[35]

ALZHEIMER'S DISEASE

Alzheimer's disease is the sixth leading cause of death in the United States, and one in three seniors dies with Alzheimer's or another dementia.[38] Alzheimer's disease is financially the costliest disease, with US$360 billion in direct costs and almost as much resulting from uncompensated informal care. It also takes a major toll on quality of life, both for the person with the disease and for their loved ones. Although the age-specific incidence of dementia has declined in recent decades,[39] the number of people affected by Alzheimer's continues to rise worldwide due to longer life expectancy. It has been estimated that delaying the onset of Alzheimer's disease by 5 years would reduce the prevalence by 50%.[40]

The development of Alzheimer's dementia occurs over a period of up to 20 years, starting with cellular changes, such as amyloid plaques, tau protein accumulation, and neurofibrillary tangles, years before the first clinical symptoms present. This provides a time window for changing the course and preventing or delaying the onset of dementia. There is growing evidence that inflammation plays an important role in the pathogenesis of Alzheimer's, through the activation of microglia.[41] The National Institute on Aging–Alzheimer's Association framework differentiates individuals with pathologic changes from those with clinical symptoms, dividing Alzheimer's disease into three stages: preclinical (i.e., pathologic changes without cognitive impairment); prodromal, or mild cognitive impairment; and Alzheimer's dementia.[42] It is not yet clear where prevention has the greatest impact along this pathway in the evolution of Alzheimer's disease.

The most recent estimate is that 45.3% of dementia worldwide is preventable.[39] The Lancet Commission on Dementia Prevention, Intervention and Care is an international group of experts who have systematically reviewed the evidence for dementia risk factors. They convened in 2017, and again in 2020 and 2024, with a progressive adjustment upward in the estimate of the proportion of preventable cases, as well as an increase in the number of identified modifiable risk factors.

The Lancet Commission concluded that risk can be reduced at any age, and divided the risk factors into the time of life in which a risk factor begins to be important and the population-attributable fraction of cases that are preventable. These are presented in Table 2.2. They further note that healthy lifestyles have been shown to delay the onset of dementia more than the increase in life expectancy, so that individuals experience more healthy years and fewer years of illness, both absolutely and proportionately;[43] in other words, there is a compression of morbidity in the last years of life.[44]

Early in life, higher educational attainment builds cognitive reserve and reduces dementia risk later in life. It has been estimated that differences in the quality of education account for about half of the disparities in dementia prevalence between racial groups in the United States. Cognitive stimulation is important in adulthood as well, with a lower risk of dementia associated with individuals who have higher

TABLE 2.2
Worldwide Population Attributable Fractions of Potentially Modifiable Dementia Risk Factors

Stage of Life	Modifiable Risk Factors for Dementia Worldwide		
	Risk Factor	Attributable Fraction for Risk Factor	Attributable Fraction for Stage
Early life	Less education	5%	5%
Midlife	Hearing loss	7%	30%
	High LDL cholesterol	7%	
	Depression	3%	
	Traumatic brain injury	3%	
	Physical inactivity	2%	
	Diabetes	2%	
	Smoking	2%	
	Hypertension	2%	
	Obesity	1%	
	Excessive alcohol	1%	
Late life	Social isolation	5%	10%
	Air pollution	3%	
	Vision loss	2%	

Source: Adapted from "Dementia Prevention, Intervention and Care": 2024 Report of the Lancet Standing Commission.[39]

cognitive stimulation at work. The impact of cognitive training in late life is less clear; a Cochrane report evaluating the impact of computerized cognitive training in cognitively healthy older adults showed limited benefit in the setting of low-quality evidence, and more research is needed to understand whether longer training interventions might have more of an impact.[45]

There is growing evidence that "what is good for the heart is good for the brain." In midlife, risk factors of LDL cholesterol (7% population attributable fraction (PAF) to dementia risk), depression (3% PAF), physical inactivity (2% PAF), diabetes (2% PAF), smoking (2% PAF), hypertension (2% PAF), obesity (1% PAF) and excessive alcohol intake[46] (1% PAF) present opportunities to reduce risk of developing dementia.[39] Addressing hearing loss (7% PAF) and preventing traumatic brain injury (3% PAF) provide additional opportunities to reduce risk.

In older adulthood, physical, cognitive and social activities attenuate the effect of neuropathology on clinical symptoms of dementia, otherwise known as increasing cognitive reserve, so that the impact of structural changes that may have accrued in midlife, including plaques and neurofibrillary tangles, may be mitigated.[47] According to the Lancet Commission, addressing social isolation (5% PAF), air pollution (3% PAF) and vision loss (2% PAF) among seniors could reduce the population risk of dementia by 10% overall.[39] Although systematic reviews have repeatedly shown social isolation leading to an increase in the risk of dementia, limited time of follow-up in studies risks reverse causation, that is, that early dementia contributes to social isolation, rather than vice versa. However, a study of over 400,000 participants in the United Kingdom, with a follow-up of 11.7 years, demonstrated a 1.26-fold risk of dementia, independent of loneliness and depression, for people with social isolation.[48] Social isolation was defined as having at least two of the following criteria: living alone, having social contacts less than monthly, and participation in social activities less than weekly.

Both fine particle air pollution (PM2.5) and particles with a diameter of $\leq 10\ \mu m$ (PM10) contribute to dementia, MCI and Alzheimer's disease, and risk is due to both indoor and outdoor air pollution. Vision loss is a risk factor for dementia that was newly added by the 2024 Lancet Commission. In a meta-analysis that included over 6 million participants in 14 prospective cohort studies, the relative risk of dementia was 1.47.[49] Intervening to reduce vision loss reduces risk; in a longitudinal cohort study of over 3,000 individuals over the age of 65, cataract extraction was associated with a 29% lower risk of developing dementia, although glaucoma surgery was not associated with benefit.[50]

OSTEOPOROSIS AND HIP FRACTURE

Osteoporosis results from a decrease in bone mineral density and bone mass, or when the structure and strength of bone changes, leading to an increased risk of fractures.[51] It is the major cause of fractures in postmenopausal women and older men. For each decade after age 50, hip fracture risk doubles, and a woman who lives to age 90 has a one in three risk of sustaining a hip fracture. Hip fractures confer a high risk of morbidity and mortality, with a 20% risk of death within the first year, and up to 50% sustaining permanent functional disability.[52,53]

Bone health is established early in life, so that fractures that occur in older adults reflect bone health throughout the lifecycle. Bone development in childhood and adolescence is key to bone health in adulthood. Bone mineral content increases 40-fold from birth to adulthood, with between 40 and 60% of adult bone mass accruing during puberty.

Peak bone mass, occurring at the end of skeletal maturity, is achieved between the ages of 25 and 30.[54] Because mineralization lags behind bone growth during adolescence, people are at increased risk of fractures during this time.[55] Between the ages of 20 and 50, bone mass remains relatively stable, and begins to decrease after age 50.[56]

Both modifiable and non-modifiable factors affect peak bone mass. Non-modifiable factors include genetic conditions, gender and ethnicity, and may account for up to 70% of bone mass variance, leaving 30% or more that is modifiable. Modifiable factors are listed in Table 2.3. A healthy diet that includes adequate calcium, vitamins D, C and K, silicon, boron, magnesium and protein is necessary for healthy bone.[55,56] Seventy percent of American children do not get adequate vitamin D, and the obesity epidemic has contributed to the prevalence of vitamin D deficiency.

TABLE 2.3
Modifiable Factors for Peak Bone Health[55,56]

Nutrition
Weight
Exercise
Medication
Hormonal status
Excess alcohol
Tobacco

Weight-bearing exercise – including walking, running and team sports such as basketball and soccer – and strength training are both essential in reaching peak bone mass. Physical activity increases bone mineral mass accumulation in both children and adolescents, but is most impactful before puberty.[55] Gains are most prominent in weight-bearing bone, such as the proximal femur, which may be protective later in life.

Higher peak bone mass protects against osteoporosis and fractures later in life. A 10% increase in peak bone mineral density (BMD) has been estimated to delay the development of osteoporosis by 13 years,[57] which would lead to a 50% reduction in risk of fracture later in life.[55] This impact is significantly greater than the impact of either the age of menopause or the rate of age-related bone loss; by comparison, a 10% increase in each of these has been estimated to delay the development of osteoporosis by 2 years.[57]

Exercise and nutrition, including adequate calcium and vitamin D, continue to be important through midlife, when bone resorption starts to occur. A study from a nationally representative sample followed 1559 women with an average age of 45 at baseline for up to 20 years and found that the more inflammatory a person's diet,[58] the higher the risk, with a 28% higher fracture risk for each standard deviation increment in inflammatory diet score.[59] A recent meta-analysis suggests that this impact persists at older ages.[60] This suggests that diets that are high in anti-inflammatory components, such as beta-carotene, fiber, green and black tea and isoflavones, and low in pro-inflammatory components, such as saturated or trans fat, overall calories and cholesterol, may be protective.[58]

A cohort study of over 30,000 people with an average age of 58, followed for 20.7 years, showed that low leisure-time physical activity, living alone, heavy work, low BMI, smoking and either no or high levels of alcohol use were predictors of fracture later in life. Every additional quintile of leisure-time physical activity was associated with lower fracture risk.[60]

Fall prevention becomes more important for reducing fracture risk in older adults, as falls occur more frequently in this age group and are more likely to result in fractures.[61] As people become more frail, the mechanism of fractures changes, putting them at higher risk for hip fractures.[62] With a decline in mobility, the trajectory of falls puts the point of impact closer to the hip, and protective responses may be slower. Interventions to improve strength and mobility and to reduce frailty may therefore be more important at this stage of life for preventing hip fractures. Lifestyle approaches to falls and bone health among older adults are addressed more fully in Chapters 23 and 25, respectively.

PROMOTING HEALTHY AGING AMONG OLDER ADULTS

Although a central goal of lifestyle medicine is a reduction of the burden of chronic disease, it is important to acknowledge that most older adults are living with chronic illness. Aside from reducing the incidence and severity of chronic disease, are there other approaches to improve health in later life? It is helpful to think about the 5Ms framework of age-friendly health care and particularly the question of "What matters most?" to older adults. In a study of primary care patients who were participating in a Medicare annual wellness visit, the most common theme expressed by patients who answered this question was relationships with family and friends, including spending time with loved ones and being able to enjoy time together.[63] This was followed by maintaining health, often through the lens of avoiding pain, not being a burden to family and being able to assist family when needed. Other themes included pursuing hobbies and interests, spirituality, mobility and function and service and contributions to others. Assessing what matters most to a patient, and intervening to promote outcomes that are of most importance to the individual, is an important step in promoting healthy aging for older adults, regardless of chronic disease burden.

CONCLUSIONS

Healthy aging is a process that starts at the earliest stages of life. Chronic disease, which develops over many years, starts with changes that occur early in life and progress over time. As a result, there are opportunities across the lifecycle to reduce chronic illness and promote healthy aging. It is useful to use a holistic definition of health, and to assess patient goals and values, in order to optimally promote healthy aging for older adults.

CLINICAL APPLICATIONS

- Clinicians have an opportunity to promote healthy aging at every stage of a patient's life.
- Addressing lifestyle pillars in childhood, adolescence and throughout adulthood can reduce the onset and progression of chronic illness.
- Chronic illnesses that are both common and lead to substantial morbidity – such as coronary artery disease, dementia and osteoporosis – have their onset early in life.

- Motivation changes throughout the life course, so it is important to ask patients what motivates them to be healthy.
- Lifestyle impacts microbiome alterations, gene expression and cellular stress and injury, leading to chronic inflammation, which in turn increases the risk of chronic disease.
- Since most older adults have chronic illnesses, understanding what matters most to the patient will help to frame approaches to promote healthy aging.

REFERENCES

1. World Health Organization. Basic Documents. World Health Organization; 2024. Accessed July 11, 2024. https://apps.who.int/gb/bd/pdf_files/BD_49th-en.pdf#page=6
2. Cosco TD, Prina AM, Perales J, Stephan BC, Brayne C. Lay perspectives of successful ageing: a systematic review and meta-ethnography. *BMJ Open*. 2013 Jun 20;3(6). doi:10.1136/bmjopen-2013-002710
3. Rowe JW, Kahn RL. Successful aging. *Gerontologist*. 1997 Aug;37(4):433–440. doi:10.1093/geront/37.4.433
4. Healthy Aging in Action: Advancing the National Prevention Strategy. 2016. *Publications and Reports of the Surgeon General*.
5. Friedman SM, Mulhausen P, Cleveland ML, et al. Healthy aging: American Geriatrics Society White paper executive summary. *J Am Geriatr Soc*. 2019 Jan;67(1):17–20. doi:10.1111/jgs.15644
6. Chronic diseases in America. US Centers for Disease Control and Prevention, 2024. Updated April 10, 2024. Accessed July 11, 2024. https://www.cdc.gov/chronic-disease/about/index.html
7. Raghupathi W, Raghupathi V. An empirical study of chronic diseases in the United States: a visual analytics approach. *Int J Environ Res Public Health*. 2018 Mar 1;15(3) doi:10.3390/ijerph15030431
8. Centers for Disease Control and Prevention NCfHS. National vital statistics system, provisional mortality on CDC WONDER online database, 2024. Accessed July 11, 2024. http://wonder.cdc.gov/mcd-icd10-provisional.html
9. Boersma P, Black LI, Ward BW. Prevalence of multiple chronic conditions among US adults, 2018. *Prev Chronic Dis*. 2020 Sep 17;17:E106. doi:10.5888/pcd17.200130
10. Freid VM, Bernstein AB, Bush M. *Multiple Chronic Conditions among Adults Aged 45 and over: Trends over the Past 10 Years*. 2012 July. https://www.cdc.gov/nchs/data/databriefs/db100.pdf
11. Fried LP, Guralnik JM. Disability in older adults: evidence regarding significance, etiology, and risk. *J Am Geriatr Soc*. 1997 Jan;45(1):92–100. doi:10.1111/j.1532-5415.1997.tb00986.x
12. National Academies of Sciences Engineering and Medicine (U.S.), Board on Health Sciences Policy. Health and Medicine Division. Board on Behavioral Cognitive and Sensory Sciences. Division of Behavioral and Social Sciences and Education. *Social Isolation and Loneliness in Older Adults: Opportunitiies for the Health Care System*. Consensus Study Report. National Academies Press; 2020:xvii, 298 pages.
13. Schroeder SA. Shattuck Lecture. We can do better – improving the health of the American people. *N Engl J Med*. 2007 Sep 20;357(12):1221–1228. doi:10.1056/NEJMsa073350

14. Walsh E. What Are Adverse Childhood Experiences (ACEs)? ACEs definition, data challenges, and resources. Regents of the University of Minnesota, 2024. Updated November 14, 2024. Accessed December 7, 2024. https://www.shadac.org/news/what-are-adverse-childhood-experiences-aces-definition-data-resources
15. About Adverse Childhood Experiences. hhs.gov, 2024. Accessed December 7, 2024. https://www.cdc.gov/aces/about/index.html
16. Social Determinants of Health. Office of Disease Prevention and Health Promotion, Office of the Assistant Secretary for Health, Office of the Secretary, U.S. Department of Health and Human Services, 2024. Accessed December 7, 2024. https://odphp.health.gov/healthypeople/priority-areas/social-determinants-health
17. Frech A. Healthy behavior trajectories between adolescence and young adulthood. *Adv Life Course Res*. 2012 Jun 1;17(2):59–68. doi:10.1016/j.alcr.2012.01.003
18. Umberson D, Crosnoe R, Reczek C. Social relationships and health behavior across life course. *Annu Rev Sociol*. 2010 Aug 1;36:139–157. doi:10.1146/annurev-soc-070308-120011
19. Waldersee V. How your motivations change as you get older. *YouGov*. 2024. Accessed December 7, 2024. https://yougov.co.uk/society/articles/21114-how-your-motivations-change-you-get-older
20. Newsom JT, Huguet N, McCarthy MJ, et al. Health behavior change following chronic illness in middle and later life. *J Gerontol B Psychol Sci Soc Sci*. 2012 May;67(3):279–288. doi:10.1093/geronb/gbr103
21. Choudry M, Ganti L. Exploration of the motivational factors that influence the maintenance of health. *Health Psychol Res*. 2024;12. doi:10.52965/001c.115356
22. Ryan RM, Deci EL. *Self-Determination Theory: Basic Psychological Needs in Motivation, Development, and Wellness*. Guilford Publications; 2017:756.
23. Bodai BI, Nakata TE, Wong WT, et al. Lifestyle medicine: a brief review of its dramatic impact on health and survival. *Perm J*. 2018;22:17–025. doi:10.7812/TPP/17-025
24. American College of Lifestyle Medicine; 2024. Accessed October 26, 2024. https://lifestylemedicine.org/
25. Vodovotz Y, Barnard N, Hu FB, et al. Prioritized research for the prevention, treatment, and reversal of chronic disease: recommendations from the Lifestyle Medicine Research Summit. *Front Med (Lausanne)*. 2020;7:585744. doi:10.3389/fmed.2020.585744
26. Ornish D, Magbanua MJ, Weidner G, et al. Changes in prostate gene expression in men undergoing an intensive nutrition and lifestyle intervention. *Proc Natl Acad Sci U S A*. 2008 Jun 17;105(24):8369–8374. doi:10.1073/pnas.0803080105
27. Duncan GE, Avery A, Thorson JLM, Nilsson EE, Beck D, Skinner MK. Epigenome-wide association study of physical activity and physiological parameters in discordant monozygotic twins. *Sci Rep*. 2022 Nov 23;12(1):20166. doi:10.1038/s41598-022-24642-3
28. Furman D, Campisi J, Verdin E, et al. Chronic inflammation in the etiology of disease across the life span. *Nat Med*. 2019 Dec;25(12):1822–1832. doi:10.1038/s41591-019-0675-0
29. Bentzon JF, Otsuka F, Virmani R, Falk E. Mechanisms of plaque formation and rupture. *Circ Res*. 2014 Jun 6;114(12):1852–1866. doi:10.1161/CIRCRESAHA.114.302721
30. Heart Disease Facts. US Centers for Disease Control and Prevention, 2024. Accessed December 10, 2024. https://www.cdc.gov/heart-disease/data-research/facts-stats/index.html#:~:text=Heart%20disease%20is%20the%20leading,lost%20productivity%20due%20to%20death.
31. Dalager S, Paaske WP, Kristensen IB, Laurberg JM, Falk E. Artery-related differences in atherosclerosis expression: implications for atherogenesis and dynamics in intima-media thickness. *Stroke*. 2007 Oct;38(10):2698–2705. doi:10.1161/STROKEAHA.107.486480

32. Fausto N. Atherosclerosis in young people: the value of the autopsy for studies of the epidemiology and pathobiology of disease. *Am J Pathol.* 1998 Oct;153(4):1021–1022. doi:10.1016/S0002-9440(10)65646-5
33. Wissler RW, Strong JP. Risk factors and progression of atherosclerosis in youth. PDAY Research Group. Pathological determinants of atherosclerosis in youth. *Am J Pathol.* 1998 Oct ;153(4):1023–1033. doi:10.1016/s0002-9440(10)65647-7
34. Lawrence EM, Mollborn S, Hummer RA. Health lifestyles across the transition to adulthood: implications for health. *Soc Sci Med.* 2017 Nov;193:23–32. doi:10.1016/j.socscimed.2017.09.041
35. Ornish D, Brown SE, Scherwitz LW, et al. Can lifestyle changes reverse coronary heart disease? The Lifestyle Heart Trial. *Lancet.* 1990 Jul 21;336(8708):129–133. doi:10.1016/0140-6736(90)91656-u
36. Ornish D, Scherwitz LW, Billings JH, et al. Intensive lifestyle changes for reversal of coronary heart disease. *JAMA.* 1998 Dec 16;280(23):2001–2007. doi:10.1001/jama.280.23.2001
37. Esselstyn CB, Jr., Gendy G, Doyle J, Golubic M, Roizen MF. A way to reverse CAD? *J Fam Pract.* 2014 Jul;63(7):356–364b.
38. Alzheimer's Disease Facts and Figures. Alzheimer's Association. 2024. Accessed December 14, 2024. https://www.alz.org/alzheimers-dementia/facts-figures?utm_source=google&utm_medium=paidsearch&utm_campaign=google_grants&utm_content=alzheimers&gad_source=1&gclid=Cj0KCQiApNW6BhD5ARIsACmEbkX9Qi9zBYSoumd5aaZssBoAm8xFjNg-A70hF3XQMrlcRxrGbfEFzewaAtTuEALw_wcB
39. Livingston G, Huntley J, Liu KY, et al. Dementia prevention, intervention, and care: 2024 report of the Lancet Standing Commission. *Lancet.* 2024 Aug 10;404(10452):572–628. doi:10.1016/S0140-6736(24)01296-0
40. Brookmeyer R, Gray S, Kawas C. Projections of Alzheimer's disease in the United States and the public health impact of delaying disease onset. *Am J Public Health.* 1998 Sep;88(9):1337–1342. doi:10.2105/ajph.88.9.1337
41. Kinney JW, Bemiller SM, Murtishaw AS, Leisgang AM, Salazar AM, Lamb BT. Inflammation as a central mechanism in Alzheimer's disease. *Alzheimers Dement (NY).* 2018;4:575–590. doi:10.1016/j.trci.2018.06.014
42. Jack CR, Jr., Bennett DA, Blennow K, et al. NIA-AA research framework: toward a biological definition of Alzheimer's disease. *Alzheimers Dement.* 2018 Apr;14(4):535–562. doi:10.1016/j.jalz.2018.02.018
43. Dhana K, Franco OH, Ritz EM, et al. Healthy lifestyle and life expectancy with and without Alzheimer's dementia: population based cohort study. *BMJ.* 2022 Apr 13;377:e068390. doi:10.1136/bmj-2021-068390
44. Fries JF. Aging, natural death, and the compression of morbidity. *N Engl J Med.* 1980 Jul 17;303(3):130–135. doi:10.1056/NEJM198007173030304
45. Gates NJ, Rutjes AWS, Di Nisio M, et al. Computerised cognitive training for 12 or more weeks for maintaining cognitive function in cognitively healthy people in late life. *Cochrane Db Syst Rev.* 2020;(2) doi:ARTN CD01227710.1002/14651858.CD012277.pub3
46. Biddinger KJ, Emdin CA, Haas ME, et al. Association of habitual alcohol intake with risk of cardiovascular disease. *JAMA Netw Open.* 2022 Mar 1;5(3):e223849. doi:10.1001/jamanetworkopen.2022.3849
47. Scarmeas N, Stern Y. Cognitive reserve: implications for diagnosis and prevention of Alzheimer's disease. *Curr Neurol Neurosci Rep.* 2004 Sep;4(5):374–380. doi:10.1007/s11910-004-0084-7

48. Shen C, Rolls ET, Cheng W, et al. Associations of social isolation and loneliness with later dementia. *Neurology*. 2022 Jul 11;99(2):e164–e175. doi:10.1212/WNL.0000000000200583
49. Shang XW, Zhu ZT, Wei W, Ha JS, He MG. The association between vision impairment and incidence of dementia and cognitive impairment. *Ophthalmology*. 2021 Aug;128(8):1135–1149. doi:10.1016/j.ophtha.2020.12.029
50. Lee CS, Gibbons LE, Lee AY, et al. Association between cataract extraction and development of dementia. *Jama Intern Med*. 2022 Feb;182(2):134–141. doi:10.1001/jamainternmed.2021.6990
51. Osteoporosis. National Inisitute of Arthritis and Musculoskeletal and Skin Diseases, 2024. Accessed December 11, 2024. https://www.niams.nih.gov/health-topics/osteoporosis
52. Friedman SM, Mendelson DA. Epidemiology of fragility fractures. *Clin Geriatr Med*. 2014 May ;30(2):175–181. doi:10.1016/j.cger.2014.01.001
53. Bischoff-Ferrari HA. Fracture epidemiology among individuals 75+. *Osteoporosis in Older Persons: Pathophysiology and Therapeutic Approach*. 2009:97–109. doi:10.1007/978-1-84628-697-1_8
54. Campbell BJ. *Healthy Bones at Every Age*. American Academy of Orthopaedic Surgeons; 2024. Accessed December 11, 2024. https://orthoinfo.aaos.org/en/staying-healthy/healthy-bones-at-every-age/#:~:text=Childhood%2C%20adolescence%2C%20and%20early%20adulthood,newer%2C%20bone%2Dforming%20medications.
55. Chevalley T, Rizzoli R. Acquisition of peak bone mass. *Best Pract Res Clin Endocrinol Metab*. 2022 Mar;36(2):101616. doi:10.1016/j.beem.2022.101616
56. Hereford T, Kellish A, Balch Samora J, Reid Nichols L. Understanding the importance of peak bone mass. *J. Pediatr Soc North Am*. 2024 May;7. doi:10.1016/j.jposna.2024.100031
57. Hernandez CJ, Beaupre GS, Carter DR. A theoretical analysis of the relative influences of peak BMD, age-related bone loss and menopause on the development of osteoporosis. *Osteoporos Int*. 2003 Oct;14(10):843–847. doi:10.1007/s00198-003-1454-8
58. Shivappa N, Steck SE, Hurley TG, Hussey JR, Hebert JR. Designing and developing a literature-derived, population-based dietary inflammatory index. *Public Health Nutr*. 2014 Aug;17(8):1689–1696. doi:10.1017/S1368980013002115
59. Shieh A, Karlamangla AS, Huang MH, Shivappa N, Wirth MD, Hebert JR, Greendale GA. Dietary inflammatory index and fractures in midlife women: study of women's health across the nation. *J Clin Endocrinol Metab*. 2023 Jul 14;108(8):e594–e602. doi:10.1210/clinem/dgad051
60. Zheng XJ, Li WH, Yan YL, Su ZJ, Huang XL. Association between the dietary inflammatory index and fracture risk in older adults: a systematic review and meta-analysis. *J Int Med Res*. 2024 May;52(5) doi:Artn 0300060524124803910.1177/03000605241248039
61. NPSD Data Spotlight, Falls: Associated Factors and Clinical Outcomes. 2023. https://www.ahrq.gov/sites/default/files/wysiwyg/npsd/data/spotlights/spotlight-falls.pdf#:~:text=Across%20most%20years%2C%20the%20relative%20percentage%20of,(960%20out%20of%201%2C666%20events)%20in%202021.&text=%2D%2015.3%%20to%2018.6%%20(3.3%%20difference)%20among%20patients%2018%2D64%20years%20old;
62. Cummings SR, Nevitt MC. A hypothesis: the causes of hip fractures. *J Gerontol*. 1989 Jul;44(4):M107–M111. doi:10.1093/geronj/44.4.m107
63. Garbarino JT, O'Connor S, Pepin RL, Aitken MS, Flaherty E. Age-friendly health care and the 4Ms in RN-led annual wellness visits. *J Am Geriatr Soc*. 2024 May;72(Suppl 2):S13–S20. doi:10.1111/jgs.18671

3 The Reality of Aging

Rebecca Masutani and Rosanne Leipzig

Everyone ages differently. With that said, familiarizing oneself with what to expect, being flexible and embracing change can help with the journey into this stage of life. In this chapter, we will discuss the 5Ms and some common physiologic and emotional changes associated with aging, focusing on the pillars of lifestyle medicine: nutrition, physical activity/movement, sleep and emotional well-being/connectedness. Notably, this review is not fully inclusive of all the changes that can occur with aging; it is intended to provide a general overview of commonly reported aging concerns.

WHAT IS AGING?

Unsurprisingly, the definition varies depending on the source. The Oxford English Dictionary defines the noun *ageing* as the "process of growing old,"[1] whereas the Encyclopedia Britannica interprets aging as "progressive physiological changes in an organism that lead to senescence, or a decline of biological functions and of the organism's ability to adapt to metabolic stress."[2] In more recent times, the National Institute of Aging defines aging as "changes in dynamic biological, physiological, environmental, psychological, behavioral, and social processes."[3] Within these definitions are terms that offer some insight into the reality of aging – process, change, grow – and words with harsher connotations – senescence, decline. In reality, aging is all of the aforementioned definitions combined, and yet it can transcend these definitions due to the very individualized experience of aging. What geriatricians and many others would argue with is the latter half of the Oxford Learner's Dictionary's definition of the adjective *ageing*, namely, "becoming older and usually less useful, safe, healthy, etc."[4] Despite negative stereotypes and cultural perceptions of aging, the truth is that aging need not be synonymous with decline or diminution.

Ageism is defined by the World Health Organization as "the stereotypes, prejudice, and discrimination towards others based on age."[5] Ageism is a serious issue that can lead to worse psychological and physical outcomes for individuals of all age groups, but older adults are at particular risk. Negative attitudes toward aging have become more prevalent globally,[6] and are fairly ubiquitous in many cultures, with older adults stereotypically displayed as cognitively disabled, unproductive or physically limited. Such inaccurate, pessimistic impressions of aging, particularly within the medical system, may portend worse outcomes for older adults. Indeed, studies have shown that health care providers, including medical students, express negative perceptions of caring for the aging population.[7] Such sentiments may lead to suboptimal care of older adults, and also contribute to the shortage of health care providers willing to care for the aging population. Ageism may also contribute to the lack of medical research on older adults. Although older adults are primary consumers of medical therapies, they are often under-represented in clinical trials.[8]

Positive perceptions of aging are associated with longer and improved quality of life in both longitudinal and cross-sectional studies. In a study published in 2022, Dr. Becca Levy found that older adults with positive self-perceptions of aging lived about 7.5 years longer than individuals with negative perceptions.[9] Other investigators found an association between positive self-perceptions of aging and a longer lifespan when matching data from the Ohio Longitudinal Study of Aging and Retirement to mortality data from the National Death Index. In addition, multiple cross-sectional studies have found that positive perceptions of aging were more strongly associated with higher quality of life.[10,11] Conversely, another study led by Dr. Levy found that participants who held more negative, discriminatory stereotypes of aging were significantly more likely to experience a cardiovascular event in the subsequent 38 years of their lives.[12] In addition, a 2020 review identified that ageism is associated with higher costs to the US health care system.[13]

The reality is that **aging is change**. The way in which this change is perceived can have profound impacts on the individual and society as a whole. Medical practitioners caring for older adults can impact individual perceptions of aging by emphasizing the positive aspects of aging and exploring the exciting new possibilities that can come with this stage of life.

WHAT ARE THE PHYSIOLOGIC CHANGES ASSOCIATED WITH AGING?

Physiologic reserves decrease with age. **Homeostenosis** is a term used to describe the inability of older adults to compensate for, and react to, external stressors due to their diminished physiologic reserves. Homeostenosis is a part of normal aging; as one ages, older adults are physiologically less able to compensate for stressful events or trauma to their bodies. For example, older people who contract influenza are more likely to require hospitalization or experience serious complications, compared to someone in their twenties.

Severe homeostenosis can result in *frailty,* a clinical state where individuals experience increased vulnerability to stressors, and ultimately a state of depleted reserve, independent of a specific disease.[14] Frail individuals are at higher risk of adverse outcomes, complications from medications and surgical procedures, and death. There are two predominant theories of frailty: phenotypic frailty and deficit accumulation. Phenotypic frailty is a distinct clinical presentation consisting of three out of the following five factors: unintentional weight loss, decreased strength, slow walking speed, low physical activity and feelings of exhaustion.[15,16] Deficit accumulation uses an aggregate of individual age-related health deficits to calculate a multi-dimensional risk state; this is referred to as a frailty index.[17,18] While there are some differences in these two definitions,[19] the bottom line is that it is crucial for medical practitioners to be aware of this syndrome and to try to prevent or attenuate it using many of the principles of lifestyle medicine like better nutrition, sleep, and exercise.

THE 5Ms: AN APPROACH TO CARING FOR OLDER ADULTS

Providers caring for aging older adults should use the Geriatric 5Ms approach, which addresses the topics outlined in Table 3.1.[20]

TABLE 3.1
The Geriatric 5Ms Framework

Matters Most
Mind
Mobility
Medications
Multicomplexity

The 5Ms offer a framework for providing holistic, comprehensive care to people who are undergoing common age-related changes in their bodies, minds and environments. They start with centering and guiding care around the individual's values (matters most); concerns about cognition and/or mood (mind); physical function and avoiding falls (mobility); appropriate use of prescribed medications and over-the-counter supplements (medications); and the interplay between medical conditions and psychosocial issues (multicomplexity).

MATTERS MOST

While each of the 5Ms is important, identifying an individual's values is the best way to provide patient centered care. Asking what is most important and taking the time to learn more about the individual beyond their medical issues not only affords providers and patients the opportunity to build meaningful relationships, but allows the patient's medical care to be aligned with their beliefs and values, resulting in individualized care plans that prioritize what is most important for that person.

Geriatric medicine, in particular, is rife with gray areas; that is, clinical scenarios that lack a distinct treatment approach due to a myriad of factors. These include a lack of evidence to help guide clinicians caring for older adults, as well as medical and psychosocial complexity that often leads to extensive discussions about the risks and benefits of medical interventions. For example, a provider may need to have a longer conversation on the risks and benefits of anti 35 coagulation, if an older adult has a history of recurrent falls due to gait instability and is at higher risk for bleeding events. In a different scenario, a frail, older adult with dementia may not be an appropriate candidate for a colonoscopy if they are unable to comply with bowel preparation or are deemed to have a high risk of peri-procedural complications. Ultimately, eliciting the principles that are most meaningful to patients can help mitigate the medical uncertainty in complex situations by allowing the patient's values to guide their care.

Mind

As individuals age, providers will oftentimes hear concerns from patients or their family members about cognition or memory loss, as well as issues pertaining to a person's mood. Cognitive changes, in particular, may cause individuals to worry about maintaining independence or autonomy in the future. While there are age-related cognitive changes that are aspects of "normal" aging, including an increased effort to learn new things, less ability to multitask, slower processing and trouble retrieving names, much remains intact. In general, skills and knowledge that individuals have acquired throughout their lives are not significantly impacted by the aging brain. Vocabulary, language comprehension and remote memory tend to remain intact. At times, individuals may experience difficulty recalling words or memories, though can identify these with various cues. Instead, the earliest signs of dementia tend to manifest as changes in executive function, or the ability to perform complex tasks. Examples include filing taxes or paying household bills.

Trained health care providers can offer cognitive evaluations for individuals who themselves report memory concerns, or have loved ones expressing concern about the individual's well-being and future. Performing cognitive assessments can help identify treatable conditions or factors (e.g., medications) impairing one's cognition. While cognitive changes are a part of aging, this does not mean that these changes should negatively impact an individual's quality of life. Importantly, cognitive assessments can also identify patient strengths and offer ways for individuals to develop compensatory strategies if they are experiencing some degree of memory loss.

Similar to cognitive changes, our moods, emotions and stressors change over time. Aging brings about different sets of changes and challenges in one's life. As a result, such changes can impact one's mood. It is important to recognize that depression is not a normal part of aging. According to the Centers for Disease Control and Prevention (CDC), it is, however, the most prevalent mental health problem among older adults, with surveillance data showing that 7.7% of adults age 50 or older reported depression, while 15.7% reported a lifetime diagnosis of depression.[21] Concerningly, studies have shown underdiagnosis and lack of treatment of depression in older adults.[22] Practitioners should identify factors associated with depression, including alcohol/substance use, medications, physical conditions and social isolation. A common concern among patients as they age is the gradual loss of friends, due to sickness, death or physical separation (e.g., friends moving out of state to be closer to their own family as they age). Practitioners should be aware of the importance of social interactions and relationships on emotions as people age. Additionally, some older adults may experience some degree of trepidation about the future. To address these concerns, older adults can benefit from different types of psychotherapy, regular exercise, as well as relaxation techniques such as yoga and meditation.

Mobility

This is defined as the ability to move freely and easily. As individuals age, changes to multiple organ systems can impact mobility and physical function. These changes impact processes from cellular repair to larger organ systems, such as the degeneration of cartilage between joints.[23] Additionally, changes in body composition, such as a decrease in lean body mass and bone mass, as well as an increase in body fat, can impact physical function and may be associated with frailty.[24,25]

Due to age-related changes in these various organ systems (i.e., cardiovascular, pulmonary, musculoskeletal), strength, coordination and balance are affected. As a result, older adults may experience slower, unsteady gait. In addition, men and women also tend to lose an average of one to three inches of height with age,[26] and as a result, may experience postural changes that can impact their physical function.

Gait speed, an important consideration in mobility and physical function, also changes as we get older. In general, older adults walk more slowly than younger adults.[27] Slower gait speed is associated with adverse events and increased mortality in the older adult population.[28-31] Sarcopenia, defined as age-related involuntary loss of muscle mass, strength, and function, can also contribute to a higher risk of falls as people age.[32] As such, geriatric medicine providers are particularly focused on gait impairment and muscle weakness/loss, as these account for some underlying risk factors for falls.[33-35] Given that falls can lead to more serious health problems, and long-term disability, providers should focus on mobility and function as people age. There are many possible etiologies for loss of mobility/gait instability, though most can be addressed by referring to specialists, including physical therapists.

MEDICATIONS

These are important to consider as older adults age. As individuals get older, drug metabolism changes and many organs become more vulnerable to the effects of medications. For example, the dose of medications normally eliminated by the kidneys may need to be modified for individuals if they develop reduced glomerular filtration rates in the setting of chronic kidney disease. Additionally, older adults are more likely to experience anticholinergic side effects of first-generation antihistamines, compared to an individual in their twenties. Adverse anticholinergic side effects, ranging from dry mouth and constipation to confusion and falls, can tremendously impact an older adult's quality of life and function. As such, medications with high anticholinergic side effect profiles are largely avoided in older adults. Since 2011, the American Geriatrics Society has published regular updates to the Beers Criteria which lists medications to avoid and/or use with caution in older adults, including those that cause anticholinergic side effects.[36] This list can be used as a helpful guide for practitioners hoping to avoid adverse drug effects in patients.

As patients age, providers can also look to deprescribing, or tapering down the dose of certain medications that were initially prescribed to treat conditions for which patients may no longer experience symptoms. For example, patients initially prescribed a proton-pump inhibitor for acid reflux may no longer require the use of this medication, and can be tapered off this medicine with close monitoring. A review of patient medication lists and careful consideration of which medications can be deprescribed is essential, given the risks of drug side effects, changes in our body metabolism with aging and, finally, the risk of interactions between drugs.

MULTICOMPLEXITY

By using the 5Ms approach, providers can be more adept at addressing geriatric syndromes – disorders such as weight loss/malnutrition, cognitive impairment, gait instability/falls, incontinence and frailty. The etiology of these geriatric syndromes is usually multifactorial in nature and largely driven by a complex interplay between multiple organ systems, the environment, and one's support systems. As mentioned previously, older adults may be more susceptible to these syndromes depending on their individual physiologic reserve (homostenosis). Similar to the foundational concepts of lifestyle medicine, the Geriatric 5Ms aim to address whole-person health in those who are transitioning to different stages in their life.

ADDITIONAL PILLARS OF LIFESTYLE MEDICINE

SOCIALIZATION

Many older adults experience full lives and a strong sense of community as they age. Yet with aging, their social circles may constrict, making them more susceptible to social isolation and loneliness. For example, death and relocation of friends or family members is more common. Physical concerns such as limited mobility may make it difficult if not impossible to leave home to attend community events. In addition, various types of sensory impairment, such as hearing or visual impairment, can also impair one's ability to interact and engage with others. Older adults with considerable hearing difficulties, for example, may feel limited in their ability to communicate with others. They may also experience challenges hearing others in loud, public settings.

A review of studies investigating the relationship of social isolation and loneliness in older adults, generally found detrimental effects on outcomes such as depression,[37] blood pressure,[38] physical activity[39] and overall sense of well-being.[40] Moreover, social isolation has been identified as a risk factor for mortality.[41] Knowing this, studies have shown effective ways to combat social isolation and loneliness in our aging population, ranging from reminiscence therapy to animal-centered interventions, including the use of robotic animals.[42–44] Involvement in religious organizations may also protect against loneliness and social isolation in older adults by offering an avenue for social networking and community-building.[45] Also, while previously limited by the lack of randomized-controlled trials and optimal methodologies, researchers have begun to focus on the impact of technology, including group videoconferencing, on perceived loneliness and social connectedness in older adults.[46,47] While socialization and connectedness are a considerable part of maintaining a quality of life as we age, it is important to also recognize that interventions to address these issues should be tailored to the individual's needs, rather than a one-size-fits-all approach. The experience of loneliness and social isolation is individualized, and therefore, interventions should focus on the individual's specific needs, goals and values, that is, **what matters most** to the person.

NUTRITION

Nutrition is important to quality of life and health with aging. Protein-calorie malnutrition is associated with increased morbidity and mortality in older adults.[48,49] A 2016 meta-analysis reported malnutrition in 3.1% of the older adult population living in the community, 6.0% in outpatient practices, 8.7% receiving home-care services, 22.0% of hospitalized older adults, 17.5% in nursing homes, 28.7% in long-term care and 29.4% in rehabilitation/sub-acute care.[50] A study published in 2010 investigated the prevalence of malnutrition in about 4,507 "old-old" adults (mean age 82.3 years). Using the Mini Nutritional Assessment, they found the overall prevalence of malnutrition in this cohort was about 22.8%; the prevalence of malnutrition in different settings was as follows: 50.5% rehabilitation, 38.7% hospital, 13.8% nursing home, 5.8% community.[51]

Poor nutrition in older adults may be due to multiple factors, including changes in appetite, medical conditions causing cachexia, impairments in mastication and the ability to prepare, digest and absorb food. One study of 563 adults aged 70 years or older found that being edentulous was an independent risk factor for significant weight loss, even after controlling for gender, income, advanced age and baseline weight.[52]

However, medical and oral issues aside, there are age-related physiologic changes that likely impact nutrition. Older age is associated with a reduced ability to detect food-related odors.[53] Given the impact of aromas on an individual's experience with tasting foods, a change in olfactory function may cause decreased enjoyment in eating. However, it can be helpful for older adults to view this change as an opportunity to explore different foods and textures that may be more palatable to them at this stage of their life. For example, patients affected by olfactory changes may benefit from trialing foods with different flavor profiles in an effort to compensate for these changes. Providers may also suggest liberalizing diets to allow individuals to maintain their food intake and nutritional status.

Maintaining adequate nutrition is a crucial aspect of aging. The breakdown of an individual's nutritional status, including specific calorie requirements, may vary depending on the individual's energy expenditures and health problems. It is, however, important to recognize physiologic changes that may impact nutrition, in order to offer realistic, lifestyle-based interventions.

SLEEP

Poor sleep is not necessarily a consequence of normal aging,[54] however, there are age-related changes in sleep and other functions that may interfere with getting a "good night's sleep." There are 5 EEG stages of sleep as shown in Table 3.2.

Studies suggest that there may be a reduction in REM sleep in both men and women.[55,56] It may take longer to fall asleep as we get older, and we tend to sleep more lightly, awakening to sounds that previously wouldn't have bothered us. Older adults may experience less slow-wave sleep compared to younger adults; this is particularly important as slow-wave sleep or "deep sleep" tends to be one of the more restorative stages of sleep. Additionally, changes in circadian rhythm, or the internal

TABLE 3.2
Stages of Sleep

Stages	Description
Wakefulness	A period characterized by mixed-frequency or alpha waves.
Stage 1	A stage of sleep that occurs when one initially falls into a light sleep; this is characterized by alpha and possibly theta waves.
Stage 2	A slightly deeper sleep that comprises about 50% of sleep time and is characterized by spine and/or K complexes.
Stage 3	A deep sleep that accounts for the most restorative stages of sleep and is characterized by theta/slow waves.
REM Sleep	A stage when one dreams; this is characterized by similar mixed-frequency amplitude EEG as when one is awake.

system regulating wakefulness and sleepiness, tend to be more common in older adults. This may cause individuals to wake up and go to sleep earlier as they age, compared to middle-aged adults.

Older adults are at increased risk for primary sleep disorders including sleep apnea and restless legs syndrome. Practitioners should also be attuned to other medical conditions such as cough, nocturia and heart failure that occur more commonly in older adults and can negatively impact sleep. Medications, such as beta-blockers and steroids, may also influence an individual's sleep pattern. While sleep patterns may change due to physiological phenomena as we age, the high rate of sleep pathology, and the consequences of sleep deprivation on memory and falls behooves practitioners to thoroughly investigate and evaluate reported sleep concerns.

CONCLUSIONS

In general, life expectancy has increased within the United States and internationally. Globally, the World Health Organization estimates life expectancy to have increased by more than 6 years between 2000 and 2019, specifically from 66.8 years in 2000 to 73.4 years in 2019.[57] Additionally, the number of people above the age of 80 years nearly tripled, from 54 million in 1990 to 143 million in 2019.[58]

While prior theories of aging tend to center on seemingly unidimensional perspectives of decline and senescence, more recent literature suggests the importance of recognizing concepts such as mental and physical resilience as a part of aging.[59-61] As patients begin to live longer and experience different stages in their lives, practitioners should remain sensitive about providing individualized, patient-centered care, and incorporate concepts such as homestenosis, frailty and other geriatric syndromes into their medical evaluations. As life expectancy increases, health systems need to support and promote healthy aging. The lived experience of patients as they move into different stages of their lives can be quite daunting; however, providers can help them navigate the uncharted waters of aging by offering practical, patient-centered recommendations informed by evidence.

CLINICAL APPLICATIONS

- Health care providers should use the 5Ms approach to provide patient-centered care to older adults.
- Consider homestenosis, frailty and geriatric syndromes when caring for older adults.
- Recognize the impact that socialization, sleep and nutrition can have on an individual's well-being, particularly as they age.
- Encourage older adults to view changes associated with aging in a positive light.

REFERENCES

1. Ageing, N. Meanings, etymology and more | Oxford English Dictionary. Accessed December 17, 2023. https://www.oed.com/dictionary/ageing_n?tl=true&tab=factsheet
2. Aging | Definition, process, & effects | Britannica. Published November 30, 2023. Accessed December 17, 2023. https://www.britannica.com/science/aging-life-process
3. Understanding the dynamics of the aging process. National Institute on Aging. Accessed December 17, 2023. https://www.nia.nih.gov/about/aging-strategic-directions-research/understanding-dynamics-aging
4. Ageing_2 adjective – definition, pictures, pronunciation and usage notes | Oxford Advanced Learner's Dictionary at OxfordLearnersDictionaries.com. Accessed December 17, 2023. https://www.oxfordlearnersdictionaries.com/us/definition/english/ageing_2
5. Ageing: Ageism. Accessed February 1, 2024. https://www.who.int/news-room/questions-and-answers/item/ageing-ageism
6. North MS, Fiske ST. Modern attitudes toward older adults in the aging world: a cross-cultural meta-analysis. *Psychol Bull*. 2015;141(5):993–1021. doi:10.1037/a0039469.
7. Elder care as "frustrating" and "boring": understanding the persistence of negative attitudes toward older patients among physicians-in-training. Accessed February 1, 2024. https://www.sciencedirect.com/science/article/abs/pii/S0890406512000552?via%3Dihub
8. Briggs R, Robinson S, O'Neill D. Ageism and clinical research. *Ir Med J*. 2012;105(9):311–312.
9. Levy BR, Slade MD, Kunkel SR, Kasl SV. Longevity increased by positive self-perceptions of aging. *J Pers Soc Psychol*. 2002;83(2):261–270. doi:10.1037/0022-3514.83.2.261.
10. Ingrand I, Paccalin M, Liuu E, Gil R, Ingrand P. Positive perception of aging is a key predictor of quality-of-life in aging people. *PLoS One*. 2018;13(10):e0204044. doi:10.1371/journal.pone.0204044.
11. Gu R, Zhang D, Jin X, et al. The self-perceptions of aging were an important factor associated with the quality of life in Chinese elderly with hypertension. *Psychogeriatrics*. 2019;19(4):391–398. doi:10.1111/psyg.12400.
12. Levy BR, Zonderman AB, Slade MD, Ferrucci L. Age stereotypes held earlier in life predict cardiovascular events in later life. *Psychol Sci*. 2009;20(3):296–298. doi:10.1111/j.1467-9280.2009.02298.x.
13. Levy BR, Slade MD, Chang ES, Kannoth S, Wang SY. Ageism amplifies cost and prevalence of health conditions. *Gerontologist*. 2020;60(1):174–181. doi:10.1093/geront/gny131.

14. Fried LP, Cohen AA, Xue QL, Walston J, Bandeen-Roche K, Varadhan R. The physical frailty syndrome as a transition from homeostatic symphony to cacophony. *Nat Aging.* 2021;1(1):36–46. doi:10.1038/s43587-020-00017-z.
15. Fried LP, Tangen CM, Walston J, et al. Frailty in older adults: evidence for a phenotype. *J Gerontol A Biol Sci Med Sci.* 2001;56(3):M146–M157. doi:10.1093/gerona/56.3.M146.
16. Bandeen-Roche K, Xue QL, Ferrucci L, et al. Phenotype of frailty: characterization in the women's health and aging studies. *J Gerontol A Biol Sci Med Sci.* 2006;61(3):262–266. doi:10.1093/gerona/61.3.262.
17. Rockwood K, Mitnitski A. Frailty in relation to the accumulation of deficits. *J Gerontol A Biol Sci Med Sci.* 2007;62(7):722–727. doi:10.1093/gerona/62.7.722.
18. Mitnitski AB, Mogilner AJ, Rockwood K. Accumulation of deficits as a proxy measure of aging. *Sci World J.* 2001;1:323–336. doi:10.1100/tsw.2001.58.
19. Blodgett J, Theou O, Kirkland S, Andreou P, Rockwood K. Frailty in NHANES: comparing the frailty index and phenotype. *Arch Gerontol Geriatr.* 2015;60(3):464–470. doi:10.1016/j.archger.2015.01.016.
20. Tip Sheet: The 5Ms of geriatrics | HealthInAging.org. Accessed December 17, 2023. https://www.healthinaging.org/tools-and-tips/tip-sheet-5ms-geriatrics.
21. OECD and World Health Organization – 2015 – Promoting Health, Preventing Disease The Economic.pdf. Accessed December 19, 2023. https://www.cdc.gov/aging/pdf/mental_health_brief_2.pdf.
22. Birrer RB, Vemuri SP. Depression in later life: a diagnostic and therapeutic challenge. *Am Fam Physician.* 2004;69(10):2375–2382.
23. Physical Changes with Aging – Geriatrics. Merck Manuals Professional Edition. Accessed December 18, 2023. https://www.merckmanuals.com/professional/geriatrics/approach-to-the-geriatric-patient/physical-changes-with-aging.
24. Reinders I, Visser M, Schaap L. Body weight and body composition in old age and their relationship with frailty. *Curr Opin Clin Nutr Metab Care.* 2017;20(1):11–15. doi:10.1097/MCO.0000000000000332.
25. Jayanama K, Theou O, Godin J, Mayo A, Cahill L, Rockwood K. Relationship of body mass index with frailty and all-cause mortality among middle-aged and older adults. *BMC Med.* 2022;20(1):404. doi:10.1186/s12916-022-02596-7.
26. Walston JD. Common clinical sequelae of aging. In: Goldman L, Schafer AI, eds. *Goldman-Cecil Medicine.* 26th ed. Elsevier; 2020:102–105.e2. doi:10.1016/B978-0-323-53266-2.00022-9.
27. Bohannon RW, Williams Andrews A. Normal walking speed: a descriptive meta-analysis. *Physiotherapy.* 2011;97(3):182–189. doi:10.1016/j.physio.2010.12.004.
28. Studenski S, Perera S, Patel K, et al. Gait speed and survival in older adults. *JAMA.* 2011;305(1):50–58. doi:10.1001/jama.2010.1923.
29. Abellan Van Kan G, Rolland Y, Andrieu S, et al. Gait speed at usual pace as a predictor of adverse outcomes in community-dwelling older people: an International Academy on Nutrition and Aging (IANA) Task Force. *J Nutr Health Aging.* 2009;13(10):881–889. doi:10.1007/s12603-009-0246-z.
30. Montero-Odasso M, Schapira M, Soriano ER, et al. Gait velocity as a single predictor of adverse events in healthy seniors aged 75 years and older. *J Gerontol A Biol Sci Med Sci.* 2005;60(10):1304–1309. doi:10.1093/gerona/60.10.1304.
31. Verghese J, Wang C, Lipton RB, Holtzer R, Xue X. Quantitative gait dysfunction and risk of cognitive decline and dementia. *J Neurol Neurosurg Psychiatry.* 2007;78(9):929–935. doi:10.1136/jnnp.2006.106914.
32. Rodrigues F, Domingos C, Monteiro D, Morouço P. A review on aging, sarcopenia, falls, and resistance training in community-dwelling older adults. *Int J Environ Res Public Health.* 2022;19(2):874. doi:10.3390/ijerph19020874.

33. Rubenstein LZ, Josephson KR. The epidemiology of falls and syncope. *Clin Geriatr Med.* 2002;18(2):141–158. doi:10.1016/S0749-0690(02)00002-2.
34. Risk factors for falls among elderly persons living in the community. *N Engl J Med.* Accessed December 19, 2023. https://www.nejm.org/doi/full/10.1056/nejm198812293192604.
35. Risk factors for recurrent nonsyncopal falls: a prospective study. *JAMA.* Accessed December 19, 2023. https://jamanetwork.com/journals/jama/article-abstract/377277.
36. American Geriatrics Society. 2023 updated AGS Beers Criteria® for potentially inappropriate medication use in older adults. *J Am Geriatr Soc.* 2023. Accessed March 25, 2024. https://agsjournals.onlinelibrary.wiley.com/doi/full/10.1111/jgs.18372.
37. Cacioppo JT, Hughes ME, Waite LJ, Hawkley LC, Thisted RA. Loneliness as a specific risk factor for depressive symptoms: cross-sectional and longitudinal analyses. *Psychol Aging.* 2006;21(1):140–151. doi:10.1037/0882-7974.21.1.140.
38. Hawkley LC, Thisted RA, Masi CM, Cacioppo JT. Loneliness predicts increased blood pressure: five-year cross-lagged analyses in middle-aged and older adults. *Psychol Aging.* 2010;25(1):132–141. doi:10.1037/a0017805.
39. Hawkley LC, Thisted RA, Cacioppo JT. Loneliness predicts reduced physical activity: cross-sectional & longitudinal analyses. *Health Psychol.* 2009;28(3):354–363. doi:10.1037/a0014400.
40. Courtin E, Knapp M. Social isolation, loneliness and health in old age: a scoping review. *Health Soc Care Community.* 2017;25(3):799–812. doi:10.1111/hsc.12311.
41. Steptoe A, Shankar A, Demakakos P, Wardle J. Social isolation, loneliness, and all-cause mortality in older men and women. *Proc Natl Acad Sci U S A.* 2013;110(15):5797–5801. doi:10.1073/pnas.1219686110.
42. Dickens AP, Richards SH, Greaves CJ, Campbell JL. Interventions targeting social isolation in older people: a systematic review. *BMC Public Health.* 2011;11:647. doi:10.1186/1471-2458-11-647.
43. Hoang P, King JA, Moore S, et al. Interventions associated with reduced loneliness and social isolation in older adults. *JAMA Netw Open.* 2022;5(10):e2236676. doi:10.1001/jamanetworkopen.2022.36676.
44. Fakoya OA, McCorry NK, Donnelly M. Loneliness and social isolation interventions for older adults: a scoping review of reviews. *BMC Public Health.* 2020;20(1):129. doi:10.1186/s12889-020-8251-6.
45. Rote S, Hill TD, Ellison CG. Religious attendance and loneliness in later life. *Gerontologist.* 2013;53(1):39–50. doi:10.1093/geront/gns063.
46. Balki E, Hayes N, Holland C. Effectiveness of technology interventions in addressing social isolation, connectedness, and loneliness in older adults: systematic umbrella review. *JMIR Aging.* 2022;5(4):e40125. doi:10.2196/40125.
47. Grey E, Baber F, Corbett E, Ellis D, Gillison F, Barnett J. The use of technology to address loneliness and social isolation among older adults: the role of social care providers. *BMC Public Health.* 2024;24(1):108. doi:10.1186/s12889-023-17386-w.
48. Malnutrition is associated with increased mortality in older adults regardless of the cause of death. *Br J Nutr.* Accessed December 18, 2023. https://www-cambridge-org.eresources.mssm.edu/core/journals/british-journal-of-nutrition/article/malnutrition-is-associated-with-increased-mortality-in-older-adults-regardless-of-the-cause-of-death/315040A95BD3AD48E274F6CEBCFA1FB9.
49. Nutritional status predicts preterm death in older people: a prospective cohort study. *Clin Key.* Accessed December 18, 2023. https://www-clinicalkey-com.eresources.mssm.edu/#!/content/playContent/1-s2.0-S0261561413001763?returnurl=null&referrer=null.

50. Nutritional status in older persons according to healthcare setting: a systematic review and meta-analysis of prevalence data using MNA®. *Clin Key.* Accessed December 18, 2023. https://www-clinicalkey-com.eresources.mssm.edu/#!/content/playContent/1-s2.0-S0261561416000996?returnurl=null&referrer=null.
51. Kaiser MJ, Bauer JM, Rämsch C, et al. Frequency of malnutrition in older adults: a multinational perspective using the Mini Nutritional Assessment. *J Am Geriatr Soc.* 2010;58(9):1734–1738. doi:10.1111/j.1532-5415.2010.03016.x.
52. Ritchie CS, Joshipura K, Silliman RA, Miller B, Douglas CW. Oral health problems and significant weight loss among community-dwelling older adults. *J Gerontol A Biol Sci Med Sci.* 2000;55(7):M366–M371. doi:10.1093/gerona/55.7.M366.
53. Rolls BJ. Do chemosensory changes influence food intake in the elderly? *Physiol Behav.* 1999;66(2):193–197. doi:10.1016/S0031-9384(98)00264-9.
54. Normal and abnormal sleep in the elderly. *Clin Key.* Accessed December 18, 2023. https://www-clinicalkey-com.eresources.mssm.edu/#!/content/playContent/1-s2.0-S0749069021000239?returnurl=null&referrer=null.
55. Redline S, Kirchner HL, Quan SF, Gottlieb DJ, Kapur V, Newman A. The effects of age, sex, ethnicity, and sleep-disordered breathing on sleep architecture. *Arch Intern Med.* 2004;164(4):406–418. doi:10.1001/archinte.164.4.406.
56. Age-related changes in slow wave sleep and REM sleep and relationship with growth hormone and cortisol levels in healthy men. *JAMA.* Accessed December 18, 2023. https://jamanetwork.com/journals/jama/fullarticle/192981.
57. GHE: Life expectancy and healthy life expectancy. *World Health Organization.* Accessed December 18, 2023. https://www.who.int/data/gho/data/themes/mortality-and-global-health-estimates/ghe-life-expectancy-and-healthy-life-expectancy.
58. World Population Prospects 2019 Highlights. United Nations Department of Economic and Social Affairs. Accessed March 25, 2024. https://population.un.org/wpp/Publications/Files/WPP2019_Highlights.pdf.
59. Smith JL, Hollinger-Smith L. Savoring, resilience, and psychological well-being in older adults. *Aging Ment Health.* 2015;19(3):192–200. doi:10.1080/13607863.2014.986647.
60. Lavretsky H. Health, resilience, and successful aging in the older US veterans. *Am J Geriatr Psychiatry.* 2021;29(3):257–259. doi:10.1016/j.jagp.2020.08.018.
61. Whitson HE, Duan-Porter W, Schmader KE, Morey MC, Cohen HJ, Colón-Emeric CS. Physical resilience in older adults: systematic review and development of an emerging construct. *J Gerontol A Biol Sci Med Sci.* 2016;71(4):489–495. doi:10.1093/gerona/glv202.

4 Confronting Ageism with Language and Lifestyle Medicine

Kaitlin Kyi

Despite mounting efforts for equity, ageism continues to be pervasive with profound implications for older adults, particularly within the realm of health care.[1] Oftentimes called one of the last socially acceptable "isms," ageism manifests as negative attitudes about older persons; while other "isms" have been more recently under scrutiny, ageism is more widely accepted, even across cultures.[2,3] Evidence of this can be found daily in "anti-aging beauty campaigns" as well as more insidious, subtle methods of infantilizing or overlooking older adults. This can be as seemingly innocuous as a joke about memory loss in aging, where older adults are described as having "senior moments." While there is certainly a higher prevalence of cognitive impairment in older adults, such "humor" can have negative outcomes if providers overlook pathologic memory loss as "normal," not to mention the negative self-image that can be engendered in older adults over time.[4] In a study looking at self-perception in older adults, individuals with increased negative age-related stereotypes were more likely to have increased cardiovascular events up to decades later; such work suggests that internalized age-related stigma can adversely affect future health outcomes.[5]

The effects of ageism become more alarming in light of stark disparities in health care access and outcomes based on age. A growing body of research indicates that older adults are less likely to be offered certain medical interventions or referred for specialized treatments compared to younger patients with similar conditions. Such discrepancy often leads to delayed and inadequate treatment.[6,7] Much of this is likely directly related to age-related stereotypes influencing health care providers' perceptions of patient function, thereby directly affecting the quality of care older patients receive. In the treatment of such diseases as cancer, older adults can have age-related toxicities, but attention to chronologic age, rather than factors such as function, resilience and treatment preference, can lead to undertreatment of older adults.[8]

Ageism in health care is further compounded by the prevalence of chronic conditions among older adults; this population is more likely to experience multiple health issues concurrently. An ageist attitude might lead health care providers to dismiss new symptoms as a natural part of aging. This was explored in the example above, wherein a patient with memory issues might be described as "having a senior moment." Rather than addressing any new or underlying medical concerns, an ageist mindset might lead to a physician dismissing memory concerns as "just part of aging." Among older adults with probable dementia, a majority were either undiagnosed or unaware of a diagnosis, which suggests ageist barriers to discussion and diagnosis of cognitive deficits between patients and providers.[9]

Aside from undertreatment and underdiagnosis, the impact of health care extends beyond individual experiences to broader health outcomes. Myriad studies demonstrate that ageism contributes to disparities in health status and mortality rates among older populations. One study found that older individuals with more positive perceptions of self and aging lived 7.5 years longer on average when compared to those with less positive perceptions of aging; this positive effect was observed even after comparing across age, gender, socioeconomic status, functional heath and perception of loneliness.[10] Perhaps unsurprisingly, older adults who perceive age-based discrimination are more likely to report poorer health outcomes, including higher rates of chronic stress, anxiety and depression.[11]

Combating ageism can begin with both patients and providers challenging stigmatizing age-based language. Within the confines of clinical care alone, ageist language can influence the management and consideration of treatments.[12] Such stigmatizing language can create a rift between providers and patients, as well as transmit bias from one clinician to another; this becomes particularly relevant as electronic health records become more accessible to patients and caregivers alike.[13] In direct communication with patients, providers can sometimes resort to "elderspeak" by exaggerating intonation and over-enunciation at a slower pace – an overall infantilizing experience for the patients themselves. Ironically, this communication strategy has actually been shown to reduce comprehension.[14]

Different ageist communication patterns have been previously described: (1) casting doubt on the patient narrative, (2) including unnecessary indicators, (3) use of disease-centered language and (4) including outdated or non-neutral word choices.[13] Awareness of these ageist communication patterns can reduce their frequency, and thus, examples will be shown for each mechanism in order to avoid bias perpetuation.

TABLE 4.1

Patterns of Stigmatizing Language and Ways in Which They Contribute to Ageist Beliefs

Stigmatizing Language Pattern	Mechanism of Propagating Ageism
Casting doubt on the patient's narrative	• Loss of patient's individual perspective
Inclusion of unnecessary indicators	• Transmission of age-related bias, for example, implication of subjective "frailty" rather than objective testing
Disease-first language	• Depersonalizing older adult and their experience
Negative terminology	• Implication of weakness or frailty • Derogatory descriptors, which can erode a patient's self-image

The first pattern of ageist communication is invoking doubt upon the patient's narrative. In older patients, this commonly occurs with a description of the older adult as a "poor historian" rather than stating why it might be difficult to provide history (e.g., illness, sedation). The next provider reading the chart might wrongly assume the patient is "unreliable" and thus not fully engage the patient in crucial decision-making, perhaps even choosing to sidestep the patient and discuss management only with family or a caregiver. Avoiding point-blank description of an older adult as a "poor historian" would allow for following providers to formulate their own timely assessment.

The next pattern of ageist communication that commonly occurs in the electronic record is the inclusion of unnecessary, subjective indicators. For example, many times, descriptions are based on the physician's perception of age, including such descriptors as "older than stated age" or "elderly." These descriptors are predicated on the assumption that older appearance is associated with poor overall health.[15] Without objective assessment, future readers of this physical description might think of patients more favorably or unfavorably; more objective assessments (such as performance status or physical testing) should be preferred.

Another ageist language choice is using disease-centered language – or using language that emphasizes their disease state (rather than their personhood). Commonly in the chart, patients can be described as a "diabetic" as opposed to a "patient" or "person with diabetes." If a patient has a diagnosis of Alzheimer's dementia, disease-first language would be labeling them "demented" rather than the preferred "person living with dementia."

Perhaps the most obvious ageist language choice is the outright usage of negative terminology. Language is ever-evolving. For older patients, even the word "elderly" has taken on connotations of weakness without specifying objective physical assessments; advocates for older patients have advised against this language choice. Similarly, usage of "frail" (commonly associated with frailty risk stratification tools) is difficult for patients viewing their own medical chart; patients who consider themselves "frail" have higher reports of feelings of inferiority.[16] Again, as patients increasingly gain access to their own health records, they have a unique opportunity to read the words of their medical providers. Aside from errors, including miscategorization of racial or ethnic identity, many patients felt the sting of stigma or were outright offended by their physicians' language. One study showed 10% of patients with access to their electronic health records felt judged or offended by their physicians' language.[17,18]

With the recognition of these most common ageist language usages, providers can regain a more neutral approach to the description of their patients in communication with others. By reframing our language surrounding age, there can be a reduction of the overall stigma around aging. Unfortunately, stigma can be a powerful catalyst for adverse patient outcomes, as with delay of diagnosis and inequity of care as previously mentioned. However, this extends to other downstream negative effects, as with denial or concealment of diagnoses (e.g., an older patient not wishing to mention memory concerns due to further stigma) and subsequent reluctance to seek care and treatment. In older adults, there are additional concerns that they may be a burden to their family or caregivers.[19]

Alongside less ageist language in medical charts, providers can extend this to everyday conversations, especially when working alongside trainees. By continuing to avoid ageist language, there can be less transmission of bias from one provider to another; this can be a powerful way to tap into the "hidden curriculum." In the world of medical training, this "hidden curriculum" refers to that set of cultural influences in medical school or clinical training environments where trainees and students imitate role models (unconsciously or consciously) in order to adapt.[20] If a clinical preceptor repeatedly uses "elderspeak" and adopts a loud, condescending manner of speech, their observing trainee might then also begin using "elderspeak," unconsciously developing ageist biases that older adults are to be infantilized. Role modeling sensitivity to ageist biases and avoidance of stigmatizing is critical in molding medical trainees in the future.

Just as thought leaders have proposed anti-racism and anti-sexism practices, perhaps anti-ageism is the next call to action; it is not enough to simply not be ageist, providers can be more proactive in improving the lives of older adults.[21]

The World Health Organization (WHO) has formulated a global campaign to "combat ageism." In their outlined goals, they hope for increased awareness and achieving a more "age-integrated society." Some of the goals are the creation of age-friendly environments and active prevention of abuse of older adults, as well as the promotion of evidence-based frameworks and strategies to tackle ageism.[22] Similarly, the FrameWorks Institute, a nonprofit organization focused on research in social science, has created a framework for changing public discourse around aging in efforts to bring awareness to ageism. Key findings from their research include challenging the notion that aging is part of an inevitable decline in independence and value. To reframe this misconception, their toolkit uses themes of dignity and inclusion, sharing stories and specific examples that demonstrate the diverse experiences of older adults. Through advocacy, educational campaigns and training for organizations, the FrameWorks Institute has built tools to combat ageism.[23] These educational campaigns from FrameWorks Institute and WHO represent a sea change in how we approach and manage the care of older adults.

The growing sector of lifestyle medicine serves as another powerful tool in combating ageism by promoting a positive view of the aging process. With an active focus on health promotion, the field highlights lifestyle factors such as nutrition, physical activity and social connections, shifting the narrative from increasing dependence and physical decline in old age. Instead, it emphasizes continued growth and vitality, directly challenging ageist stereotypes that older age is a period of decline and frailty.[24]

With an emphasis on self-care, lifestyle medicine also empowers older adults to take a more active role in their health and well-being. Providing education, resources and support for making healthy lifestyle choices, enables individuals to regain a sense of control over their health outcomes. This is in direct contrast to assumptions that older adults are passive recipients of care, unable to manage their health.[25] In this same vein, lifestyle medicine also embraces a personalized approach to individual health needs. This personalized approach directly challenges the idea of older adults as a monolithic entity; by taking a personalized approach to health

TABLE 4.2
Tenets of Lifestyle Medicine and How Each Guides Anti-Ageist Practice

Lifestyle Medicine Tenet	Mechanism of Challenging Ageism
Self-care	• Regain a sense of control for older adults
Personalized approach	• Providers tailor intervention to older adults' specific needs and values
Social inclusion	• Bolster lifestyle factors, for example, physical activity, sleep • Refute the assumption that older adults are disconnected within their communities
Normalization of the aging process	• Celebrates strengths and contributions of older adults • Increased inclusion and respect

promotion, health care providers are encouraged to tailor interventions to the specific needs and value preferences of older adults.[26] By respecting older adults as individuals with diverse experiences forming different functionalities and values, ageism is directly confronted head-on. There is no room for stereotypes or prejudice in this scenario.

Lifestyle medicine also emphasizes the importance of social connections and community engagement. Social inclusion can challenge ageist assumptions that older adults are disconnected from society and within communities. Such social supports can additionally bolster other lifestyle factors (physical activity, sleep).[27]

Perhaps the most potent tenet of lifestyle medicine is the way in which it normalizes the aging process. Rather than generalizing aging, lifestyle medicine emphasizes that aging is a natural and diverse experience. By celebrating the strengths and contributions of older adults, it counters negative stereotypes that portray aging as a uniform experience characterized by decline and dependency. This normalization of aging promotes a more inclusive and respectful view of older adults in society.[28]

Overall, lifestyle medicine plays a crucial role in combating ageism by promoting an empowered, personalized view of aging. By emphasizing health promotion, empowerment and personalized care, lifestyle medicine helps create a culture that treats older adults as integral members of society.

Addressing ageism in health care requires a nuanced, multi-pronged approach. From challenging ageist language and biases within the medical record to the actual implementation of evidence-based interventions and educational campaigns, there are growing movements to combat ageism and promote a more inclusive and respectful health care environment for older adults. Initiatives such as lifestyle medicine can be transformative for older adults, celebrating their diversity and normalizing the aging process. By embracing personalized care, promoting social connection and fostering a positive view of aging, lifestyle medicine and similar approaches can lead the way toward a future where older adults are more globally valued as integral members of society.

CLINICAL APPLICATIONS

Using the above text, clinicians can:

- Recognize and challenge age-related stigma when they observe it in clinical interactions in order to improve patient-provider communications.
- Adopt a personalized approach to the care of older adults, considering physical function, resilience and treatment preferences rather than narrowly focusing on chronological age.
- Advocate for older adults to ensure equitable care with medical work-ups and management.
- Educate other health care providers and trainees about the downstream effect of ageism in efforts to foster increased inclusivity for our older adult patients.
- Encourage older adults to be more active in addressing health concerns, including lifestyle modifications, particularly nutrition, physical activity and social connections.
- Normalize and celebrate the aging process, thereby promoting a culture of respect in health care for older adults.

REFERENCES

1. Bodner E, Palgi Y, Wyman MF. Ageism in mental health assessment and treatment of older adults. In: Ayalon L, Tesch-Römer C, eds. *Contemporary Perspectives on Ageism.* International Perspectives on Aging. Springer; 2018, vol. 19. doi:10.1007/978-3-319-73820-8_15.
2. Weir K. Ageism is one of the last socially acceptable prejudices. Psychologists are working to change that. *Monitor Psychol.* 2023;54(2). Accessed March 1, 2023. https://www.apa.org/monitor/2023/03/cover-new-concept-of-aging.
3. Boduroglu A, et al. Age-related stereotypes: a comparison of American and Chinese cultures. *Gerontology.* 2006;52(5):324–333.
4. Gendron TL, Welleford EA, Inker J, White JT. The language of ageism: why we need to use words carefully. *Gerontologist.* 2016;56(6):997–1006. doi:10.1093/geront/gnv066.
5. Levy BR, Zonderman AB, Slade MD, Ferrucci L. Age stereotypes held earlier in life predict cardiovascular events in later life. *Psychol Sci.* 2009;20(3):296–298. doi:10.1111/j.1467-9280.2009.02298.x.
6. Peake MD, Thompson S, Lowe D, Pearson MG; Participating Centres. Ageism in the management of lung cancer. *Age Ageing.* 2003;32(2):171–177.
7. Haigney E, Morgan R, King D, Spencer B. Breast examinations in older women: questionnaire survey of attitudes of patients and doctors. *BMJ.* 1997;315(7115):1058–1059. doi:10.1136/bmj.315.7115.1058.
8. DuMontier C, Loh KP, Bain PA, et al. Defining undertreatment and overtreatment in older adults with cancer: a scoping literature review. *J Clin Oncol.* 2020;38(25):2558–2569.
9. Amjad H, Roth DL, Sheehan OC, Lyketsos CG, Wolff JL, Samus QM. Underdiagnosis of dementia: an observational study of patterns in diagnosis and awareness in US older adults. *J Gen Intern Med.* 2018;33(7):1131–1138. doi:10.1007/s11606-018-4377-y.

10. Levy BR, Slade MD, Kunkel SR, Kasl SV. Longevity increased by positive self-perceptions of aging. *J Pers Soc Psychol.* 2002;83(2):261–270. doi:10.1037//0022-3514.83.2.261.
11. Kang H, Kim H. Ageism and psychological well-being among older adults: a systematic review. *Gerontol Geriatr Med.* 2022;8:23337214221087023. doi:10.1177/23337214221087023.
12. Ben-Harush A, Shiovitz-Ezra S, Doron I, et al. Ageism among physicians, nurses, and social workers: findings from a qualitative study. *Eur J Ageing.* 2016;14(1):39–48. doi:10.1007/s10433-016-0389-9.
13. Kyi K, Gilmore N, Kadambi S, Loh KP, Magnuson A. Stigmatizing language in caring for older adults with cancer: common patterns of use and mechanisms to change the culture. *J Geriatr Oncol.* 2023;14(8):101593. doi:10.1016/j.jgo.2023.101593.
14. Shaw CA, Ward C, Gordon J, Williams KN, Herr K. Elderspeak communication and pain severity as modifiable factors to rejection of care in hospital dementia care. *J Am Geriatr Soc.* 2022;70(8):2258–2268.
15. Hwang SW, Atia M, Nisenbaum R, Pare DE, Joordens S. Is looking older than one's actual age a sign of poor health? *J Gen Intern Med.* 2011;26(2):136–141.
16. Durepos P, et al. Older adults' perceptions of frailty language: a scoping review. *Can J Aging.* 2022;41(2):193–202.
17. Yemane L, Mateo CM, Desai AN. Race and ethnicity data in electronic health records-striving for clarity. *JAMA Netw Open.* 2024;7(3):e240522. doi:10.1001/jamanetworkopen.2024.0522.
18. Himmelstein G, Bates D, Zhou L. Examination of stigmatizing language in the electronic health record. *JAMA Netw Open.* 2022;5(1):e2144967.
19. Newheiser AK, Barreto M. Hidden costs of hiding stigma: ironic interpersonal consequences of concealing a stigmatized identity in social interactions. *J Exp Soc Psychol.* 2014;52:58–70.
20. Lempp H, Seale C. The hidden curriculum in undergraduate medical education: qualitative study of medical students' perceptions of teaching. *BMJ.* 2004;329(7469):770–773.
21. Morrow-Howell N, Kunkel S, Gendron T, Jarrott SE, Andreoletti C. Anti-ageism for gerontologists. *J Aging Soc Policy.* 2023 Mar 29:1–11. doi:10.1080/08959420.2023.2194816.
22. Officer A, de la Fuente-Núñez V. A global campaign to combat ageism. *Bull World Health Organ.* 2018;96(4):295–296. doi:10.2471/BLT.17.202424.
23. Rippe JM. Lifestyle medicine: the health-promoting power of daily habits and practices. *Am J Lifestyle Med.* 2018;12(6):499–512. doi:10.1177/1559827618785554.
24. Frameworks Institute. Gaining momentum: a FrameWorks Communication Toolkit. 2020. Accessed March 25, 2024. https://www.frameworksinstitute.org.
25. Symington E, El-Osta A, Birrell F. Supported self-care is integral to lifestyle medicine: can Virtual Group Consultations promote them both? *Lifestyle Med.* 2021;2:e43. doi:10.1002/lim2.43.
26. Burnes D, et al. Interventions to reduce ageism against older adults: a systematic review and meta-analysis. *Am J Public Health.* 2019;109(8):e1–e9.
27. Holt-Lunstad J. Positive social connection: a key pillar of lifestyle medicine. *J Fam Pract.* 2022;71(1):S38–S40.
28. Friedman SM. Lifestyle (medicine) and healthy aging. *Clin Geriatr Med.* 2020;36(4):645–653. doi:10.1016/j.cger.2020.06.007.

5 Climate Change, Lifestyle Medicine and Older Adults

Matthew Nelson and Jennifer Muniak

INTRODUCTION

Climate change is becoming more difficult to ignore. Between 2011 and 2020, global surface temperatures reached 1.1°C above 1850–1900 averages, primarily driven by human activity resulting in greenhouse gas emissions.[1] If we (humans) do not change our collective lifestyle in the next decade, particularly our reliance on fossil fuels, we are projected to exceed the goal of warming below 1.5°C set by the Paris Climate Agreement. An increase of this magnitude or greater will lead to irreparable harm to our biosphere and those who depend on it, ourselves included.[1]

Numerous health and well-being considerations are intertwined with the effects of climate change. This includes heat-related, respiratory and mental health disorders, infectious diseases and food insecurity.[2] Furthermore, environmental degradation due to climate change has the potential to negate gains made in the last several decades owing to improved medicines and technologies.[2,3] According to the Lancet Commission, the consequences of climate change could reverse the health gains achieved by the past 50 years of global economic development by 2050.[4] The medical field has begun to understand the magnitude of this challenge. The American College of Lifestyle Medicine, the American Medical Association and the American Academy of Pediatrics are among the signatories of the *U.S. Call to Action on Climate, Health, and Equity: A Policy Action Agenda*, which outlines ten priority action items that it calls on government, business and civil society leaders and candidates for elected office to address.[5] Notably, the American Geriatrics Society is not listed among its many signers. This is unfortunate as the global population is both aging and carrying a greater burden of chronic diseases that are exacerbated by climate change-related health effects.[6]

As a means of framing this textbook's discussion of lifestyle medicine in a geriatric context, this chapter will attempt to answer the call for increased attention to climate change in health care by reviewing the impact of the health care system on climate change, the unique vulnerability of older adults and the unique potential of lifestyle medicine as a climate-conscious approach to geriatric medicine. Ultimately, the authors wish to convey the congruence that exists between lifestyle medicine,

Climate Change, Lifestyle and Older Adults

geriatric medicine and climate concern, and to encourage increased and urgent attention to this topic.

THE HEALTH CARE SYSTEM AND CLIMATE CHANGE

The health care industry, due to its scale and reliance on fossil fuels, contributes a great deal to greenhouse gas emissions. Health care is responsible for 4.4% of emissions (two gigatons of carbon dioxide equivalent) which, put into perspective, is equivalent to the annual greenhouse gas emissions from 514 coal-fired power plants.[7] Said another way, if the global health care system was a country, it would be the *fifth largest emitter* on the planet.[7] In short, this means that decarbonizing the health care system is a significant part of mitigating climate change.

To consider how health care may need to evolve, it is helpful to understand the distribution of greenhouse gas emissions within the global health care system. It is uneven, with the United States, China and the collective countries of the European Union carrying 56% of the world's health care climate footprint.[7] The United States (US) health sector is by far the biggest emitter in both absolute and per capita terms.[7] Specifically, the US health care system is responsible for approximately 10% of national greenhouse gas emissions.[8] This is on par with emissions from the US agricultural industry, often cited as one of the biggest contributors to greenhouse gas emissions.[9] The oversized impact of Western and industrialized health care systems, particularly in the United States, informs our focus on the US health care sector in this section.

Greenhouse gas emissions within a given sector can be broken up into "scopes," a globally accepted and standardized framework developed by the Greenhouse Gas Protocol.[10]

- *Scope 1* refers to emissions directly from facilities, which in the case of health care refers to hospitals, outpatient offices, post-acute and long-term care facilities, health care-owned vehicles and other medical infrastructure such as administrative offices.[7]
- *Scope 2* refers to indirectly generated emissions, primarily the purchasing and consumption of energy from the national grid (electricity, steam, cooling and heating).[7,11]
- *Scope 3* is the supply chain – the production, transportation and disposal of goods and services (such as pharmaceuticals and other chemicals), food and agricultural products, medical devices, hospital equipment and instruments.[7]

Each scope accounts for a certain percentage of a sector's carbon footprint, with the distribution for the US health care system summarized in Figure 5.1. Scope 3 – the supply chain – accounts for the vast majority of emissions both in the United States (82%) and globally (71%), although sources vary on the exact percentages for emissions by scope.[7,11] The most important takeaway here is that the carbon footprint of the US health care sector is large, much larger than any individual's carbon footprint,

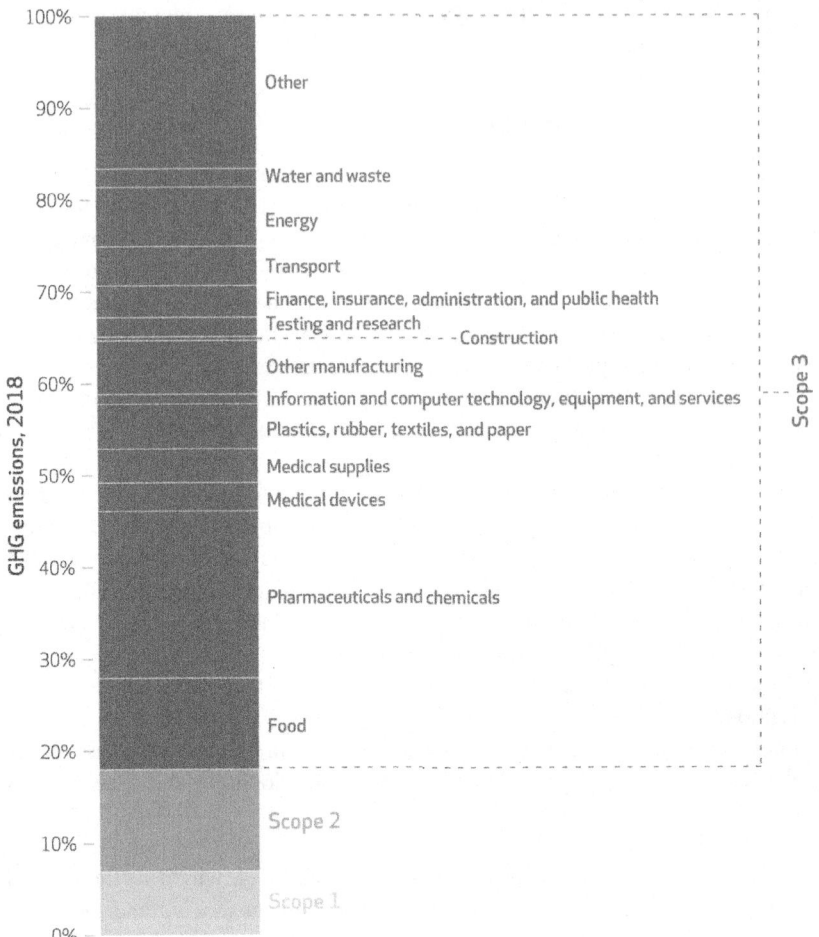

FIGURE 5.1 US health sector greenhouse gas emissions by Greenhouse Gas (GHG) Protocol scope using 2018 data. (Reprinted from Eckelman et al. Health Care Pollution and Public Health Damage in the United States: An Update. 2020. Exhibit 2.[12])

and inextricably intertwined with global reliance on fossil fuels which power supply chains, build hospitals, grow food for patients and produce pharmaceuticals. That said, many individuals taking collective lifestyle action, such as shifting to plant-based diets and less reliance on emissions-heavy travel, is incredibly important and needs to occur in lock-step with the decarbonization of our health care system.[12]

GERIATRIC MEDICINE AND CLIMATE CHANGE

Most humans living in industrialized consumer societies are reliant on industries powered by fossil fuels, the health care sector included. Older adults particularly

Climate Change, Lifestyle and Older Adults

so given their increased reliance on the health care system. This population is also growing, with the US population of those aged 65 expected to double over the next 30 years, from 43.1 million in 2012 to an estimated 83.7 million in 2050.[13] Geriatric medicine is dedicated to the health care challenges that come with aging, and must now take into consideration the needs of its growing target population from within an unsustainable health care system. In addition to their increased reliance on the health care system, this population is uniquely vulnerable to the health impacts of climate change. These are summarized in Figure 5.2 and discussed below.

Older adults are less able to compensate for the health impacts of environmental hazards such as air pollution and are more likely to have health conditions that make them more sensitive to these climate hazards.[14,15] Extreme weather

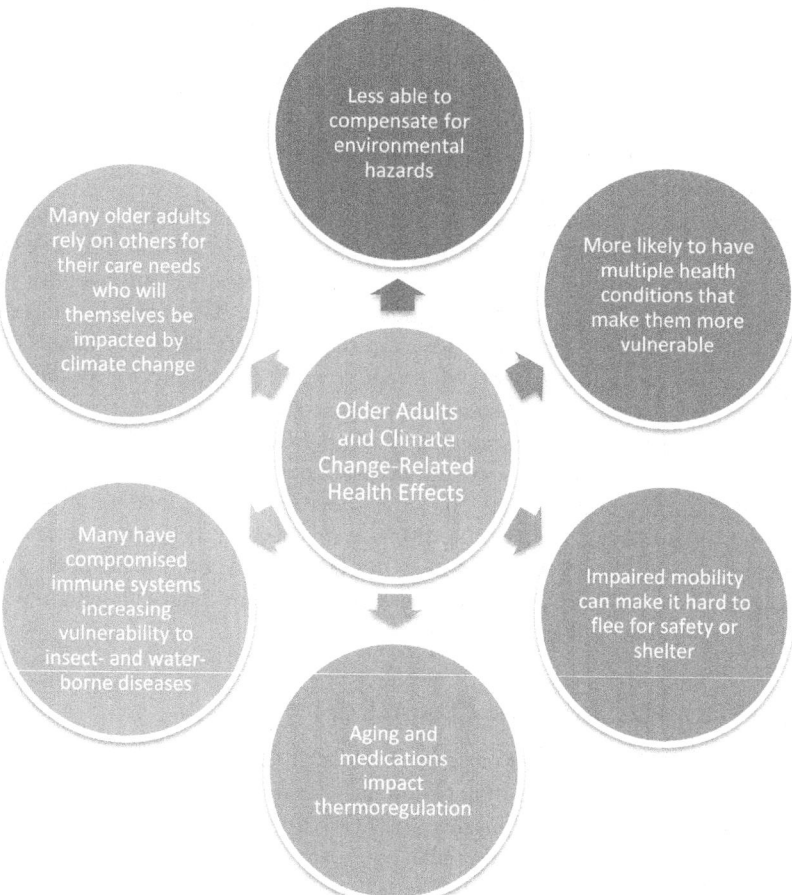

FIGURE 5.2 Climate change–related health effects on older adults. (Derived from the United States Environmental Protection Agency. Climate Change and the Health of Older Adults. 2022.[14])

events, such as storms, flooding or wildfires may require one to find shelter and/or flee to safety, which is a challenge for many older adults who are functionally limited or immobile.[14] The psychological impact and disorientation due to the chaos created in either sheltering or fleeing is also worse for those with cognitive impairments.[15] In the event of property destruction, the loss of treasured family memorabilia can be particularly distressing to older adults who rely on them for solace.[15] Disruptions in care caused by extreme weather can also impact life-saving equipment, and medications that many older adults rely on may not be available in a temporary shelter or due to supply chain disruptions.[15] Regarding heat waves, aging and common medications impact the body's ability to respond to heat effectively.[14] In fact, older adults account for an estimated 80% of heat-related deaths, which is likely an underestimation.[16] Furthermore, aging, medications and certain diseases common in older adults contribute to compromised immune systems, raising older adult's vulnerability to climate-linked insect- and water-borne diseases.[14] Finally, the climate crisis also impacts caregivers. Older adults, especially frail older adults, are more dependent on others for their medical care and assistance in daily life. The above climate-related health impacts affect everyone, caregivers included, potentially disrupting older adults' support systems and social connections.[14]

Fortunately, geriatric medicine is rooted in a model of care that is remarkably compatible with climate action in medicine. The Institute for Healthcare Improvement's (IHI) call to create Age-Friendly Health Systems focuses on four evidence-based elements of high-quality care for older adults – the 4Ms. These are: *What Matters, Medications, Mentation* and *Mobility*.[13] On the one hand, climate change and its downstream effects on our planet will directly impact our health care system's ability to care for older adults at the standards proposed by organizations such as the IHI. This is already known to some extent based on the COVID-19 pandemic – when the fault lines of our health care system are exposed, older adults are disproportionately harmed.[17,18] Furthermore, climate change is inevitably intertwined with our ability to consider the 4Ms as we age; the 4Ms are much more difficult to achieve in a degraded environment. At the same time, the 4Ms inform geriatric medicine's focus on deprescribing and lifestyle-based interventions that are congruent with more sustainable health care, as described below.

LIFESTYLE MEDICINE AND CLIMATE CHANGE

Lifestyle medicine applied to the care of older adults reflects the urgent need to integrate adaptation and mitigation of climate change into medical practice. The six pillars of lifestyle medicine – physical activity, nutrition, avoiding risky substances, sleep, stress management, social connection – are all directly impacted by climate change *and* are all connected to climate action. Like the 4Ms, the best practices of lifestyle medicine are both threatened in a changing climate and synergistic with reducing our carbon footprint. This section explores each pillar from this perspective in more detail.

Climate Change, Lifestyle and Older Adults

LIFESTYLE MEDICINE INTERVENTIONS AND CLIMATE CHANGE

There are several lifestyle medicine interventions that, on an individual level, provide co-benefits for targeting unhealthy lifestyle habits *and* act as effective climate mitigation strategies. The most frequently discussed of these are moving to a plant-based diet (beef, dairy, poultry and eggs contribute significantly more to greenhouse gas emissions than plant-based protein sources) and going car-free (with the idea of cycling or walking to work or in your community instead).[6,19–22] In fact, all six pillars of lifestyle medicine can be implemented through a climate lens. This was most recently examined by Drs. Neha Pathak and Amanda McKinney in the *American Journal of Lifestyle Medicine* in a paper titled "Planetary Health, Climate Change, and Lifestyle Medicine: Threats and Opportunities."[6] What follows is a distillation of this important work, focusing on the climate and health impacts, adaptations and actions relevant to each pillar. Readers are directed to the article by Drs. Pathak and McKinney[6] for a more thorough overview.

PHYSICAL ACTIVITY

Impact:

- Extreme weather events, increase in heat waves and worsening air pollution make it challenging (and dangerous) to exercise outdoors.[23–29]

Climate-friendly adaptation:

- Cycling, running or walking instead of driving reduces chronic disease and mortality, and reduces the individual's carbon footprint.[2,30]
- Exercising indoors helps avoid extreme weather conditions (requires access to indoor facilities and consideration of energy usage).

Action:

- Lobbying for active transport infrastructure (promoting walking or cycling, reducing transportation-related emissions).[30]
- Increasing access to indoor spaces for exercise that is energy efficient and relies less on the national grid (heat pumps, geothermal, solar).[31]

NUTRITION

Impact:

- Supply chain disruptions and risk of crop loss from extreme weather events reduce the reliability of healthy foods.[32]
- Increase in atmospheric CO_2 decreases protein and other mineral concentrations in a variety of foods.[32–34]

- Meat and dairy industry release significant greenhouse gas emissions.[35-38]
- Agricultural and food industries (especially highly processed food) contribute to deforestation, soil erosion, intensive water and energy use and pollution.[4,29,35,36,39]

Climate-friendly adaptation:

- Shifting to whole food plant-based diet not only increases health and nutritional benefits but is also environmentally more sustainable.[32,40]

Action:

- Bringing whole food plant-based diets into the exam room (reference diets available including Planetary Health Diet, Menus of Change and Reset the Table).[41-43]
- Advocating at the political level for increasing government subsidies for plant-based food sources.[44]

AVOIDING RISKY SUBSTANCES

Impact:

- Toxic pollutants in air, water, soil and consumer products are a modifiable burden of disease globally contributing significantly to chronic disease burden and mortality.[32,45-54]
- Increase in substance abuse is a maladaptive, but very real, coping strategy to climate distress.[2,55,56]

Climate-friendly adaptation:

- Avoid certain products high in pollutants such as personal care products and plastic food containers.[45]
- Avoid exposure to outdoor air on poor air quality days, utilizing respirator masks as appropriate, air purifiers and high-quality water filters.[57,58]

Action:

- Screening patients who have experienced extreme-weather events or suffered climate-related displacement for mental illness and substance use.[2,55,56]
- Lobbying for increased transparency, regulation and elimination of implicated chemicals and pesticides (recent modeling suggests targeting greenhouse gas emissions from energy, transport and agriculture sectors to achieve Paris Agreement and UN Sustainable Development Goals could result in 1.18 million avoided deaths from reduction in particulate air pollution alone[30]).

SLEEP

Impact:

- Restorative sleep is disrupted by extreme weather events.
- Restorative sleep is disrupted by noise and light pollution – common in urban settings which are often in close proximity to polluting industrial and manufacturing facilities (often socioeconomically disadvantaged and minority communities).[59,60]
- Increase in average temperatures impacts the body's ability to obtain restorative sleep.[61]
- Higher rates of sleep deprivation result in more psychological and physiological distress (worse for those living in urban tropical islands).[61]

Adaptation/Action (adaptations and actions indistinct for restorative sleep):

- Increase tree canopies and green space, which has been shown to result in better overall sleep time.[62]
- Shift toward more sustainable energy sources and electric vehicles is both an adaptation (electric vehicles and machinery have reduced noise levels) and helps mitigate environmental degradation.[6]

STRESS MANAGEMENT

Impact:

- Eco-anxiety (distress about future events from climate change) and solastalgia (distress about climate change in the home environment) are new terms among many others used to describe the way people are feeling about mounting climate-related disasters and environmental degradation.[56,63]
- Higher average temperatures increase the risk of causing and exacerbating rates of depression, anxiety, substance abuse and suicide.[56]

Climate-friendly adaptation:

- Build resilience in the face of ever-mounting, ever-increasing threats to individual and planetary health.
- Mind–body therapies such as yoga, meditation and mindfulness along with cognitive behavioral therapy are a selection of proposed resilience-building strategies.[64,65]

Action:

- Nature-based therapies offer both an adaptation and a climate mitigation strategy (improve resiliency, well-being and social cohesion, and promote carbon capture through tree planting and forests).[66-76]

- Collective action to halt climate change shown to have a positive impact on stress levels.[32,76]

SOCIAL CONNECTION

Impact:

- Rising global temperatures, unstable weather patterns and other associated climate-related effects strain social connections and cohesion.[2]

Climate-friendly adaptation:

- Bolstering our social connections and networks to build individual and community resilience in the face of climate change (community groups, faith communities, other social activities).[77]

Action:

- Protecting natural environments and building green spaces that can function as sacred spaces, build social cohesion and mitigate effects of climate change.[32,76]
- Using positive psychology interventions and discussing them with patients (gratitude, forgiveness, finding purpose) to help build and strengthen individual and community resilience in the face of mounting climate instability.[6,64]
- In turn, people are more likely to feel capable of being part of local efforts to anticipate and mitigate the effects of climate change.[6]

This brief review outlines the ways in which individuals' ability to practice the six pillars of lifestyle medicine is threatened by climate change and, at the same time, when thoughtfully implemented, the majority of these interventions can be climate actions in and of themselves. Of note, these are not the only and not necessarily the most impactful climate actions on the individual scale. Having one fewer child and avoiding airplane travel are evidence-based and high-impact individual climate mitigation strategies, but are acknowledged as less relevant to care providers in the course of a patient encounter.[19,20] That said, these two actions coupled with plant-based diets and going car-free have been shown to have a significantly greater individual impact on reducing greenhouse gas emissions than more commonly promoted strategies such as recycling (four times less effective than a plant-based diet) or changing household light bulbs (eight times less effective).[20]

There is an important perspective here, relevant to both climate action and lifestyle medicine. In clinical decision making it is important to know not only what interventions are available, but which are effective. Geriatric medicine, for example, has pioneered medication deprescribing in older adults to target the negative health effects of polypharmacy.[78] In so doing, the clinician is effectively stripping away *ineffective* (and oftentimes, potentially harmful) pharmacologic interventions in favor of focusing on more evidence-based and *effective* interventions for older adults. So too, when it comes to lifestyle interventions, identifying the most effective and evidence-based interventions to focus efforts on is paramount. This is especially true for climate change since the consequences of inaction *and* focusing on only low-impact behaviors (e.g., recycling) are severe. With this in mind, it is important to reiterate that climate-conscious behavior change at the individual level is an important part of the process people must go through, especially when done as part of collective action, but it is equally important not to lose sight of the larger systems-level changes that need to take place to bring carbon emissions down to zero and move from an extractive way of living to a regenerative one.

—

Don't forget to breathe. The trouble with writing (or reading) a chapter on climate change is that part of our "lifestyle" comes from the news we encounter, in which we consume fear with no reprieve, pause or help to process. If we are to be effective clinicians and care providers in this time of great upheaval, we must begin to turn toward the fear, loss, helplessness and love for the world we feel. This pause in a chapter on climate change is an invitation to breathe and feel. Eco-philosopher Joanna Macy is a wonderful guide in this:

> This is a dark time, filled with suffering and uncertainty. Like living cells in a larger body, it is natural that we feel the trauma of our world. So don't be afraid of the anguish you feel, or the anger or fear, because these responses arise from the depth of your caring and the truth of your interconnectedness with all beings.[79]

This concludes the review of the connections between climate change and health care as a whole, as well as climate change as it relates to geriatric and lifestyle medicine. The remainder of the chapter discusses how the choices made at end of life present an ethical dilemma for the climate-conscious clinician, with broader implications for lifestyle medicine.

—

LIFESTYLE MEDICINE, GERIATRIC MEDICINE AND CLIMATE CHANGE

Lifestyle medicine and geriatric medicine have a shared ethos around the compression of comorbidities or "squaring the curve." A focus on primary prevention strategies such as avoiding cigarettes or participating in physical activity (i.e., lifestyle medicine interventions) offers the greatest chance at compressing the period of our lives spent living with disability and chronic illness before death.[80,81] In this way, both approaches aim for better care and healthier lives with less aggressive

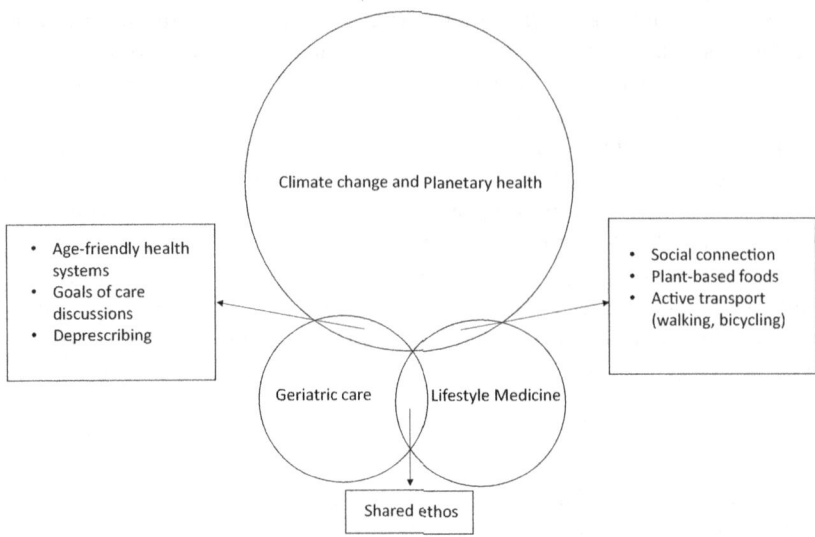

FIGURE 5.3 The shared ethos (e.g., patient-centered care, compression of morbidity, less intervention-intensive / higher quality-of-life focused care) of lifestyle and geriatric medicine ultimately work to positively impact both our own health and planetary health.

interventions. This is relevant to the kinds of larger-scale behavior change needed to develop a sustainable health care sector. The next section will touch on the ethical dilemma of resource utilization at end of life and how an environmental ethic might follow from medical decision-making that respects and values the dying patient, and so too with lifestyle medicine practices that give more respect, value and autonomy to older adults.

RESOURCE UTILIZATION AT END OF LIFE

In clinical medicine discussions at or near end of life, there are commonly used phrases to describe two distinct pathways, or philosophies, of care. There are the "aggressive interventions," which generally refer to utilizing ICU-level care, intubations, ventilators, feeding tubes, costly and energy-intensive testing (e.g., MRI and CT scans) and costly and toxic medications (e.g., chemotherapy and broad-spectrum antibiotics). Alternatively, there are the "palliative" or "comfort measures" care pathways that prioritize quality of life and patient comfort (i.e., treat in place and treat symptoms). Patients, families and even at times health care workers often interpret a nudge in the latter direction as providers restricting or withdrawing care. This makes sense, given the life-saving and life-prolonging capability of many of these interventions, and our cultural discomfort (at least in the United States) with death and dying.[82] However, emphasizing less aggressive intervention for the purposes of improving quality of life, as is common in lifestyle and geriatric medicine, is intensive in a different way. For example, hospice patients often require incredibly comprehensive care as they are attended by a nurse or family at home 24 hours a day, 7 days a week. The dying patient requires a multidisciplinary team with close monitoring of pain, anxiety, agitation, secretions, delirium, in addition to dressing, diaper and linen changes, and bereavement and support services for the family. Similarly, making a lifestyle change, whether that is transitioning to a plant-based diet or avoiding toxins such as cigarettes, is an intensive process in its own right and often difficult to accomplish without the help of a care provider (often multiple, with the help of behavioral health experts) and support from family and friends. Whether dealing with a patient at the end of life or a community-dwelling older adult, the shared ethos of lifestyle and geriatric medicine is reduced reliance on costly, energy-intensive medical intervention in favor of a holistic, meaning-centered approach to well-being in older age. Many in both fields have argued this approach to care produces better outcomes in terms of patient and family satisfaction and better quality of life near end of life than a more resource-intensive approach to care.[81,83] The authors also suggest that this approach to end-of-life care informs a climate-conscious approach to medicine.

Christine Vatovec,[84] an environmental health social scientist at the University of Vermont, asks a provocative question in her book *Dying Green: A Journey through End-of-Life Medicine in Search of Sustainable Healthcare*. She wonders whether we are harming human health on a global scale in our pursuit of improved and highly individualized care for each patient. She asks this question through the lens of care models for terminally ill cancer patients, but it reverberates outward into the broader question of an environmentally sustainable health care sector. How might we respect patient autonomy while also respecting planetary boundaries? How might we acknowledge the impossibility of unlimited resource-intensive medical care in a climate-changed world, and adapt to this possibility in advance?

In fact, movement away from highly individualized and resource-intensive care may benefit both people and the planet. Vatovec suggests that, "by promoting practices that encourage the dignity, autonomy, and inherent value of dying patients, we may actually create the circumstances under which a more ecologically sustainable health care system can emerge." In other words, we may not need to impose an environmental ethic on end-of-life care. Instead, such an ethic may be the natural outcome of centering the unique human experience of dying. For example, an increase in goals-of-care discussions at end of life, in particular with palliative care experts, or when hospice is specifically discussed, leads to an increase in hospice enrollment.[85,86] This in turn shifts the care at end of life away from aggressive, energy-intensive, pharmaceutical-intensive and environmentally toxic care toward comfort-focused, energy-limited, pharmaceutically limited and, ultimately, more climate-friendly care. Let us emphasize that this is not an argument for environmental concerns overriding respect for patient autonomy, but that there is a simple yet profound implication to respecting patient autonomy and dignity that has the potential to result in less environmental degradation. Beyond end-of-life care, it is possible to imagine an environmental ethic that emerges naturally from increased focus on the importance of lifestyle and behavioral changes, rather than "silver bullet" or pharmaceutically forward solutions. For example, a diet heavy in red meat and highly processed carbohydrates leads to an increased risk of high blood pressure, heart disease and diabetes, all of which, once developed, require intensive medical management and resources to keep under control. This is not only bad for our individual health, but for the impact on our climate and environment. By contrast, a diet that includes more plant-forward food sources and whole foods instead of heavily processed foods not only leads to better health outcomes on an individual level, but also reduces greenhouse gas emissions and improves planetary health. Given humans are living longer than ever before, these sorts of lifestyle interventions are necessary for us as a species to continue to age well because, as a result, our planet will age well too.

CONCLUSIONS

The benefits offered by both lifestyle medicine and geriatric medicine are inevitably intertwined with and enriched by a healthy planetary ecosystem, and a healthy planetary ecosystem is ultimately the natural extension of the shared ethos of both fields. The current state and structure of the global health care system is adding to climate change and environmental degradation. It is therefore incumbent on all of us to keep climate impact at the forefront of medical decision-making, all the way from the systems level down to the individual.

Ultimately, the challenge ahead of us is not just how to introduce more plant-based protein sources in our diets or to sign onto more pledges and calls to action, but rather how to transition from adding 51 billion tons of greenhouse gas emissions into the atmosphere every year down to zero in a 30-year window.[87] This will require innovations and efforts from every sector (energy, transportation, industry, agriculture, etc.). Health care is not separate or isolated from helping to solve the climate crisis, which will affect all of us, doctors and patients, care providers and the cared-for, alike. Drs. Pathak and McKinney[88] propose a call to action for their fellow lifestyle medicine colleagues to "use your time, talent, knowledge, and influence for dedicated, collective action to help solve the human and planetary challenges we face." The authors would include our colleagues in geriatric medicine in this shared call to action. Older adults, while not a homogenous population by any means, face exceedingly difficult hurdles and challenges to their health care in a climate-changed world. If health care as a system does not take the time to reflect on this and make the necessary changes, it will remain complicit in harming our future on this planet. Ultimately, if we are to fully engage with our important role as healers in this time of great upheaval and global environmental degradation, integrating our understanding of climate change into our work is imperative.

CLINICAL APPLICATIONS

- Bring these conversations into the exam room; many are dealing with varying levels of solastalgia and eco-anxiety, which should be discussed with a care provider.

- Plant-based diets and car-free travel have the best evidence base for lifestyle changes that act synergistically to improve our overall health and reduce our individual carbon footprints.
- Reference diets to have in the exam room include: Planetary Health Diet, Menus of Change, and "Reset the Table."
- Physician/provider as activist – we need to lobby collectively at the political level for system-wide changes to occur in the exam room and beyond.

REFERENCES

1. IPCC. *Climate Change 2023: Synthesis Report*. IPCC; 2023.
2. Patz JA, Frumkin H, Holloway T, Vimont DJ, Haines A. Climate change: challenges and opportunities for global health. *JAMA*. 2014;312(15):1565–1580. doi:10.1001/jama.2014.13186.
3. Whitmee S, Haines A, Beyrer C, et al. Safeguarding human health in the Anthropocene Epoch: report of the Rockefeller Foundation – Lancet Commission on planetary health. *Lancet*. 2015;386(10007):1973–2028. doi:10.1016/s0140-6736(15)60901-1.
4. Swinburn BA, Kraak VI, Allender S, et al. The global syndemic of obesity, undernutrition, and climate change: the Lancet Commission report. *Lancet*. 2019;393(10173):791–846. doi:10.1016/s0140-6736(18)32822-8.
5. Climatehealthaction.org. U.S. call to action on climate, health, and equity: a policy action agenda. 2019. Accessed March 25, 2024. https://climatehealthaction.org/cta/climate-health-equity-policy/
6. Pathak N, McKinney A. Planetary health, climate change, and lifestyle medicine: threats and opportunities. *Am J Lifestyle Med*. 2021;15(5):541–552. doi:10.1177/15598276211008127.
7. ARUP and Healthcare without Harm. Healthcare's climate footprint. 2019. Accessed March 25, 2024. https://www.arup.com/perspectives/publications/research/section/healthcares-climate-footprint
8. Ways and Means Commission Democrats. Health care and the climate crisis: preparing America's health care infrastructure. 2022. Accessed March 25, 2024. https://democrats-waysandmeans.house.gov/health-care-and-climate-crisis-preparing-americas-health-care-infrastructure
9. United States Environmental Protection Agency. Sources of greenhouse gas emissions. 2021. Accessed March 25, 2024. https://www.epa.gov/ghgemissions/sources-greenhouse-gas-emissions
10. Greenhouse Gas Protocol. Accessed March 25, 2024. https://ghgprotocol.org/
11. Seervai SG, Abrams MK. How the U.S. health care system contributes to climate change. *Explainer, the Commonwealth Fund*. 2022.
12. Eckelman MJ, Huang K, Lagasse R, Senay E, Dubrow R, Sherman JD. Health care pollution and public health damage in the United States: an update. *Health Affairs*. 2020;39(12):2071–2079. doi:10.1377/hlthaff.2020.01247.
13. Institute for Healthcare Improvement. What is an age-friendly health system? 2023. Accessed March 25, 2024. https://www.ihi.org/Engage/Initiatives/Age-Friendly-Health-Systems/Pages/default.aspx

14. United States Environmental Protection Agency. Climate change and the health of older adults. 2022. Accessed March 25, 2024. https://www.epa.gov/climateimpacts/climate-change-and-health-older-adults
15. Cooper R. Climate change and older adults: planning ahead to protect your health. *National Council on Aging.* 2022. Accessed March 25, 2024. https://www.ncoa.org/article/climate-change-and-older-adults-planning-ahead-to-protect-your-health
16. Kenny GP, Yardley J, Brown C, Sigal RJ, Jay O. Heat stress in older individuals and patients with common chronic diseases. *CMAJ.* 2010;182(10):1053–1060. doi:10.1503/cmaj.081050.
17. Morrow-Howell N, Galucia N, Swinford E. Recovering from the COVID-19 pandemic: a focus on older adults. *J Aging Soc Policy.* 2020;32(4–5):526–535. doi:10.1080/08959420.2020.1759758.
18. Luker S, Laver K, Lane R, et al. 'Put in a room and left': a qualitative study exploring the lived experiences of COVID-19 isolation and quarantine among rehabilitation inpatients. *Ann Med.* 2023;55(1):198–206. doi:10.1080/07853890.2022.2155698.
19. Bernstein A, Katz DL. Lifestyle medicine and climate change: the role of providers in addressing a public health challenge. *Am J Lifestyle Med.* 2022;16(2):251–253. doi:10.1177/15598276211017097.
20. Wynes S, Nicholas KA. The climate mitigation gap: education and government recommendations miss the most effective individual actions. *Environ Res Lett.* 2017;12(7):074024. doi:10.1088/1748-9326/aa7541.
21. Esteve-Llorens X, Darriba C, Moreira MT, Feijoo G, González-García S. Towards an environmentally sustainable and healthy Atlantic dietary pattern: life cycle carbon footprint and nutritional quality. *Sci Total Environ.* 2019;646:704–715. doi:10.1016/j.scitotenv.2018.07.264.
22. González-García S, Esteve-Llorens X, Moreira MT, Feijoo G. Carbon footprint and nutritional quality of different human dietary choices. *Sci Total Environ.* 2018;644:77–94. doi:10.1016/j.scitotenv.2018.06.339.
23. Haines A, Ebi K. The imperative for climate action to protect health. *N Engl J Med.* 2019;380(3):263–273. doi:10.1056/NEJMra1807873.
24. Heaney AK, Carrión D, Burkart K, Lesk C, Jack D. Climate change and physical activity: estimated impacts of ambient temperatures on bikeshare usage in New York City. *Environ Health Perspect.* 2019;127(3):37002. doi:10.1289/ehp4039.
25. Lanza K, Stone B, Chakalian PM, et al. Physical activity in the summer heat: how hot weather moderates the relationship between built environment features and outdoor physical activity of adults. *J Phys Act Health.* 2020;17(3):261–269. doi:10.1123/jpah.2019-0399.
26. United States Environmental Protection Agency. Ground-level ozone basics. Published January 14, 2021. Accessed January 29, 2024. https://www.epa.gov/ground-level-ozone-pollution/ground-level-ozone-basics#formation
27. Stieb DM, Shutt R, Kauri LM, et al. Cardiorespiratory effects of air pollution in a panel study of winter outdoor physical activity in older adults. *J Occup Environ Med.* 2018;60(8):673–682. doi:10.1097/jom.0000000000001334.
28. An R, Zhang S, Ji M, Guan C. Impact of ambient air pollution on physical activity among adults: a systematic review and meta-analysis. *Perspect Public Health.* 2018;138(2):111–121. doi:10.1177/1757913917726567.
29. Salas RN, Lester PK, Hess JJ. Lancet Countdown on health and climate change policy brief for the United States of America. 2020. Accessed January 29, 2024. https://www.lancetcountdownus.org/2020-lancet-countdown-u-s-brief/

30. Hamilton I, Kennard H, McGushin A, et al. The public health implications of the Paris agreement: a modelling study. *Lancet Planet Health.* 2021;5(2):e74–e83. doi:10.1016/s2542-5196(20)30249-7.
31. Abu-Omar K, Gelius P, Messing S. Physical activity promotion in the age of climate change. *F1000Res.* 2020;9:349. doi:10.12688/f1000research.23764.2.
32. Myers S, Frumkin H. *Planetary Health: Protecting Nature to Protect Ourselves.* Island Press; 2020.
33. Myers SS, Zanobetti A, Kloog I, et al. Increasing CO_2 threatens human nutrition. *Nature.* 2014;510(7503):139–142. doi:10.1038/nature13179.
34. Zhu C, Kobayashi K, Loladze I, et al. Carbon dioxide (CO_2) levels this century will alter the protein, micronutrients, and vitamin content of rice grains with potential health consequences for the poorest rice-dependent countries. *Sci Adv.* 2018;4(5):eaaq1012. doi:10.1126/sciadv.aaq1012.
35. Watts N, Amann M, Arnell N, et al. The 2019 report of the Lancet countdown on health and climate change: ensuring that the health of a child born today is not defined by a changing climate. *Lancet.* 2019;394(10211):1836–1878. doi:10.1016/s0140-6736(19)32596-6.
36. Crippa M, Solazzo E, Guizzardi D, Monforti-Ferrario F, Tubiello FN, Leip A. Food systems are responsible for a third of global anthropogenic GHG emissions. *Nat Food.* 2021;2(3):198–209. doi:10.1038/s43016-021-00225-9.
37. de Vries M, de Boer IJM. Comparing environmental impacts for livestock products: A review of life cycle assessments. *Livest Sci.* 2010;128(1):1–11. doi:10.1016/j.livsci.2009.11.007.
38. Scarborough P, Appleby PN, Mizdrak A, et al. Dietary greenhouse gas emissions of meat-eaters, fish-eaters, vegetarians and vegans in the UK. *Clim Change.* 2014;125(2):179–192. doi:10.1007/s10584-014-1169-1.
39. Tilman D, Clark M. Global diets link environmental sustainability and human health. *Nature.* 2014;515(7528):518–522. doi:10.1038/nature13959.
40. Willett W, Rockström J, Loken B, et al. Food in the Anthropocene: The EAT-lancet commission on healthy diets from sustainable food systems. *Lancet.* 2019;393(10170):447–492. doi:10.1016/s0140-6736(18)31788-4.
41. EAT. The Planetary Health Diet. Accessed March 18, 2025. https://eatforum.org/learn-and-discover/the-planetary-health-diet/
42. Menus of Change. Accessed March 18, 2025. https://www.menusofchange.org/
43. The Rockefeller Foundation. Reset the table: meeting the moment to transform the US food system. 2020 Accessed March 18, 2025. https://www.rockefellerfoundation.org/wp-content/uploads/2020/07/RF-Reset-the-Table-FULL-PAPER_July-28_FINAL.pdf
44. Hayes J. USDA livestock subsidies top $59 billion. Environmental Working Group. 2023. Accessed March 18, 2025. https://www.ewg.org/news-insights/news/2023/08/usda-livestock-subsidies-top-59-billion.
45. Landrigan PJ, Fuller R, Acosta NJR, et al. The Lancet Commission on pollution and health. *Lancet.* 2018;391(10119):462–512. doi:10.1016/s0140-6736(17)32345-0.
46. Global, regional, and national life expectancy, all-cause mortality, and cause-specific mortality for 249 causes of death, 1980–2015: a systematic analysis for the Global Burden of Disease Study 2015. *Lancet.* 2016;388(10053):1459–1544. doi:10.1016/s0140-6736(16)31012-1.
47. Global, regional, and national comparative risk assessment of 79 behavioural, environmental and occupational, and metabolic risks or clusters of risks, 1990–2015: a systematic analysis for the Global Burden of Disease Study 2015. *Lancet.* 2016;388(10053):1659–1724. doi:10.1016/s0140-6736(16)31679-8.
48. Schraufnagel DE, Balmes JR, Cowl CT, et al. Air pollution and noncommunicable diseases: a review by the Forum of International Respiratory Societies' Environmental Committee, part 1: the damaging effects of air pollution. *Chest.* 2019;155(2):409–416. doi:10.1016/j.chest.2018.10.042.

49. Schraufnagel DE, Balmes JR, Cowl CT, et al. Air pollution and noncommunicable diseases: a review by the Forum of International Respiratory Societies' Environmental Committee, part 2: air pollution and organ systems. *Chest.* 2019;155(2):417–426. doi:10.1016/j.chest.2018.10.041.
50. World Health Organization. Ambient (outdoor) air pollution. 2018. Accessed March 18, 2025. https://www.who.int/news-room/fact-sheets/detail/ambient-(outdoor)-air-quality-and-health.
51. Cohen AJ, Brauer M, Burnett R, et al. Estimates and 25-year trends of the global burden of disease attributable to ambient air pollution: an analysis of data from the Global Burden of Diseases Study 2015. *Lancet.* 2017;389(10082):1907–1918. doi:10.1016/s0140-6736(17)30505-6
52. Portier CJ, Tart KT, Carter S, et al. A human health perspective on climate change: a report outlining the research needs on the human health effects of climate change. Published 2010. Accessed March 18, 2025. https://www.niehs.nih.gov/health/materials/a_human_health_perspective_on_climate_change_full_report_508.pdf
53. Yang Q, Zhang X, Almendinger JE, et al. Climate change will pose challenges to water quality management in the St. Croix River Basin. *Environ Pollut.* 2019;251:302–311. doi:10.1016/j.envpol.2019.04.129
54. Kim KH, Kabir E, Kabir S. A review on the human health impact of airborne particulate matter. *Environ Int.* 2015;74:136–143. doi:10.1016/j.envint.2014.10.005
55. Bulbena A, Sperry L, Cunillera J. Psychiatric effects of heat waves. *Psychiatr Serv.* 2006;57(10):1519. doi:10.1176/ps.2006.57.10.1519
56. Cianconi P, Betrò S, Janiri L. The impact of climate change on mental health: a systematic descriptive review. *Front Psychiatry.* 2020;11:74. doi:10.3389/fpsyt.2020.00074
57. Schraufnagel DE, Balmes JR, De Matteis S, et al. Health benefits of air pollution reduction. *Ann Am Thorac Soc.* 2019;16(12):1478–1487. doi:10.1513/AnnalsATS.201907-538CME
58. Centers for Disease Control and Prevention. Drinking water: choosing home water filters & other water treatment systems. Published 2023. Accessed March 18, 2025. https://www.cdc.gov/healthywater/drinking/home-water-treatment/water-filters.html
59. NAACP. Environmental & climate justice. Published 2023. Accessed March 18, 2025. https://naacp.org/issues/environmental-justice/
60. Casey JA, James P, Morello-Frosch R. Urban noise pollution is worst in poor and minority neighborhoods and segregated cities. *Conversation.* Published 2017. Accessed March 18, 2025. https://theconversation.com/urban-noise-pollution-is-worst-in-poor-and-minority-neighborhoods-and-segregated-cities-81888
61. Obradovich N, Migliorini R, Mednick SC, Fowler JH. Nighttime temperature and human sleep loss in a changing climate. *Sci Adv.* 2017;3(5):e1601555. doi:10.1126/sciadv.1601555
62. Mayne SL, Morales KH, Williamson AA, et al. Associations of the residential built environment with adolescent sleep outcomes. *Sleep.* 2021;44(6). doi:10.1093/sleep/zsaa276
63. Goldmann E, Galea S. Mental health consequences of disasters. *Annu Rev Public Health.* 2014;35:169–183. doi:10.1146/annurev-publhealth-032013-182435
64. Vodovotz Y, Barnard N, Hu FB, et al. Prioritized research for the prevention, treatment, and reversal of chronic disease: recommendations from the Lifestyle Medicine Research Summit. *Front Med (Lausanne).* 2020;7:585744. doi:10.3389/fmed.2020.585744
65. Oral R, Ramirez M, Coohey C, et al. Adverse childhood experiences and trauma informed care: the future of health care. *Pediatr Res.* 2016;79(1–2):227–233. doi:10.1038/pr.2015.197

66. Gotsch SG, Draguljić D, Williams CJ. Evaluating the effectiveness of urban trees to mitigate storm water runoff via transpiration and stemflow. *Urban Ecosyst.* 2018;21(1):183–195. doi:10.1007/s11252-017-0693-y
67. Nowak DJ, Greenfield EJ, Hoehn RE, Lapoint E. Carbon storage and sequestration by trees in urban and community areas of the United States. *Environ Pollut.* 2013;178:229–236. doi:10.1016/j.envpol.2013.03.019
68. Ward Thompson C, Roe J, Aspinall P, Mitchell R, Clow A, Miller D. More green space is linked to less stress in deprived communities: evidence from salivary cortisol patterns. *Landscape Urban Plan.* 2012;105(3):221–229. doi:10.1016/j.landurbplan.2011.12.015
69. Maas J, van Dillen SME, Verheij RA, Groenewegen PP. Social contacts as a possible mechanism behind the relation between green space and health. *Health Place.* 2009;15(2):586–595. doi:10.1016/j.healthplace.2008.09.006
70. Yeager R, Riggs DW, DeJarnett N, et al. Association between residential greenness and exposure to volatile organic compounds. *Sci Total Environ.* 2020;707:135435. doi:10.1016/j.scitotenv.2019.135435
71. Beyer KM, Kaltenbach A, Szabo A, Bogar S, Nieto FJ, Malecki KM. Exposure to neighborhood green space and mental health: evidence from the survey of the health of Wisconsin. *Int J Environ Res Public Health.* 2014;11(3):3453–3472. doi:10.3390/ijerph110303453
72. Fong KC, Hart JE, James P. A review of epidemiologic studies on greenness and health: updated literature through 2017. *Curr Environ Health Rep.* 2018;5(1):77–87. doi:10.1007/s40572-018-0179-y
73. James P, Banay RF, Hart JE, Laden F. A review of the health benefits of greenness. *Curr Epidemiol Rep.* 2015;2(2):131–142. doi:10.1007/s40471-015-0043-7
74. Aspinall P, Mavros P, Coyne R, Roe J. The urban brain: analysing outdoor physical activity with mobile EEG. *Br J Sports Med.* 2015;49(4):272–276. doi:10.1136/bjsports-2012-091877
75. Threlfall CG, Mata L, Mackie JA, et al. Increasing biodiversity in urban green spaces through simple vegetation interventions. *J Appl Ecol.* 2017;54(6):1874–1883. doi:10.1111/1365-2664.12876
76. Roe JJ, Thompson CW, Aspinall PA, et al. Green space and stress: evidence from cortisol measures in deprived urban communities. *Int J Environ Res Public Health.* 2013;10(9):4086–4103. doi:10.3390/ijerph10094086
77. Hikichi H, Aida J, Matsuyama Y, Tsuboya T, Kondo K, Kawachi I. Community-level social capital and cognitive decline after a natural disaster: a natural experiment from the 2011 Great East Japan Earthquake and Tsunami. *Soc Sci Med.* 2020;257:111981. doi:10.1016/j.socscimed.2018.09.057
78. Kaldy J. Drive to deprescribe journey: just getting started. *Caring for the Ages.* 2022;23(6):11. doi:10.1016/j.carage.2022.06.021
79. Macy J, Gahbler N. *Pass It On: Five Stories That Can Change the World.* Parallax Press. 2006.
80. Hubert HB, Bloch DA, Oehlert JW, Fries JF. Lifestyle habits and compression of morbidity. *J Gerontol A Biol Sci Med Sci.* 2002;57(6):M347–M351. doi:10.1093/gerona/57.6.m347
81. Friedman SM. Lifestyle (medicine) and healthy aging. *Clin Geriatr Med.* 2020;36(4):645–653. doi:10.1016/j.cger.2020.06.007
82. Gawande A. *Being Mortal: Medicine and What Matters in the End.* Metropolitan Books; 2014.
83. Fulmer T, Reuben DB, Auerbach J, Fick DM, Galambos C, Johnson KS. Actualizing better health and health care for older adults. *Health Affairs.* 2021;40(2):219–225. doi:10.1377/hlthaff.2020.01470

84. Vatovec C. *Dying Green: A Journey through End-of-Life Medicine in Search of Sustainable Healthcare.* Rutgers University Press. 2023.
85. Starr LT, Ulrich CM, Junker P, Appel SM, O'Connor NR, Meghani SH. Goals-of-care consultation associated with increased hospice enrollment among propensity-matched cohorts of seriously ill African American and White patients. *J Pain Symptom Manage.* 2020;60(4):801–810. doi:10.1016/j.jpainsymman.2020.05.020
86. Gustafson A, Sharma M, Wong T, Eaton KD. Goals of care discussion and hospice enrollment. *J Clin Oncol.* 2019;37(27_suppl):229–229. doi:10.1200/JCO.2019.37.27_suppl.229
87. Breakthrough Energy. Getting to Zero: the most ambitious innovation effort in human history. https://breakthroughenergy.org/our-approach/getting-to-zero/
88. Pathak N, Pollard KJ, McKinney A. Lifestyle medicine interventions for personal and planetary health: the urgent need for action. *Am J Lifestyle Med.* 2022;16(5):589–593. doi:10.1177/15598276221090887

6 Lifestyle Medicine in a Geriatric Primary Care Practice

Kamal Wagle

CARING FOR COMMUNITY-DWELLING OLDER PATIENTS: AN INTRODUCTION

In the 2022 US census, 57.8 million adults were 65 and older, comprising 17.3% of the population.[1] This is projected to grow to 22% by 2040.[1] A total of 93.5% of older adults live in communities.[1] About 28% of older adults living in communities live alone.[1] The majority of community-dwelling older adults receive their primary care from outpatient primary care centers. A fraction of homebound older adults receive primary care from home-based primary care programs, and a fraction of community-dwelling older adults who need nursing-level care are cared for by a program called Program of All-Inclusive Care for the Elderly (PACE) at PACE centers. Whether it is a home-based primary care program, primary care office-based program, or through a PACE center, the primary care team is key in health promotion, management of chronic illnesses and rehabilitation programs for older adults. There are also various models of primary care: the traditional fee-for-service model, value-based care model, direct primary care or concierge primary care program. Care of older adults can be complex, due to their unique health challenges ranging from multimorbidities, evolving social determinants of health and potential changes in function and cognition; hence common facets of geriatric health care teams regardless of type of primary care practice are: person-centered care, interdisciplinary team and caregiver support.[2]

GERIATRIC PRIMARY CARE TEAM

The geriatric primary care provider is a core member of the primary care team, and can be an internist, family physician, geriatrician, nurse practitioner or physician assistant. Other core team members are medical assistants, office supporting staff and the primary care office manager. Important extended members of the primary care team include the social worker, pharmacist, nurse, physical therapist, occupational therapist, speech therapist, nutritionist, behavioral health therapist and a patient navigator. A practice that is well integrated with lifestyle medicine may

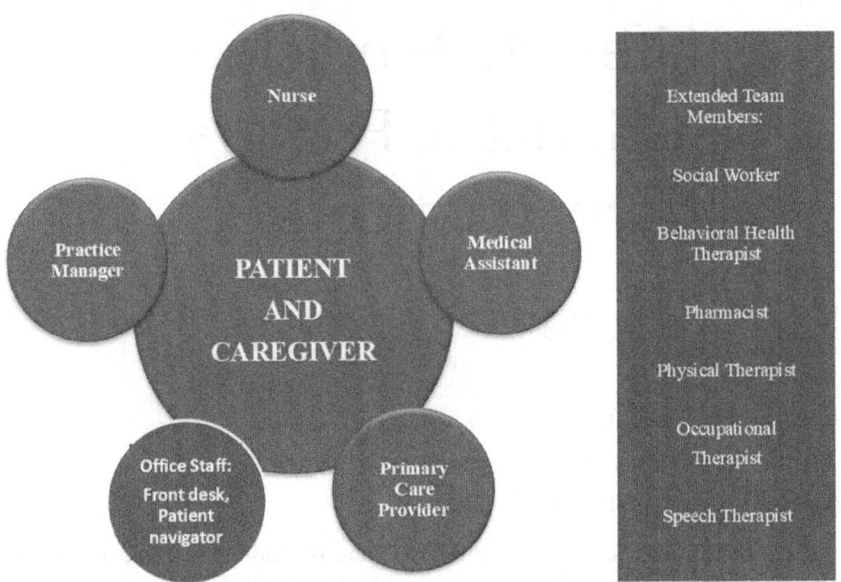

FIGURE 6.1 The core and extended primary care team members for older adults (core members appear in circles, and extended members appear in the box).

also include a health coach and a personal trainer as extended team members. Some programs have all disciplines co-located whereas a typical geriatric primary care program has to collaborate with multiple disciplines at different times and locations rather than during an older adult's primary care visit. Given multimorbidities, and complex health concerns, most older adults may also need periodic evaluation by specialist physicians. Figure 6.1 depicts the core and extended members of the primary care team for older adults.

Older adults are major consumers of hospital services and emergency department visits and often they go through transitions from hospital to rehabilitation or hospital to home with home health services. Specialty care and transitions of care are all coordinated by the primary care office of the older adult. The role of a geriatric primary care center is depicted in Figure 6.2, which illustrates coordination with hospitals, post-acute care centers, community-based organizations, and local resources.

It is important to highlight a few key components of a highly efficient primary care team, as that is even more important in the care of vulnerable populations such as older adults. These include clear and well-defined team roles, professional responsibilities and shared team goals. A well-functioning team will follow active listening, consistent communication strategies and ongoing team huddles to do pre-visit planning, review barriers and changes in processes and review the quality and outcomes of teamwork.[3–5]

A patient with a complex problem may need to be evaluated by multiple disciplines for recommendations. These disciplines may not necessarily interact to make a common plan when providing multidisciplinary care. On the other hand, if multiple

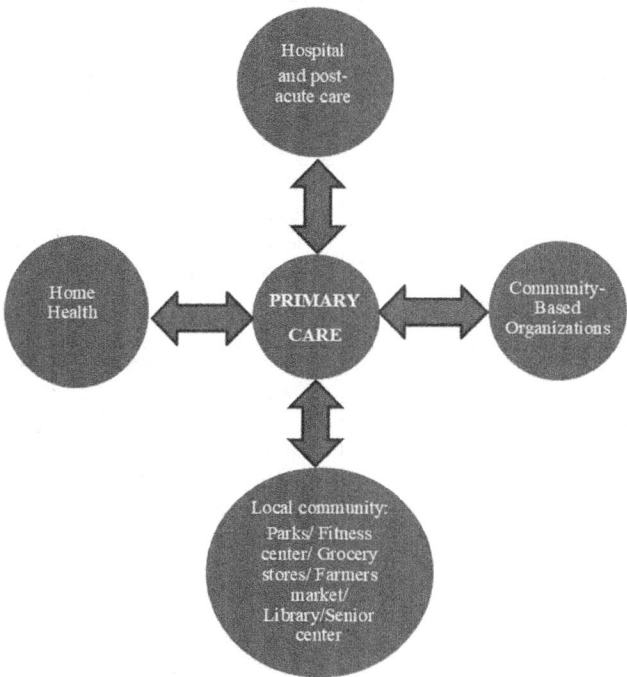

FIGURE 6.2 Geriatric primary care practices coordinate with various other stakeholders to support the care of their patients.

disciplines evaluate patients independently but communicate and make common care plans, it is referred to as an interdisciplinary team. A well-functioning geriatric primary care team is interdisciplinary, where team members work independently at the top of each team member's scope of practice, with full collaboration, seamless communication and shared decision-making in creating care plans for patients.[6]

COMPREHENSIVE GERIATRICS ASSESSMENT AND 5Ms OF GERIATRICS

In Chapter 1, we discussed comprehensive geriatric assessment and the 5Ms model of geriatric care. The primary care team of an older adult conducts geriatric assessments and screens for the geriatric syndromes. The age-friendly health system initiative provides guidance on how the geriatric assessment can be incorporated in various sites including primary care sites. It starts with understanding what matters to the older adult, how the care can be aligned with patient priorities, whether the patient's medication is age-friendly, the mental and cognitive health of the patient and the limitations on the patient's mobility.[7] Various tools are utilized for geriatric assessment and these assessments also integrate various lifestyle pillars. This is summarized in Table 6.1.

TABLE 6.1
Geriatric Assessment Tool, in Relation to 5Ms and Lifestyle Pillars

Tools	Components	Comments on Lifestyle and Geriatrics	Which of the 5Ms?
Katz Index for ADLs[21]	• Bathing • Dressing • Toileting • Transferring • Continence • Feeding	ADLs assessment gives a foundation upon which one can do lifestyle assessment and recommendations	• Multicomplexity • Mobility • Matters Most
The Lawton Instrumental Activities of Daily Living (IADL) Scale[22]	• Food preparation • Housekeeping • Telephone use • Transportation • Managing medications • Managing finances • Shopping and laundry	IADLs assessment gives a foundation upon which one can understand the ability to access healthy foods, social activities, transportation to safe places and to exercise	• Multicomplexity • Matters Most
Vision and Hearing Screening Vision: Snellen Chart, Confrontation Test Hearing: Whispered Voice Test, Finger Rub Test	• Screening and appropriate referrals for vision and hearing loss	Vision and hearing correction are important to optimize communication and function, which are important for addressing lifestyle pillars	• Multicomplexity
Nutrition Screening Nutritional Health Checklist [23,24] 24-Hour Dietary Recall	• Intake of adequate servings of vegetables, fruits, whole grains and fiber while avoiding excess high saturated fat and processed foods	Food access is a part of the nutrition pillar	• Multicomplexity
Timed Up and Go Test[25]	• Gait assessment	Relevant for exercise pillar	• Mobility
Mini-Cog, MMSE, MOCA[26]	• Various cognitive domains	Foundational for LM assessment and plan	• Mind
PHQ-9, GAD-7[27]	• Mood assessment	Foundational for LM assessment and plan	• Mind

(Continued)

TABLE 6.1 (Continued)

Tools	Components	Comments on Lifestyle and Geriatrics	Which of the 5Ms?
Tobacco / Alcohol/ Substance Screening	• Tobacco, alcohol substance abuse	Lifestyle pillar of avoidance of high-risk behavior	• Mind • Multicomplexity
AGS Beer's Criteria START/STOPP[28,29]	• Screening for appropriate indications and potentially harmful medications	Optimizing lifestyle pillars fosters deprescribing	• Medications
Advance Care Planning Documents	• Health Care Representative • Living Will • Power of Attorney • Physician Orders for Life-Sustaining Treatment (POLST)	Important considerations before making lifestyle recommendations	• Matters Most

ASSESSMENT OF LIFESTYLE PILLARS IN PRIMARY CARE

A geriatric primary care practice needs to integrate lifestyle medicine practice into each step of the clinic flow. Figure 6.3 illustrates a clinic process map and incorporation of lifestyle medicine strategies in practice, which is discussed in subsequent sections.

LIFESTYLE VITAL SIGNS

Screening for lifestyle pillars is important as this can provide information about modifiable risk factors for chronic health conditions. Given the importance of assessing and documenting this information, they are often referred to as "lifestyle vital signs."[8] Incorporating lifestyle vital signs along with routine vital signs during a patient's assessment in primary care practice is feasible and recommended.[9] Assessing lifestyle vital signs allows the primary care team to see the trend of lifestyle factors for the patient and their influence on the disease states, and enables the primary care team to continue to provide relevant lifestyle recommendations in every visit. Table 6.2 provides sample screening questions to get an understanding of lifestyle vital signs.

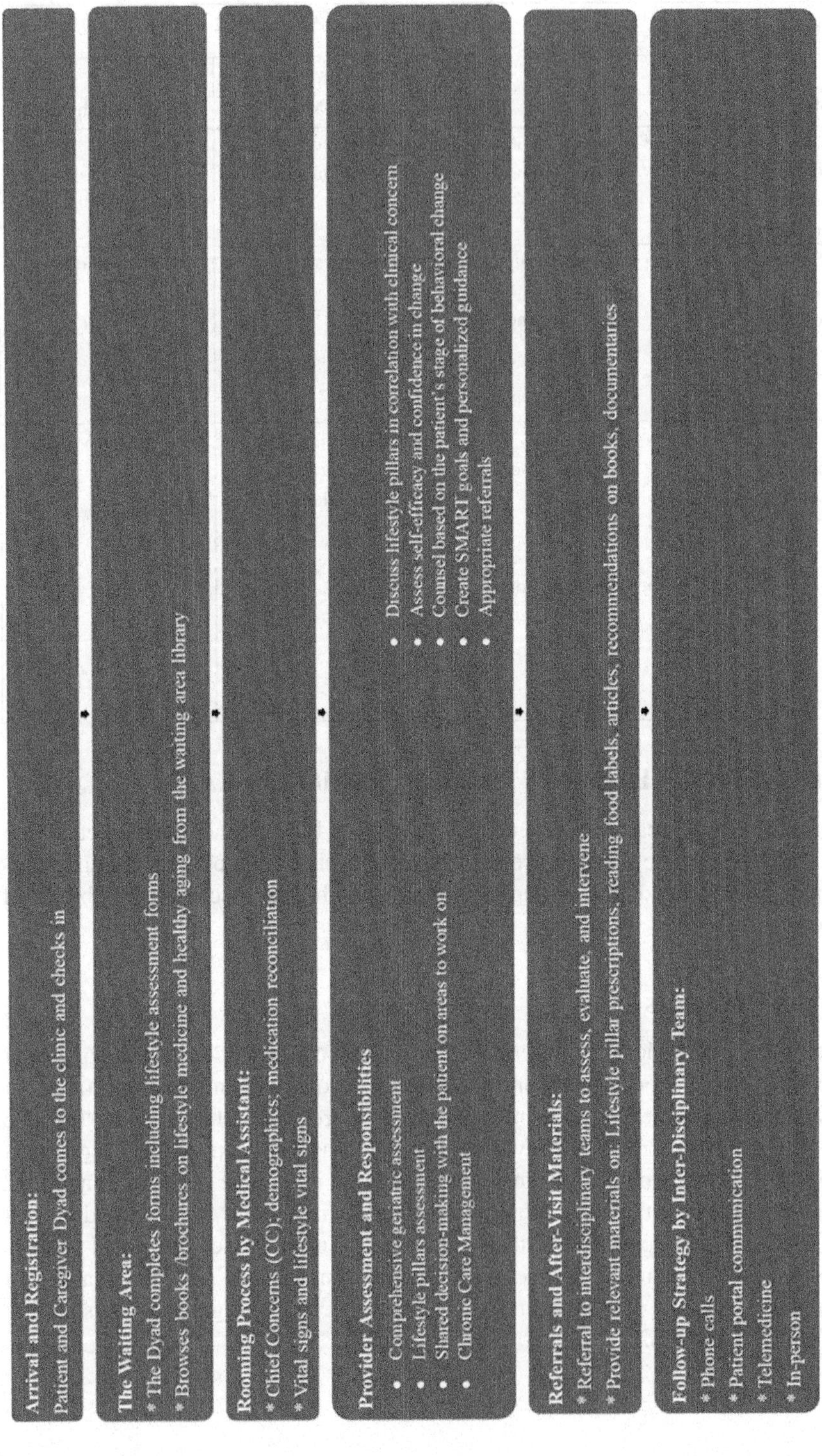

Arrival and Registration:
Patient and Caregiver Dyad comes to the clinic and checks in

The Waiting Area:
* The Dyad completes forms including lifestyle assessment forms
* Browses books/brochures on lifestyle medicine and healthy aging from the waiting area library

Rooming Process by Medical Assistant:
* Chief Concerns (CC); demographics; medication reconciliation
* Vital signs and lifestyle vital signs

Provider Assessment and Responsibilities
- Comprehensive geriatric assessment
- Lifestyle pillars assessment
- Shared decision-making with the patient on areas to work on
- Chronic Care Management

- Discuss lifestyle pillars in correlation with clinical concern
- Assess self-efficacy and confidence in change
- Counsel based on the patient's stage of behavioral change
- Create SMART goals and personalized guidance
- Appropriate referrals

Referrals and After-Visit Materials:
* Referral to interdisciplinary teams to assess, evaluate, and intervene
* Provide relevant materials on: Lifestyle pillar prescriptions, reading food labels, articles, recommendations on books, documentaries

Follow-up Strategy by Inter-Disciplinary Team:
* Phone calls
* Patient portal communication
* Telemedicine
* In-person

FIGURE 6.3 Integration of lifestyle medicine in a geriatric primary care practice.

TABLE 6.2
Lifestyle Vital Signs

Lifestyle Pillars	Lifestyle Vital Sign Questions	Tool Example
Nutrition	• "Tell me what is your typical breakfast, lunch, dinner, snack, beverages, and when do you eat them?" • "Who prepares the food?" • "Can you share how you prepare meals?" • "Tell me your understanding of reading food labels?"	• 24-Hour Dietary Recall[30] • MEDAS[31] • Rapid Diet Assessment Screening Tool[32] • ACLM Diet Screener[11,33]
Exercise	• "On average, how many days per week and how much each time, do you engage in moderate to vigorous physical activity (like a brisk walk)?" • "Where do you exercise and if there is a companion, with whom? • "How often do you have to walk in your daily life?" • "What household chores do you do on a daily and weekly basis?"	• Self-Reported Two-Question Exercise Screening[34] • International Physical Activity Questionnaire Short Form (IPAQ-SF)[35] • FITT-P Principle (Frequency, Intensity, Time, Type, Progression) for Exercise Counseling[34]
Sleep	• "Out of 7 nights last week, how many nights did you sleep well?" • "Do you feel your sleep is adequate?"	• Pittsburgh Sleep Quality Index (PSQI)[36]
High-Risk Behavior	• Review of tobacco, alcohol and substance use	• CAGE Questionnaire[37] • AUDIT-C[38] • Tobacco, Alcohol, Prescription Medication, and Other Substance Use (TAPS) Tool[39]
Stress Management	• "Rate your stress level: mild, medium or high" • "What is your strategy to cope with stress?"	• Perceived Stress Scale[40] • The brief COPE[41]
Healthy Social Relationship	• "How often do you see other people?" • "How often do you feel lonely?" • "Who are the people you can count on to discuss topics that are important to you?"	• Berkman–Syme Social Network Index[42,43] • Network Index • Three-Item UCLA Loneliness Scale[43,44]

Synthesizing Information from Lifestyle Medicine Vital Signs and the Geriatric 5Ms

Once lifestyle pillars and 5Ms are assessed, primary care providers can then discuss what lifestyle pillars to work on to address relevant geriatric problems that are of utmost importance for the patient. Tools are available for the primary care team for further evaluation of each lifestyle pillar,[10,11] and the team can decide which tool is most helpful and feasible for the patient and which tool is achievable to incorporate into their practice. Providers will present why addressing geriatric syndromes aligns with a patient's goals in health and what lifestyle pillars to work on to address the geriatric syndromes.

Shared Decision-Making

Shared decision-making is one of the important strategies in taking care of older adults.[12] This process involves understanding the patient's priorities and coming to an agreement about the proposed recommendations before incorporating them into the care plan. The shared decision-making process makes the patient and clinical team both highly engaged in the care plan and it likely improves adherence to the recommendations. Once lifestyle assessment and geriatric assessments are done, discussing the findings within the context of the patient's health concerns helps both the patient and caregiver understand the importance of those interventions.

Assessing the Stage of Change

The transtheoretical model of change is used to assess a patient's stage of behavioral change to optimize their lifestyle and this helps the primary care team plan an appropriate approach to lifestyle counseling.[9,13] A person can be in various stages of behavioral change:

1. *Precontemplation:* When the patient is not thinking about the change;
2. *Contemplation:* When the patient is weighing in benefits and costs associated with the change;
3. *Preparation:* When the patient is taking small steps toward making a change;
4. *Action:* When the patient is adopting change behavior;
5. *Maintenance:* When the patient has implemented and is maintaining the change; and
6. *Relapse:* When the patient falls back to old habits.

After understanding which stage a patient is at in behavioral change, providers also need to assess how likely patients feel they are to make a change (self-efficacy) and how confident they are in change (confidence for change). This helps set the stage for counseling patients appropriately.[13,14] Table 6.3 provides examples of approaches for counseling depending upon a person's stage of change.

TABLE 6.3
Stage of Behavioral Change and Approach to the Patient

Stage in Transtheoretical Model of Change	Models of Counseling for Change
Precontemplation (not thinking about the change)	Eliciting perceived barriers and understanding of the rationale, providing education to cue action
Contemplation (weighing benefits and costs of change)	Eliciting perceived barriers, utilizing cues to action, motivational interviewing
Preparation (trying small changes)	Understanding what needs to happen to make a leap or more changes, utilizing motivational interviewing
Action (taking definite changes)	Anticipating potential challenges/relapse and ways to overcome them, creating social support, cognitive behavioral therapy
Maintenance (maintaining changes over a period)	Anticipating potential challenges/relapse and ways to overcome them, continuous reinforcement, creating social support, cognitive behavioral therapy
Relapse (falling back to old habit)	Going back to the above stage, counseling accordingly, exploring social support, and reflecting on what happened

STRATEGIES FOR INTEGRATING LIFESTYLE MEDICINE TOOLS IN PRIMARY CARE

PREPARING INTERDISCIPLINARY TEAM MEMBERS TO PROMOTE LIFESTYLE PILLARS

As discussed above, a high-quality primary care team would include interdisciplinary team members working together for a single shared goal. Integrating lifestyle medicine in primary care starts with coaching and training interdisciplinary team members on the importance of lifestyle pillars in optimizing health and best practice strategies in using the tools in primary care without burning out the team. Traditionally, teams and practices are not attuned to incorporating lifestyle assessment as a foundation of the practice; this paradigm change can be confusing to the staff who are not used to doing those assessments. To facilitate this change, there should be a leader in the team who can be available to support and lead the program. The lifestyle medicine leader can be from any discipline within the team and can work with all disciplines from the front desk to the back desk of the practice in making the process seamless for the patients and their caregivers as well as for staff. Implementation of lifestyle medicine programs in practice may require a series of lunch-and-learn programs to learn about lifestyle pillars and to discuss how to continue to make the integration of lifestyle medicine better and seamless.

TEAM HUDDLES

Primary care team huddles are integral parts of primary care practice. This can also be a time to discuss a patient's barriers in optimizing lifestyle and brainstorm among various disciplines in matching appropriate resources for the patient. Huddles also provide time and space to check in with the team daily on what went well and how to improve on daily processes.

Resources for Patients and Caregivers

It is important to understand a patient's preferred way of learning. Some individuals would like to read printed materials; for others, it could be a documentary or a community event where the lifestyle pillars are discussed. Some patients may be interested in scientific papers and journals as well. It is helpful to have some books, journals, magazines and brochures in the waiting room. Some lifestyle medicine practices have libraries in the practice where patients can borrow recommended books.

Lifestyle Prescriptions

Clearly written recommendations go a long way in helping patients to stick to them. The proposed goals should be Specific, Measurable, Achievable, Relevant and Time-bound (SMART).[15] These can be written or typed up on a prescription pad and handed to the patient.[9] An example of such recommendations could be: "Start walking with your spouse, in the morning, in the neighborhood, for 20 minutes, 4 days a week for a month until next follow-up" (physical activity prescription); "add 1 cup of cooked bean soup – alternating between navy and pinto beans, three times a week on Monday, Wednesday and Friday during dinner for 2 months until the next follow-up" (diet prescription); or "attend book club in your local library on the second and fourth Tuesday of the month" (social prescription).

Community Resources

As highlighted in Figure 6.2, primary care teams often need to coordinate with community resources to support patient needs. This is crucial for the integration of lifestyle strategies. Interdisciplinary teams can support or brainstorm on appropriate community resources for patients depending on where they live. This can be events from local area agencies on aging, senior centers, township activities, fitness centers, insurance-supported programs, farmer's markets, parks and libraries.

Follow-Ups

Any lifestyle modification needs close follow up and this is achieved with various approaches. In-person follow-up may be difficult for patients or from an access/availability point of view. This can be addressed by utilizing other approaches as follows:

1. *Phone calls:* This can be incorporated by designating a support staff to make phone calls to patients to follow up on changes made;
2. *Patient portal messaging:* With the HITECH Act of 2009, electronic health records are increasingly utilizing secure patient portal messaging programs and this can be utilized for following up with the patient on lifestyle changes;[16]
3. *Telemedicine follow-ups:* Interactive audio-video platforms have been utilized much more since the COVID-19 pandemic and still can be utilized to follow up on lifestyle modifications and coaching;

4. *In-person visits with interdisciplinary teams:* Patients may follow up with one of the disciplines in the team for lifestyle changes follow up;
5. *In-person provider follow-up:* These also need to be incorporated at an appropriate frequency to follow up and support during optimization of lifestyle.

It is particularly important to follow-up on whether lifestyle changes are bringing the desired outcomes in geriatric syndromes and to assess whether this provides any deprescribing opportunities, and so on.

REGISTRY AND METRICS REVIEW

Registry and review of metrics are integral parts of practice management in primary care. In particular to lifestyle, measuring and looking at trends of lifestyle vital signs, as well as pertinent patient biometrics such as lipid profile, hemoglobin A1c, blood pressure, weight trends, and so on, are equally important. Besides progress notes, lifestyle pillars can be documented in sections of electronic health records that are readily available to the interdisciplinary team. In all the common Electronic Health Records (EHR), there is a snapshot view of the patient which tells us the patient's vital signs, medical history, allergies, medicines and key screening questions such as depression and falls. In the same section, lifestyle vital signs can be integrated.

REIMBURSEMENT

The primary care team should be familiar with billing and coding of lifestyle medicine-specific encounters, and they can also incorporate lifestyle assessment and counseling in common primary care encounters.[17,18] The American College of Lifestyle Medicine is a resource for primary care teams to look for tools and reimbursement resources.[11] Primary care practices can also do shared medical appointments with groups of patients to deliver lifestyle medicine services to foster peer learning and group coaching and these can be feasible from an access and reimbursement point of view.[19]

BARRIERS AND SOLUTIONS

There are various potential barriers to the integration of lifestyle medicine strategies in geriatric primary care but there are also possible solutions for them. These are summarized in Table 6.4.

Barriers include:

1. Time management
2. Lack of interdisciplinary team members
3. Communication challenges
4. Access to follow-up
5. Resource availability
6. Reimbursement

TABLE 6.4
Barriers and Potential Solutions for Integration of Lifestyle Medicine in a Geriatric Primary Care Practice

Barriers	Solutions
Time management	Use user-friendly tools in practice Create a highly efficient team and leverage team members for assessment of the lifestyle vitals and geriatric assessments Often, lifestyle questionnaires can be completed by patients in the waiting room or can be mailed to the patient to complete before the visit
Lack of multi-disciplinary team	Collaborate across locations: Often, geriatric primary care teams may not have extended team members in the same location or same day of patient care, and it is helpful to develop relationships with various disciplines in the health system or in the community and not necessarily located in the clinic in the same space
Communication	Establish well-defined team roles; revisit them in team huddles
Access for follow-ups	Schedule follow-up with multiple disciplines Schedule various approaches such as phone/video visits, secure patient portal messaging or visits with interdisciplinary team members
Resources	Connect to available community resources Connect to community lifestyle programs Connect to virtual lifestyle training and education programs
Reimbursement	The model of practice may be a barrier to providing or developing sustainable integration of lifestyle medicine in geriatric practice. However, there are various lifestyle-related diagnoses (ICD codes) that can be billed for the visit Similarly, shared medical appointments can be another feasible option in practice[22]

These barriers can be addressed by incorporating best practices in team building, looking for collaborations with various team members outside the primary care practice and in the community, utilizing electronic health records, leveraging all team members for follow-up, and exploring community resources. Shared medical appointments are growing in the nation in providing group visits for chronic diseases and lifestyle medicine.[19,20] With rapid practice improvement projects, lifestyle medicine tools and strategies can be incorporated into geriatric primary care practice over time.

CONCLUSION/SUMMARY

Lifestyle medicine strategies are important components of the prevention and treatment of multimorbidity and multiple geriatric syndromes. Management of multiple morbidities and geriatric syndromes includes optimizing lifestyle pillars as a key strategy. Hence integration of lifestyle medicine in geriatric primary care practice is crucial. It is also feasible. The first and foremost step is to prepare the primary care team to incorporate lifestyle medicine assessments in practice. Integration of lifestyle medicine in primary care practice requires team building, regularly scheduled team huddles and revising process mapping of the practice. This intentional approach, along with enhancing collaboration with disciplines within and outside practice, and collaborating with community partners, are some of the strategies to overcome those barriers. Although there are challenges to incorporating lifestyle medicine in geriatric primary care, a continuous effort at various levels – practice, health system and advocacy in professional organizations and communities, can gradually make it a more seamless process.

CLINICAL APPLICATIONS

- Interdisciplinary planning in each step of the patient/caregiver journey through the practice, from check-in to check-out, will make the integration of lifestyle medicine in geriatrics possible.
- Collaboration with multiple disciplines within and outside the practice, as well as community-based organizations, is key to providing holistic care to older adults, thereby improving their health outcomes.
- Primary care teams can utilize SMART lifestyle prescriptions, recommend patient supporting materials for lifestyle modification and counsel as per the patient's stage of behavioral change, to effectively help patients make and sustain lifestyle changes.

REFERENCES

1. Administration on Aging (AoA), part of the Administration for Community Living (ACL), an operating division of the U.S. Department of Health and Human Services. 2023 Profile of Older Americans. 2024. https://acl.gov/sites/default/files/Profile%20of%20OA/ACL_ProfileOlderAmericans2023_508.pdf.
2. McNabney MK, Green AR, Burke M, et al. Complexities of care: common components of models of care in geriatrics. *J Am Geriatr Soc.* 2022;70(7):1960–1972. doi:10.1111/jgs.17811
3. Pimentel CB, Snow AL, Carnes SL, et al. Huddles and their effectiveness at the frontlines of clinical care: a scoping review. *J Gen Intern Med.* 2021;36(9):2772–2783. doi:10.1007/s11606-021-06632-9
4. Warde CM, Giannitrapani KF, Pearson ML. Teaching primary care teamwork: a conceptual model of primary care team performance. *Clin Teach.* 2020;17(3):249–254. doi:10.1111/tct.13037
5. Stewart EE, Johnson BC. Improve office efficiency in mere minutes. *Fam Pract Manag.* 2007;14(6):27–29.
6. Martin AK, Green TL, McCarthy AL, Sowa PM, Laakso EL. Healthcare teams: terminology, confusion, and ramifications. *J Multidiscip Healthc.* 2022;15:765–772. doi:10.2147/JMDH.S342197
7. Mate K, Fulmer T, Pelton L, et al. Evidence for the 4Ms: interactions and outcomes across the care continuum. *J Aging Health.* 2021;33(7–8):469–481. doi:10.1177/08982643 21991658
8. Rozanski A, Sakul S, Narula J, Berman D. Assessment of lifestyle "vital signs" in healthcare settings. *Prog Cardiovasc Dis.* 2023;77:107–118. doi:10.1016/j.pcad.2023.02.002

9. Grega ML, Shalz JT, Rosenfeld RM. American College of Lifestyle Medicine expert consensus statement: lifestyle medicine for optimal outcomes in primary care. *Am J Lifestyle Med*. 2024;18(2):269–293. doi:10.1177/15598276231202970
10. American Academy of Family Physicians. Tools for the lifestyle medicine team. Accessed December 20, 2024. https://aafp.s3.amazonaws.com/2021-lifestyle-medicine/pdfs/additional-tools.pdf
11. American College of Lifestyle Medicine. Tools and resources. Accessed December 17, 2024. https://lifestylemedicine.org/tools-and-resources/
12. American Geriatrics Society Expert Panel on the Care of Older Adults with Multimorbidity. Guiding principles for the care of older adults with multimorbidity: an approach for clinicians. *J Am Geriatr Soc*. 2012;60(10):E1–E25. doi:10.1111/j.1532-5415.2012.04188.x
13. Prochaska JO, Velicer WF. The transtheoretical model of health behavior change. *Am J Health Promot AJHP*. 1997;12(1):38–48. doi:10.4278/0890-1171-12.1.38
14. Zimmerman GL, Olsen CG, Bosworth MF. A "stages of change" approach to helping patients change behavior. *Am Fam Physician*. 2000;61(5):1409–1416.
15. White ND, Bautista V, Lenz T, Cosimano A. Using the SMART-EST goals in lifestyle medicine prescription. *Am J Lifestyle Med*. 2020;14(3):271–273. doi:10.1177/1559827620905775
16. Han HR, Gleason KT, Sun CA, et al. Using patient portals to improve patient outcomes: systematic review. *JMIR Hum Factors*. 2019;6(4):e15038. doi:10.2196/15038
17. Gobble J, Donohue D, Grega M. Reimbursement as a catalyst for advancing lifestyle medicine practices. *J Fam Pract*. 2022;71(Suppl 1):eS105–eS109. doi:10.12788/jfp.0255
18. American Academy of Family Physicians. Reimbursement and coding for lifestyle medicine-related services. Accessed December 17, 2024. https://aafp.s3.amazonaws.com/2021-lifestyle-medicine/pdfs/reimbursement-and-coding.pdf
19. Freeman K, Bidwell J. Lifestyle medicine: shared medical appointments. *J Fam Pract*. 2022;71(Suppl 1):S62–S65. doi:10.12788/jfp.0278
20. Kirsh SR, Aron DC, Johnson KD, et al. A realist review of shared medical appointments: how, for whom, and under what circumstances do they work? *BMC Health Serv Res*. 2017;17(1):113. doi:10.1186/s12913-017-2064-z
21. Katz S, Downs TD, Cash HR, Grotz RC. Progress in development of the index of ADL. *Gerontologist*. 1970;10(1):20–30. doi:10.1093/geront/10.1_part_1.20
22. Lawton MP, Brody EM. Assessment of older people: self-maintaining and instrumental activities of daily living. *Gerontologist*. 1969;9(3):179–186.
23. Elsawy B, Higgins KE. The geriatric assessment. *Am Fam Physician*. 2011;83(1):48–56.
24. Barrocas A, Bistrian BR, Blackburn GL, et al. Appropriate and effective use of the NSI checklist and screens. An update on caring for the elderly by preventing malnutrition. *J Am Diet Assoc*. 1995;95(6):647–648. doi:10.1016/s0002-8223(95)00177-8
25. CDC STEADI. https://www.cdc.gov/steadi/media/pdfs/STEADI-Assessment-TUG-508.pdf
26. Falk N, Cole A, Meredith TJ. Evaluation of suspected dementia. *Am Fam Physician*. 2018;97(6):398–405.
27. Neulinger B, Ebert C, Lochbühler K, Bergmann A, Gensichen J, Lukaschek K. Screening tools assessing mental illness in primary care: a systematic review. *Eur J Gen Pract*. 2024;30(1):2418299. doi:10.1080/13814788.2024.2418299
28. American Geriatrics Society Beers Criteria Update Expert Panel. 2023 Updated AGS Beers Criteria for potentially inappropriate medication use in older adults. *J Am Geriatr Soc*. 2023;71(7):2052–2081. doi:10.1111/jgs.18372
29. O'Mahony D, Cherubini A, Guiteras AR, et al. STOPP/START criteria for potentially inappropriate prescribing in older people: version 3. *Eur Geriatr Med*. 2023;14(4):625–632. doi:10.1007/s41999-023-00777-y

30. Subar AF, Kirkpatrick SI, Mittl B, et al. The automated self-administered 24-hour dietary recall (ASA24): a resource for researchers, clinicians, and educators from the National Cancer Institute. *J Acad Nutr Diet.* 2012;112(8):1134–1137. doi:10.1016/j.jand.2012.04.016
31. Schröder H, Fitó M, Estruch R, et al. A short screener is valid for assessing Mediterranean diet adherence among older Spanish men and women. *J Nutr.* 2011;141(6):1140–1145. doi:10.3945/jn.110.135566
32. Vadiveloo M, Lichtenstein AH, Anderson C, et al. Rapid diet assessment screening tools for cardiovascular disease risk reduction across healthcare settings: a scientific statement from the American Heart Association. *Circ Cardiovasc Qual Outcomes.* 2020;13(9):e000094. doi:10.1161/HCQ.0000000000000094
33. Karlsen MC, Staffier KL, Pollard KJ, et al. Piloting a brief assessment to capture consumption of whole plant food and water: version 1.0 of the American College of Lifestyle Medicine Diet Screener (ACLM Diet Screener). *Front Nutr.* 2024;11:1356676. doi:10.3389/fnut.2024.1356676
34. Young. Lifestyle medicine: physical activity. *J Fam Pract.* 2022;71(1 Suppl). doi:10.12788/jfp.0253
35. Lee PH, Macfarlane DJ, Lam TH, Stewart SM. Validity of the International Physical Activity Questionnaire Short Form (IPAQ-SF): a systematic review. *Int J Behav Nutr Phys Act.* 2011;8:115. doi:10.1186/1479-5868-8-115
36. Buysse DJ, Reynolds CF, Monk TH, Berman SR, Kupfer DJ. The Pittsburgh Sleep Quality Index: a new instrument for psychiatric practice and research. *Psychiatry Res.* 1989;28(2):193–213. doi:10.1016/0165-1781(89)90047-4
37. Ewing JA. Detecting alcoholism. The CAGE questionnaire. *JAMA.* 1984;252(14):1905–1907. doi:10.1001/jama.252.14.1905
38. Bush K, Kivlahan DR, McDonell MB, Fihn SD, Bradley KA. The AUDIT alcohol consumption questions (AUDIT-C): an effective brief screening test for problem drinking. Ambulatory Care Quality Improvement Project (ACQUIP). Alcohol Use Disorders Identification Test. *Arch Intern Med.* 1998;158(16):1789–1795. doi:10.1001/archinte.158.16.1789
39. McNeely J, Wu LT, Subramaniam G, et al. Performance of the Tobacco, Alcohol, Prescription Medication, and Other Substance Use (TAPS) tool for substance use screening in primary care patients. *Ann Intern Med.* 2016;165(10):690–699. doi:10.7326/M16-0317
40. Cohen S, Kamarck T, Mermelstein R. A global measure of perceived stress. *J Health Soc Behav.* 1983;24(4):385–396.
41. Carver CS. You want to measure coping but your protocol's too long: consider the brief COPE. *Int J Behav Med.* 1997;4(1):92–100. doi:10.1207/s15327558ijbm0401_6
42. Berkman LF, Syme SL. Social networks, host resistance, and mortality: a nine-year follow-up study of Alameda County residents. *Am J Epidemiol.* 1979;109(2):186–204. doi:10.1093/oxfordjournals.aje.a112674
43. National Academies of Sciences, Engineering, and Medicine; Division of Behavioral and Social Sciences and Education; Health and Medicine Division; Board on Behavioral, Cognitive, and Sensory Sciences; Board on Health Sciences Policy; Committee on the Health and Medical Dimensions of Social Isolation and Loneliness in Older Adults. *Social Isolation and Loneliness in Older Adults: Opportunities for the Health Care System.* National Academies Press; 2020. Accessed December 23, 2024. http://www.ncbi.nlm.nih.gov/books/NBK557974/
44. Hughes ME, Waite LJ, Hawkley LC, Cacioppo JT. A short scale for measuring loneliness in large surveys: results from two population-based studies. *Res Aging.* 2004;26(6):655–672. doi:10.1177/0164027504268574

Section 2

Lifestyle Medicine Pillars as Applied to Older Adults

7 Why Exercise? *Sedentarism, Physical Activity and Exercise among Older Adults*

Jorge C. Mora and Willy Marcos Valencia

Physical activity and exercise are fundamental for healthy aging. Despite the clear benefits of exercise and the current understanding and ongoing research about how exercise may positively modulate biological aging, data from the CDC indicates that physical inactivity increases with age. More than 1 in 4 (26.9%) older adults aged 65 to 74, and more than 1 in 3 (35.3%) of older adults aged 75 and older, self-report as being physically inactive. In addition to chronologic age, chronic conditions, low educational levels, and higher BMIs are also associated with greater physical inactivity.[1]

Although sedentary behavior was once considered synonymous with inactivity by the medical community, we now understand that they are quite different. Distinguishing between sedentary behaviors and inactivity can help tailor interventions for older adults, especially for those living with chronic diseases. A person can be medically classified as both sedentary and physically active (Figure 7.1). Although the effects of sedentary behavior and physical inactivity may have the same negative outcomes, *excessive* sedentary behavior may have adverse effects even in the presence of aerobic exercise. For example, a study of more than 1,000,000 individuals concluded that 60 to 75 minutes of daily physical activity is required to offset the risk of dying among individuals who are sedentary (e.g., sitting), but it does not completely reverse the associated risks if that time is spent being highly sedentary, such as when watching TV.[2]

People are considered physically inactive if they engage in less than 150 minutes a week of moderate to vigorous physical exercise, or less than 75 minutes a week of vigorous physical activity. Sedentary behavior is defined as when a person spends more than 9.5 hours a day being sedentary.[2] People engaging in sedentary behavior perform activities that require a metabolic cost of less than 1.5 metabolic equivalents (METs), and this has been associated with accelerated biological aging. In addition, sedentary behavior is associated with a higher risk of cardiovascular disease, cancers, mobility issues, cognitive issues, falls and chronic disease. The combination of light physical activity (1.6–2.9 METs) with moderate or vigorous exercise (>3 METs) slows down the effects of aging, and significantly reduces all-causes of mortality.[3]

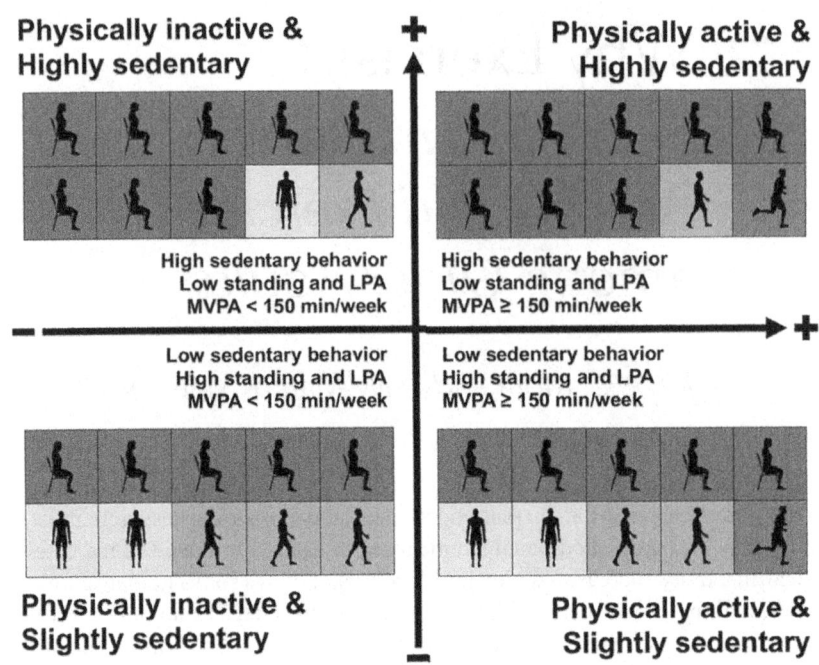

FIGURE 7.1 Sedentary behavior and physical activity.

PHYSIOLOGICAL EFFECTS OF SUSTAINED SEDENTARY BEHAVIOR

Sedentary behavior and physical inactivity increase inflammation and oxidative stress and reduce glucose tolerance. The lack of mechanical workload in the skeletal muscles reduces muscle remodeling, decreases energy turnover, shifts toward glycolytic fibers, decreases lipid use, increases glucose use and decreases mitochondrial density and oxidative capacity. These changes lead to decreased insulin sensitivity, muscle atrophy, fat accumulation, decreased oxidative capacity and increased VLDL production. As a result, there can be an increase in adipose tissue at the central and the peripheral levesl, worsening inflammation and creating an environment for metabolic syndrome[4] (Table 7.1).

BENEFITS OF EXERCISE

Overall

Regular physical activity improves quality of life, including a person's feeling of well-being and physical function, and reduces overall cardiovascular mortality risk. Patients who engage in activities that burn more than 1,000 calories per week have a 30% reduction in overall mortality. Physical activity also reduces cancer risk, risk for falls, anxiety and depression.[6]

Why Exercise?

TABLE 7.1
Activity METs and Intensity

Activity	METs	Intensity[5]
Seating quietly	1.0	No exertion at all
Walking slowly	2.0	Easy
Walking, 2 mph	2.5	Easy
Housework light	2.5	Easy
Stretching exercises, yoga	2.5	Easy
Playing a piano	2.5	Easy
Dancing, ballroom slow	2.9	Easy
Walking, 3 mph	3.3	Moderate
Bicycling, leisurely	3.5	Moderate
Gardening, active	4.0	Moderate
Tai Chi	4.0	Moderate
Pickleball	4.1	Moderate
Walking, 4 mph	5.0	Moderate
Swimming recreational	6.0	Moderate
Tennis	7.0	Vigorous
Jogging 12 min/mile	8.0	Vigorous

Notes: Moderate Intensity: You can talk but not sing during the activity. Vigorous Intensity: You will not be able to say more than a few words without pausing for a breath.

CARDIOVASCULAR AND PULMONARY SYSTEMS

Physical activity reduces cardiovascular disease risk, heart failure, heart attacks, blood pressure, peripheral vascular disease and risk of stroke. The vascular and pulmonary benefits are due to an increase in heart rate variability, improvement in endothelial reactivity and a reduction of arterial stiffness. Physical activity is known to reduce inflammatory markers such as cytokines, improve muscle function and adaptation to oxidative stress, enhance gas exchange and improve mitochondrial function. It also improves cellular integrity, vascular health and release of exerkines. Regular exercise induces chronic changes in the coronary vascular system resulting in an increased size of the coronary arteries and luminal diameter, an increase in the number of collateral blood vessels and in their vasodilatory capacity as well as a decrease in wall thickness and stiffness. And regular exercise reduces the risk of fatal arrhythmia in the presence of prolonged coronary occlusion by inducing cardiac preconditioning – which is the cardioprotective response to normal brief periods of chronic myocardial ischemia while doing regular exercise.[7] In addition, exercise reduces plasma norepinephrine, plasma renin and systemic vascular resistance, which are important factors in cardiac health and remodeling. For example, 30 to 60 minutes of regular exercise per week is enough to reduce both systolic and diastolic BP by as much as 5–7 mmHg in patients with hypertension and a further benefit is seen in those who exercise 61 to 90 min/week.[8,9] Aerobic exercise is effective for reducing blood pressure in those with high blood pressure and in those with normal blood pressure. Moreover, the positive effects of exercise on blood pressure are not related to losing weight. Additionally, while dynamic resistance training and static isometric exercise show blood pressure-lowering effects, neither surpasses the benefits of aerobic exercise.[10,11]

In patients with peripheral vascular disease and heart failure, physical activity improves exercise tolerance by providing an extended time for claudication. Exercise improves respiratory muscle function and reduces dyspnea.

IMMUNOLOGICAL

Regular exercise reduces systemic markers of inflammation and the risk of many common cancers including colon, breast, prostate, lung and endometrial cancer.[12]

A recent literature review highlighted the progress of successful cancer immunotherapies and concluded that exercise and physical activity can reduce incidences and improve outcomes in cancer patients, as an adjuvant therapy.[13] Another review postulated a connection between the intestinal microbiome composition, biodiversity, dysbiosis and inflammation; and within the muscle system, a connection between protein deposition and muscle function. Researchers concluded that this "gut-muscle axis" could be regulated by exercise.[14] A follow-up review by this team discussed the health benefits arising from biodiversity and functionality of intestinal microbiota, and how epidemiological evidence indicates an association between physical activity and fitness as indicated by the gut microbiota composition in older adults.[15]

NEUROLOGICAL

Physical activity is one of the top interventions to reduce the risk of mild cognitive impairment and improve cognition in patients already diagnosed with dementia. Regular exercise improves memory, attention and reaction time, visual-spatial orientation and proprioception and sleep. Routine physical exercise promotes structural changes and connectivity between areas of the brain important for memory and executive function by increasing brain-derived neurotrophic factor (BDNF), insulin-like growth factor 1 and vascular endothelial growth factor (VEGF),[16] which are known factors to mediate cell growth, proliferation and differentiation. Regular exercise also reduces the levels of homocysteine which is linked with improved cognition. For example, a 6-month aerobic training program has been shown to increase hippocampal volume among older adults.[17]

Aerobic exercise improves executive function, verbal and visual memory, communication, global cognition and episodic memory. Combining aerobic exercise with strength exercise produces the strongest positive effects on cognitive function.[18]

MUSCULOSKELETAL

Regular physical exercise improves muscle mass, increases the synthesis of collagen in ligaments and tendons, improves mitochondrial function and preserves and improves bone mass. It also reduces the risk of osteoporosis and fracture, sarcopenia and frailty, and improves long-term physical function. Exercise improves pain tolerance and physical function in patients with osteoarthritis and musculoskeletal pain, including back pain. For patients with severe osteoporosis, balance training and resistance exercise may be more important in reducing the risk of falls and fractures.[19]

Exercise, along with pharmacological interventions, is an integral component of the treatment of osteoporosis. A recent review described how moderate exercise increases bone formation by stimulating the secretion of anti-inflammatory cytokines and myohormones by mediating apoptosis and autophagy. In addition, exercise mediates epigenetic processes involved in bone metabolism. These mechanisms favor osteogenic differentiation and increased expression of osteogenic genes.[20] However, exercise alone cannot prevent osteoporosis, sarcopenia and age-related loss in muscular function.[21,22]

Endocrine and Metabolism

Regular exercise improves insulin sensitivity and glucose homeostasis, decreases inflammatory cytokines and other markers of systemic inflammation, increases basal metabolic rate and decreases bad cholesterol. Therefore, an exercise prescription should be included for any patient suffering from hyperglycemia, diabetes, metabolic syndrome, hyperlipidemia and obesity-related conditions. For example, a combination of aerobic and resistance training of at least 150 minutes/week of moderate exercise (or the equivalent of 530–600 MET/min per week) has been associated with a reduction of Hba1c levels of −0.3 to −0.4%. This reduction in HbA1c can lead to an approximate 5% reduction in cardiovascular disease risk and a 12% reduction in risk of microvascular complications.[23]

Patients suffering from obesity benefit from regular exercise to increase their energy expenditure and improve physical function (mobility) and quality of life (self-esteem). In older adults suffering from obesity and already at risk for negative body composition changes, adiposity and sarcopenia, exercise prescriptions should emphasize weight loss as an added benefit.[24] Considering the efficacy of glucagon-like peptide 1 receptor agonists (GLP-1 RAs) to induce weight loss, multiple studies have addressed the role of concomitant exercise interventions in improving health outcomes. A randomized clinical trial of 195 adults confirmed the benefits of combining exercise and GLP-1RA treatment.[25] The researchers found improved reductions of metabolic syndrome severity, abdominal obesity and inflammation, when adults adhered to exercise with GLP-1RA, more than with individual treatments alone. More clinical trials are needed in the older adult population, although it is anticipated that the evidence will continue to favor the implementation of exercise in older adults, especially resistance exercise.

Psychological

All modes of regular exercise are beneficial to treat symptoms of depression, anxiety and psychological distress, and reactivity to stress. Exercise also has been effective in improving sleep quality in older adults. Several types of exercise, including aerobic walking, stretching, strengthening and activities such as dancing have shown benefits in reducing psychological distress and improving quality of life. Moderate-to high-intensity exercise tends to be more effective than low-intensity exercise.[26,27]

FALLS

Regular exercise along with balance and strength training reduces the risk of falls, fall-related injuries and fear of falling. For patients at risk of falls, exercise programs that include gait training and strength training provide additional benefits in reducing falls. However, patients who have serious balance problems may need to be enrolled in a supervised physical therapy program.[28]

PHYSICAL ACTIVITY AND GERIATRIC CARE

COMMON INJURIES

Older adults are at an increased risk of common injuries, especially with repetitive and high-impact exercises. At the same time, fear of injury is frequently expressed as a barrier that inhibits older adults from starting and maintaining a regular exercise program. The consequences of injuries among older adults can be devastating, primarily by reducing mobility, function and quality of life, and increasing the risk of disability.

Approximately, 70% of all injuries among older adults are due to overuse.[29] Older individuals have decreased functional reserve and at the same time, their injuries take a longer time to heal. The most common injuries among older adults are acute strains, strains due to overuse, sprains, falls, fractures and bursitis.[30] As people grow older, tendons and ligaments show decreased compliance and vascularity. Therefore, repetitive macro trauma increases stiffness in tendons making them more prone to inflammation, chronic damage and tears. Meniscus and articular cartilage lose the ability to dissipate high-stress impacts and produce cartilage damage. Therefore, arthritis is commonly seen due to trauma and overuse. Aging is also associated with a decrease in the number of muscle fibers, decreased mitochondrial volume, changes associated with types of muscle fibers and increased collagen content. These changes reduce the ability of the muscle to adapt to high levels of weight loading, increasing the likelihood of muscle tears, strains and weakness. Older adults also show an increase in osteophyte formation, a decrease in the amounts of lubricin, an increase in collagen cross-linking and fiber separation and calcification of tendons, causing pain, reduction in mobility and the destruction of joints. Adhesive capsulitis, especially in patients with type 2 diabetes, increases the risk of joint injury and reduction in movement.[31]

PREVENTION OF INJURIES

Although there are no specific guidelines restricting the intensity of exercise for older adults, all exercise prescriptions should minimize the risk of injury.

TABLE 7.2
Common Injuries among Older Adults[32,33]

Diagnosis	Cause	Clinical Presentation
Tendinitis	• Decreased compliance • Decreased vascularity • Repetitive microtrauma • Increase collagen cross-linking	• Insidious onset of pain • Limitation on ROM • Swelling join • Unstable joint
Arthritis	• Trauma • Osteophyte formation • Decrease lubricin • Decreased proprioception	• Pain and inflammation • Limited ROM • Joint destruction • Chondromalacia • Calcification of joint tissues • Decreased water content in the cartilage
Muscle injuries	• Decreased number of muscle fibers Decreased mitochondrial volume • Increased collagen content • Decreased flexibility	• Muscle weakness • Localized stiffness • Swelling • Pain and tenderness
Fall and fractures	• Decreased proprioceptionChanges in the vestibular system • Vision changes • Age-related changes in the bone and soft tissues • Concomitant diseases: e.g., Parkinson's	• Acute pain • Disability • Reduction ROM

Recommendations to reduce risk of injury:[32]

- Increase the intensity of exercise gradually. Sudden increases are associated with injury.
- Multimodal exercises (endurance, flexibility, strength and balance) are preferred to prevent overuse injuries.
- Warm-up is more beneficial among older adults than in younger adults to reduce the risk of injury.
- Stretching as part of the warm-up may reduce the risk of musculotendinous injuries.
- Use of protective equipment: helmets, external joint supports and protective vests.
- Use of technically efficient equipment, for example, sports shoes.
- Avoid contact sports or practice modified team sports to avoid body contact (Figure 7.2).

Although there are numerous studies looking at the risk of injury of older adults when performing exercise, many of them focus on a single outcome or risk factor. Indeed, there are many factors that can increase the likelihood of injury or harm in a

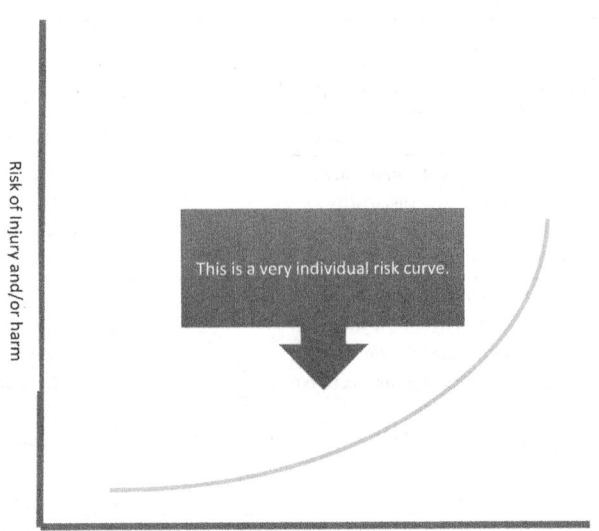

FIGURE 7.2 Predictive factors of injury or harm with exercise among older adults.

person. These factors are very individualized. Intensity, type and frequency of exercise are factors that play a role in the risk of injury. Also, baseline fitness level, age, presence of chronic conditions, polypharmacy and environmental factors have been also implicated in the risk of injury and harm.[32,34] Therefore, health care providers should identify which factors may play a more important role for a given individual and plan a prescription of exercise accordingly. For example, the prescribed exercise regimen for a 70-year-old frail person with multiple medications and a high risk for falls should be different from the one prescribed to a 70-year-old person with no frailty and no medications.

MEDICATION MANAGEMENT

Older adults are more likely to be suffering from chronic conditions and use prescribed and over-the-counter medications to treat their illnesses. Ninety percent of all older adults take at least one prescribed medication. Therefore, when discussing exercise prescriptions among older adults, providers need to consider the potential impact of medications on exercise performance and negative outcomes or complications. For example, non-selective beta-blockers can reduce tolerance to exercise and can produce exacerbation of exercise-induced bronchospasm or asthma. They can impair left ventricular function, producing a reduction of VO_2 max and causing early fatigue. Thiazides, a common hypertensive medication, can induce urinary loss of potassium and magnesium, increasing the risk of muscle cramping, rhabdomyolysis and arrhythmias. Metformin can increase the heart rate and increase concentrations of lactate during exercise. Nevertheless, there are some studies showing that metformin can enhance mitochondrial oxidation and therefore improve exercise performance in the long term.[35]

Steroids and quinolones can increase the risk of tendonitis and tendon ruptures.[36] Medications such as omeprazole and other proton-pump inhibitors (PPIs) can reduce levels of magnesium, increasing the risk of muscle cramps weakness and arrhythmias.[37] Antihistamines and selective serotonin reuptake inhibitors – SSRIs can reduce reaction time and decrease visual discrimination, increasing the risk of falls and accidents.[38] Statins may alter muscle metabolism during exercise, increasing fatigue, muscle weakness and pain.[39] NSAIDs can increase the risk of renal insufficiency, especially in patients who do not hydrate during exercise.[40]

Common over-the-counter medications such as turmeric can increase the risk of arrhythmias. Saw Palmetto (used for BPH) can increase the risk of tachycardia arrhythmias and fatigue. Melatonin can decrease reaction time and therefore increase the risk of falling. St. John's Wort can increase the risk of fatigue, common muscle and joint pain and spasms.[41] On the other hand, there is a pharmacological benefit from persistent physical activity and exercise. Gerofit is a long-duration, multicenter, clinical program to improve physical activity and exercise in thousands of veterans which is offered at 33 different VA Healthcare Systems around the country.[42] Within this project, an analysis of 453 participants demonstrated that after one year of exercise interventions, there were significant reductions in medications: 47% for those requiring opioids, 42% in mental health medications, 45% in cardiac medications, 25% in diabetes medications and 22% for those taking lipid-lowering medications.[43] When patients successfully adhere to physical activity and exercise interventions, providers should be aware of the potential impact on conditions that require pharmacologic treatments and proactive interventions. For instance, a diabetic patient exercising may be at risk for hypoglycemia, and it is best to offer closer monitoring, and reduce the pertinent dosages. This could be a good opportunity for patient education and motivation. Many older patients accumulate chronic conditions that inevitably may lead to polypharmacy. There is enough evidence that exercise improves chronic conditions, and providers should feel comfortable enough to counsel patients about the effects of exercise on medication reduction.

CHRONIC DISEASE AND EXERCISE

For all adults experiencing a higher prevalence of chronic disease, an exercise prescription should be included as part of their medical management. Although there are general guidelines and recommendations for exercise, one-size-fits-all programs are not always recommended for older adults. The intensity of an exercise prescription should be individualized, and the provider should consider matching it with the patient's exercise baseline performance, the presence of chronic conditions, patient preferences and potential physical capability. Exercise prescriptions among older adults should consider the potential improvement of health outcomes, mobility and slowing any age-associated health problems while minimizing the risk of injury.[44] *Physical activity and exercise guidelines for older adults is discussed in more detail in the next chapter.*

Although following the exercise guidelines is generally safe for all adults, there may be some circumstances when they should consult a medical provider before starting an exercise program. For example, there are absolute contraindications for exercise among patients with a recent acute ischemic event, unstable angina and uncontrolled heart failure, severe aortic stenosis, uncontrolled cardiac arrhythmia, acute pericarditis and dissecting aneurysm. These patients should not engage in any physical activity until consulting a health care provider. Many of these patients may need a supervised environment to safely perform exercises. There are some relative contraindications which may require additional assessments to clear patients to exercise. These include moderate aortic stenosis, severe arterial hypertension, hypertrophic cardiomyopathy, high degree atrioventricular block, ventricular aneurysm, uncontrolled electrolyte imbalance and left main coronary artery stenosis.[45]

Frailty

Physical exercise is one of the strategies to treat frailty. After the age of 25, aerobic capacity decreases with age, and there is a decrease in muscle strength and muscle mass, with an approximate 30% reduction of strength between the ages of 50 to 70 years of age.[46,47] However, there is a more pronounced decline in physical strength after the age of 70.[48] Although sarcopenia is one of the risk factors for frailty, sarcopenia and frailty are two different conditions. Progressive decline of muscle mass, especially on lower extremities, alters mobility in a very significant way, increasing the risk for frailty. Progressive resistance exercises improve muscle mass and muscle strength. Exercise along with good nutrition seems to reduce frailty by reducing age-related oxidative damage and inflammation, improving mitochondrial function and myokine profile, improving insulin sensitivity and increasing muscle protein synthesis.[49,50]

On the other hand, the current obesity epidemic now includes treatments with multifactorial interventions, including newer pharmacologic interventions, that are successful in facilitating weight loss. However, diet-induced weight loss can lead to fat, muscle and bone mass loss, and further exacerbate age-related sarcopenia and frailty in older adults.[51]

Barriers and Motivations to Exercise

Why do people fail to exercise knowing that being active is good for their health? In a systematic review addressing the barriers and motivators of physical activity participation in middle-aged and older adults, it was discovered that for older adults, the key motivators were peer encouragement and having fun, social interactions involving physical activity, and the support of health care providers. Older adults identified physical activity as a social motivator and an opportunity to be busy. Key barriers to participating in physical activity identified by researchers included the lack of belief in one's capabilities to perform exercises (physical and mental health problems, fear of falling, fears about safety to carry out physical activity and feeling that one is too old), environmental factors and lack of support from their social area of influence such as family and friends. Lack of guidance from health care providers was another key factor that was identified among older adults that prevented them from exercising.[52]

A 12-month follow-up study delivered a 12-week physical training program for 214 adults aged 58.8 ± 11.9, 71% women, 62% with hypertension, 64% with dyslipidemia and 15% with impaired glucose tolerance.[53] At the end of follow-up, 48% reported long-term adherence.

The main predictor was baseline sports activities (4.22, 1.72–10.4). More recently, a 2-arm RCT compared a 12-week physical activity intervention combined with municipal and sports resources with added social support and social participation strategies and usual medical care combined with social education meetings.[54] The goal was to assess adherence over a 15-month period. The average age in the groups was 69.5 ± 8.4 and 68.2 ±8.9 years. The participants were overweight, had hypertension (65%, and 55%), diabetes (26.4% and 25.2%), myocardial infarction (12.3% and 11.9%), heart failure (9.5% and 9.4%) and osteoarthritis (44.5% and 45%). Again, higher adherence was associated with higher baseline physical activity, and in this case, with social support.

CONCLUSIONS

Exercise prescriptions should be patient-centered. Individualized exercise programs need to include the type, intensity, duration and frequency of the exercise. At the same time, providers need to address the patients' needs and interests which are necessary for long-term adherence. The presence of multidisciplinary teams, supervision and the use of technology tracking devices have also been shown to contribute to increased adherence to exercise programs. Enjoyment of physical activity is crucial to improve adherence to physical exercise. Patients are more likely to adhere to these programs when their basic needs regarding autonomy, competence and relatedness are satisfied. Other factors that improve adherence to an exercise routine are the integration of exercise in daily living, and belonging to a group (relatedness), for example, yoga club.[55]

CLINICAL APPLICATIONS

- Providers should offer support and guidance, and identify patient needs and interests to increase long-term adherence to an exercise program.
- Providers should identify the predictive factors involving the risk of exercise injury before prescribing exercise.
- Providers should consider the potential impact of medications on exercise performance and any negative outcomes or complications when prescribing exercise to older adults with chronic conditions.
- Providers should consider the potential impact of exercise on the number and dosages of medications that a patient has been prescribed, and discuss this with their patient.
- Providers should consider a patient's chronic conditions, patient preferences and capabilities when offering exercise prescriptions.

REFERENCES

1. Centers for Disease Control and Prevention. *Physical Inactivity among Adults 50 Years and Older.* Updated September 2016. Accessed June 5, 2024. https://www.cdc.gov/physicalactivity/inactivity-among-adults-50plus/mmwr-data-highlights.pdf
2. Pinto AJ, Bergouignan A, Dempsey PC, et al. Physiology of sedentary behavior. *Physiol Rev.* 2023;103(4):2561–2622. doi:10.1152/physrev.00022.2022
3. Raffin J, de Souto Barreto P, Le Traon AP, Vellas B, Aubertin-Leheudre M, Rolland Y. Sedentary behavior and the biological hallmarks of aging. *Ageing Res Rev.* 2023;83:101807. doi:10.1016/j.arr.2022.101807
4. Valenzuela PL, Ruilope LM, Santos-Lozano A, et al. Exercise benefits in cardiovascular diseases: from mechanisms to clinical implementation. *Eur Heart J.* 2023;44(21):1874–1889. doi:10.1093/eurheartj/ehad170
5. Centers for Disease Control and Prevention. *Measuring Physical Activity Intensity.* Updated June 2022. Accessed June 5, 2024. https://www.cdc.gov/physicalactivity/basics/measuring/index.html
6. Mora JC, Valencia WM. Exercise and older adults. *Clin Geriatr Med.* 2018;34(1):145–162. doi:10.1016/j.cger.2017.08.007
7. Valenzuela PL, Ruilope LM, Santos-Lozano A, et al. Exercise benefits in cardiovascular diseases: from mechanisms to clinical implementation. *Eur Heart J.* 2023;44(21):1874–1889. doi:10.1093/eurheartj/ehad170
8. Ishikawa-Takata K, Ohta T, Tanaka H. How much exercise is required to reduce blood pressure in essential hypertensives: a dose–response study. *Am J Hypertens.* 2003;16(8):629–633. doi:10.1016/S0895-7061(03)00895-1
9. Hegde SM, Solomon SD. Influence of physical activity on hypertension and cardiac structure and function. *Curr Hypertens Rep.* 2015;17(10):77. doi:10.1007/s11906-015-0588-3
10. Whelton PK, Carey RM, Aronow WS, et al. 2017 ACC/AHA/AAPA/ABC/ACPM/AGS/APhA/ASH/ASPC/NMA/PCNA guideline for the prevention, detection, evaluation, and management of high blood pressure in adults: a report of the American College of Cardiology/American Heart Association task force on clinical practice guidelines. *Hypertension.* 2018;71(6):e13–e115. doi:10.1161/HYP.0000000000000065
11. Arnett DK, Blumenthal RS, Albert MA, et al. 2019 ACC/AHA guideline on the primary prevention of cardiovascular disease: executive summary: a report of the American College of Cardiology/American Heart Association task force on clinical practice guidelines. *Circulation.* 2019;140(11):e563–e595. doi:10.1161/CIR.0000000000000677
12. Kruk J, Aboul-Enein HY. Physical activity in the prevention of cancer. *Asian Pac J Cancer Prev.* 2006;7:11–21.
13. Gustafson MP, Wheatley-Guy CM, Rosenthal AC, Gastineau DA, Katsanis E, Johnson BD, et al. Exercise and the immune system: taking steps to improve responses to cancer immunotherapy. *J Immunother Cancer.* 2021;9(7):e001872. doi:10.1136/jitc-2020-001872
14. Ticinesi A, Lauretani F, Tana C, Nouvenne A, Ridolo E, Meschi T. Exercise and immune system as modulators of intestinal microbiome: implications for the gut-muscle axis hypothesis. *Exerc Immunol Rev.* 2019;25:84–95.
15. Strasser B, Wolters M, Weyh C, Krüger K, Ticinesi A. The effects of lifestyle and diet on gut microbiota composition, inflammation, and muscle performance in our aging society. *Exerc Immunol Rev.* 2019;25:84–95.
16. Sanders LMJ, Hortobágyi T, Karssemeijer EGA, Van der Zee EA, Scherder EJA, van Heuvelen MJG. Effects of low- and high-intensity physical exercise on physical and cognitive function in older persons with dementia: a randomized controlled trial. *Alzheimers Res Ther.* 2020;12(1):28. doi:10.1186/s13195-020-00597-3

17. Bossers WJ, van der Woude LH, Boersma F, Hortobágyi T, Scherder EJ, van Heuvelen MJ. A 9-week aerobic and strength training program improves cognitive and motor function in patients with dementia: a randomized, controlled trial. *Am J Geriatr Psychiatry*. 2015;23(11):1106–1116. doi:10.1016/j.jagp.2014.12.191
18. Cai H, Li G, Hua S, Liu Y, Chen L. Effect of exercise on cognitive function in chronic disease patients: a meta-analysis and systematic review of randomized controlled trials. *Clin Interv Aging*. 2017;12:773–783. doi:10.2147/CIA.S135700
19. Garber CE, Blissmer B, Deschenes MR, et al. American College of Sports Medicine position stand. Quantity and quality of exercise for developing and maintaining cardiorespiratory, musculoskeletal, and neuromotor fitness in apparently healthy adults: guidance for prescribing exercise. *Med Sci Sports Exerc*. 2011;43(7):1334–1359. doi:10.1249/MSS.0b013e318213fefb
20. Zhang L, Zhen YL, Wang R, Wang XQ, Zhang H. Exercise for osteoporosis: a literature review of pathology and mechanism. *Front Immunol*. 2022;13:1005665. Published 2022 Sep 9. doi:10.3389/fimmu.2022.1005665
21. Bilsky J, Pierzchalski P, Szczepanik M, Bonior J, Zoladz J. Multifactorial mechanism of sarcopenia and sarcopenic obesity. Role of physical exercise, microbiota, and myokines. *Cells*. 2022;11(1):160. doi:10.3390/cells11010160.
22. Skolnick A. It's important, but don't bank on exercise alone to prevent osteoporosis, experts say. *JAMA*. 1990;263(13):1751–1752. doi:10.1001/jama.1990.03440130021005.
23. Church TS, Blair SN, Cocreham S, et al. Effects of aerobic and resistance training on hemoglobin A1c levels in patients with type 2 diabetes: a randomized controlled trial [published correction appears in JAMA. 2011 Mar 2;305(9):892]. *JAMA*. 2010;304(20):2253–2262. doi:10.1001/jama.2010.1710.
24. Valencia WM, Stoutenberg M, Florez H. Weight loss and physical activity for disease prevention in obese older adults: an important role for lifestyle management. *Curr Diab Rep*.
25. Sandsdal RM, Juhl CR, Jensen SBK, Lundgren JR, Janus C, Blond MB, et al. Combination of exercise and GLP-1 receptor agonist treatment reduces severity of metabolic syndrome, abdominal obesity, and inflammation: a randomized controlled trial. *Cardiovasc Diabetol*. 2023;22(1):41. doi:10.1186/s12933-023-01765-z.
26. Singh B, Olds T, Curtis R, et al. Effectiveness of physical activity interventions for improving depression, anxiety, and distress: an overview of systematic reviews. *Br J Sports Med*. 2023;57(18):1203–1209. doi:10.1136/bjsports-2022-106195.
27. Awick EA, Ehlers DK, Aguiñaga S, Daugherty AM, Kramer AF, McAuley E. Effects of a randomized exercise trial on physical activity, psychological distress, and quality of life in older adults. *Gen Hosp Psychiatry*. 2017;49:44–50. doi:10.1016/j.genhosppsych.2017.06.005.
28. Vinik AI, Camacho P, Reddy S, Valencia WM, Trence D, Matsumoto AM, et al. Aging, diabetes, and falls. *Endocr Pract*. 2017;23(9):1117–1139. doi:10.4158/EP171794.RA. Epub 2017 Jul 13.
29. Kannus P, Niittymäki S, Järvinen M, Lehto M. Sports injuries in elderly athletes: a three-year prospective, controlled study. *Age Ageing*. 1989;18(4):263–270. doi:10.1093/ageing/18.4.263.
30. Little RM, Paterson DH, Humphreys DA, Stathokostas L. A 12-month incidence of exercise-related injuries in previously sedentary community-dwelling older adults following an exercise intervention. *BMJ Open*. 2013;3(6):e002831. Published 2013 Jun 20. doi:10.1136/bmjopen-2013-002831.
31. McCarthy MM, Hannafin JA. The mature athlete: aging tendon and ligament. *Sports Health*. 2014;6(1):41–48.

32. Kostka T, Kostka J. Injuries in sports activities in older people. In: Michel JP, et al, eds. *Oxford Textbook of Geriatric Medicine*. 3rd ed. Oxford University Press; 2017: online edn, Oxford Academic. Accessed December 5, 2024. https://doi.org/10.1093/med/9780198701590.003.0077_update_001.
33. Mora JC, Valencia WM. Physical activity and exercise for older adults. In: Busby-Whitehead J, Durso SC, Arenson C, Elon R, Palmer MH, Reichel W, eds. *Reichel's Care of the Elderly: Clinical Aspects of Aging*. Cambridge University Press; 2022:64–80.
34. Kallinen M, Markku A. Aging, physical activity, and sports injuries: an overview of common sports injuries in the elderly. *Sports Med*. 1995;20(1):41–52. doi:10.2165/00007256-199520010-00004.
35. Niedfeldt MW. Managing hypertension in athletes and physically active patients. *Am Fam Physician*. 2002;66(3):445–452.
36. van der Linden PD, Sturkenboom MCJM, Herings RMC, Leufkens HMG, Rowlands S, Stricker BHC. Increased risk of Achilles tendon rupture with quinolone antibacterial use, especially in elderly patients taking oral corticosteroids. *Arch Intern Med*. 2003;163(15):1801–1807. doi:10.1001/archinte.163.15.1801.
37. Florentin M, Elisaf MS. Proton pump inhibitor-induced hypomagnesemia: A new challenge. *World J Nephrol*. 2012;1(6):151–154. doi:10.5527/wjn.v1.i6.151.
38. Gebara MA, Lipsey KL, Karp JF, Nash MC, Iaboni A, Lenze EJ. Cause or effect? Selective serotonin reuptake inhibitors and falls in older adults: a systematic review. *Am J Geriatr Psychiatry*. 2015;23(10):1016–1028. doi:10.1016/j.jagp.2014.11.004.
39. Parker BA, Thompson PD. Effect of statins on skeletal muscle: exercise, myopathy, and muscle outcomes [published correction appears in *Exerc Sport Sci Rev*. 2013 Jan;41(1):71]. *Exerc Sport Sci Rev*. 2012;40(4):188–194. doi:10.1097/JES.0b013e31826c169e.
40. Nelson DA, Marks ES, Deuster PA, O'Connor FG, Kurina LM. Association of nonsteroidal anti-inflammatory drug prescriptions with kidney disease among active young and middle-aged adults. *JAMA Netw Open*. 2019;2(2):e187896. doi:10.1001/jamanetworkopen.2018.7896.
41. Mora JC, Valencia WM. Physical activity and exercise for older adults. In: Busby-Whitehead J, Durso SC, Arenson C, Elon R, Palmer MH, Reichel W, eds. *Reichel's Care of the Elderly: Clinical Aspects of Aging*. Cambridge University Press; 2022:64–80.
42. Morey MC, Lee CC, Castle S, et al. Models of geriatric care, quality improvement, and program dissemination: should structured exercise be promoted as a model of care? Dissemination of the Department of Veterans Affairs Gerofit Program. *J Am Geriatr Soc*. 2018;66(5):1009–1016.
43. Pepin MJ, Valencia WM, Bettger JP, et al. Gerontology & geriatric medicine. *Gerontol Geriatr Med*. 2020;6:1–6.4.
44. McPhee JS, French DP, Jackson D, Nazroo J, Pendleton N, Degens H. Physical activity in older age: perspectives for healthy ageing and frailty. *Biogerontology*. 2016;17(3):567–580. doi:10.1007/s10522-016-9641-0.
45. Nelson ME, Rejeski WJ, Blair SN, Duncan PW, Judge JO, King AC, et al. Physical activity and public health in older adults: recommendations from the American College of Sports Medicine and the American Heart Association. *Circulation*. 2007;116(9):1094–1105.
46. Hollenberg M, Yang J, Haight TJ, Tager IB. Longitudinal changes in aerobic capacity: implications for concepts of aging. *J Gerontol A Biol Sci Med Sci*. 2006;61(8):851–858. doi:10.1093/gerona/61.8.851.
47. Keller K, Engelhardt M. Strength and muscle mass loss with aging process. *Muscles Ligaments Tendons J*. 2014;3(4):346–350.

48. Siparsky PN, Kirkendall DT, Garrett WE Jr. Muscle changes in aging: understanding sarcopenia. *Sports Health*. 2014;6(1):36–40. doi:10.1177/1941738113502296.
49. Aguirre LE, Villareal DT. Physical exercise as therapy for frailty. *Nestle Nutr Inst Workshop Ser*. 2015;83:83–92. doi:10.1159/000382065.
50. Angulo J, El Assar M, Álvarez-Bustos A, Rodríguez-Mañas L. Physical activity and exercise: strategies to manage frailty. *Redox Biol*. 2020;35:101513. doi:10.1016/j.redox.2020.101513.
51. Colleluori G, Villareal DT. Aging, obesity, sarcopenia and the effect of diet and exercise intervention. *Exp Gerontol*. 2021;155:111561. doi:10.1016/j.exger.2021.111561.
52. Spiteri K, Broom D, Bekhet AH, de Caro JX, Laventure B, Grafton K. Barriers and motivators of physical activity participation in middle-aged and older adults: a systematic review. *J Aging Phys Act*. 2019;27(4):929–944. Published 2019 Sep 1. doi:10.1123/japa.2018-0343.
53. Saida TGRH, Sørensen TJ, Langberg H. Long-term exercise adherence after public health training in at-risk adults. *Ann Phys Rehabil Med*. 2017;60(4):237–243.
54. Martín-Borràs C, Giné-Garriga M, Puig-Ribera A, Martín C, Solà M, Cuesta-Vargas A. A new model of exercise referral scheme in primary care: is the effect on adherence to physical activity sustainable in the long term? A 15-month randomized controlled trial. *BMJ Open*. 2018 Mar 3;8(3):e017211.
55. Collado-Mateo D, Lavín-Pérez AM, Peñacoba C, et al. Key factors associated with adherence to physical exercise in patients with chronic diseases and older adults: an umbrella review. *Int J Environ Res Public Health*. 2021;18(4):2023. doi:10.3390/ijerph18042023.

8 Physical Activity and Exercise Recommendations among Older Adults

Jorge C. Mora, and Edgar Ramos Vieira

EXERCISE IS MEDICINE

Exercise is a structured form of physical activity. Other forms of physical activity include most sports, walking as a means of transportation, games and recreational activities involving significant amounts of body movement such as dancing, and even sex. Increased levels of physical activity are associated with improved quality of life, reduced stress, increased longevity, a decreased risk of non-communicable and chronic diseases, improved mobility, improved cognition and positive mental status, and it has many other established health benefits.[1]

EXERCISE GUIDELINES

Physical exercise and physical activity are important to help older adults age well. Regular physical exercise reduces age-related problems and helps to preserve functional capacity. Data from the Centers for Disease Control and Prevention shows that physical inactivity increases as we age, and many older adults in the United States do not meet the minimum recommendations for physical activity. Hispanics, Blacks and adults with low levels of education are most likely to be inactive.[2] The World Health Organization also states that physical inactivity is one of the leading causes of non-communicable diseases including type 2 diabetes, hypertension, some cancers and falls[3]. According to the Centers for Disease Control and the World Health Organization, older adults need at least 150 minutes of moderate physical activity (MPA), or 75 to 150 min/week of vigorous physical activity (VPA) a week, or an equivalent combination of both. Older adults should also engage in activities to improve the strengthening of their muscle flexibility and to improve balance.[4,5] However, there is data showing that the lowest mortality is achieved by performing 300 minutes of VPA a week or about 600 minutes a week of MPA.[6] Approximately 8% of deaths among those 70 and older can be attributed to not meeting the aerobic physical guidelines.[7]

TABLE 8.1
Exercise Recommendations for Older Adults

	Exercise Recommendations and Examples	
Exercise Type	Recommendation	Example
Aerobic	150–300 minutes a week of moderate physical activity, or 75–150 minutes a week of vigorous physical activity Additional health benefits when engaging in physical activity beyond the 300 minutes a week	Moderate Exercise[8] • Brisk walking (at least 2.5 miles per hour) • Water aerobics • Dancing (ballroom or social) • Gardening • Tennis (doubles) • Biking slower than 10 miles per hour Vigorous Exercise • Hiking uphill or with a heavy backpack • Running • Swimming laps • Vigorous aerobic dancing • Heavy yard work such as continuous digging or hoeing • Tennis (singles) • Cycling 10 miles per hour or faster • Jumping rope
Strengthening	Two times a week involving all major muscle groups, moderate-vigorous intensity There is no recommendation for the duration of the session.	Weightlifting or exercises with bands
Balance	For recurrent falls, or for individuals with a high risk for falls and mobility problems	Tai Chi, Otago exercises or chair yoga
Flexibility	Activities designed to preserve or increase range of motion. During one warm-up or cooldown activity. It does not count towards aerobic or resistance guidelines.	Neck stretch, back stretch or calf stretch

Physical exercise and physical activity do not need to be strenuous to improve health outcomes. Low-intensity exercise programs can improve exercise capacity and help older adults stay physically active, especially among those suffering from musculoskeletal disorders.[9] In addition, older adults may further benefit from combining several types of exercise, minimizing injury and improving function, and/or reducing the rate of functional decline.

There has been much more emphasis on the cardiovascular benefits of exercise compared to other health benefits. However, there is growing evidence involving multi-component exercise to improve the performance of Activities of Daily Living (ADLs), especially among the frail and cognitively impaired, particularly in reducing disability and improving quality of life (QOL).[10,11] Furthermore, the implementation of functional exercise programs (FXT) along with pharmacological agents to prevent or reverse functional limitations involved with aging may lead to better outcomes in terms of function and mobility among vulnerable older adults.[12] In fact, FXTs for older adults which include progressive resistance strength training (PRT) of multiple muscle groups two to three times a week along with balance, speed and power exercises improved physical functioning in older people, resulting in better functioning for simple and complex activities such as climbing stairs, rising from a chair, getting out of a car, etc.[13]

PHYSICAL FUNCTION AND ACTIVITY IN DAILY LIFE

There are many tests and activities that relate to daily life and function and should be considered to identify physical decline and help plan medical interventions. Ecologically valid tests of physical function which relate to daily living tasks are important and include evaluating, for example, the ability to go from sitting to standing (e.g., 30-second sit-to-stand test);[14] walk (e.g., timed up-and-go test); get up from the floor;[15] and putting on socks and shoes and tying the laces. Exercise can help maintain such abilities and has many health benefits. However, not everybody is able to exercise due to their medical, physical, mental and/or emotional states. Instead of talking about exercise and diet, it may be more effective and productive to talk about "moving more and eating better," especially for older adults who have a harder time changing life-long behaviors and habits. Physical activity levels can be increased by small changes. For example, if someone likes to watch TV, they can be instructed to sit and stand ten times during commercial breaks.[16]

EXERCISE PRESCRIPTION FOR OLDER ADULTS

Practitioners must evaluate the risks involved in initiating an exercise program for older adults with multiple comorbidities. While the overall risk of cardiovascular events is generally low, it is crucial to consider the individual's baseline level of physical activity, personal goals and motivation when starting a new program, and to identify absolute contraindications to exercise.

ROLE OF PROVIDERS

Primary care settings are ideal for promoting physical activity due to their ability to reach a wide range of patients. However, many health care providers do not routinely assess exercise habits or prescribe physical activity during patient visits. A cross-sectional survey that randomly selected primary care physicians in the United States found that most providers did not offer appropriate counseling to their patients regarding physical activity. Some of them mentioned time constraints, lack of reimbursement and insufficient knowledge or experience as reasons why counseling was not offered.[19]

TABLE 8.2
Absolute Contraindications to Regular Exercise in Older Adults

Absolute	Cardiovascular[17]
No activity is advised for conditioning purposes for these patients. The primary focus should be on treating the patient and stabilizing their health conditions	• Unstable ischemia • Severe and symptomatic valvular stenosis or regurgitation • Congenital heart disease • Uncontrolled heart failure • Acute pulmonary embolism • Recent acute ischemic event • Dissecting aneurysm • Acute pericarditis
	Musculoskeletal[18] • Low back pain due to fracture, infection, cancer, or cauda equina syndrome

The Affordable Care Act promotes physical activity screening and counseling, particularly for older adults. As part of its national health priorities to reduce disability and manage chronic conditions, "The US Preventive Services Task Force (USPSTF) recommends (as a grade B) offering or referring adults with cardiovascular disease risk factors to behavioral counseling interventions to promote a healthy diet and physical activity."[20] Unfortunately, it does not recommend routine counseling of exercise (as a grade C) for adults without known cardiovascular disease (CVD) risk factors, affecting reimbursement.[21] Insurance companies will only pay for services for adults that have a rating of "A" or "B" in the current USPSTF recommendations[22] To be reimbursed, providers should assess activity levels and make exercise recommendations and referrals, using them as tools to manage chronic conditions such as high blood pressure, type 2 diabetes, obesity or depression. To address this gap, primary care physicians need to collaborate with community partners to support physical activity among their patients.

HEALTH COACHES AND EXERCISE

Physical inactivity increases with aging.[23] Therefore, health care providers and health systems need to explore innovative ways of promoting active lifestyles to reduce the burden of chronic disease while maximizing the independence of older adults in the community. Therefore, health coaches play a pivotal role in encouraging healthier behaviors while incorporating accountability. Health coaches educate and help patients set their own goals by identifying patient beliefs, values, and readiness for change.[24] A systematic review of randomized controlled trials found that health coaches were an effective intervention for increasing physical activity in people 60 years and older independent of health status. In addition, face-to-face interventions were more effective than telephone interventions.[25]

PHYSICAL ACTIVITY MONITORS

Pedometers and wearable trackers can be effective tools that can help older adults track and monitor their physical activity. This information can be useful for health care providers to discuss individual targets and accountability. At least in the short term, the use of these activity monitors is associated with increased physical activity.[26] In general, healthy older adults average 2,000–9,000 steps a day. Older adults living with disability and/or chronic illnesses average 1,200–8,800 steps a day. Pedometer-based interventions increase activity by 775 to 2,215 steps a day. When averaged over a week, 150 minutes of moderate-to-vigorous physical activity is equivalent to 7,100 steps/day.[27]

NUTRITION AND EXERCISE

Most of the emphasis on exercise and nutrition is directed toward older adults with sarcopenia and frailty. However, aging brings unique changes in physiology and nutritional needs compared to younger populations, which may lead to an increased risk of adverse events or even injuries when starting a new exercise program. In fact, approximately 25% of older adults are malnourished or at risk of malnutrition.[28]

Exercise increases caloric needs and some micronutrient requirements, including B vitamins, vitamin C and several minerals. At the same time, older adults have

TABLE 8.3
Micronutrient and Exercise Performance[32]

Micronutrient	Optimal Levels – Not Necessarily through Supplementation
Vitamin D	Increase muscle power and stamina, and reduce the risk of stress fractures and tissue inflammation
Vitamin B1	Improves exercise tolerance
Vitamin B2	Improves exercise tolerance
Vitamin B3	Improves exercise tolerance
Vitamin B6	Improves exercise tolerance
Vitamin B12	Improves exercise tolerance, improves brain functioning and maintenance of focus, especially during long bouts of exercise
Vitamin C	Reduces fatigue and helps with the integrity of joints and muscles
Iron	Helps regulate body temperature (especially in hot weather), and exercise tolerance
Calcium	Improves exercise performance, muscle strength, recovery time and delays the onset of muscle soreness
Potassium	Reduces the amount of lactic acid and muscle cramping
Magnesium	Reduces fatigue and improves exercise performance Decreases risk of arrhythmias
Zinc	Boosts aerobic performance, reduces inflammation, accelerates recovery time
Selenium	Boosts performance and reduces inflammation

decreased perceptions of thirst leading them to dehydration and syncope. Therefore, adjustments of vitamin supplementation, dietary counseling and encouragement of hydration should be part of the discussion when advising older adults about exercise. The protein requirement for older adults who are exercising is not clear. While some have recommended up to 1.5 gm/kg/day, this carries with it an increase in risk of some adverse medical outcomes, such as chronic kidney disease and cancer. Recent data have shown little or no impact of additional protein above the 0.8 gm/kg/day recommended for young and middle-aged adults.[29-31]

SPECIAL CONSIDERATIONS FOR EXERCISE

Arthroplasty of the hip and knee are common surgeries among older adults. In general, these procedures improve joint function, decrease pain and increase quality of life in a relatively short time.[33] After surgery, patients are expected to engage in regular exercise within 3 to 6 months after the procedure. Although most patients will be able to return to normal physical exercise after surgery, the type of exercise can impact physical wear and tear. Therefore, it is very important for health providers to counsel patients on the type of exercises that will prolong the life of the prosthesis.[34,35]

EXERCISE IN FALL PREVENTION

Falls are the number one cause of injury-related deaths in older adults and the rates of falls-related deaths are increasing.[38] Falls are not a normal part of aging. Physical function, gait, balance and lower limb strength are related to falls, and declines in these abilities are associated with aging. However, the effects of aging, such as sarcopenia (reduced muscle mass and strength), reduced range of motion and impaired

TABLE 8.4
Guidelines for Exercise after Hip and Knee Arthroplasty[36,37]

Recommended	Sports to Avoid
• Cycling	• High-impact aerobics
• Golf	• Football
• Doubles tennis	• Soccer
• Walking	• Handball
• Low-impact aerobics	• Squash
• Elliptical	• Taekwondo
• Ballroom dancing	• Martial arts
• Rowing	• Volleyball
• Tai Chi	• Singles tennis
• Bowling	• Gymnastics
• Stair climber	• Racquetball
• Weights	• Jogging

mobility and balance, can be prevented, treated and even reversed through exercise.[39] These declines often trigger the vicious cycle illustrated in Figure 8.1.

Fear of falls and prior falls lead to decreased mobility, community participation and social isolation. People who were able to walk to grocery stores and church and/or social gatherings, for example, are no longer able to do that because of increased fatigue, or because they have injuries resulting from falls and/or because they no longer feel safe in walking by themselves. That then leads to the next factor depicted in Figure 8.1 – deconditioning and depression. These changes and declines in multiple domains accelerate the physiological changes we described at the beginning of the cycle. Therefore, this cycle needs to be broken. This can be done at any stage and in multiple ways, one of them being by increasing physical activity and exercise.[40]

Preventative strategies need to be in place to reduce the risk of falls among older adults. Proper nutrition plays a big role. Older people need to ingest sufficient high-quality protein to counteract the effects of sarcopenia, sustain muscle mass and protect the joints and body against the potential effects of fall-related impacts. Protein also has an important role in osteoporosis and bone strength. Adequate sleep is needed to maintain attention during the day. Hydration and fluid intake schedules are important to establish to minimize the number of trips to the bathroom required

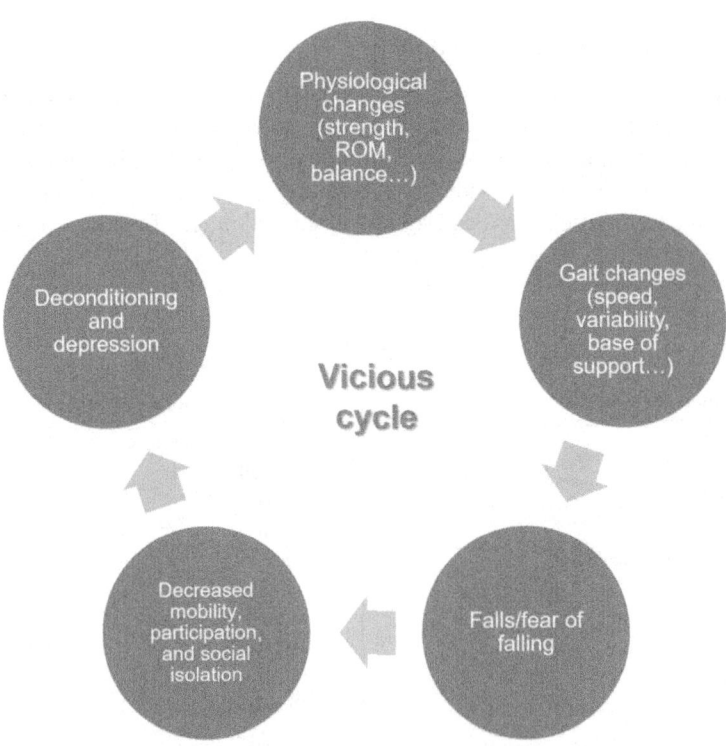

FIGURE 8.1 The vicious cycle of falls, deconditioning and gait changes.

during the night, and to address issues related to postural hypotension. Among many other factors, the following "4Es" also need to be considered:

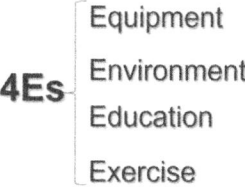

1. *Equipment:* Older adults' gait needs to be assessed, and proper assistive devices need to be prescribed and used in case they are needed to reduce the risk of falls and sustain mobility.
2. *Environment:* Changes and adaptations to the environment need to be considered. Steps and stairs can be a challenge for older adults; ramps and/or stairlifts may need to be considered. Rugs should be removed; handrails and bars need to be properly placed. Adequate lighting is required.
3. *Education:* Awareness of the risk factors and preventative measures are needed to reduce falls. Older people need to understand the need for proper nutrition and hydration as discussed. Adequate footwear and anti-slip socks may need to be worn.
4. *Exercise:* Finally, exercise can increase muscle mass, improve strength and balance, and significantly reduce the risk of falls. Exercise has been found to be the most effective intervention to prevent falls in older adults.

EXERCISE AND FRAILTY

As defined by the American Geriatrics Society, frailty is an "excess vulnerability to stressors with a reduced ability to maintain or regain homeostasis after a destabilizing event."[41] Therefore, frailty represents compromised self-regulatory and recovery ability. It is a state of susceptibility to external factors with the lack of endurance and strength to overcome challenges. Physical frailty impacts body weight, strength, fatigue, activity levels, mobility, balance and walking capacity. Physical frailty is associated with aging, chronic conditions, diet and sedentary lifestyle.

Exercise improves physical performance, and prevents and reverses frailty and mobility-related disability.[42,43] However, the decline in physical capacities may be too prominent to allow frail older adults to practice regular exercise. Often a combination of increased protein intake with physical therapy and progressive resistance exercise may be required before regular physical activity can be resumed. Small increments in physical activity levels and the practice of movements are often the best strategies to start to counteract the deleterious effect of frailty on physical function. Simple, low-intensity physical activities such as the Otago exercise program for fall prevention,[44] Tai Chi[45] and chair yoga[46] can be a good starting point. As an example, the Otago Exercise Program (OEP) is a 6-month program developed by the Falls Prevention Research Group at the University of Otago Medical School in New

Zealand. It is an individually tailored, low-intensity exercise program delivered by a nurse or physical therapist within the older adult's home. Based on its history of success, OEP was adopted by the Centers for Disease Control and Prevention and translated for use in the United States in 2012. The program includes a series of 17 strength (n = 5) and balance (n = 12) exercises, and participants are encouraged to engage in a self-led walking program.

EXERCISE AS A PART OF LIFE

The effects of engaging in physical activity are long-lasting. For example, a physical activity and behavioral maintenance program improved and sustained physical function in older adults over a 24-month period.[47] Considering all the benefits and protective effects, physical activity/exercise needs to be practiced on a regular basis throughout life for healthy aging, longevity, and sustained quality of life.

SMART goals can be used as a strategy.[48] SMART is an acronym for Specific (including what, where and when); Measurable (repetitions, duration and progression are tracked); Achievable (the activity is challenging enough, but possible to complete safely); Relevant/Realistic (the activity includes practices that will improve daily life function such as the ability to move from sitting to standing, walking and or picking up objects) and Time-bound (the activity has a timeline of expected effect such as you will practice these skills for 10 minutes a day for 15 days with reassessments in order to progress to the next stage as needed). Teaching, establishing and revising the SMART exercise/physical activity goals from time to time can empower older adults to play an important role in their health and "health care."

EXERCISE, DISABILITY AND SOCIAL CONNECTIONS

Older adults are more likely to exercise alone than younger adults. Although exercising alone provides older adults with significant health benefits, doing exercise with others can provide extra health benefits. For example, older adults who exercised with others decreased their risk for cognitive impairment by 29.2% compared to 15.1% for those who exercised alone.[49] Social relationships may explain the extra benefits of exercising with others. In addition to social connections, exercising with others enhances exercise adherence and reduces the incidence of functional disability.[50,51]

CLINICAL APPLICATIONS

- Assess and document patients' physical activity levels during routine visits to identify at-risk individuals.
- Counsel patients on exercise recommendations tailored to age, comorbidities and functional abilities.
- Incorporate SMART goals and specific exercise prescriptions into care plans to ensure adherence and progress tracking.
- Collaborate with community programs, physical therapists or health coaches to enhance patient engagement and support.

- Use wearable activity monitors to track progress and motivate patients toward achieving fitness goals.
- Screen for contraindications to exercise in patients with multiple comorbidities and provide tailored guidance.
- Educate patients on the role of exercise in fall prevention and frailty reversal, emphasizing balance and strength training.
- Integrate nutrition counseling, including protein and hydration advice, into exercise discussions to maximize benefits and minimize risks.

REFERENCES

1. Tao D, Awan-Scully R, Ash GI, et al. Health policy considerations for combining exercise prescription into noncommunicable diseases treatment: a narrative literature review. *Front Public Health*. 2023;11:1219676. doi:10.3389/fpubh.2023.1219676.
2. Centers for Disease Control and Prevention. Many older adults in the United States do not meet physical activity guidelines. Updated April 23, 2024. Accessed November 20, 2024. https://www.cdc.gov/physical-activity/php/reports/adults-50-and-older.html.
3. World Health Organization. Physical activity: fact sheet. Updated June 26, 2024. Accessed November 20, 2024. https://www.who.int/news-room/fact-sheets/detail/physical-activity.
4. Centers for Disease Control and Prevention. Physical activity guidelines for older adults. Updated December 22, 2023. Accessed November 20, 2024. https://www.cdc.gov/physical-activity-basics/guidelines/older-adults.html.
5. World Health Organization. Physical activity: fact sheet. Updated June 26, 2024. Accessed November 20, 2024. https://www.who.int/news-room/fact-sheets/detail/physical-activity.
6. Lee DH, Rezende LFM, Joh HK, et al. Long-term leisure-time physical activity intensity and all-cause and cause specific mortality: a prospective cohort of US adults. *Circulation*. 2022;146(7):523–534. doi:10.1161/CIRCULATIONAHA.121.058162.
7. Carlson SA, Adams EK, Yang Z, Fulton JE. Percentage of deaths associated with inadequate physical activity in the United States. *Prev Chronic Dis*. 2018;15:E38. doi:10.5888/pcd18.170354.
8. American Heart Association. Recommendations for physical activity in adults. Updated January 19, 2024. Accessed November 20, 2024. https://www.heart.org/en/healthy-living/fitness/fitness-basics/aha-recs-for-physical-activity-in-adults.
9. De Maio M, Bratta C, Iannaccone A, et al. Home-based physical activity as a healthy aging booster before and during COVID-19 outbreak. *Int J Environ Res Public Health*. 2022;19(7):4317. doi:10.3390/ijerph19074317.
10. Lau LK, Tou NX, Jabbar KA, et al. Effects of exercise interventions on physical performance and activities of daily living in oldest-old and frail older adults: a review of the literature. *Am J Phys Med Rehabil*. 2023;102(10):939–949. doi:10.1097/PHM.0000000000002246.
11. Venegas-Sanabria LC, Cavero-Redondo I, Martínez-Vizcaino V, Cano-Gutierrez CA, Álvarez-Bueno C. Effect of multicomponent exercise in cognitive impairment: a systematic review and meta-analysis. *BMC Geriatr*. 2022;22(1):617. doi:10.1186/s12877-022-03302-1.
12. Reid KF, Storer TW, Bhasin S. Functional exercise training plus promyogenic therapy: a winning formula for preventing and treating mobility-disability? *J Am Geriatr Soc*. 2023;71(6):2017–2022. doi:10.1111/jgs.18293.

13. Liu CJ, Latham NK. Progressive resistance strength training for improving physical function in older adults. *Cochrane Database Syst Rev.* 2009;2009(3):CD002759. doi:10.1002/14651858.CD002759.pub2.
14. McAllister LS, Palombaro KM. Modified 30-second sit-to-stand test: reliability and validity in older adults unable to complete traditional sit-to-stand testing. *J Geriatr Phys Ther.* 2020;43(3):153–158.
15. Bergland A, Laake K. Concurrent and predictive validity of "getting up from lying on the floor." *Aging Clin Exp Res.* 2005;17:181–185.
16. Vieira ER, Richard L, da Silva RA. Perspectives on research and health practice in physical and occupational therapy in geriatrics during and post COVID-19. *Phys Occup Ther Geriatr.* 2020;38(3):199–202.
17. Fletcher GF, Ades PA, Kligfield P, et al. Exercise standards for testing and training: a scientific statement from the American Heart Association. *Circulation.* 2013;128(8):873–934. doi:10.1161/CIR.0b013e31829b5b44.
18. Hoffmann TC, Maher CG, Briffa T, et al. Prescribing exercise interventions for patients with chronic conditions. *CMAJ.* 2016;188(7):510–518. doi:10.1503/cmaj.150684.
19. Abramson S, Stein J, Schaufele M, Frates E, Rogan S. Personal exercise habits and counseling practices of primary care physicians: a national survey. *Clin J Sport Med.* 2000;10(1):40–48. doi:10.1097/00042752-200001000-00008.
20. U.S. Preventive Services Task Force. Healthy diet and physical activity for cardiovascular disease prevention in adults with cardiovascular risk factors: behavioral counseling interventions. Published November 24, 2020. Accessed November 20, 2024. https://www.uspreventiveservicestaskforce.org/uspstf/recommendation/healthy-diet-and-physical-activity-counseling-adults-with-high-risk-of-cvd.
21. U.S. Preventive Services Task Force. Healthy diet and physical activity for cardiovascular disease prevention in adults without cardiovascular disease risk factors: behavioral counseling interventions. Published July 26, 2022. Accessed November 20, 2024. https://www.uspreventiveservicestaskforce.org/uspstf/recommendation/healthy-lifestyle-and-physical-activity-for-cvd-prevention-adults-without-known-risk-factors-behavioral-counseling.
22. Kaiser Family Foundation. Preventive services covered by private health plans under the Affordable Care Act. Published February 28, 2024. Accessed November 20, 2024. https://www.kff.org/womens-health-policy/fact-sheet/preventive-services-covered-by-private-health-plans/.
23. Hallal PC, Andersen LB, Bull FC, et al. Global physical activity levels: surveillance progress, pitfalls, and prospects. *Lancet.* 2012;380(9838):247–257. doi:10.1016/S0140-6736(12)60646-1.
24. Huffman MH. Health coaching: a fresh, new approach to improve quality outcomes and compliance for patients with chronic conditions. *Home Healthc Nurse.* 2009;27(8):490–498. doi:10.1097/01.NHH.0000360924.64474.04.
25. Oliveira JS, Sherrington C, Amorim AB, Dario AB, Tiedemann A. What is the effect of health coaching on physical activity participation in people aged 60 years and over? A systematic review of randomised controlled trials. *Br J Sports Med.* 2017;51(19):1425–1432. doi:10.1136/bjsports-2016-096943.
26. Bravata DM, Smith-Spangler C, Sundaram V, et al. Using pedometers to increase physical activity and improve health: a systematic review. *JAMA.* 2007;298(19):2296–2304. doi:10.1001/jama.298.19.2296.
27. Tudor-Locke C, Craig CL, Aoyagi Y, et al. How many steps/day are enough? For older adults and special populations. *Int J Behav Nutr Phys Act.* 2011;8:80. doi:10.1186/1479-5868-8-80.
28. Dent E, Wright ORL, Woo J, Hoogendijk EO. Malnutrition in older adults. *Lancet.* 2023;401(10380):951–966. doi:10.1016/S0140-6736(22)02612-5.

29. Deutz NE, Bauer JM, Barazzoni R, et al. Protein intake and exercise for optimal muscle function with aging: recommendations from the ESPEN Expert Group. *Clin Nutr.* 2014;33(6):929–936. doi:10.1016/j.clnu.2014.04.007.
30. American College of Sports Medicine, Sawka MN, Burke LM, et al. American College of Sports Medicine position stand. Exercise and fluid replacement. *Med Sci Sports Exerc.* 2007;39(2):377–390. doi:10.1249/mss.0b013e31802ca597.
31. Manore MM. Exercise and the Institute of Medicine recommendations for nutrition. *Curr Sports Med Rep.* 2005;4(4):193–198. doi:10.1097/01.csmr.0000306206.72186.00.
32. Ghazzawi HA, Hussain MA, Raziq KM, et al. Exploring the relationship between micronutrients and athletic performance: a comprehensive scientific systematic review of the literature in sports medicine. *Sports (Basel).* 2023;11(6):109. doi:10.3390/sports11060109.
33. Jones CA, Voaklander DC, Johnston DW, Suarez-Almazor ME. The effect of age on pain, function, and quality of life after total hip and knee arthroplasty. *Arch Intern Med.* 2001;161(3):454–460. doi:10.1001/archinte.161.3.454.
34. Papalia R, Del Buono A, Zampogna B, Maffulli N, Denaro V. Sport activity following joint arthroplasty: a systematic review. *Br Med Bull.* 2012;101:81–103. doi:10.1093/bmb/ldr009.
35. Wylde V, Livesey C, Blom AW. Restriction in participation in leisure activities after joint replacement: an exploratory study. *Age Ageing.* 2012;41(2):246–249. doi:10.1093/ageing/afr180.
36. Jassim SS, Douglas SL, Haddad FS. Athletic activity after lower limb arthroplasty: a systematic review of current evidence. *Bone Joint J.* 2014;96-B(7):923–927. doi:10.1302/0301-620X.96B7.31585.
37. Golant A, Christoforou DC, Slover JD, Zuckerman JD. Athletic participation after hip and knee arthroplasty. *Bull NYU Hosp Jt Dis.* 2010;68(2):76–83.
38. Kendrick P, Kelly YO, Baumann MM, Kahn E, Compton K, Schmidt C, Sylte DO, Li Z, La Motte-Kerr W, Daoud F, Ong KL. Mortality due to falls by county, age group, race, and ethnicity in the USA, 2000–19: a systematic analysis of health disparities. *The Lancet Public Health.* 2024 Aug 1;9(8):e539–550.
39. Beckwée D, Delaere A, Aelbrecht S, Baert V, Beaudart C, Bruyere O, de Saint-Hubert M, Bautmans I. Exercise interventions for the prevention and treatment of sarcopenia: a systematic umbrella review. *J Nutr Health Aging.* 2019;23(6):494–502. doi:10.1007/s12603-019-1196-8.
40. Sherrington C, Fairhall N, Wallbank G, Tiedemann A, Michaleff ZA, Howard K, Clemson L, Hopewell S, Lamb S. Exercise for preventing falls in older people living in the community: an abridged Cochrane systematic review. *Br J Sports Med.* 2020 Aug 1;54(15):885–891.
41. Walston J, Hadley EC, Ferrucci L, et al. Research agenda for frailty in older adults: toward a better understanding of physiology and etiology: summary from the American Geriatrics Society/National Institute on Aging Research Conference on Frailty in Older Adults. *J Am Geriatr Soc.* 2006;54(6):991–1001. doi:10.1111/j.1532-5415.2006.00745.x.
42. Kidd T, Mold F, Jones C, Ream E, Grosvenor W, Sund-Levander M, Tingström P, Carey N. What are the most effective interventions to improve physical performance in pre-frail and frail adults? A systematic review of randomised control trials. *BMC Geriatr.* 2019 Dec;19:1–1.
43. Pérez-Zepeda MU, Martínez-Velilla N, Kehler DS, Izquierdo M, Rockwood K, Theou O. The impact of an exercise intervention on frailty levels in hospitalised older adults: secondary analysis of a randomised controlled trial. *Age Ageing.* 2022 Feb;51(2):afac028.
44. Campbell J, Robertson C. *Otago exercise programme to prevent falls in older adults.* University of Otago Medical School; Accident Compensation Corporation (ACC);

2007. ISBN: 9780478251944. Funded by ACC, the Health Research Council of New Zealand, and the New Zealand Lottery Grants Board. Published under Creative Commons Attribution 4.0 License.
45. Zhong D, Xiao Q, Xiao X, et al. Tai Chi for improving balance and reducing falls: an overview of 14 systematic reviews. *Ann Phys Rehabil Med.* 2020;63(6):505–517. doi:10.1016/j.rehab.2019.12.008.
46. Loewenthal J, Innes KE, Mitzner M, Mita C, Orkaby AR. Effect of yoga on frailty in older adults: a systematic review. *Ann Intern Med.* 2023 Apr;176(4):524–535.
47. Stathi A, Greaves CJ, Thompson JL, Withall J, Ladlow P, Taylor G, Medina-Lara A, Snowsill T, Gray S, Green C, Johansen-Berg H. Effect of a physical activity and behaviour maintenance programme on functional mobility decline in older adults: the REACT (Retirement in Action) randomised controlled trial. *Lancet Public Health.* 2022 Apr 1;7(4):e316–326.
48. Doran GT. There's a SMART way to write management's goals and objectives. *Manag Rev.* 1981;70(11).
49. Nagata K, Tsunoda K, Fujii Y, Jindo T, Okura T. Impact of exercising alone and exercising with others on the risk of cognitive impairment among older Japanese adults. *Arch Gerontol Geriatr.* 2023;107:104908. doi:10.1016/j.archger.2022.104908.
50. Kanamori S, Kai Y, Kondo K, et al. Participation in sports organizations and the prevention of functional disability in older Japanese: the AGES Cohort Study. *PLoS One.* 2012;7(11):e51061. doi:10.1371/journal.pone.0051061.
51. Kanamori S, Takamiya T, Inoue S, Kai Y, Kawachi I, Kondo K. Exercising alone versus with others and associations with subjective health status in older Japanese: the JAGES Cohort Study. *Sci Rep.* 2016;6:39151. doi:10.1038/srep39151.

9 Nutrition Care for the Older Adult

Melissa Bernstein and Alison Reyes

INTRODUCTION

Lifestyle behaviors, including healthy eating patterns early in life, can have a dramatic and lasting impact on disease burden, and promote healthy aging. The goal of nutrition recommendations for the aging population is the maintenance of a nutrient-dense diet to promote optimal health and prevent nutrition-related complications that can contribute to disease burden, mental and cognitive decline, functional dependency and frailty. Unfortunately, the poor diet quality of older Americans continues to have a negative impact on healthy aging. From 2001 to 2018, the proportion of older adults with poor diet quality increased from 50.9% to 60.9% and those with an ideal diet stayed consistently low at 0.4%.[1] Similar to other age groups, the actual average daily intakes of fruits, vegetables, dairy foods, nuts, legumes and seafood falls below recommended intake ranges and exceeds limits for added sugar, saturated fat and meats in the United States.[2]

DIETARY GUIDANCE FOR OLDER ADULTS

Healthy eating throughout life can lower the risk of chronic diseases associated with aging. The Dietary Guidelines for Americans, 2020–2025, now emphasize the importance of specific eating patterns for each stage of life from birth through older adulthood.[3] Older adults are encouraged to follow the same healthy dietary pattern as the general adult population with an emphasis on nutrient density and lower calories.[3] Examples of healthy dietary patterns defined by the Dietary Guidelines include a "Healthy Vegetarian Eating Pattern and the Healthy Mediterranean–Style Eating Patterns" the Mediterranean diet.[3] The USDA MyPlate food guide provides recommendations for older adults which are tailored to address the unique needs of individuals over the age of 60. These guidelines include nutrition tips that address common barriers to a healthy diet and resources to help older adults make better choices. The USDA MyPlate for older adults emphasizes:[4]

- Consuming a variety of nutrient-dense foods rich in protein, vegetables, fruits, whole grains, healthy oils and low-fat dairy choices.
- Drinking water often to stay hydrated.

- Choosing foods with little or no added sugar, saturated fat and sodium.
- Maintaining a healthy body weight.
- Regular physical activity.
- Food safety.

Lifestyle medicine is defined by the American College of Lifestyle Medicine (ACLM) as "a medical specialty that uses therapeutic lifestyle interventions as a primary modality to treat chronic conditions including, but not limited to, cardiovascular diseases, type 2 diabetes, and obesity."[5] The nutrition pillar of lifestyle medicine encourages a whole food plant-predominant diet (WFPPD) based on a variety of unprocessed plant foods, including vegetables, fruits, whole grains, legumes, nuts and seeds.[5,6] The WFPPD is an impactful strategy to help individuals make meaningful lifestyle changes and improve health outcomes. The aim of the lifestyle medicine nutrition pillar is to empower individuals at any age to choose a sustainable dietary pattern that promotes health including the prevention, treatment and reversal of chronic diseases such as obesity, heart disease, diabetes.[6]

BLUE ZONES

Healthy aging can be studied by identifying populations across the globe whose inhabitants live exceptionally long lives. The Blue Zones were identified in the early 2000s as the world's healthiest, longest-living and happiest communities. The five original Blue Zones include Okinawa, Japan; Ikaria, Greece; Sardinia, Italy; Nicoya, Costa Rica; and Loma Linda, CA as areas of the world that produced the most centenarians.[7,8] Native inhabitants of these Blue Zones are ten times more likely to reach 100 years of age compared to the United States overall. All five Blue Zones support the notion that longevity and health benefits can be achieved by following healthy lifestyle behaviors and underlying dietary principles that include consuming a WFPPD, avoiding processed foods, a marked reduction or absence of animal protein and in most cases a reduction in total calories consumed (Table 9.1). [7,8]

SPECIFIC NUTRIENT RECOMMENDATIONS AND REQUIREMENTS FOR OLDER ADULTS

Healthy aging is dependent upon appropriate caloric intake supported by an adequate consumption of macro- and micronutrients. Numerous benefits of a WFPPD have been identified; however, careful attention to ensure sufficient intakes of protein, healthy fats and select nutrients such as vitamin B12, folate, vitamin D, magnesium and zinc should be considered in older adults. Simply removing animal products from the diet (i.e., a vegan diet) does not equate to a healthy dietary pattern especially if a person is consuming a diet of mainly highly refined grains, added sugars and processed vegetable fats. Older adults with chronic health conditions and those at risk for malnutrition should be monitored closely for dietary adequacy. To ensure a healthy dietary pattern, patients with nutrition-related concerns and conditions should be encouraged to consult with a Registered Dietitian Nutritionist (RDN) who

TABLE 9.1
Key Dietary Features of the Blue Zones

Blue Zone	Okinawa	Nicoya	Ikaria	Sardinia	Loma Linda
Unique Practice	• Calorie restriction is a common practice with a ritual called Hara hachi bu where they stop eating when they are 80% full	• Consume little to no processed foods, plant-based proteins are considered a major contributor to their longevity history	• Regular but moderate consumption of antioxidant-rich Ikarian red wine is thought to contribute to their longevity	• Meat is reserved for Sundays or special occasions practice Time-restricted eating, which decreases their overall daily caloric intake	• Seventh Day Adventist community who fasts every Saturday which reduces the total calories consumed
Dietary Pattern	• WFPB Diet	• WFPB Diet	• Mediterranean Diet	• WFPB Diet	• WFPB Diet – Vegan or Vegetarian
Beverages	• Ooitabi Extract	• Drinking Water – Rich in Mg and Calcium	• Ikarian Red Wine, Greek Coffee • Sideritis Sipylea (Medicinal Tea)	• Cannonau Wine	• No Alcohol
Common Foods	• Alpinia Zerumbet (Ginger)	• Tropical fruits • Beans • Squash • Corn	• Olives • Avocados • Chorta (wild greens)	• Kombu Seaweed • Goyas	• Beans • Lentils • Chickpeas

Abbreviation: WFPB Diet = Whole food plant-based diet.

will assess and make individualized recommendations to promote healthy aging.[9] A summary of key nutrients that require special attention with advancing age is listed in Table 9.3.

TOTAL ENERGY

In general, older adults have lower calorie needs but similar or even increased nutrient needs compared to younger adults; therefore, the overall nutrient density of the dietary pattern is particularly important for this age group.[3] Lower caloric energy requirements result from decreased energy expenditure, losses in lean body mass and reduced physical activity. Older adults who do not reduce their caloric intake to balance a decrease in energy expenditure are at risk for excessive weight gain, obesity, metabolic consequences and comorbidities. Eating nutrient-dense foods without overconsuming calories can be challenging for patients with functional dependence, frailty and illness. Encouraging the consumption of a whole food plant predominant dietary pattern will ensure an abundance of naturally occurring nutrients that minimize added fat, sugar, sodium and excess calories, and can support a higher quality of life as individuals age.[6]

CARBOHYDRATES AND FIBER

Carbohydrate requirements should be met with fiber-rich fruits, vegetables, beans, nuts, seeds and legumes. Limiting processed foods, such as baked goods, white bread and pasta, and other refined carbohydrates is advised because they are typically higher in added sugar, fat and calories, lower in nutrients and could crowd-out more nutrient-rich food options.

Dietary fiber can aid in the prevention and management of age-related diseases including diabetes, neurodegenerative diseases, cardiovascular diseases and cancer.[10] Dietary sources such as fruits, vegetables, beans and whole grains, legumes, nuts and seeds contain both soluble and insoluble fiber. Soluble fiber can be helpful in the management of diarrhea and high cholesterol and promotes a favorable gut microbiome. Insoluble fiber is important for bowel health, regularity and managing constipation. Constipation, although multifactorial, affects one-third of older adults.[11] Therefore, it is important that older adults consume adequate amounts of dietary fiber to lower the prevalence of constipation. To reduce the adverse effects of a high-fiber diet, foods high in dietary fiber should be added slowly and fluid intake increased.[12] Many fiber-rich foods delay gastric emptying, resulting in the sensation of fullness, which although beneficial for weight loss, blood glucose control and GI health, can be a problem for frail and underweight older adults who are struggling to consume adequate calories and meet nutritional requirements.

FAT

Older adults should be encouraged to choose foods that are higher in healthy fats including monounsaturated and polyunsaturated sources, lower in saturated fat sources and free from trans fats.[13] Dietary patterns that are predominantly rich in healthy fats, such as the Mediterranean diet, are associated with the preservation of brain health including slower rates of cognitive decline and reduced risk of dementia and Alzheimer's disease.[14–16] Omega-3 fatty acids may have benefits for reducing the risk of cognitive decline potentially treating age-related memory disorders, major depressive disorder (MDD), minimizing neuroinflammation, maintaining muscle performance and enhancing immune function.[17–21] The optimal ratio of omega-6:3 is not fully understood; however, populations who consume higher amounts of omega-3 fatty acids coupled with a healthy diet, show a reduction in bodily inflammation.[21] Foods rich in omega-3 fatty acids include fatty fish (salmon, mackerel, fresh tuna, sardines), flaxseed oil and ground flaxseed, walnuts and chia seeds.

PROTEIN

Nutrition guidance for older adults emphasizes adequate high-quality dietary protein to meet metabolic and physiologic needs and prevent age-related loss of lean muscle mass that commonly accompanies aging.[22,23] Some experts believe the current protein recommendation may not be adequate even as a minimum level for older adults and recommend moderate increases in protein intake to enhance muscle protein metabolism and provide a mechanism for reducing progressive muscle loss.[22] Fifty percent of women and 30% of men ages 71 and older fall short of consuming adequate protein due to a reduced appetite, functional and social limitations and economic hardship.[3] Including more protein-rich plant foods such as beans and legumes throughout the day can help meet protein requirements and provide additional health benefits.[24] Plant proteins are rich in dietary fiber, antioxidants and phytochemicals, lower in saturated fat and cholesterol and, at the same time, are affordable and easy to prepare. Past research shows that plant proteins are associated with an overall reduction in all-cause mortality and animal proteins are associated with an overall increase in all-cause mortality.[24] Additionally, older adults who followed a vegan diet experienced a 58% decrease in the number of prescribed medications, compared with those who followed a non-vegetarian diet.[25] If concern exists regarding the nutritional quality of dietary protein, then intake can be closely monitored by an RDN for older adults following a predominantly plant-based diet.

FLUIDS

Aging results in physiological changes that increase the risk of dehydration.[26] Dehydration can be further exacerbated by common medications such as laxatives and diuretics, polypharmacy and cognitive impairment which may lead to a decrease in fluid consumption.[27] Older adults may also voluntarily restrict fluids due to incontinence, fear of incontinence, social isolation, dysphagia and decline in physical function.[27] Fluid requirements should be individualized based on coexisting medical conditions such as congestive heart failure, liver or renal diseases.[26] Dehydration is the most common fluid and electrolyte disturbance in older adults and commonly occurs among institutionalized elderly individuals.[26] Evidence suggests that institutionalized residents will increase fluid consumption when offered a variety of beverage choices accompanied by staff encouragement and assistance throughout the day.[26] Foods that have high water content such as vegetables, fruits and broth-based soups can contribute to total fluid intake while simultaneously helping to achieve plant-predominant diet recommendations. Additional strategies include encouraging 180 ml with medications, providing drinks between meals, happy hours with non-alcoholic beverages and the use of larger drinking vessels.[26]

MICRONUTRIENTS: VITAMINS AND MINERALS

Age-related changes in food intake, nutrient absorption and metabolism along with acute and chronic medical conditions and polypharmacy can contribute to vitamin and mineral deficiencies. Recommended intakes of vitamins and minerals for older adults should take into consideration the variability in requirements and individual health status among this age group and provide specific recommendations for older adults ages 51 to 70 years and 70 and older.[28] Although chronological age is used as a cutoff for the Dietary Reference Intakes, actual nutrient requirements may be wide-ranging in older adults due to the significant heterogeneity in this population.[28] Additionally, micronutrient malnutrition is thought to play an essential role in cognitive decline and physical frailty which can further contribute to aging.[29]

B6, B12 AND FOLATE

Chronic and acute nutrient deficiencies including B vitamins can damage the DNA in brain cells and contribute to cognitive decline.[29,30] Vitamin B12 deficiency is characterized by central nervous system abnormalities, peripheral neuropathy, decreased muscle strength and functional disability. Worldwide prevalence of a vitamin B12 deficiency is estimated to be 6% and 10–19% in older adults particularly those who are institutionalized.[31] The cause of vitamin B12 insufficiency/deficiency in older adults is multifactorial and may be the result of an inadequate diet alone or in combination with physiological changes. The ability to absorb vitamin B12 decreases due to age-related changes in the GI tract such as lower gastric acid, lack of intrinsic factor, atrophic gastritis and small bowel bacterial overgrowth. As a result, it may be easier for older adults to absorb synthetic vitamin B12 from supplements and fortified foods than naturally occurring vitamin B12 from food.[32,33] Folate deficiencies have also been associated with mild cognitive impairment and mental health deterioration. Plasma total homocysteine reflects the functional status of B12, folate and B6 and should therefore be considered when screening for these cognitive-related deficiencies.[34] Early intervention with B-vitamin supplementation for a minimum of 12 months in duration may slow or prevent cognitive decline.[33]

Vitamin D

Vitamin D insufficiency and deficiency is common in the older population resulting from low dietary intake, limited sunlight exposure, decreased skin synthesis and a decline in renal production of vitamin D.[35] Older adults who are deficient in vitamin D are at higher risk for osteomalacia, osteoporosis and muscle weakness.[35] Additionally, vitamin D regulates neurotransmitters and is associated with brain health, decreased inflammation and antioxidant properties.[36] Furthermore, emerging evidence suggests that vitamin D may prevent cognitive decline, dementia and Alzheimer's disease.[37] Vitamin D deficiency may lead to declines in mobility, physical performance and function, hip fractures, diabetes, cancer, heart disease, arthritis, depression, cognition, frailty and overall poor health. Low-fat dairy and dairy alternatives (almond, cashew, soy and pea protein milk products) can be good sources of calcium, Vitamin D and protein and are low in calories and fat, making them beneficial for older adults. It can be challenging for older adults to consume the recommended amounts of vitamin D from food alone; therefore, supplementation may be needed for this population. Vitamin D repletion should be considered to prevent cognitive decline and frailty.[35,37]

Sodium

Ninety-four percent of older males and 72% of older females exceed the recommended daily limit of 2,300 mg sodium.[3] Approximately 70% of the sodium in the typical US diet comes from processed, packaged and restaurant foods, with almost 50% of the sodium in the US diet from mixed dishes.[38] In addition to sodium, ultra-processed foods contribute to increased consumption of sugar and unhealthy fats, adding excess calories while crowding out more nutrient-dense plant-based foods.

Older adults with hypertension should be advised to follow the DASH plan to reduce dietary sodium and lower the risk of cardiovascular disease and stroke.[39] The DASH diet is high in vegetables, fruits, low-fat dairy products, whole grains, poultry, fish, beans and nuts, and low in sweets, sugar-sweetened beverages and red meats. The DASH diet is also lower in sodium than the typical US diet and low in saturated fats while rich in potassium, calcium, magnesium, dietary fiber and protein.[39] Dietary intake in older adults who are prescribed a low-sodium diet should be monitored regularly. Although sodium restriction has been shown to lower blood pressure, it may contribute to a bland diet, decrease food intake and negatively impact nutritional status in older adults at risk of malnutrition.

Antioxidants

To reduce oxidative stress and inflammation associated with many common chronic conditions, older adults should follow an eating pattern that emphasizes minimally processed plant foods. The Mediterranean–DASH Intervention for Neurodegenerative Delay (MIND) diet is a neuroprotective dietary pattern aimed specifically at protecting the brain, reducing dementia, and preventing declines in brain health associated with age.[40–42] (Table 9.2)

TABLE 9.2
MIND Diet

- Encourages minimally processed plant foods such as vegetables, specifically green leafy vegetables, berries, nuts, olives, whole grains and beans, as well as olive oil, fish and poultry.
- Limits foods from animal sources and foods high in saturated fat including butter and margarine, cheese, red meat, fried foods, pastries, sweets, processed desserts and wine (< 1 glass daily)

Research on the MIND diet in older adults has encouraging findings for those seeking to preserve brain health, slow cognitive decline and reduce the risk of Alzheimer's dementia with aging.[40–42] For the most beneficial effects, older adults should aim to boost their food sources of naturally occurring antioxidants such as minimally processed grains, fruits and vegetables.

MAGNESIUM

Magnesium deficiencies are also prevalent with aging due to decreased intake, impaired absorption and renal magnesium wasting.[43] Mild magnesium deficiency may be asymptomatic or associated with symptoms which have multiple etiologies such as constipation, nausea, fatigue and abnormal heart rhythms.[43] More advanced magnesium deficiencies can cause generalized weakness, sleep disorders, cognitive decline and emotional problems. Magnesium deficiency is also associated with cardiovascular diseases, hypertension, stroke, diabetes, asthma, mental illness, Alzheimer's disease, osteoporosis and cancer.[43] Magnesium status should be assessed, and optimized throughout life especially with the aging population by encouraging foods such as whole grains, dark green leafy vegetables, nuts, beans and legumes.

ZINC

Zinc is necessary in multiple pathways and evidence suggests that optimal intake can reduce neurodegenerative decline found in Alzheimer's Disease and other forms of dementia as well as vascular diseases, sleep disorders and cancer.[44] Zinc deficiency has also been associated with oxidative stress and premature aging.[44] Additionally, zinc plays a crucial role as an antioxidant that targets oxidative stress and optimizing serum zinc levels will strengthen the immune system.[44] Serum zinc levels declines with age and deficiencies have been found to be more severe in patients with Alzheimer's disease. Furthermore, ensuring adequate zinc has been shown to decrease inflammation and reduce plaque deposition in this patient population.[44]

TABLE 9.3
Key Nutrient Requirements for Older Adults

Nutrient	Daily Recommendation	Considerations	Suggested Food Sources
Calories	Females ages 60+: 1,600 to 2,200 calories Males ages 60+: 2,000 to 2,600 calories	Dietary guidance for many older adults focuses on meeting nutrient recommendations while simultaneously reducing calories to maintain a healthy weight	Nutrient dense foods
Carbohydrates	Males & Females age 51+: 45 – 65% total calories	Older adults should aim to meet their carbohydrate needs by choosing predominantly whole and minimally processed vegetables, fruits, and whole grains	Fruits, vegetables, legumes, beans, nuts, seeds, whole grains
Fiber	Females age 51+: 22 grams Males age 51+: 28 grams	Regular consumption of fruits, vegetables, beans, and seeds should ensure older adults are consuming sufficient fiber	Fruits, vegetables, legumes, beans, nuts, seeds, whole grains, flax
Fat	<30% Total calories 5 – 6% SFA Minimize TFA	Fat is a valuable source of concentrated energy for frail and underweight older adults struggling to maintain healthy body weight Dietary fat provides a necessary source of essential fatty acids which may have the potential to prevent and reduce comorbidities and lower mortality Dietary patterns that are predominantly plant-based and rich in healthy fats and Omega 3 FA are recommended	Avocados, nuts, seeds, olives, fatty fish (salmon, mackerel, tuna, sardines)
Protein	0.8 g/kg body weight to 2.0 g/kg body weight	An even distribution of protein-rich foods throughout the day is suggested to help older adults consume adequate dietary protein	Beans, nuts, seeds, tofu, quinoa, fish, low-fat dairy, dairy alternatives – cashew milk/yogurt, pea protein

(Continued)

TABLE 9.3 (Continued)
Key Nutrient Requirements for Older Adults

Nutrient	Daily Recommendation	Considerations	Suggested Food Sources
Fluid/Water	25 – 35 mL/kg body weight or 1 mL/kcal ingested	Aging results in physiological changes including a decrease in thirst sensation, a decrease in urine concentration by the kidneys, and a decrease in total body water leading to an increased risk of dehydration. Adverse effects of poor hydration include cognitive decline, increased rates of hospital admissions, poor recovery, decreased quality of life, and increased medical costs. Opportunities to offer more fluids throughout the day increase fluid consumption	Water, soda water, fruits, vegetables
Vitamin B12 & Folate	Males & Females age 51+: 2.4 mcg B12/day 400 mcg Folate	Older adults are encouraged to meet the recommendations for protein foods, a common source of Vitamin B12, and include foods fortified with Vitamin B12 such as breakfast cereals in a healthy eating pattern and a supplement when indicated	B12-enriched foods, tempeh, mushrooms, nutritional yeast, nori Folate – Leafy greens, enriched foods, lentils, broccoli, asparagus
Vitamin D	Males & Females age 51+: 600 IUs	Vitamin D insufficiency and deficiency are common in the older population putting them at risk for numerous acute and chronic conditions and overall poor health calcium and vitamin D supplementation may be needed in this population due the challenges in meeting these requirements through food alone.	Low-fat dairy, milk alternatives, fortified and enriched foods

(Continued)

TABLE 9.3 (Continued)

Nutrient	Daily Recommendation	Considerations	Suggested Food Sources
Antioxidants	Males and females age 51+: Vitamin A: 900 mcg (M) and 700 mcg (F) Vitamin C: 90 mg (M) and 75 mg (F) Vitamin E: 15 mg for both M and F	Antioxidants are necessary to prevent age-related diseases including atherosclerosis, cognitive decline, cancer, and diabetes they target free radicals and reduce oxidative stress which is a major contributor to disease.	Fruits, vegetables, dark chocolate, nuts, beans
Magnesium	320 mg (M) 420 mg (F)	Magnesium deficiencies are prevalent with aging due to decreased intake, impaired absorption and renal magnesium Early and advanced magnesium deficiencies are associated with a wide range of symptoms and diseases	Dark chocolate, avocados, nuts, seeds, brown rice, tofu
Zinc	11 mg (M) 8 mg (F)	Zinc levels naturally decline with age and can contribute to neurodegenerative decline, vascular diseases, sleep disorders and cancer	Tofu, oatmeal, low-fat dairy, nuts, seeds, enriched foods, berries, fish

ALCOHOL

Consumption of alcohol can crowd-out essential nutrients, decrease appetite, alter taste perception and interfere with the absorption, utilization and nutritional balance in older adults who may have difficulty meeting nutritional recommendations and are at risk for malnutrition.[45] Alcohol may interfere with prescription and over-the-counter medications and increase the risk for falls and alcohol-related injuries in older adults. For older adults who choose to drink alcohol, the Dietary Guidelines for Americans recommends that adults limit consumption to two drinks or less per day for men and one drink or less per day for women.[3]

DIETARY SUPPLEMENTS

Approximately 84% of older adults use dietary supplements for a variety of reasons including overall wellness, disease prevention, pain reduction and as an adjunct to conventional medical treatments.[46] Increased supplement usage is associated with older age (75+ years), female sex, higher education, daily alcohol use, arthritis, regular medication use and physical activity. The most commonly reported supplements are multivitamins, vitamin D, fish oil, calcium, vitamin C and vitamin B12.[46] To the extent possible, older adults should aim to get their required nutrients from food as part of a healthy plant predominant diet rather than from dietary supplements.[47] For older adults who find it difficult to eat enough nutrient-dense foods to meet their needs, supplementation may be indicated to prevent deficiency or insufficiency and maintain health and body weight.[46] Providers need to be aware that many adults do not discuss supplement use with their health care provider because they do not think of them as medications. Furthermore, unnecessary supplement use can contribute to polypharmacy and drug interactions, needless financial expense and create a false sense of nutritional well-being.[46,47]

PROMOTING NUTRITION AND HEALTHY LIFESTYLES FOR OLDER ADULTS

Eighty-five percent of noninstitutionalized older adults have at least one chronic health condition that could be improved with proper nutrition.[48] Sixty-six percent of all health care dollars in the United States are spent on managing chronic conditions in older adults.[49] A WFPPD is the cornerstone of health and longevity and an important prescriptive tool to help patients achieve a better quality of life as they age.

Like most Americans however, many older adults are not consuming an optimal dietary pattern for many reasons including physical and medical limitations, poor food choices and/or food insecurity associated with lower socioeconomic status. Individualized and interdisciplinary patient care is essential because the nutritional needs and challenges are as unique as the older adults themselves. Including an RDN, in the care of older adults can ensure that patients are screened for food insecurity on a regular basis and provided with assistance long before negative health outcomes develop.[50] RDNs are highly educated, knowledgeable and well-trained to help patients make healthier choices, which can positively affect outcomes. Most RDNs have advanced degrees and are experienced food and nutrition professionals. RDNs can assist provider care teams with conditions that impact older adult populations and bring a multidimensional skill set with demonstrated value to the

TABLE 9.4
Reasons to Consult an RDN for Older Adult Patients

• Medical condition that requires specialized food or a modified diet plan	• New diagnosis or presence of a chronic disease such as hypertension, prediabetes and obesity
• Inability to prepare one's own meals	• Assistance with weight gain or loss
• Requires specially prepared meals and/or needs assistance obtaining them	• Food and/or nutrition insecurity (unable to purchase nutritious food on an ongoing basis)
• Lives in a food desert without means to obtain healthy foods	• End-of-life nutrition and hydration

interprofessional care team. RDNs are qualified to conduct nutrition screening and assessments, identify nutrition problems, implement medical nutrition therapy, evaluate diet histories, identify barriers to food access, provide nutrition education to patients and family members and suggest community support and resources such as food as medicine programming, medically tailored meals produce prescriptions, culinary medicine and food pantry guidance. Medical nutrition therapy (MNT) provided by RDNs has been demonstrated to improve clinical outcomes, reduce costs related to PCP time, decrease medication usage and reduce hospital admissions for individuals with obesity, diabetes and other chronic diseases[51,52] (Table 9.4).

CONCLUSIONS

Good nutrition is a fundamental component of healthy aging. It can be difficult for older adults to meet their nutritional needs due to increased nutrient requirements, lower energy needs and numerous health and lifestyle barriers to adequate food intake. The maintenance of good health for the growing population of older adults requires approaches that recognize multiple levels of influence on the individual medical, social, cultural, environmental, organizational and personal factors. Older adults should be encouraged to consume a variety of predominantly plant-based, wholesome, minimally processed and nutrient-dense foods as the cornerstone to healthy aging. Services provided by the RDN as part of an interprofessional team focused on nutrition and lifestyle behaviors at every age are vital for making a positive impact on the quality of life for older adults to promote health and longevity.

CLINICAL APPLICATIONS

- The goal for nutritional health in adults at every age should be to preserve physical and mental well-being and maintain a high quality of life.
- Consumption of a high-quality, predominantly minimally processed whole food plant-based diet is essential to optimize health and well-being at any age.
- Dietary intake and requirements are influenced by overall health and factors that may occur naturally with aging, or due to illness or environment. This can create a challenge for an older adult to meet their nutritional needs, especially when calorie needs are reduced.
- Routine screening for nutrition-related chronic and acute medical conditions, malnutrition, frailty, sarcopenia and sarcopenic obesity can lead to early intervention and prevention of worsening health outcomes.

REFERENCES

1. Long T, Zhang K, Chen Y, Wu C. Trends in diet quality among older US adults from 2001 to 2018. *JAMA Netw Open.* 2022 Mar 1;5(3):e221880. doi:10.1001/jamanetworkopen.2022.1880.
2. Roberts SB, Silver RE, Das SK, et al. Healthy aging-nutrition matters: start early and screen often. *Adv Nutr.* 2021;12(4):1438–1448. doi:10.1093/advances/nmab032.
3. U.S. Department of Agriculture and U.S. Department of Health and Human Services. *Dietary Guidelines for Americans, 2020–2025.* 9th ed. Updated 2020. Accessed March 3, 2023. DietaryGuidelines.gov.
4. U.S. Department of Agriculture. *MYPlate. Older Adults.* Accessed March 3, 2023. https://www.myplate.gov/life-stages/older-adults.
5. Tips J. American College of Lifestyle Medicine announces dietary lifestyle position statement for treatment and potential reversal of disease. PRWeb. 2018. Accessed June 27, 2020. https://www.prweb.com/releases/american_college_of_lifestyle_medicine_announces_dietary_lifestyle_position_statement_for_treatment_and_potential_reversal_of_disease/prweb15786205.htm.
6. American College of Lifestyle Medicine. The benefits of plant-based nutrition longevity and quality of life. Accessed October 10, 2024. https://lifestylemedicine.org/articles/benefits-plant-based-nutrition-longevity/.
7. Pes GM, Dore MP, Tsofliou F, Poulain M. Diet, and longevity in the Blue Zones: a set-and-forget issue? *Maturitas.* 2022;164:31–37. doi:10.1016/j.maturitas.2022.06.004.
8. Buettner D, Skemp S. Blue Zones: lessons from the world's longest lived. *Am J Lifestyle Med.* 2016;10(5):318–321. doi:10.1177/1559827616637066.
9. LoBuono DL, Milovich M Jr. A scoping review of nutrition health for older adults: Does technology help? *Nutrients.* 2023 Oct 17;15(20):4402. doi:10.3390/nu15204402.
10. Niero M, Bartoli G, De Colle P, Scarcella M, Zanetti M. Impact of dietary fiber on inflammation and insulin resistance in older patients: a narrative review. *Nutrients.* 2023;15(10):2365. doi:10.3390/nu15102365.
11. National Institute on Aging. Concerned about constipation? Accessed October 10, 2024. https://www.nia.nih.gov/health/constipation/concerned-about-constipation#:~:text=Nearly%20everyone%20becomes%20constipated%20at,not%20serious%20and%20is%20treatable.
12. American Family Physician. Management of constipation in older adults. Accessed October 10, 2024. https://www.aafp.org/pubs/afp/issues/2015/0915/p500.html#afp20150915p500-b2.
13. American Heart Association. Saturated fat. Accessed October 10, 2024. https://www.heart.org/en/healthy-living/healthy-eating/eat-smart/fats/saturated-fats#:~:text=AHA%20Recommendation,of%20saturated%20fat%20per%20day.
14. Flanagan E, Lamport D, Brennan L, et al. Nutrition and the ageing brain: moving towards clinical applications. *Ageing Res Rev.* 2020;62:101079. doi:10.1016/j.arr.2020.101079.
15. Liu Y, Gao X, Na M, Kris-Etherton PM, Mitchell DC, Jensen GL. Dietary pattern, diet quality, and dementia: a systematic review and meta-analysis of prospective cohort studies. *J Alzheimers Dis.* 2020;78(1):151–158. doi:10.3233/JAD-200499.
16. Barbaresko J, Lellmann AW, Schmidt A, et al. Dietary factors and neurodegenerative disorders: an umbrella review of meta-analyses of prospective studies. *Adv Nutr.* 2020;11(5):1161–1173. doi:10.1093/advances/nmaa053.
17. Muscaritoli M. The impact of nutrients on mental health and well-being: insights from the literature. *Front Nutr.* 2021 Mar 8;8:656290. doi:10.3389/fnut.2021.656290.

18. Appleton KM, Voyias PD, Sallis HM, Dawson S, Ness AR, Churchill R, Perry R. Omega-3 fatty acids for depression in adults. *Cochrane Database Syst Rev.* 2021 Nov 24;11(11):CD004692. doi:10.1002/14651858.CD004692.pub5.
19. Mischoulon D, Dunlop BW, Kinkead B, et al. Omega-3 fatty acids for major depressive disorder with high inflammation: a randomized dose-finding clinical trial. *J Clin Psychiatry.* 2022;83(5):21m14074. doi:10.4088/JCP.21m14074.
20. Moradi S, Moloudi J, Moradinazar M, Sarokhani D, Nachvak SM, Samadi M. Adherence to healthy diet can delay Alzheimer's disease development: a systematic review and meta-analysis. *Prev Nutr Food Sci.* 2020;25(4):325–337. doi:10.3746/pnf.2020.25.4.325.
21. Djuricic I, Calder PC. Beneficial outcomes of omega-6 and omega-3 polyunsaturated fatty acids on human health: an update for 2021. *Nutrients.* 2021;13(7):2421. doi:10.3390/nu13072421.
22. Volpi E, Campbell WW, Dwyer JT, et al. Is the optimal level of protein intake for older adults greater than the recommended dietary allowance? *J Gerontol A Biol Sci Med Sci.* 2013;68(6):677–681. doi:10.1093/gerona/gls229.
23. Paddon-Jones D, Rasmussen B. Dietary protein recommendations and the prevention of sarcopenia. *Curr Opin Clin Nutr Metab Care.* 2009;12(1):86–90. doi:10.1097/MCO.0b013e32831cef8b.
24. Baum JI, Kim I, Wolfe RR. Protein consumption and the elderly: What is the optimal level of intake? *Nutrients.* 2016;8(6):359. doi:10.3390/nu8060359.
25. Kahleova H, Levin S, Barnard ND. Plant-based diets for healthy aging. *J Am Coll Nutr.* 2021;40(5):478–479. doi:10.1080/07315724.2020.1790442.
26. Dos Santos H, Gaio J, Durisic A, Beeson WL, Alabadi A. The Polypharma Study: association between diet and amount of prescription drugs among seniors. *Am J Lifestyle Med.* 2021;155982762110488. doi:10.1177/15598276211048812.
27. Bruno C, Collier A, Holyday M, Lambert K. Interventions to improve hydration in older adults: a systematic review and meta-analysis. *Nutrients.* 2021;13(10):3640. doi:10.3390/nu13103640.
28. Beck AM, Seemer J, Knudsen AW, Munk T. Narrative review of low-intake dehydration in older adults. *Nutrients.* 2021;13(9):3142. doi:10.3390/nu13093142.
29. Institute of Medicine. *Dietary Reference Intakes: Vitamins.* National Academies. Accessed February 27, 2022. https://www.nationalacademies.org/hmd/~/media/Files/Activity%20Files/Nutrition/DRIs/DRI_Vitamins.pdf.
30. Mustafa Khalid N, Haron H, Shahar S, Fenech M. Current evidence on the association of micronutrient malnutrition with mild cognitive impairment, frailty, and cognitive frailty among older adults: a scoping review. *Int J Environ Res Public Health.* 2022;19(23):15722. doi:10.3390/ijerph192315722.
31. Wang Z, Zhu W, Xing Y, Jia J, Tang Y. B vitamins and prevention of cognitive decline and incident dementia: a systematic review and meta-analysis. *Nutr Rev.* 2022 Mar 10;80(4):931–949. doi:10.1093/nutrit/nuab057.
32. Nalder L, Zheng B, Chiandet G, Middleton LT, de Jager CA. Vitamin B12 and folate status in cognitively healthy older adults and associations with cognitive performance. *J Nutr Health Aging.* 2021;25(3):287–294. doi:10.1007/s12603-020-1489-y.
33. Porter KM, Hoey L, Hughes CF, et al. Associations of atrophic gastritis and proton-pump inhibitor drug use with vitamin B-12 status, and the impact of fortified foods, in older adults. *Am J Clin Nutr.* 2021;114(4):1286–1294. doi:10.1093/ajcn/nqab193.
34. Elangovan R, Baruteau J. Inherited and acquired vitamin B12 deficiencies: Which administration route to choose for supplementation? *Front Pharmacol.* 2022;13:972468. doi:10.3389/fphar.2022.972468.
35. Smith AD, Refsum H, Bottiglieri T, Fenech M, Hooshmand B, McCaddon A, Miller JW, Rosenberg IH, Obeid R. Homocysteine and dementia: an international consensus statement. *J Alzheimers Dis.* 2018;62(2):561–570. doi:10.3233/JAD-171042.

36. Giustina A, Bouillon R, Dawson-Hughes B, et al. Vitamin D in the older population: a consensus statement. *Endocrine.* 2023;79(1):31–44. doi:10.1007/s12020-022-03208-3.
37. Cui X, Eyles DW. Vitamin D and the central nervous system: causative and preventative mechanisms in brain disorders. *Nutrients.* 2022 Oct 17;14(20):4353. doi:10.3390/nu14204353.
38. Sultan S, Taimuri U, Basnan SA, et al. Low vitamin D and its association with cognitive impairment and dementia. *J Aging Res.* 2020;2020:6097820. doi:10.1155/2020/6097820.
39. American Heart Association. How much sodium should I eat per day? Accessed October 10, 2024. https://www.heart.org/en/healthy-living/healthy-eating/eat-smart/sodium/how-much-sodium-should-i-eat-per-day#:~:text=Because%20the%20average%20American%20eats,foods%20%E2%80%94%20not%20the%20salt%20shaker.
40. National Heart, Lung, and Blood Institute. *Description of the DASH eating plan.* Accessed February 27, 2022. http://www.nhlbi.nih.gov/health/health-topics/topics/dash.
41. van den Brink AC, Brouwer-Brolsma EM, Berendsen AAM, van de Rest O. The Mediterranean, Dietary Approaches to Stop Hypertension (DASH), and Mediterranean-DASH Intervention for Neurodegenerative Delay (MIND) diets are associated with less cognitive decline and a lower risk of Alzheimer's disease: a review. *Adv Nutr.* 2019 Nov 1;10(6):1040–1065. doi:10.1093/advances/nmz054.
42. Hosking DE, Eramudugolla R, Cherbuin N, Anstey KJ. MIND not Mediterranean diet related to 12-year incidence of cognitive impairment in an Australian longitudinal cohort study. *Alzheimers Dement.* 2019;15(4):581–589. doi:10.1016/j.jalz.2018.12.011.
43. Devranis P, Vassilopoulou E, Tsironis V, et al. Mediterranean diet, ketogenic diet, or MIND diet for aging populations with cognitive decline: a systematic review. *Life (Basel).* 2023;13(1):173. doi:10.3390/life13010173.
44. Barbagallo M, Veronese N, Dominguez LJ. Magnesium in aging, health, and diseases. *Nutrients.* 2021 Jan 30;13(2):463. doi:10.3390/nu13020463.
45. Sun R, Wang J, Feng J, Cao B. Zinc in cognitive impairment and aging. *Biomolecules.* 2022;12(7):1000. doi:10.3390/biom12071000.
46. Butts M, Sundaram VL, Murughiyan U, Borthakur A, Singh S. The influence of alcohol consumption on intestinal nutrient absorption: a comprehensive review. *Nutrients.* 2023;15(7):1571. doi:10.3390/nu15071571.
47. Tan EC, Eshetie TC, Gray SL, et al. Dietary supplement use in middle-aged and older adults. *J Nutr Health Aging.* 2022;26(2):133–138. doi:10.1007/s12603-022-1732.
48. Bernstein M, Munoz N. Position of the Academy of Nutrition and Dietetics: food and nutrition for older adults: promoting health and wellness. *J Acad Nutr Diet.* 2012;112(8):1255–1277.
49. National Institute on Aging. Supporting older patients with chronic conditions. Accessed October 10, 2024. https://www.nia.nih.gov/health/supporting-older-patients-chronic-conditions#:~:text=Approximately%2085%25%20of%20older%20adults,conditions%20is%20a%20real%20challenge. Updated 2022.
50. Population Reference Bureau. Fact sheet: aging in the United States 2019. Accessed October 10, 2024. https://www.prb.org/resources/fact-sheet-aging-in-the-united-states/.
51. Gahche JJ, Arensberg MB, Weiler M, Dwyer JT. Opportunities for adding undernutrition and frailty screening measures in US national surveys. *Adv Nutr (Bethesda, Md).* 2021;12(6):2312–2320. doi:10.1093/advances/nmab056.
52. Academy of Nutrition and Dietetics. The National Resource Center on Nutrition and Aging: medical nutrition therapy works for seniors: a resource guide for registered dietitian nutritionists and senior nutrition program advisors. Accessed September 30, 2024. https://www.eatrightpro.org/-/media/files/eatrightpro/career/mnt/mnt-works-for-seniors-toolkit.pdf?rev=df549af9beb54af1abec6b133db16955&hash=24BC523A0C7A510757E7B58AC122FD3A.

10 Malnutrition in Older Adults
A Lifestyle Medicine Approach

Susan M. Friedman, Melissa Bernstein and Alison Reyes

INTRODUCTION

Since 2010, diet has been identified as the leading risk factor for both mortality and disability-adjusted life years in the United States, overtaking tobacco.[1] Globally, the recognition of the significant adverse impact of malnutrition led to the UN declaring 2016–2025 as the Decade of Action on Nutrition.[2] Despite this, diet quality was noted to decline from 2001 to 2018, and more than half of older adults in the United States have poor diet quality, putting them at risk for malnutrition.[3] Malnutrition is common among older adults and can contribute to the onset of geriatric syndromes, in addition to increasing the risk for morbidity and mortality. The previous chapter outlined the importance of nutrition for healthy aging. In this chapter, we will summarize issues related to malnutrition – what it is, outcomes, causes and approaches to treatment.

WHAT IS MALNUTRITION?

Malnutrition has been defined as "an imbalance between the growth and breakdown of body tissues and nutrient stores, resulting in loss of muscle and organ mass, diminished physical and mental functioning, and impaired clinical outcomes."[4] Although the traditional phenotype is one of wasting, and most clinical studies of malnutrition are in fact studying undernutrition, increasingly, this imbalance and its consequences can result from both overnutrition and undernutrition. As such, the World Health Organization (WHO) describes malnutrition as "deficiencies, excesses or imbalances in a person's intake of energy and/or nutrients."[5] Issues related to overnutrition and obesity are discussed in Chapter 24, and so the focus of this chapter will be on undernutrition.

Three terms relevant to malnutrition should be defined. The first is protein-calorie malnutrition, also known as protein-energy malnutrition or protein-energy undernutrition. This occurs "when food and nutrient intake is unable to meet protein, energy and nutrient requirements over time leading to a disruption of homeostasis in lean tissues, body weight and physical function."[6]

The second is sarcopenic obesity. Sarcopenic obesity is characterized by the simultaneous presence of excess adipose tissue and reduced muscle mass and function, and reinforces the importance of evaluating muscle function and mass separately from weight.[7] Patients with sarcopenic obesity thus have concerns related to both overnutrition and undernutrition. With rising rates of obesity and sedentary lifestyles amid the aging population, the prevalence of sarcopenic obesity is expected to increase. The combined impact of excess adipose tissue with loss of skeletal muscle puts patients at risk for a wide range of adverse clinical outcomes, including metabolic dysfunction, geriatric syndromes, multiple comorbidities, disability and higher health care utilization.[8,9]

The third term relevant to a discussion of malnutrition in older adults is anorexia of aging, which is defined as the loss of appetite and/or a decrease in food intake later in life.[10] A more complete discussion of the anorexia of aging is presented in the section on causes of malnutrition below.

EPIDEMIOLOGY OF MALNUTRITION

Malnutrition is a condition that affects people in every country, and it has been estimated that nearly one in three people globally have at least one form of malnutrition.[11] The WHO estimates that approximately 390 million adults are underweight and 890 million are living with obesity.[5]

The prevalence of malnutrition varies by age, place of residence, health status and specific medical conditions. The criteria used to define malnutrition also impact prevalence estimates. For example, women are more likely than men to be categorized as malnourished as defined by low BMI, but gender differences are not as pronounced when using the criteria of weight loss.[12] The prevalence of malnutrition among independent, healthy older adults is low, estimated at 1%, and up to 15% in non-institutionalized older adults overall, but the prevalence of malnutrition is higher in long-term care facilities (estimates ranging from 23% to 60%), acute hospital settings (12–50%) and inpatient rehabilitation units (30–50%).[2,13,14] Overall, the prevalence of malnutrition is higher in women, individuals living in rural areas, those over age 80, those with chronic illness and among community dwellers living in low- or middle-income countries vs those living in Europe or Asia.[2]

Worldwide, the rates of undernutrition have declined during this century.[15] Although considerable progress has been made in improving the nutritional status of other populations, including infant, young child and maternal nutrition, the estimates are that, overall, approximately one-quarter of adults aged 65 and older are malnourished or at risk of malnutrition.[2] Additionally, the rise in obesity has led to an increased risk for a nutrient-poor, excess-calorie diet and its outcomes.

Older adults are more prone to nutritional deficiencies due to aging changes, the presence of disease and social circumstances. In addition to age, a systematic review identified several risk factors that predicted the onset of malnutrition.[14] These include

TABLE 10.1
Predictors of Malnutrition in Older Adults*

Age
Physical
• Frailty
• Taking ten or more medications
• Functional decline, loss of handgrip strength
• Difficulty walking or climbing stairs
• Decline in cognition, dementia
• Parkinson's disease
• Constipation
• Poor or moderate self-reported health status
Mouth and feeding
• Poor oral hygiene
• Dysphagia
• Poor appetite
• Needing assistance to eat
Psychological
• Loss of interest in life
Social, health utilization
• Being unmarried, separated or divorced
• Living in an institution
• Previous or incident hospitalization

*Adapted from Favaro-Moreira et al. and Streicher et al.[14,16]

physical factors, such as frailty, polypharmacy, functional and cognitive decline, Parkinson's disease, constipation and poor or moderate self-reported health status. Several eating-related characteristics, such as dysphagia, poor oral hygiene, loss of appetite and needing assistance with feeding, were noted to be predictors. Loss of interest in life was the psychological factor in this review associated with the onset of malnutrition. Finally, living in an institution was also noted to be a risk factor. In a meta-analysis of determinants of onset of malnutrition in community-dwelling older adults, being unmarried, separated or divorced; previous or incident hospitalization; and difficulty walking or climbing stairs were the strongest predictors[16] (Table 10.1). Identifying these characteristics in older adults can help target those who are at increased risk for developing malnutrition, so as to institute early screening and treatment.

Malnutrition is associated with worsening clinical outcomes including higher risk of infections, chronic illness, frailty, osteoporosis, poor immune function, pressure sores, impaired wound healing, and death. [2,18] Malnutrition is also associated with poorer outcomes after traumatic injury, and higher health care costs and utilization, including hospital readmission. Protein-energy malnutrition is associated with loss of muscle mass and strength, which in turn lead to functional decline and frailty.[12]

Functional recovery from weight loss due to malnutrition is unlikely, due to loss of skeletal muscle mass, even with full nutritional support.[2]

In summary, malnutrition is both an outcome of declining health, as well as a cause. This can lead to a vicious cycle, with outcomes of increasing morbidity and a higher risk of mortality.

CAUSES OF MALNUTRITION

Multiple pathways can lead to the outcome of malnutrition. Malnutrition can result from either an inadequate *amount* of food (insufficient intake of food, calories and nutrients) or poor *quality* of food (insufficient intake of macro- or micro-nutrients). In addition to issues with adequate intake, malnutrition can result from increased nutrient requirement, poor nutrient absorption or increased nutrient loss.[13] In a recent review of malnutrition in adults, Cederholm and Bosaeus provide a framework for understanding causality,[4] which is adapted here for an older adult population.

AGING CHANGES

Loss of appetite and/or decreased food intake is seen often later in life, and this phenomenon is termed the "anorexia of aging."[10] The prevalence of anorexia of aging

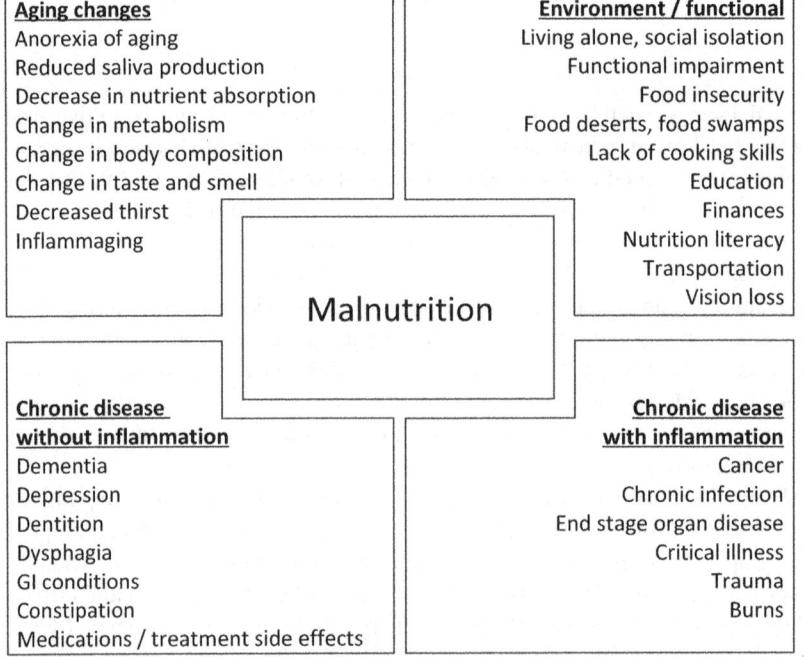

FIGURE 10.1 Framework for causes of malnutrition in older adults, with examples.

ranges from 25% in community-dwelling older adults, to 62% in the hospital and 85% in nursing homes,[19] with higher rates among women and with increasing age.[20] Anorexia of aging has a multifactorial etiology that includes a decrease in hunger, altered control of satiety and age-related gastrointestinal motility changes. Change in appetite regulation occurs through alterations in several gastrointestinal hormones, including a decrease in ghrelin and an increase in cholecystokinin.[7,20,21] A decrease in pleasure associated with eating palatable foods can also contribute to anorexia of aging. With aging, there is a decrease in gastric compliance, leading to more rapid antral filling, which, in turn, leads to earlier satiety. Early satiety contributes to a decrease in intake of protein, fiber, whole grains and fruits and vegetables.[19] In addition, aging leads to an increase in colonic transit time, increased intestinal permeability and a change in intestinal microbiota.[7,21] These changes may start around the fourth decade of life and are seen frequently by age 75.[21]

Approximately one-third of people over the age of 65 have reduced saliva production.[20] Age-related reduction in saliva may lead to a decreased ability to tolerate certain foods. Additionally, changes in smell and taste occur, and both senses are important in stimulating appetite. Older adults often have a decreased perception of salt and sugar, which can lead to choosing more unhealthy foods, a decrease in overall intake or a less varied diet.[10] The inability to detect food aromas may increase the risk of eating spoiled food. The number of taste buds declines over time, and this can be compounded by the effect of medications, smoking and environmental exposures.

Energy needs are a function of physical activity and body composition.[22] Over time, lean body mass decreases and body fat increases, with a concomitant decrease in resting energy expenditure.[22] The thermic effect of food (the energy expenditure needed after meals to digest, absorb and store nutrients) is reduced in older adults, reducing caloric needs. A reduction in physical activity, which is common among older adults, can contribute to a decrease in caloric needs as well.

The absorption of several micronutrients decreases with age. Vitamin B12 absorption is dependent on pepsin and acid secretion, which is lower in older adults, leading to an increased risk of deficiency. Calcium and vitamin D absorption also decline with aging.[21]

Aging itself leads to low-grade chronic inflammation (termed "inflammaging"), which in turn can lead to malnutrition.[7] Inflammaging has been defined as "ageing-associated chronic inflammation that results from combined genetic, epigenetic and metabolic dysfunction in different cell types and organs."[23] Chronic inflammation can lead to the depletion of several minerals, such as iron, zinc and manganese,[7] and contributes to many of the chronic diseases found commonly in older adults, as well as to the aging process itself.[7,24]

Chronic Illness

Older adults have a high prevalence of chronic illness, which can increase the risk of malnutrition both through inadequate intake or reduced absorption of nutrients, or through chronic inflammation. In the United States, 23.9% of adults over the age of 65 have one chronic condition, and 63.7% have two or more.[25] A few common chronic conditions and their contributions to malnutrition are highlighted here.

Depression is common, affecting 32% of older adults worldwide.[26] Depression can lead to either an increase or decrease in intake, as can the medications used to treat it. Depression can also result in increased or decreased appetite, lack of interest in preparing meals, skipping meals and an increased desire for sweet foods. In one study, the presence of depression was associated with a 2.9-fold risk of malnutrition.[27] Conversely, inadequate intake of a variety of nutrients, including certain amino acids, omega-3 fatty acids, folate, vitamin B12, selenium and magnesium, increases the risk of depression.[28]

Dementia is seen increasingly with age. Approximately 10% of older adults in the United States have dementia, and 22% have mild cognitive impairment.[29] A recent meta-analysis reported that 32.5% of older adults with dementia worldwide had malnutrition, and 46.8% had a risk of malnutrition.[30] Dementia may lead to a loss of appetite, difficulty with planning and making meals and difficulty with feeding or swallowing. All of these can decrease food intake. Issues with wandering or with agitation can increase energy expenditure. Both a decrease in intake and an increase in energy expenditure contribute to the risk of malnutrition. Additionally, dementia can impact food safety in a variety of ways, including forgetting to turn off the stove or letting food spoil before eating it.

Dysphagia, or difficulty swallowing, is increasingly common with aging. It can occur with neurological diseases, such as dementia, Parkinson's disease, stroke or multiple sclerosis; problems with the esophagus, such as achalasia or gastro-esophageal reflux disease; or oral issues, such as certain cancers and their treatment. It is reported that 39.2% of people with dysphagia are at risk of malnutrition.[31]

Older adults are at risk for tooth loss due to multiple factors, including lack of dental care coverage, medication side effects, and decreased access to oral health care. Globally, approximately 30% of adults aged 65–74 are edentulous. Although dental health among older adults in the United States has been improving overall in recent decades, improvements have been limited to those who are not living in poverty. Overall, approximately 45% of US adults over the age of 65 lack functional dentition (more than 20 permanent teeth, excluding the third molars), with 11% being edentulous. Individuals with poor dentition are less likely to eat fruits and vegetables, nuts and cooked meats.[32] In a study of 563 community-dwelling adults aged 70 and older, individuals with edentulousness were twice as likely to have a 10% weight loss as those without.[33]

Many gastrointestinal issues can alter nutrient absorption. Most nutrient absorption occurs in the small intestine, so conditions that affect this portion of the intestine warrant nutritional monitoring. Absorption can be impacted by wide-ranging conditions, such as inflammatory bowel disease (Crohn's disease and ulcerative colitis); autoimmune diseases, such as celiac disease; lactose intolerance; and small intestinal bacterial overgrowth. A history of GI surgery should alert the clinician to evaluate for malnutrition as well.

Constipation is increasingly common with age, as colonic motility decreases with time.[21] In community-dwelling older adults 30–40%, and more than 50% of those residing in nursing homes, have chronic constipation.[34] Often multifactorial in etiology, multiple comorbidities, impaired mobility, decreased intake of fiber, fluid restriction and side effects of medications are common contributors to constipation.[34] In a systematic review of risk factors for malnutrition, constipation was associated with a 2.5-fold risk for developing malnutrition.[14]

Many of the most prevalent chronic diseases are driven by chronic inflammation, and inflammation-driven malnutrition eventually occurs in the final stages of most chronic diseases of major organ systems.[4] Diseases such as chronic obstructive pulmonary disease (COPD), heart failure, chronic kidney disease and cancer induce upregulation of inflammatory cytokines.[2] This leads to an increase in resting energy expenditure and skeletal muscle protein breakdown. The process is not regulated by nutrient requirements and continues even with sufficient intake of protein and calories.[4]

Treatments for chronic disease can inadvertently have iatrogenic consequences. For example, although sodium restriction has been shown to lower blood pressure, it may contribute to a bland diet which could decrease food intake and negatively impact nutritional status in older adults at risk of malnutrition.

The medications used to treat chronic diseases can also contribute to malnutrition in older adults. Many medications alter appetite, either increasing or suppressing it. Medications can change taste, which can impact intake or reduce absorption of nutrients. Medications may also have side effects such as xerostomia, which may alter the consistency of food. The association between polypharmacy and risk of malnutrition is significant. Almost 90% of older adults take at least one prescription medication, almost 80% regularly take at least two and 36% take at least five different prescription medications.[35] This data does not include over-the-counter medications and dietary supplements.

FUNCTIONAL/ENVIRONMENTAL

Food provides more than just nourishment throughout life, especially as we age. Meals contribute to a sense of security, add meaning and structure to the day, provide an opportunity for socialization and boost psychological well-being. Social, psychological, functional, economic and behavioral factors influence food intake, and several factors can simultaneously influence food choices, making the task of maximizing nutrition in older adults challenging and complex.

As eating is a social experience, loneliness and social isolation, common in older adults, put them at risk for developing malnutrition. Lack of social integration, social support and companionship may all impact food and fluid intake. After adjusting for other variables, a study of 1,200 older adults showed that social isolation was associated with a 1.58-fold risk of malnutrition, and loneliness was associated with a 1.15 odds ratio of malnutrition.[36]

Food choices and preparation methods are often deeply entrenched in a person's cultural, ethnic and religious background. These ties have significant emotional connections, and may be challenging to adjust, despite health implications. An understanding of these issues is essential when working with patients to make culturally sensitive changes that can reduce malnutrition.

Economic circumstances can impact dietary behaviors and put patients at risk in multiple ways. Food insecurity, lack of finances to purchase high-quality foods, health and nutritional literacy and limited cooking skills are common risk factors for malnutrition. The main factors influencing food insecurity include barriers to acquiring and preparing nutritious food, lack of food quality due to limited funds, anxiety related to food access and preparation and adherence to social norms or acceptance.[37] Where a person lives can also impact access to food, such as living in food deserts and food swamps. Individuals who are dependent on others for transportation may have reduced access as well.

Alcohol use disorder is an increasingly common issue among older adults that is often undiagnosed, underreported or overlooked.[38] Approximately 15% of community-dwelling individuals aged 65 and over endorse symptoms of alcohol abuse and dependence, and rates are substantially higher in medical settings. Alcohol use disorder can contribute to malnutrition through a variety of mechanisms, including displacing nutrient-rich food, association with disease, change in food intake and changes in metabolism, with decreased nutrient absorption.[39]

Functional and cognitive decline can also contribute to the risk of developing malnutrition. Tasks such as food shopping, food preparation and cooking and cleaning up after a meal can become overwhelming, leading to progressive worsening of nutritional status.

All of these issues can lead to poor diet quality. From 2001 to 2018, the proportion of older adults in the United States with poor diet quality increased from 50.9% to 60.9%, as measured by the primary American Heart Association score, where those with ideal diet quality remained consistently low at 0.4%.[3] Intake of fruits and vegetables decreased from 3.9 to 2.5 servings a day, consumption of legumes decreased from 0.37 to 0.31 servings per day, and the consumption of processed meat, sugar-sweetened beverages and saturated fat increased. These findings suggest the need for food and nutrition programs and services aimed at meeting the unique and multifactorial challenges that affect older adults.

EVALUATION AND MANAGEMENT OF MALNUTRITION

Depending on the definition used, the prevalence of malnutrition remains a significant problem reported with high frequency in older adults. Due to underlying disease, as well as economic, social, functional and physical barriers, older adults are frequently malnourished or at risk of becoming malnourished, therefore, early identification of nutritional risks and malnutrition is critical.[7] Unfortunately, one-fourth of patients at risk of malnutrition do not receive nutritional support or counseling, even when they have been in contact with health care professionals.[14] Consulting with a Registered Dietitian Nutritionist (RDN) ensures that a comprehensive nutrition assessment including anthropometric, biochemical, clinical, neurological, social and dietary parameters is performed when a potential risk has been identified. Conducted by an RDN, a nutrition-focused physical exam (NFPE) follows a systematic whole-body approach with observation and palpation techniques and uses physical assessment findings to help determine nutrition status and diagnose malnutrition.[40] The NFPE also provides opportunities to assess for macro and micronutrient losses and deficiencies.

Screening for nutritional inadequacies, malnutrition, food security and other diet and nutrition-related health disparities linked to malnutrition which could worsen patient health and add complexity to care should be included as part of routine nutrition evaluation for all older adults. This is particularly important for those who are frail, undernourished, overweight or obese.[37,41] The Malnutrition Quality Improvement Initiative (MQII) is an evidence-based resource for interdisciplinary health care professionals to promote optimal nutrition standards of care and eliminate malnutrition.[17] MQII uses food insecurity as a hunger vital sign along with nutrition risk, as the presence of food insecurity leads to multiple negative health outcomes.

One of the greatest challenges is that currently there is no universally accepted definition of malnutrition. In order to address this, the Global Leadership Initiative on Malnutrition (GLIM), drawing from more than 70 national scientific societies, published criteria to identify malnutrition, considering global variations in screening and assessment.[42-44] It is a minimum set of practicable indicators for characterizing patients as malnourished, with a flexible framework that allows for different phenotypes and etiology criteria to promote use in different environments. Validation of this framework, presented in Table 10.2, is ongoing.[7]

Numerous tools have been developed to screen for malnutrition in older adults.[45] A widely used and studied tool is the Mini Nutritional Assessment, which has both a long and short form and is recommended for malnutrition assessment in older adults living in both the community and long-term care.[46] The Subjective Global Assessment (SGA) is recommended if the MNA is not feasible.

Nutritional status has a significant and direct impact on the trajectory of aging and disease, and therefore, careful analysis of all underlying diseases and conditions and appropriate individualized medical nutrition therapy (MNT) is crucial to the

---

TABLE 10.2
GLIM Criteria for Diagnosis of Malnutrition: Presence of at Least One Phenotypic and One Etiologic Criterion Is Needed for Diagnosis

Criteria	
Phenotypic	
Unintentional weight loss	>5% within the past 6 months, or >10% beyond 6 months
Low body mass index (BMI; kg/m^2)	< 20 kg/m^2 for < 70 years (<18.5 for Asian); < 22 kg/m^2 for >70 years (< 20 for Asian)
Reduced muscle mass	Validated body composition techniques
Etiologic	
Reduced food intake or assimilation	<=50% of energy requirements >1 week, or any reduction for >2 weeks, or any chronic GI condition that limits food assimilation/absorption
Inflammation	Acute disease/injury or chronic disease-related

successful nutritional management of older adults. Options such as oral nutrition supplements, home-delivered and congregate meals and food fortification should be considered.[46] Treatment should be initiated based on the mechanism(s) underlying the malnutrition. Table 10.3 gives examples of the breadth of approaches that can be used, depending on underlying causes. This is not meant to be an exhaustive list, but rather to demonstrate that interventions can vary greatly depending on etiology.

For older adults experiencing poor appetite, it is important to assess food preferences to help optimize intake. Calorically dense foods, and favoring liquid over solid textures, such as smoothies, can increase intake of both macro- and micronutrients. Physical activity can improve well-being and may improve appetite.[20]

There is a divergence in recommendations for supplementation by different organizations. The American Geriatrics Society's "Choosing Wisely" campaign

TABLE 10.3
Causes of Malnutrition and Potential Interventions

Cause of Malnutrition	Possible Interventions
Decreased appetite	Assess food preferences; smaller, calorically dense foods, for example, smoothies; increased physical activity
Changes in taste and smell	Increase use of herbs and spices; adjust recipes
Decreased thirst	Scheduled intake of fluids; prompting
Dry mouth	Regular sips of water; avoid hard dry foods; use saliva replacement products; review of medications
Poor dentition	Dental evaluation; dental extraction; dentures as needed; altered food consistency
Dysphagia	Change in food and drink consistency; discussion of goals including feeding tube
Constipation	Increase in intake of fiber; optimize hydration; increase physical activity
Dementia	Assistance with meal preparation; assistance with feeding; use of finger foods; early discussion of goals
Depression	Treatment of depression; social support
History of GI surgery	Evaluate for nutrient absorption
Inflammatory condition	Treat underlying condition
Medications/polypharmacy	Evaluation of medications for drug-drug and drug-nutrient interactions; efforts at deprescribing
Social isolation	Informal social support; congregate housing; social coaching
Inexperience with cooking	Cooking classes; meal preparation service; meals on wheels
Food desert or food swamp	Transportation to grocery store; food delivery; use of frozen or canned foods, root vegetables and grains
Limited finances	Education; plant-based diet; cooking classes; cookbooks

recommends against "using prescription appetite stimulants or high-calorie supplements for treatment of anorexia or cachexia in older adults," and instead recommends optimizing social supports, stopping medications that may interfere with eating, providing food that is appealing, with assistance if necessary, and clarifying patient goals and expectations.[47] A systematic review and meta-analysis of oral nutritional supplementation found no beneficial effects for body weight or BMI changes, or for muscle strength, functional outcomes (activities of daily living and timed Up&Go), quality of life or mortality; however, quality of evidence was very low due to risk of bias and small sample size.[48] On the other hand, the 2023 Academy of Nutrition and Dietetics guidelines for malnutrition in older adults concluded with "high" expert confidence based on developing available evidence that oral nutrition supplements one to two times per day are likely to increase calorie and protein intake, promote weight maintenance or desired weight gain and improve nutrition status for older adults with or at risk of malnutrition.[46] Additionally, the Academy of Nutrition and Dietetics Evidence Analysis Library recommends oral nutrition supplementation for hospitalized patients diagnosed or at risk for malnutrition. In the hospital setting, oral nutritional supplementation has been shown to reduce mortality, particularly in those with established malnutrition, compared to patients at nutritional risk, and has also been associated with a reduction in non-elective hospital readmission.[49] Given these different recommendations, it is prudent to individualize care based on patient circumstances and goals. A "food first" approach provides many benefits over supplementation, but may not always be practical for meeting the nutritional needs of many older adults.

For those who experience changes in taste and smell, adjustment of recipes, with an increase in the use of herbs and spices – such as pepper, onion, garlic, tomato, sweet pepper, basil, parsley, thyme, celery, lime, chili, rosemary, curry, coriander and lemon – can improve the eating experience. A decrease in the sense of thirst can be addressed through prompting or scheduling the intake of fluids. Similarly, dry mouth as an etiology can be addressed through regular sips of water, avoiding dry foods, use of saliva replacement products and review of medications for side effects of dry mouth.

Patients who suffer from dysphagia may benefit from a formal swallow evaluation, which can elicit food and drink consistencies that are better tolerated or advise on optimal positioning. For underlying conditions that are progressive, a discussion of goals of care is warranted, including the potential consequences of placing a feeding tube.

Constipation may be improved by increasing fiber intake, which is found in whole plant foods. Hydration should be optimized, and physical activity should be encouraged.

In the earlier stages of dementia, patients may need assistance with shopping and meal preparation. As dementia progresses, the use of finger foods or assistance with feeding may help preserve intake. Early discussion of goals of care is necessary, to provide care that is consistent with patient wishes. For patients with depression, treatment of the depression and provision of social support may be helpful. Patients with a history of GI surgery should have an evaluation for nutrient status that is based on the site of their surgery, with targeted supplementation as indicated. As inflammatory conditions can lead to malnutrition that is resistant to treatment, early treatment of the underlying condition is targeted, with the goal of delaying or preventing the onset of malnutrition.

Because medications can impact nutritional status, over-the-counter and prescription medications and dietary/herbal supplement use should be regularly evaluated for potential side effects and drug-nutrient interactions. Lifestyle medicine, emphasizing a minimally processed, whole food plant-predominant diet, can successfully support safe deprescription of pharmaceuticals, reducing medication burden and side effects, and improving patient outcomes and quality of life.[50] Eating a vegan diet has been found to be associated with a 58% lower number of pills in adults age 60 and older, when compared to non-vegetarians.[51]

Social connection is another pillar of lifestyle medicine that can be leveraged to improve nutritional well-being. Loneliness and social isolation as sources of malnutrition can be addressed through providing informal social support, congregate housing or social coaching. For those who are not experienced with cooking, do not enjoy cooking or are unable to cook, cooking classes, meal preparation services and Meals on Wheels can fill the gap. Since the COVID-19 pandemic, more cooking classes are available online, providing easier access for many particularly when leaving home is a barrier.

Reliable, safe and affordable transportation to grocery stores may be challenging and not available on a regular basis. Food delivery services are increasingly available in cities, but at a cost. Judicious use of frozen and canned foods, root vegetables and grains, which are longer lasting, can be suggested. Community farmer's markets, mobile produce markets and surplus food programs can also be recommended when available.

Poverty is a significant cause of malnutrition. There is a widely held belief that eating a healthy diet is expensive; however, a recent study demonstrated that eating a whole food plant-based diet led to significant cost savings.[52] Many of the staples of a whole food plant-based diet, such as grains, beans and root vegetables, are inexpensive relative to processed food and animal products. Resources are available for ways to make inexpensive, healthy meals. For example, "Good and Cheap," by Leanne Brown, is available in Spanish and English free of charge for download.[53] Buying fruits and vegetables may help SNAP (Supplemental Nutrition Assistance Program) dollars go further, as many states have a program to double the value of SNAP dollars when fruits and vegetables are purchased.[54]

Addressing the pillars of lifestyle medicine has a theoretical basis for preventing and treating malnutrition in older adults. Promoting a healthful diet throughout life, that focuses on whole plant-based sources, and minimizes processed food, can help reduce chronic inflammation,[55] and thus has a rationale for reducing the prevalence of malnutrition. More research on this approach is warranted. Screening for and treating alcohol use disorder can address this as a root cause of malnutrition. Adopting a lifestyle that promotes activity, social connection, good sleep hygiene and managing stress at any age can support optimal nutrition and thereby promote longevity and healthy aging.

The prevalence of obesity among men and women aged 60 and older is almost 43%.[8,56] Additionally, the simultaneous occurrence of both under- and overnutrition is an important red flag to monitor for malnutrition. Sarcopenic obesity is frequently undiagnosed and could be mitigated with early identification and intervention.[8,57] Optimizing nutritional intake with high-quality protein and antioxidants in particular are nutritional priorities for older adults with sarcopenia and sarcopenic obesity. Interventions that combine physical exercise, specifically progressive resistance strength training, along with dietary strategies can minimize sarcopenia in older adults.[8]

Dietary interventions for older adults should aim to complement medical treatment, respect aging body systems, preserve quality of life, support patient goals and promote overall well-being.[8,57] Given the prevalence and significant impact of malnutrition among older adults, a high level of awareness of risk should be accompanied by a low threshold for screening. As the causes of malnutrition in older adults are myriad, interventions should be targeted toward addressing those causes.

CLINICAL APPLICATIONS

- Malnutrition can be driven by aging-related changes, chronic disease with or without inflammation and functional and environmental circumstances.
- It is important to identify the cause(s) of malnutrition in order to develop a patient-centered, individualized approach to treatment.
- Malnutrition that results from inflammation is not regulated by nutrient requirements and continues even with sufficient intake of protein and calories.
- Consulting with a Registered Dietitian Nutritionist (RDN) ensures that a comprehensive nutrition assessment, including anthropometric, biochemical, clinical, neurological, social and dietary parameters, is performed when a potential risk has been identified.
- A lifestyle medicine approach has a theoretical role in preventing and addressing malnutrition – whether over- or undernutrition – through implementing a healthy diet, promoting socialization, managing stress, avoiding risky substances and promoting sleep and exercise, which in turn can reduce chronic inflammation, polypharmacy and chronic disease burden.

REFERENCES

1. Murray CJ, Atkinson C, Bhalla K, et al. The state of US health, 1990–2010: burden of diseases, injuries, and risk factors. *JAMA*. 2013 Aug 14;310(6):591–608. doi:10.1001/jama.2013.13805.
2. Dent E, Wright ORL, Woo J, Hoogendijk EO. Malnutrition in older adults. *Lancet*. 2023 Mar 18;401(10380):951–966. doi:10.1016/S0140-6736(22)02612-5.
3. Long T, Zhang K, Chen Y, Wu C. Trends in diet quality among older US adults from 2001 to 2018. *JAMA Netw Open*. 2022 Mar 1;5(3):e221880. doi:10.1001/jamanetworkopen.2022.1880.

4. Cederholm T, Bosaeus I. Malnutrition in adults. *N Engl J Med.* 2024 Jul 11;391(2):155–165. doi:10.1056/NEJMra2212159.
5. World Health Organization (WHO). Malnutrition. Accessed August 29, 2024. https://www.who.int/news-room/questions-and-answers/item/malnutrition.
6. Marshall S. Protein-energy malnutrition in the rehabilitation setting: evidence to improve identification. *Maturitas.* 2016 Apr;86:77–85. doi:10.1016/j.maturitas.2016.01.014.
7. Norman K, Hass U, Pirlich M. Malnutrition in older adults – recent advances and remaining challenges. *Nutrients.* 2021 Aug 12;13(8). doi:10.3390/nu13082764.
8. Donini LM, Busetto L, Bischoff SC, et al. Definition and diagnostic criteria for sarcopenic obesity: ESPEN and EASO consensus statement. *Clin Nutr.* 2022 Apr;41(4):990–1000. doi:10.1016/j.clnu.2021.11.014.
9. Prado CM, Batsis JA, Donini LM, Gonzalez MC, Siervo M. Sarcopenic obesity in older adults: a clinical overview. *Nat Rev Endocrinol.* 2024 May;20(5):261–277. doi:10.1038/s41574-023-00943-z.
10. Landi F, Calvani R, Tosato M, et al. Anorexia of aging: risk factors, consequences, and potential treatments. *Nutrients.* 2016 Jan 27;8(2):69. doi:10.3390/nu8020069.
11. World Health Organization (WHO). The double burden of malnutrition: policy brief. Accessed September 17, 2024. https://iris.who.int/bitstream/handle/10665/255413/WHO-NMH-NHD-17.3-eng.pdf?sequence=1.
12. Wolters M, Volkert D, Streicher M, et al. Prevalence of malnutrition using harmonized definitions in older adults from different settings – a MaNuEL study. *Clin Nutr.* 2019 Oct;38(5):2389–2398. doi:10.1016/j.clnu.2018.10.020.
13. Evans C. Malnutrition in the elderly: a multifactorial failure to thrive. *Perm J.* 2005 Summer;9(3):38–41. doi:10.7812/TPP/05-056.
14. Favaro-Moreira NC, Krausch-Hofmann S, Matthys C, et al. Risk factors for malnutrition in older adults: a systematic review of the literature based on longitudinal data. *Adv Nutr.* 2016 May;7(3):507–522. doi:10.3945/an.115.011254.
15. Webb P, Stordalen GA, Singh S, Wijesinha-Bettoni R, Shetty P, Lartey A. Hunger and malnutrition in the 21st century. *BMJ.* 2018 Jun 13;361:k2238. doi:10.1136/bmj.k2238.
16. Streicher M, van Zwienen-Pot J, Bardon L, et al. Determinants of incident malnutrition in community-dwelling older adults: a MaNuEL multicohort meta-analysis. *J Am Geriatr Soc.* 2018 Dec;66(12):2335–2343. doi:10.1111/jgs.15553.
17. Malnutrition Quality Improvement Initiative. Malnutrition care process. Academy of Nutrition and Dietetics Avelere. Accessed September 18, 2024. https://malnutritionquality.org/malnutrition-care-process/.
18. The Malnutrition Quality Collaborative. National Blueprint: Achieving Quality Malnutrition Care for Older Adults, 2020 Update. 2020.
19. Cox NJ, Ibrahim K, Sayer AA, Robinson SM, Roberts HC. Assessment and treatment of the anorexia of aging: a systematic review. *Nutrients.* 2019 Jan 11;11(1). doi:10.3390/nu11010144.
20. Pilgrim AL, Robinson SM, Sayer AA, Roberts HC. An overview of appetite decline in older people. *Nurs Older People.* 2015 Jun;27(5):29–35. doi:10.7748/nop.27.5.29.e697.
21. Kassis A, Fichot MC, Horcajada MN, et al. Nutritional and lifestyle management of the aging journey: a narrative review. *Front Nutr.* 2022;9:1087505. doi:10.3389/fnut.2022.1087505.
22. Palmer AK, Jensen MD. Metabolic changes in aging humans: current evidence and therapeutic strategies. *J Clin Invest.* 2022 Aug 15;132(16). doi:10.1172/JCI158451.
23. Sutherland JM, McLaughlin EA. Ovarian aging: Where are we now? And where to next? *Curr Opin Endocrinol Metab.* 2021;18:29–34.
24. Esposto J, Balendra V. Chapter 3. Brief about hallmarks of aging. In: *Anti-aging Drug Discovery on the Basis of Hallmarks of Aging.* Academic Press; 2022:41–60.

25. Boersma P, Black LI, Ward BW. Prevalence of multiple chronic conditions among US adults, 2018. *Prev Chronic Dis.* 2020 Sep 17;17:E106. doi:10.5888/pcd17.200130.
26. Zenebe Y, Akele B, M WS, Necho M. Prevalence and determinants of depression among old age: a systematic review and meta-analysis. *Ann Gen Psychiatry.* 2021 Dec 18;20(1):55. doi:10.1186/s12991-021-00375-x.
27. Rodriguez-Tadeo A, Wall-Medrano A, Gaytan-Vidana ME, Campos A, Ornelas-Contreras M, Novelo-Huerta HI. Malnutrition risk factors among the elderly from the US-Mexico border: the "one thousand" study. *J Nutr Health Aging.* 2012 May;16(5):426–431. doi:10.1007/s12603-011-0349-1.
28. Rao TS, Asha MR, Ramesh BN, Rao KS. Understanding nutrition, depression and mental illnesses. *Indian J Psychiatry.* 2008 Apr;50(2):77–82. doi:10.4103/0019-5545.42391.
29. Manly JJ, Jones RN, Langa KM, et al. Estimating the prevalence of dementia and mild cognitive impairment in the US: the 2016 health and retirement study harmonized cognitive assessment protocol project. *JAMA Neurol.* 2022 Dec 1;79(12):1242–1249. doi:10.1001/jamaneurol.2022.3543.
30. Arifin H, Chen R, Banda KJ, et al. Meta-analysis and moderator analysis of the prevalence of malnutrition and malnutrition risk among older adults with dementia. *Int J Nurs Stud.* 2024 Feb;150:104648. doi:10.1016/j.ijnurstu.2023.104648.
31. Ueshima J, Momosaki R, Shimizu A, et al. Nutritional assessment in adult patients with dysphagia: a scoping review. *Nutrients.* 2021 Feb 27;13(3). doi:10.3390/nu13030778.
32. Dye BA, Weatherspoon DJ, Lopez Mitnik G. Tooth loss among older adults according to poverty status in the United States from 1999 through 2004 and 2009 through 2014. *J Am Dent Assoc.* 2019 Jan;150(1):9–23.e3. doi:10.1016/j.adaj.2018.09.010.
33. Ritchie CS, Joshipura K, Silliman RA, Miller B, Douglas CW. Oral health problems and significant weight loss among community-dwelling older adults. *J Gerontol A Biol Sci Med Sci.* 2000 Jul;55(7):M366–371. doi:10.1093/gerona/55.7.m366.
34. Gallagher P, O'Mahony D. Constipation in old age. *Best Pract Res Clin Gastroenterol.* 2009;23(6):875–887. doi:10.1016/j.bpg.2009.09.001.
35. Ruscin JM, Linnebur SA. Aging and medications. In: *Merck Manual.* Merck & Co.; 2021. Accessed November 4, 2024. https://www.merckmanuals.com/home/older-people%E2%80%99s-health-issues/aging-and-medications/aging-and-medications.
36. Boulos C, Salameh P, Barberger-Gateau P. Social isolation and risk for malnutrition among older people. *Geriatr Gerontol Int.* 2017 Feb;17(2):286–294. doi:10.1111/ggi.12711.
37. Gahche JJ, Arensberg MB, Weiler M, Dwyer JT. Opportunities for adding undernutrition and frailty screening measures in US national surveys. *Adv Nutr.* 2021 Dec 1;12(6):2312–2320. doi:10.1093/advances/nmab056.
38. Bommersbach TJ, Lapid MI, Rummans TA, Morse RM. Geriatric alcohol use disorder: a review for primary care physicians. *Mayo Clin Proc.* 2015 May;90(5):659–666. doi:10.1016/j.mayocp.2015.03.012.
39. Klein S, Iber FL. Alcoholism and associated malnutrition in the elderly. *Nutrition.* 1991 Mar–Apr;7(2):75–79.
40. Gordon B, RDN, LD. *What Is the Nutrition Focused Physical Exam?* Academy of Nutrition and Dietetics. Accessed November 4, 2024. https://www.eatright.org/health/health-conditions/malnutrition-and-deficiencies/what-is-the-nutrition-focused-physical-exam.
41. Gkiouras K, Cheristanidis S, Papailia TD, Grammatikopoulou MG, Karamitsios N, Goulis DG, Papamitsou T. Malnutrition and food insecurity might pose a double burden for older adults. *Nutrients.* 2020 Aug;12(8). doi:10.3390/nu12082407.
42. Cederholm T, Jensen GL, Correia M, et al. GLIM criteria for the diagnosis of malnutrition – a consensus report from the global clinical nutrition community. *Clin Nutr.* 2019 Feb;38(1):1–9. doi:10.1016/j.clnu.2018.08.002.

43. Jensen GL, Cederholm T, Correia M, et al. GLIM criteria for the diagnosis of malnutrition: a consensus report from the global clinical nutrition community. *JPEN J Parenter Enteral Nutr.* 2019 Jan;43(1):32–40. doi:10.1002/jpen.1440.
44. Global Leadership Initiative on Malnutrition (GLIM): a framework for diagnosing adult malnutrition. The European Society for Clinical Nutrition and Metabolism. Updated September 5, 2023. Accessed November 14, 2024. https://www.nutritioncare.org/uploadedFiles/Documents/Malnutrition/Global%20Leadership%20Initiative%20on%20Malnutrition%20(GLIM)%20A%20Framework%20for%20Diagnosing%20Adult%20Malnutrition.pdf.
45. Skipper A, Coltman A, Tomesko J, et al. Position of the Academy of Nutrition and Dietetics: malnutrition (undernutrition) screening tools for all adults. *J Acad Nutr Diet.* 2020 Apr;120(4):709–713. doi:10.1016/j.jand.2019.09.011.
46. Malnutrition in Older Adults. Academy of Nutrition and Dietetics. Accessed November 14, 2024. Accessed September 15, 2024 https://www.andeal.org/topic.cfm?menu=6064.
47. AGS Health in Aging Foundation. Choosing Wisely.
48. Correa-Perez A, Abraha I, Cherubini A, et al. Efficacy of non-pharmacological interventions to treat malnutrition in older persons: a systematic review and meta-analysis. The SENATOR project ONTOP series and MaNuEL knowledge hub project. *Ageing Res Rev.* 2019 Jan;49:27–48. doi:10.1016/j.arr.2018.10.011.
49. Gomes F, Baumgartner A, Bounoure L, et al. Association of nutritional support with clinical outcomes among medical inpatients who are malnourished or at nutritional risk: an updated systematic review and meta-analysis. *JAMA Netw Open.* 2019 Nov 1;2(11):e1915138. doi:10.1001/jamanetworkopen.2019.15138.
50. Bradley MD, Arnold ME, Biskup BG, et al. Medication deprescribing among patients with type 2 diabetes: a qualitative case series of lifestyle medicine practitioner protocols. *Clin Diabetes.* 2023 Spring;41(2):163–176. doi:10.2337/cd22-0009.
51. Dos Santos H, Gaio J, Durisic A, Beeson WL, Alabadi A. The polypharma study: association between diet and amount of prescription drugs among seniors. *Am J Lifestyle Med.* 2021 Oct 20. doi:10.1177/15598276211048812.
52. Campbell EK, Taillie L, Blanchard LM, et al. Post hoc analysis of food costs associated with Dietary Approaches to Stop Hypertension diet, whole food, plant-based diet, and typical baseline diet of individuals with insulin-treated type 2 diabetes mellitus in a nonrandomized crossover trial with meals provided. *Am J Clin Nutr.* 2024 Mar;119(3):769–778. doi:10.1016/j.ajcnut.2023.12.023.
53. Brown L. All about good and cheap. Accessed September 15, 2024. https://leannebrown.com/good-and-cheap-2/.
54. Fair Food Network. Get double the fruits and veggies. https://doubleupamerica.org/.
55. Menzel J, Jabakhanji A, Biemann R, Mai K, Abraham K, Weikert C. Systematic review and meta-analysis of the associations of vegan and vegetarian diets with inflammatory biomarkers. *Sci Rep.* 2020 Dec 10;10(1):21736. doi:10.1038/s41598-020-78426-8.
56. Naseeb MA, Volpe SL. Protein and exercise in the prevention of sarcopenia and aging. *Nutr Res.* 2017 Apr;40:1–20. doi:10.1016/j.nutres.2017.01.001.
57. Heuberger RA. Geriatric nutrition. In: Bernstein M, McMahon K, eds. *Nutrition Across Life Stages.* Jones & Bartlett Learning, LLC; 2018:chap 15.

11 Sleep and Older Adults

Brian House

INTRODUCTION

Sleep disturbance is one of the primary issues which impact the older adult population and will likely continue to increase in prevalence as the older adult population continues to grow. Sleep disturbance in older adults has been associated with increased fall and injury risk, decreased quality of life, worsening depression and anxiety, fatigue and cognitive impairment.[1] By the year 2050, it is projected that the global population over the age of 60 will reach about 2 billion. In the United States, according to US 2020 census data, the growth rate of the US older adult population has increased approximately five times faster than that of the rest of the US population, a large portion of which is attributed to the baby boomer cohort, those born between the years 1946 and 1964.[2] Today, adults over the age of 65 account for approximately 55.8 million people in the United States, comprising 16.8% of the total US population. Within the older adult population, it is estimated that about 50% will experience difficulty with either initiation or maintenance of sleep.[3] In fact, the prevalence of insomnia in the United States has been found to be the highest among the older adult population, with an incidence of approximately 5% per year.[4]

There are a variety of sleep disorders which impact the ability of older adults to both achieve as well as maintain a restful night's sleep. Additionally, physiologic changes which come naturally with aging may serve to further undermine the achievement of restful sleep even without the presence of a primary sleep disorder. It should be noted however that age in and of itself is not a risk factor, but rather the risk for sleep disturbance results from the changes which come with age such as increased prevalence of comorbid conditions, a decrement in socialization, increased inactivity and changes in sleep architecture.[5] Given the volume of older adults grappling with sleep impairment, over the last several decades it is not surprising that there has been an uptrend in the market for over-the-counter products targeted towards older adults suffering from sleep disturbance. As shown in the National Follow-Up Survey of Self-Care and Aging, approximately 65.9% of older adult participants used over-the-counter medications for arthritis-related pain, most commonly to relieve pain-associated disruptions in sleep.[6] Additionally, this survey found that approximately 20% of participants used a bedtime hypnotic several times per week with the desired goal of improving sleep. Unfortunately, many of these over-the-counter drugs frequently act on anticholinergic pathways to achieve their marketed effect and have been found to be associated with an increased risk of adverse side effects such as falls, confusion, urinary retention and constipation.[1] Given the changes which occur with pharmacokinetic processing, older adults in particular may be more susceptible to adverse side effects from the administration of these non-prescription medications, resulting in an increased risk for adverse outcomes with their use.[1] In part as a consequence of these known adverse outcomes, non-pharmacological interventions are increasingly being utilized as a first-line treatment to help reduce sleep disturbance and promote the restoration and maintenance of an appropriate normative sleep–wake cycle in older adults in place of pharmacologic treatment.[7] In this chapter, the age-related physiologic changes that occur in the sleep–wake cycle will be discussed and non-pharmacologic strategies to help mitigate and treat sleep disturbance in older adults will be reviewed.

AGE-RELATED CHANGES IN SLEEP

In order to understand the challenges inherent in managing sleep disorders in older adults, it is important to first recognize the normative changes that occur to the sleep–wake cycle that come with natural aging.[8] Sleep architecture is a term used as a means by which to classify and frame sleep into objectively measurable stages through analysis of EEG brain wave patterns, muscle tone and eye movements.[9] As shown in Table 11.1, EEG wave patterns can be used to differentiate stages of sleep, thus creating a framework to classify normative sleep architecture throughout the natural human lifecycle. Through studying sleep architecture, sleep researchers have been able to identify the quantifiable changes that occur with aging. Sleep stages may be divided into non-REM sleep, with sub-stages referred to as N1, N2 and N3 as well as REM sleep.[1] REM sleep is more commonly known as the stage during which dreams occur. Within non-REM sleep, the N1 and N2 stages are classified as a more shallow form of sleep during which it is easier to have nighttime awakenings. In contrast, the N3 stage of non-REM sleep is a deeper stage of sleep, meaning waking is more difficult to achieve. With the aging process, a greater proportion of time is spent in non-REM sleep, particularly in the N1 and N2 stages, with a proportional decrement in the amount of time spent in the deeper N3 stage.[1] As a result of this normative age transition in sleep architecture, there is a corresponding increase in the frequency of nocturnal awakenings as a greater proportion of time is allocated to shallow sleep. Table 11.2 below outlines the physiologic changes in

TABLE 11.1

EEG Findings Associated with the Various Stages of Sleep

Sleep Stages	EEG Waveform
Stage W (Wakeful)	Some Alpha waves, mixed frequency pattern
N1	Some Theta waves, no Alpha waves
N2	K-complexes +/– Spindles
N3	Theta waves
REM	REM-Dreaming

TABLE 11.2
Expected Sleep Changes Found in Older Adults Associated with Aging

1. Increased duration of N1 and N2 sleep
2. Decreased duration of N3 and REM sleep
3. Decline in sleep efficiency
4. Increased frequency of daytime napping
5. Increased disruption in sleep maintenance
6. Advancement to earlier bedtime and waking times
7. Shortened duration of sleep
8. Increased time spent awake following sleep onset

sleep architecture that come with normative aging. Indeed, older adults have been shown to have the lowest total sleep duration, averaging approximately 8.1 hours per night.[10] Comparatively, middle-aged adults have been shown to attain a total sleep duration averaging 9.1 hours per night, while younger adults achieve the greatest total sleep duration, averaging approximately 10.5 hours per night. The National Sleep Foundation recommends that older adults over the age of 65 should strive to maintain a target sleep duration approximating about 7 to 8 hours of sleep per night.[1]

With aging, the time to onset of sleep initiation, known as "sleep latency" proportionally increases steadily following the age of 50.[10] In addition to and in part as a consequence of increased sleep latency, sleep efficiency in older adults correspondingly decreases. Sleep efficiency is defined "as the percentage of time in bed spent sleeping compared with the total time spent in bed."[1] As shown, in Table 11.2, with aging comes an increase in the amount of time spent in shallow N1/N2 sleep, an increase in time onset to sleep, as well as a decrement in sleep efficiency, all of which may contribute to increased risk of developing maladaptive sleep behaviors. This subsequently may lead to the creation of a positive feedback cycle, resulting in sleep–wake cycle dysregulation and an increased risk for the development of sleep disturbance and sleep disorders.[5] Since a greater proportion of time is spent in N1 and N2 non-REM sleep, this results in a greater propensity for nighttime awakenings and fragmented sleep time, resulting in a decrement in sleep efficiency. As there is a decrement in the amount of restorative sleep achieved, daytime fatigue may become more prominent resulting in compensatory strategies such as increased frequency of daytime naps, especially in the early evening.[5] Older adults residing at institutions or those with cognitive impairment are a particularly vulnerable subgroup who have been shown to be at heightened risk for sleep disturbance. Another contributing factor to sleep disturbance among older adults relates to the removal of time cues, known as Zeitgebers, a German word meaning "time givers."[1] Socialization, meal timing, exercise, light exposure and work schedules are examples of time cues utilized by the body, and are factors which typically change with aging.[1] Located within the anterior hypothalamus, the Suprachiasmatic Nucleus (SCN) in part relies on Zeitgebers, as stimuli to help guide and regulate circadian rhythms, and as these cues change over the lifecycle, so too does the associated input to the SCN.[8] Neuronal density has also been shown to decline with age, which may further serve to undermine the ability of the SCN to regulate these cues.[11] A consequence of this alteration of external stimuli is that older adults on average will awaken earlier in the morning and go to sleep earlier in the evening compared to their middle-aged or younger adult peers. This advancement of the sleep–wake cycle is reflective of the change in circadian rhythm associated with aging.

COMMON SLEEP DISORDERS

Although some changes to the sleep–wake cycle are physiologic and thus normative with aging, there are a variety of sleep disorders that are pathologic and impact the older adult population. Some examples include Obstructive Sleep Apnea (OSA), Restless Legs Syndrome (RLS) and Periodic Limb Movement Disorder (PLMD), to name but a few.[6]

OSA is one of the most commonly diagnosed sleep disorders across all age groups and is defined as episodic partial or complete upper airway obstruction while asleep. These episodes of obstruction lead to a decrement of oxygen binding to hemoglobin, resulting in nocturnal awakening and sleep disruption. Studies have shown that older adults in particular have a high prevalence of OSA. The Osteoporotic Fractures in Men (MrOS) sleep study found the prevalence of OSA in older adult men, over 80 years of age, to be three times greater compared to middle-aged men. Although some evidence suggests that estrogen may have a protective role against the development of OSA, post-menopausal women have been found to have a similar risk for developing OSA compared to their age-matched male counterparts.[12] A diagnosis of OSA requires both positive polysomnography testing in tandem with symptoms such as apneic episodes or excessive fatigue. Alternatively, a diagnosis of OSA can also be made with positive polysomnography in the setting of known comorbid disease such as hypertension, coronary artery disease, stroke, diabetes or atrial fibrillation.[12]

Restless Legs Syndrome (RLS) is another condition which can negatively impact sleep, and which is more common in prevalence among older adults. RLS is characterized by a desire to move the lower extremities, particularly between the knees and lower ankles and especially during the late evening hours and times of prolonged inactivity.[13] Patients who suffer from RLS frequently feel the urge to get up and walk to experience relief, a form of coping behavior referred to as "Night-Walker's Syndrome," which results in loss of sleep.[13] Although the pathophysiology of RLS is not well understood, there does seem to be an association with iron deficiency, particularly in the CNS, as well as with uremia in patients with renal failure requiring dialysis. Several classes of medications including antihistamines (such as hydroxyzine and diphenhydramine), antidepressants (such as mirtazapine) and anti-dopaminergic agents (such as metoclopramide and prochlorperazine) have been found to be associated with RLS, but it remains unclear whether such medications may serve to worsen or lead to the onset of RLS.[13]

Periodic Limb Movements of Sleep (PLMS) is a term given to the repetitive limb movements of patients with RLS, although these repetitive movements may also exist in the absence of a diagnosis of RLS. PLMS are also found in other conditions such as OSA as well as Parkinson's disease and the prevalence of PLMS has been found to increase with age. Although PLMS may have no impact on nocturnal awakenings, should these repetitive movements result in sleep disturbance without an alternative identifiable cause then Periodic Limb Movement Disorder (PLMD) may be diagnosed. It is important to note that PMLD is therefore a diagnosis of exclusion requiring polysomnography and may not be diagnosed in patients who have concurrent sleep disorder diagnoses.

Non-pharmacologic strategies are an important component of the treatment of certain sleep disorders in older adults and, if utilized appropriately, may serve to reduce adverse side effects and harmful outcomes which oftentimes are an inherent risk in the use of pharmacologic treatment modalities as previously discussed.[7]

Approximately one-fifth of older adults report Excessive Daytime Sleepiness (EDS), which is not a part of the physiologic aging process and may stem directly from poor duration and quality of sleep in the setting of sleep disorders.[9] EDS frequently coexists with a host of comorbid diagnoses such as cardiovascular disease, neurological disorders and endocrinopathies, in addition to sleep disorders such as OSA. Indeed, sleep disturbance in the older adult population is known to be associated with higher rates of depression, increased fall risk, increased progression of cognitive decline, increased all-cause mortality, as well as worsening control of chronic medical conditions and increased morbidity from acute medical illness. As a result, sleep disturbance can directly lead to a decrement in quality of life for older adults as well as poorer health outcomes, while also increasing the cost to the medical system.[7,14]

EVALUATION AND TREATMENT OF SLEEP DISTURBANCE

In order to effectively intervene in sleep disturbance, it is important to first differentiate between physiologic changes in sleep architecture that occur with aging from the development of a true sleep disorder. The *Diagnostic and Statistical Manual-5* (DSM-5) criteria for the diagnosis of insomnia disorder include, "dissatisfaction with sleep quantity or quality, associated with one or more of the following: difficulty initiating sleep, difficulty maintaining sleep, or early morning awakening with inability to return to sleep."[1] Further criteria to meet for a diagnosis of insomnia per the DSM-5 guidelines includes "clinically significant distress or impairment" and sleep disturbances which occurs at least 3 nights per week, for at least 3 months while having the opportunity for sleep.[1] Finally, the sleep disturbance must not be substance induced nor secondary to a comorbid psychiatric or medical illness. This differs somewhat from the International Statistical Classification of Diseases and Related Health Problems-10 (ICD-10) classification system for defining sleep disturbance, which states that a sleep disturbance requires one month of symptoms unexplained by illicit drug use, coexisting medical condition or psychiatric impairment.[7] In the older adult population, it has been estimated that insomnia symptoms are present in as much as 50% of older adults.[15] However, a diagnosis of insomnia is present in only approximately 12 to 20% of older adults.[7] Interestingly, women have higher rates of sleep disturbance compared to their age-matched male counterparts.[5] In part, this difference may be due to reporting bias, as women have been found to be more likely than men to seek out treatment for sleep disorders, and have been found to be more likely to report symptoms compared to males. Importantly for older adults, primary insomnia cannot be diagnosed if dissatisfaction with sleep quantity or quality may be predominantly explained by a coexisting psychiatric or medical illness. In clinical practice, this may be difficult to tease apart as older adults frequently do have diagnoses which may be significantly impacting their sleep such as chronic pain, movement disorders, cancer, COPD, GERD, thyroid disorders, depression/anxiety, nicotine/alcohol use disorder or sleep apnea to name but a few.[10] These conditions have been found to have a bidirectional relationship with sleep disorders and thus it is paramount for the provider to not view sleep complaints in isolation, but rather as part of a comprehensive geriatric assessment.[6] Working to help optimize and manage these chronic conditions may help to improve the degree of sleep impairment in older adults. If, upon completion of a comprehensive geriatric assessment, it is determined that these chronic comorbidities are optimized, yet sleep disturbance persists, then non-pharmacologic interventions may be appropriate to implement.

Spielman's 3P model can be used as a lens through which to view the development of insomnia.[5] With normal aging comes physiologic changes which may serve to increase the predisposition for the development of insomnia. In Spielman'a 3P model, declining functional status with or without concurrent comorbid disease may precipitate the advent of sleep disorders. With sleep impairment comes the development of associations which serve to solidify, perpetuate and worsen sleep disturbance. For example, when having difficulty initiating sleep, older adults may develop an association with this inability to sleep with their bed, bedroom or bedtime, leading to more wakefulness in bed, strengthening the association, which subsequently leads to even more anxiety and frustration and increased activation of the sympathetic nervous system further decreasing the likelihood of sleep onset.[5] Additionally, older adults may develop compensatory behaviors as a means by which to cope with impaired sleep. Unfortunately, many of these compensatory behaviors are often detrimental and lead to the creation of a positive feedback cycle which exacerbates sleep disturbance. For example, due to excessive fatigue from their sleep disorder, older adults may begin to take naps throughout the day, which then leads to a decreased level of physical activity and exercise during the daytime hours, which over time may lead to worsening functional status and increased frailty. Higher physical activity levels are also independently associated with improved sleep health, and reducing daily physical activity may increase the risk of poor sleep. Reduced light exposure, increased social isolation and increased caffeine consumption all serve to perpetuate the development of sleep impairment, creating a positive feedback cycle promoting sleep dysregulation.[10] Table 11.3 lists examples of factors which serve to increase the risk for the development of insomnia.[15]

TABLE 11.3
Factors Associated with an Increased Risk for the Development of Insomnia

1. Sleep Environment (noise, habitation change, institutions, excess cold/heat, ambient light)
2. Socialization Change (retirement, death of family/friends, job transitions)
3. Behavioral (lack of routine sleep pattern, alcohol/nicotine/caffeine use, daytime napping)
4. Female Sex
5. Medical Comorbidities (hypertension, cardiovascular disease, sleep apnea, chronic pain)
6. Medication Side Effects (corticosteroids, opioids, antihistamines, antihypertensives)

COGNITIVE BEHAVIORAL THERAPY FOR INSOMNIA

The aim of non-pharmacological treatment for sleep disorders is in part to break these positive feedback cycles by removing negative associations and replacing established maladaptive compensatory strategies.[5] Once identified, one of the primary non-pharmacologic treatments for insomnia is the use of Cognitive Behavioral Therapy for Insomnia (CBT-I). This treatment should be implemented as part of a multi-modal approach and consists of approximately six to ten sessions over the course of several weeks.[7] There are several domains of focus which CBT-I uses to achieve the goal of removing negative emotions and replacing maladaptive compensatory strategies. These domains include Sleep Hygiene Education (SHE), Relaxation Techniques (RT), Stimulus Control Therapy (SCT), Sleep Restriction Therapy (SRT) and Cognitive Therapy (CT).[5] As seen in Table 11.4, there are a variety of behaviors that may interfere with sleep[1]. Sleep hygiene education seeks to inform older adults of these behaviors with the goal of altering these behaviors when applicable. Lack of a daily routine, frequent daytime napping, performing stimulating activities around or close to bedtime and use of stimulating chemicals such as nicotine or caffeine too close to bedtime are but a few examples of such behaviors which promote poor sleep hygiene and increase the risk for the development of sleep disturbance.[1] Frequently, when sleep disturbance is present, maladaptive behaviors emerge as a compensatory response such as increased screen time

TABLE 11.4
Examples of Activities Associated with Poor Sleep Hygiene

Activities Which Interfere with Practicing Good Sleep Hygiene
1. Daytime napping
2. Lack of regimented sleep–wake routine
3. Chemical stimulant use at bedtime (nicotine or caffeine)
4. Using bed/bedroom for non-sleep activities (television, reading, smartphone/tablets)
5. Poor bedroom environment (excessive cold or warm temperatures, noise, light)
6. Performing stimulating or stress-inducing activities (exercise, work, bills, projects)
7. Frequently spending non-sleep time in bed

via watching television, use of smartphones, tablets, etc.[16] In addition to serving as a wakefulness-promoting stimulus, when these devices are used in the bedroom, with time an inadvertent connection may emerge in which the brain associates the use of such devices with the bedroom itself. This unintended association then serves to further promote sleep disturbance as the bedroom then becomes associated with non-sleep-related activities.

It is important to note that the recognition and promotion of sleep hygiene alone has not been shown to have efficacy on reducing sleep disturbance, but rather should be utilized as part of a multi-modal approach to treat insomnia to have a measurable effect.[16] Once undesirable activities have been identified, then implementing interventions to limit the behavior is appropriate. To this end, important questions to ask when discussing sleep might include: When do you go to bed? Do you have a bedtime routine? Do you feel rested the following day? Do you feel the need to nap? Do you own pets, and if so do they sleep with you or interfere with your sleep? Are there any environmental factors which may impact your sleep, such as lights in the bedroom or surrounding ambient noise? How close to bedtime do you consume fluids, and do you wake from sleep to urinate? Any use of alcohol or caffeine or nicotine, and if so how much, how often, and how close to bedtime?[9] The answers to these questions will better serve to help guide and frame further discussions surrounding sleep.

Should patterns emerge which are consistent with poor sleep hygiene, then interventions may be planned accordingly. Some examples include limiting caffeine consumption to earlier in the day for those who are identified to be consuming caffeine in the afternoon or evening hours. Similarly, limiting daytime naps which occur past the noon-time hour as well as maintaining a regular regimented sleep schedule to help promote a scheduled sleep–wake cycle and maintain Zeitgebers is important. Additionally, limit activities or substances such as nicotine and caffeine which may promote sympathetic nervous system activation, especially within 2 hours of bedtime.[1] Indeed, while exercise is an important component in the reduction of cardiovascular disease and associated morbidity, exercise routines should ideally also be completed at least 2 hours prior to planned sleep. Limiting or eliminating the use of over-the-counter sleep aids, and avoiding spending greater than 20 minutes awake in bed at a time are also important elements of good sleep hygiene. Table 11.5 demonstrates examples of commonly recommended sleep hygiene practices which may serve to help promote improved sleep quality among older adults.[4]

Relaxation techniques to help reduce stress and ease muscle tension are also used as part of CBT-I.[5] Meditation, yoga and stretching exercises serve to ease stress and promote relaxation. In one RCT looking at the effects of Tai Chi in older adult females with insomnia, the authors found that compared to the control group, the group who practiced Tai Chi demonstrated statistically significantly improved sleep efficiency, as well as demonstrated a reduction in wake time following sleep onset, a measurement for the total amount of time an individual spends awake following the initial onset of sleep.[17] Additionally, an Israeli study looking at the effect of practicing yoga in classes twice weekly over the course of 3 months demonstrated

TABLE 11.5
Examples of Behaviors Associated with the Promotion of Good Sleep Hygiene

Sleep Hygiene Strategies
1. Avoid excessive time in bed when not sleeping, no more than 10 minutes
2. Practice maintenance of regular sleeping and waking times
3. Avoid napping close to bedtime
4. If unable to fall asleep in bed, remove yourself from the bedroom until sleepy
5. Strive for regular exercise, but avoid exercising close to bedtime
6. Limit consumption of liquids close to bedtime
7. Limit caffeine, alcohol and nicotine intake, especially close to bedtime

that older adults over the age of 60 with insomnia who participated in yoga had subjective improvement in overall sleep quality, sleep efficiency, sleep latency, stress, fatigue, tension, anxiety and depression.[18] Another study, looking at the impact of aerobic activity and sleep hygiene education on sleep, mood and quality of life in older adults with chronic insomnia found that the physical activity group demonstrated improvement in sleep quality, sleep latency, daytime dysfunction and sleep efficiency compared to the control group.[19] Thus, it can be seen that there is evidence that through incorporating relaxation techniques into daily practice, older adults may achieve improvements in sleep disturbance.

Stimulus Control Therapy (SCT) is another set of behavioral interventions through which improvement in sleep disturbance may be attained as part of a CBT-I approach to care.[16] As shown in Table 11.6, SCT focuses on the performance of a sequence of steps to help promote a healthy sleep–wake cycle. The purpose of stimulus control therapy is to diminish the strength of association between learned behaviors linking the bed with activities other than sleep such as watching television or reading while simultaneously strengthening the association between the bed

TABLE 11.6
Stimulus Control Therapy (SCT) Strategies

Stimulus Control Instruction Examples
1. Only go to sleep when feeling sleepy
2. Avoid being in bed, except for sleep or sex
3. Restrict daytime napping
4. Regiment alarms to promote routine
5. Restrict television, reading, tablets, use of phones in bed
6. If unable to sleep within 10 minutes, leave the bedroom – do not return until sleepy
7. Upon return to bed, if unable to sleep, repeat #6

and/or bedroom with sleep.[7] Sleep Restriction Therapy (SRT) is another component of CBT-I which seeks to improve sleep efficiency, a term which refers to "the ratio of total sleep time to time in bed."[9] SRT achieves this by limiting the amount of time spent in bed in an effort to gradually improve fidelity to time spent sleeping.[7] Unfortunately, older adults with insomnia have an increased tendency to remain in bed for longer periods of time, resulting in increased difficulty falling asleep at an appropriate and/or desired bedtime. Although SRT may be performed on its own as a non-pharmacologic treatment modality for insomnia, it is typically utilized as part of a multifaceted CBT-I approach over the course of several weeks and involves the use of a sleep diary to closely track time spent in bed in order to ultimately enhance sleep efficiency.[3] The final component of CBT-I is Cognitive Therapy, the goal of which is to target the maladaptive thoughts and beliefs of worry and anxiety that become intertwined with as well as a driver for insomnia.[16] This is achieved over the course of several weeks during which these thoughts and beliefs are identified and during which sleep expectations are normalized. Once this has been achieved, a framework is then implemented to replace these maladaptive thoughts with better adaptive strategies in order to overcome negative beliefs, thereby breaking the positive feedback cycle.[5]

MEDICATIONS AND SLEEP

Although the focus of this chapter does not include a discussion of the pharmacologic treatment of sleep disorders, sleep is impacted by a variety of medication classes, and it is, therefore, important to perform a thorough medication review and reconciliation to identify any potential contributory prescription or non-prescription medications which may be impacting sleep.[9] Based on National Sleep Foundation poll data, it is estimated that approximately 24% of older adults have four or more chronic health conditions.[6] Additionally, a review of Medicare data shows that approximately 44% of US community-dwelling older adults take approximately five or more medications.[6] Sleep may be impacted by both the prescribing of new medications as well as the deprescribing of pre-existing medications; therefore it is important to take into account any recent medication changes when discussing sleep concerns. Another factor to consider when reviewing multiple medications is any potential drug–drug interactions.[1] Polypharmacy is commonly seen in the older adult population as new medications are added to treat symptoms which may unknowingly be a side effect of a prior prescription medication. When reviewing older adults' medication lists it is therefore also important to take note of any non-prescription medications that are being taken over the counter as well as the timing that both prescription and non-prescription medications are being administered as this may also impact the sleep–wake cycle directly, but also indirectly by causing adverse side effects which then disrupt normative sleep.[6] Some identifiable classes of medications which may contribute to sleep disturbance include: stimulants, sedatives, antihistamines, antidepressants, antihypertensives, anti-epileptics, benzodiazepines, steroids, opioids and antispasmodics.[1] Table 11.7, contains a list of some medications which have been found to be associated with sleep pattern alteration. Substance use, both illegal

TABLE 11.7
Medications Associated with Sleep Disturbance

Drug Class	Examples
Antihypertensives	Benazepril, Lisinopril, Fosinopril, Enalapril, Captopril
Beta-Blockers	Carvedilol, Atenolol, Metoprolol, Propranolol
Calcium Channel Blockers	Amlodipine, Felodipine, Diltiazem, Verapamil
Antihistamines	Loratadine, Fexofenadine, Cetirizine
Opioids	Oxycodone, Hydromorphone, Codeine
Corticosteroids	Prednisone, Methylprednisolone
Antidepressants	SSRIs (Escitalopram, Sertraline, Fluoxetine) and SNRIs (Duloxetine, Venlafaxine)
Acetylcholinesterase Inhibitors	Donepezil, Rivastigmine

as well as legal, has also been shown to contribute to sleep disturbance. As a result, screening older adults to identify the frequency, timing and quantity of substance use is helpful in order to determine an effective treatment plan. Caffeine, alcohol and nicotine are three legal substances which have also been shown to contribute to sleep disturbance and in the case of caffeine and alcohol may even be utilized by older adults as a modality of self-treatment for underlying sleep disorders. Unfortunately, this may further serve to alter the normative sleep–wake cycle leading to the perpetuation of sleep disruption. Screening of alcohol, tobacco and caffeine product use when discussing sleep concerns is therefore important as modifying intake may help to treat sleep disturbance and can unmask related substance use disorders which may be contributing to impaired sleep.

COMORBID CONDITIONS AFFECTING SLEEP

In addition to screening for underlying substance use disorders, attaining optimum control of comorbid diseases is another important treatment for underlying sleep disorders. Sleep Disordered Breathing (SDB) is a frequently encountered comorbid condition which shares a high degree of fidelity with insomnia in older adults.[5] SDB prevalence increases with age, with prevalence of between 22 to 54.9% among older adults.[5,6] Some proposed mechanisms of action include decreased neck and throat muscle tone from sleep deprivation, sleep loss from frequent nocturnal desaturations, and nighttime urination causing increased nighttime awakenings.[5] Therefore, if there is any clinical suspicion of SDB, including symptoms such as excessive daytime fatigue, apneic episodes, snoring, morning headaches and/or memory/concentration impairment, consider referral for overnight polysomnography for further workup and evaluation.

OSA is considered to be the most commonly diagnosed form of SDB and when considering OSA on the differential, there are several screening tools which may be of assistance, two of the most common being the STOP-BANG questionnaire and the Epworth Sleepiness Scale.[12] In validation studies, the negative predictive value of the STOP-BANG questionnaire was found to be as high as 90.2% with a sensitivity of 92.9% for moderate OSA. Therefore, when using the STOP-BANG, scores less than 3 are helpful to rule out OSA while scores greater than 5 are helpful to rule in OSA. The Epworth Sleepiness Scale is a questionnaire evaluating a patient's proclivity to fall asleep in various situations with a score profile range from 0–24, with scores greater than 10 being reflective of EDS with a sensitivity of 94% and specificity of 100%.[12] Physical exam findings such as a BMI >30 kg/m^2, neck circumference >43 cm in males or >40.6 cm in females, macroglossia, tonsillar hypertrophy or small oral cavity may all serve to support a diagnosis of OSA. Once diagnosed, the treatment of OSA is directed towards the reduction of the upper airway critical closing pressure, thereby ensuring airway integrity. Weight loss, avoidance of alcohol and other CNS depressants, ensuring alleviation of nasal congestion and non-invasive positive pressure ventilation should all be considered when implementing a treatment plan for OSA.[12]

Should SDB persist undiagnosed, this can further lead to cardiovascular complications such as hypertension, cardiac remodeling and even heart failure given sufficient ongoing duration. The symptoms from these comorbid conditions may additionally act to increase the risk of developing sleep disorders in older adults. Additionally, if cardiovascular comorbidities are present, the medications used to treat these conditions, such as diuretics and antihypertensives in and of themselves may serve to promote the development of sleep disorders and separately increase the risk profile for susceptible older adults for the development of pathologic sleep impairment. Indeed, this increased risk has even been demonstrated with certain advanced procedural interventions. For example, patients who received ICD implantation were found to have an association with sleep disruption and an increased risk for the development of insomnia.[5] This was theorized to be secondary to the development of associated negative emotions such as anxiety and fear surrounding the possibility of ICD malfunction.

CONCLUSIONS

Ultimately, sleep disorders in older adults are known to be associated with adverse health outcomes. It is therefore important to view sleep disturbance in the context of comprehensive geriatric assessment, considering functional status, activity level, medications, behaviors, comorbid medical and/or psychiatric disease, environmental influences, as well as a thorough sleep history. When appropriate, non-pharmacological modalities should be utilized as a first-line treatment over pharmacologic treatments, which frequently carry an increased risk for adverse effects and drug–drug interactions among the older adult population.

CLINICAL APPLICATIONS

- Consider screening for secondary causes of insomnia in older adults, and recognize that comorbid disease and sleep have a bidirectional relationship.
- When appropriate, consider CBT-I as a first-line treatment for insomnia in place of prescription medications.
- Always perform a thorough medication review in older adult patients as several classes of medications are known to adversely impact the natural sleep cycle.

REFERENCES

1. Cohen ZL, Eigenberger PM, Sharkey KM, Conroy ML, Wilkins KM. Insomnia and other sleep disorders in older adults. *Psychiatr Clin North Am.* 2022 Dec;45(4):717–734.
2. Caplan Z. U.S. Older population grew from 2010 to 2020 at fastest rate since 1880 to 1890. *US Census Bureau.* May 23, 2023. https://www.census.gov/library/stories/2023/05/2020-census-united-states-older-population-grew.html
3. Wennberg A, et al. Sleep disturbance, cognitive decline, and dementia: a review. *Semin Neurol.* 2017 Aug;37(4):395–406.
4. Roepke S, Ancoli-Israel S. Sleep disorders in the elderly. *Indian J Med Res.* 2010 Feb;131:302–310.
5. Williams J, Roth A, Vatthauer K, McCrae CS. Cognitive behavioral treatment of insomnia. *CHEST.* 2013 Feb 1; 143(2):554–565.
6. Vaz Fragoso CA, Gill TM. Sleep complaints in community-living older persons. *J Am Geriatr Soc.* 2007 Nov;5(11):1853–1866.
7. Patel D, Steinberg J, Patel P. Insomnia in the elderly: a review. *J Clin Sleep Med.* 2018 June 15;14(6):1017–1024.
8. Gulia KK. Sleep disorders in the elderly: a growing challenge. *Psychogeriatrics.* 2018 May;18(3):155–165.
9. Feinsilver SH. Normal and abnormal sleep in the elderly. *Clin Geriatr Med.* 2021 Aug; 37(3):377–386.
10. Li J, Vitiello MV, Gooneratne N. Sleep in normal aging. *Sleep Med Clin.* 2018 Mar;13(1):1–11.
11. Wennberg A, et al. Optimizing sleep in older adults: treating insomnia. *Maturitas.* 2014 Nov;76(3):247–252.
12. Foldvary-Schaefer NR, Waters TE. Sleep disordered breathing. *Continuum.* 2017 Aug;23(4, Sleep Neurology):1093–1116.
13. Ekbom K, Ulfberg J. Restless leg syndrome. *J Intern Med.* 2009 Nov;266(5):419–431.
14. Abad V, Guilleminault C. Insomnia in elderly patients: recommendations pharmacological management. *Drugs Aging.* 2018 Sep;35(9):291–817.
15. Brewster, et al. Insomnia in the older adult. *Sleep Med Clin.* 2018 Mar;13(1):13–19.
16. Dopheide JA. Insomnia overview: epidemiology, pathophysiology, diagnosis and monitoring, and nonpharmacologic therapy. *Am J Manag Care.* 2020 Mar;26(4 Suppl): 876–884.
17. Siu P, et al. Effects of Tai Chi or exercise on sleep in older adults with insomnia. *JAMA Netw Open.* 2021 Feb 1;4(2):1–14.
18. Halpern J, Cohen M, Kennedy G, Reece J, Cahan J, Baharav A. Yoga for improving sleep quality and quality of life for older adults. *Altern Ther Health Med.* 2014 May–Jun;20(3):37–46.
19. Reid KJ, Baron KG, Lu B, Naylor E, Wolfe L, Zee PC. Aerobic exercise improves self-reported sleep and quality of life. *Sleep Med.* 2010 Oct;11(9):934–940.

12 Social Connection
An Essential Lifestyle Pillar for Older Adults

Susan M. Friedman

INTRODUCTION

"We are called to build a movement to mend the social fabric of our nation. It will take all of us – individuals and families, schools and workplaces, health care and public health systems, technology companies, governments, faith organizations, and communities – working together to destigmatize loneliness and change our cultural and policy response to it. It will require reimagining the structures, policies, and programs that shape a community to best support the development of healthy relationships."

– Vivek Murthy, MD, MBA, Surgeon General of the United States[1]

Humans are inherently social beings. Social connection is an essential part of life, not just adding to well-being, but to resilience, physical health and even longevity. We have a biological need to interact with others, and our interdependence has been essential to our survival as a species. On a community level, social connection contributes not only to population health, but to a community's safety and prosperity.[1]

In a recent study in which older adults were asked what mattered most to them, relationships with family, spouse, children, grandchildren, friends and loved ones were mentioned most often – almost twice as often as health, and more than ten times as often as being alive or living a long time.[2] In the original Blue Zones – areas around the world where people are reported to live the longest and have low rates of chronic illness – five of the nine common themes in these communities are social in nature.[3] Social connection and engagement have been recognized by the American College of Lifestyle Medicine as one of its six pillars[4] and as one of three key components in Rowe and Kahn's model of successful aging.[5]

There is an increasing global recognition of, and concern for, the impact of social isolation and loneliness on older adults.[6] The COVID-19 pandemic moved something that was previously seen largely as a personal issue into the realm of public health, as the fallout from months of social distancing and the resulting isolation became apparent. In May 2023, the Surgeon General issued a General Advisory, labeling loneliness, isolation and lack of connection as a public health crisis.[1] This issue is gaining attention globally; both the United Kingdom and Japan have created ministries of loneliness to address this public health challenge.

SOCIAL CONNECTION, LONELINESS AND SOCIAL ISOLATION

Social connection is a term with three distinct dimensions, namely, structure, function and quality.[1,7] Structure refers to the number of relationships, their variety and frequency of interactions. It includes marital/partnership status and living arrangement, as well as friend circle size. Function describes the degree to which others can be relied on for various needs, including both emotional and material support. Quality refers to the degree to which relationships are positive, helpful or satisfying, and the degree to which one feels included or excluded. Structural and functional measures are only weakly correlated[7] so that their impact may be cumulative, and there may be different interventions that can improve outcomes. Social connection is multifaceted, including relationships and interactions with family, friends, neighbors and colleagues; one's digital environment; and neighborhood, school and workplace.

Loneliness and social isolation are distinct concepts that relate to social connection. One can be socially isolated but not lonely; lonely but not socially isolated; or both. Social isolation is an objective measure that refers to being alone or having few or infrequent social contacts, and with limited social roles or group memberships (see Table 12.1). It is a measure of integration and meaningful ties to friends, family and community.[8] Social isolation is most commonly experienced by individuals, but for some groups, for example, migrant communities, social isolation may impact the entire community.[9]

Loneliness encompasses the subjective and distressing feelings stemming from a discrepancy between one's desired and actual social connections. It may include a perception of social isolation, a lower level of contact than is desired or the absence of a specific desired companion.[10] With loneliness, there is a perceived unmet need, which may involve feelings of disconnectedness or not belonging. Interestingly, both loneliness and social isolation appear to have a genetic influence, with 38% of the former and 40% of the latter accounted for by genes.[11,12]

EPIDEMIOLOGY

Social connection has been an evolving issue for the better part of a century. In his groundbreaking book, *Bowling Alone*, published in 2000, Robert Putnam made the case that the previous half century had seen a significant decline in community participation, from membership in volunteer organizations, to faith groups, to sports leagues, to the PTA.[13] Although his focus was on civic engagement, this deterioration in group participation has impacted social connection broadly. In 2018, only 16% of Americans reported feeling very attached to their local community.[1]

Social networks are getting smaller, and the time spent in social activities is declining, with increasing time spent alone.[1] From 2003 to 2020, social isolation increased and time spent with non-household family and friends decreased, further

TABLE 12.1
Social Isolation versus Loneliness

	Loneliness	Social Isolation
Definition	• The subjective and distressing feelings stemming from a discrepancy between one's desired and actual social connection; perceived unmet need	• Being alone or having few or infrequent social connections, with limited social roles or group memberships
Perspective	• Subjective	• Objective
Genetic influence	• 38%	• 40%
Frequency in older adults	• 43%	• 24%
Who is at risk?	• Women • Young adults and older adults • Lower socioeconomic status • Smoking • More comorbid conditions • Functional impairment • Less alcohol use • Less frequent physical activity • Rural • Living alone • Immigrants • Identifying as LGBTQ+	• Men • Older • White • Widowed, separated, divorced or never married • Lower education • Lower income • Immigrant communities • LGBTQ+ • Family caregivers • Medical conditions – dementia, COPD, incontinence, CVA, DM • Rural
Potential outcomes	• Higher mortality, functional decline/loss of independence, more chronic conditions (e.g., heart disease, stroke, hypertension, diabetes), decreased immune function, more hospitalizations, higher health care costs, depression, anxiety, more cognitive decline, more deaths, frailty, from overdose and suicide, lower QOL	
Screening question	• How often do you feel lonely?	• Looking back over the last year, who are the people you talked to most often about important things?
Screening tool	• UCLA Loneliness Scale	• Berkman–Syme Social Network Index

exacerbated by the pandemic.[14] Household family social engagement also declined during that time, but was not made worse by the pandemic. Forty-nine percent of Americans reported three or fewer close friends in 2021, up from 27% in 1990.[1] Overall, the average size of core social networks has decreased by a third since 1985, with less diversity of networks and less inclusion of non-kin.[7]

The last several decades have seen other significant societal changes that impact social connection. Family and household structures have changed. For example, the proportion of Americans aged 25 to 49 who were living with their spouse and one or more children has gone from 67% in 1970 to 37% in 2021. The proportion of US adults who have never married has gone from 17 to 31% in that timeframe.[15] Married Americans tend to have larger social networks, more satisfying social lives and greater satisfaction in their personal health.[16] Furthermore, the rate of single-person households in the United States has gone from 13% in 1960 to 29% in 2022.[1] All of these can impact social connection later in life. Women are having fewer children, which has the potential to change social connections and social support across the lifecycle.[15]

We live in an aging society. While that potentially is a source of opportunities for social support and connection (e.g., multi-generational families, volunteerism, etc.), there are potential barriers, discussed below, that limit social connection in the later stages of life. The prevalence of loneliness has been shown to increase with age,[17] and social networks shrink with age, with personal and friendship networks declining throughout adulthood.[18]

We also live in an increasingly digital age, with pervasive use of social media, the internet, smartphones and the growing use of remote work, virtual reality, artificial intelligence and assistive technologies. Americans spend 6 hours per day on average on digital media.[1] Digital technology has facilitated communication in many ways, including connecting people who live far away from each other, and providing opportunities for participation and community for individuals with disabilities and those from marginalized groups. There has been a generational shift in reliance on social media for communication and interaction, often replacing face-to-face interactions. In a review of loneliness and social internet use, Nowland et al. concluded that when the internet is used to enhance existing relationships and develop new social connections, it can reduce loneliness. However, when it is used to avoid the social pain of interaction, loneliness increases.[19] In a systematic review by Chen and Schulz, information and communication technology was found to positively affect social support and connectedness, and reduce isolation for older adults, although the results for loneliness were less conclusive.[20] The generational differences in the use of digital technologies are likely to impact social connection as today's teenagers and young adults become older.

In the midst of these social and demographic trends, we are seeing more loneliness and social isolation. In the United States, 24% of community-dwelling older adults are socially isolated, and 4% are severely so.[21] In a nationally representative study of adults aged 60 and over, 43% reported feeling lonely, with 32% reporting a lack of companionship, 25% reporting feelings of being left out and 18% reporting feeling isolated at least some of the time. About a third of those reported having these feelings often.[22] Together, loneliness and social isolation are more prevalent than obesity, inactivity and smoking.[1,7]

Both young adults and older adults are at risk of being lonely.[23] Loneliness is associated with being female, lower socioeconomic status, living alone, smoking, having more comorbid conditions, more functional impairment, lower alcohol use and less frequent physical activity, being an immigrant, or identifying as LGBTQ+.[1,22,23] Older adults with social isolation are more likely to be male, White, unmarried (widowed, separated, divorced or never married) and have lower education and income.[21] Older adults living in rural areas have a higher prevalence of both loneliness and social isolation compared to their urban counterparts.[24]

Although lonely individuals are more likely to live alone than those who are not lonely, the majority of lonely people live with someone.[22] Among married couples, three out of ten relationships are severely discordant,[7] highlighting the importance not only of the presence of relationships, but of quality as well.

BARRIERS TO CONNECTION

There are many potential barriers to connection that become more common with age. Social connection is dependent on individual, community and societal factors[9] (Figure 12.1).

Sensory impairment becomes increasingly common with age. About one-third of older adults have hearing impairment,[25] and more than one in four have vision impairment.[26] Sensory impairment has been linked to social isolation, with mechanisms including impact on daily functioning and mobility, disengagement and ability to communicate. In a cohort study of Medicare beneficiaries aged 65 and older, hearing impairment was predictive of a 38% greater odds of having no social participation in the past month, when surveyed 8 years later. Vision impairment (44%) and dual sensory impairment (54%) were also associated with a higher risk, although this did not reach statistical significance, likely due to lower prevalence.[27] In another study, sensory impairment was associated with loneliness but not social isolation.[24]

Aging is accompanied by an increased risk of chronic disease, which in turn can increase a person's risk of social isolation or loneliness.[23,28] About one-fourth of

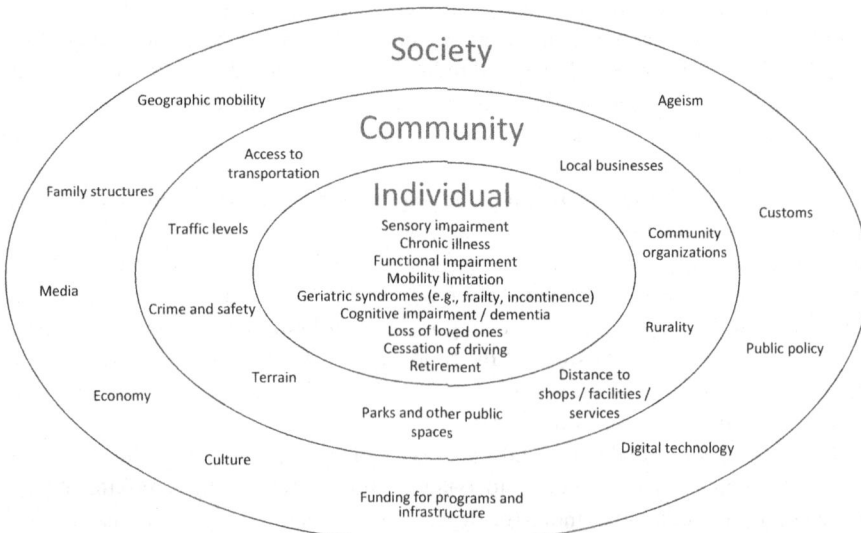

FIGURE 12.1 Theoretical framework for the impact of social isolation and loneliness on health outcomes.

adults over the age of 65 have one chronic condition, and almost two-thirds have two or more.[29] Chronic illness puts individuals at risk of functional/mobility impairment, which can also contribute to social isolation or loneliness.[30] In addition to chronic illness, aging is associated with a higher risk of geriatric syndromes, such as frailty, incontinence and dementia, which can contribute to social isolation and loneliness.[28]

Retirement leads to a change in routine, role perception and opportunities for interaction with others. Loss of loved ones, including a spouse, friend or sibling, is also increasingly common with age, with similar outcomes of reducing social connection and increasing the risk of loneliness.[28] Cessation of driving, especially in areas that do not have alternative options for transportation, can limit social connection.[28]

We live in a mobile society. Although the rate of moving has decreased over recent years, Americans move 11.7 times on average in their lifetime. In 2022, 235,000 Americans moved to retire.[31] Depending on the circumstances, a move can lead to a significant disruption of one's social network. As people age, an increasing percentage of people who move do so to live closer to family; 35% of people aged 65–69 and 53% of people aged 75 or more who move do so to be closer to family.[32] This is likely to change the makeup of the individual's social circle, but may also increase the level of support. The likelihood of living in a multi-generational household increases with age, and Asians, Hispanics and Blacks are more likely than Whites to live in a multi-generational household.[33]

Community structure can also facilitate or impede social connection. This may encompass a wide range of issues, including access to public or private transportation; traffic levels; crime and safety; local businesses; community organizations; rurality;[23] distance to shops, facilities and services; terrain; and access to parks and other public spaces.[1,9]

In addition to individual and community-based barriers, societal factors can impact social connection. Ageism may impact the value placed on connections with older adults. Customs and culture may impact the role of older adults and how people perceive their place in society.[28] The media can promote age discrimination, or fear of crime greater than is warranted.[9] Political decisions and public policy, whether local or national, impact funding that can bolster both infrastructure and programs that foster connection.

FUNCTIONAL, EMOTIONAL AND MEDICAL CONSEQUENCES

In a meta-analysis that included data from more than 300,000 participants, individuals with stronger social relationships had a 50% greater likelihood of survival.[34] This finding applies consistently across different ages, gender, causes of death and country of origin.[28] Similarly, a meta-analysis assessing the association of loneliness with all-cause mortality found a 22% increased risk overall, with an effect that was more pronounced among men.[35] Social connection has been demonstrated to have a comparable or greater impact on mortality than smoking,[7,28] alcohol,[1] physical activity,[7,28] obesity,[7,28,36] hypertension[36] and hyperlipidemia,[36] and the effect is independent of age and initial health status.[28]

Social isolation and loneliness independently increase a person's risk for poor health.[30,37] This includes a greater risk of functional decline[22] and several chronic conditions, such as heart disease,[30,38] stroke,[23,30,38] hypertension[1,39] and diabetes.[37] Furthermore, social isolation, but not loneliness, predicts mortality for those who have had a heart attack or stroke.[38] People with social isolation or loneliness are more susceptible to viruses and have less ability to mount an effective immune response to vaccines, leading to an increased risk of infectious disease.[30] Socially isolated patients have higher medical costs, higher hospitalization rates and worse clinical outcomes.[30]

Social isolation and loneliness have been shown to increase the risk of depression,[23,37,40] anxiety,[23,28,30] cognitive decline, dementia[23,41,42] and death from overdose or suicide.[28,30] In-person contacts and perceived adequacy of relationships appear to have the largest impact on depression and anxiety.[28] Men and women with loneliness, and men with social isolation are at higher risk of developing frailty,[43] which puts them at risk of other adverse outcomes.

These outcomes may result from both biological and functional pathways.[44] Inflammatory markers, such as C-reactive protein and IL-6, can be impacted by social isolation and loneliness, as can markers of immune function, such as natural killer cells.[44] Loneliness has been associated with higher levels of amyloid and tau protein – pathological changes seen in Alzheimer's disease.[28] On the other hand, more social connections can improve biomarkers of cardiovascular functioning, such as cardiovascular reactivity and oxidative stress.[1] Social connection may impact lifestyle and medical adherence, which in turn impacts outcomes such as blood pressure, gene expression and neuroendocrine function.[45] It also promotes engagement in preventive health services.[46] A wide variety of instrumental mechanisms have the potential to impact medical outcomes. These could include stimulation through social interaction; transportation to medical appointments; early recognition of a decline that needs evaluation; advocacy to obtain timely and effective care; association with health-related behaviors such as exercise and sleep; self-care, including cooking and eating a healthy diet, or medication compliance; or assistance with activities of daily living or instrumental activities of daily living.

EVALUATION

There are many measurement tools to assess social isolation and loneliness, but most of them have been developed for research purposes.[28] Social integration, corresponding to the absence of social isolation, can be measured by the 4-Item Berkman–Syme Social Network Index for Social Connection.[7,47] This tool has been used for several national surveys and has been recommended by the Institute of Medicine for inclusion in electronic medical records.[28] Scores range from 0 to 4, with one point each for being married or living with a partner; averaging 3 or more interactions per week with others by phone or in person; attending church or religious services 4 or more times per year; and belonging to a club or organization.[36]

Measurement tools have been described and compared based on their evaluation of structure versus function of social contacts, and on the degree of subjectivity asked of respondents.[28] The 6-Item Lubben Social Network Scale evaluates the social network of older adults in terms of size, closeness and frequency of contact with relatives and friends.[48,49] The Interpersonal Support Evaluation List provides

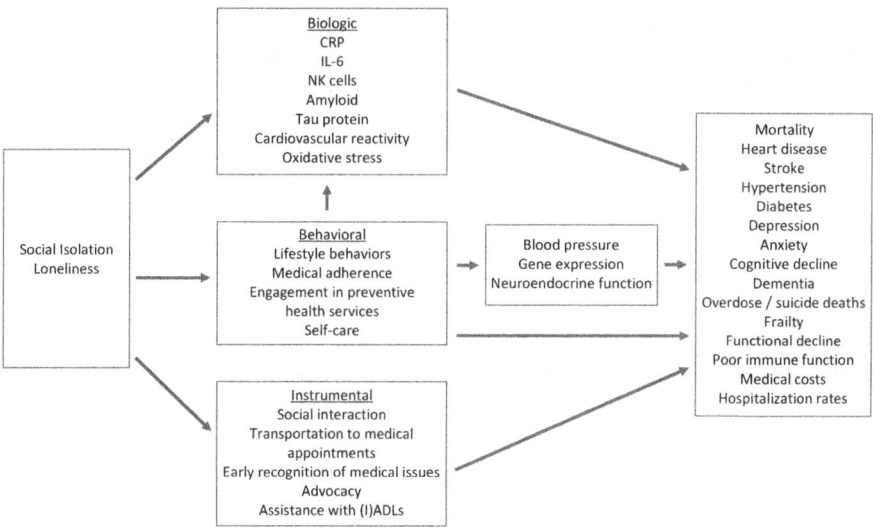

FIGURE 12.2 A framework for barriers to connection among older adults. (Adapted from Bristol City Council Report, 2014.[9])

a more functional and subjective evaluation of support; the original tool contains 40 statements about the perceived availability of different social resources, such as someone to help in a crisis, watch the house if one goes away, go to dinner with, get advice from or share worries. Shorter forms have been developed and validated.[50]

The UCLA Loneliness Scale is a widely used tool to assess loneliness, with a validated 3-item version.[49] This scale asks "How often do you feel that you lack companionship?" "How often do you feel left out?" and "How often do you feel isolated from others?" Each question can be answered hardly ever, some of the time, or often, and is scored 1, 2 or 3, respectively, yielding an overall score ranging from 3 (low) to 9 (high).

INTERVENTIONS

Interventions to address loneliness and social isolation can range from the individual, to systems, to society at large. A wide variety of interventions have been developed, including social skills development or social cognitive training; offering activities, such as social or physical programs; providing support, through counseling, therapy or education; internet training; home visits; providing regular contacts, care or companionship; and increasing opportunities for social interaction, such as through online chat rooms, telephone befriending, or a "companion robot" or virtual pet companion.[28,51] Goals of these interventions include facilitating social bonding, enhancing coping with loneliness, and preventing loneliness. Several reviews have focused on technology-based interventions. A recent scoping review concluded that there was not a one-size-fits-all approach due to the individuality of the experience, so that interventions need to be tailored to suit the needs of the individual or groups being treated. Additionally, the heterogeneity of interventions, including setting, group versus individual delivery and study population, limit their usefulness for driving policy.[6] The authors note that for some, social isolation is a risk for developing loneliness, so interventions that address social isolation may also help to alleviate loneliness; however, since not all lonely individuals are isolated, this is not an approach that would impact all who have loneliness.

From a conceptual standpoint, since the barriers listed in the section above can adversely impact loneliness and social isolation, addressing them may improve these outcomes. As an example, a 1999 US survey of 2,300 hearing-impaired adults age 50 and older found that only 32% of those who had untreated hearing loss participated regularly in social activities, compared to 42% of those who wore hearing aids.[52] In this survey, more than half of hearing aid users reported improvement in their relationships and over a third reported improvement in their social life. Other approaches to reducing barriers include improving access to transportation through ride-hailing apps, and piloting voice-controlled technology to foster connection to individuals and their community.[53]

Psychosocial interventions have been shown to improve downstream health outcomes. In a meta-analysis of randomized studies targeting patients, interventions had a positive impact on depression when the spouse was included and, in some cases, impacted mortality. For family members, these interventions reduced caregiver burden, depression and anxiety.[54] A meta-analysis of family-based interventions addressing family relationships or psychoeducation demonstrated small but significant benefits to the physical and mental health of the patient, as well as for the family members' health.[54]

Psychosocial interventions provided in the health care setting – particularly those promoting health behaviors – showed improvements in survival, with a 29% increased probability of survival compared to controls.[55] Holt-Lunstad and Perissonotto recommend using the "EAR" framework (Educate, Assess, Respond) to

TABLE 12.2
EAR Framework for Addressing Social Isolation and Loneliness

Educate	• Social connection is a component of a healthy lifestyle • Social isolation and loneliness increase risk of illness and death • Social connection helps patients maintain health, manage medical conditions and adhere to medical treatment
Assess	• Use the EMR to document social support, isolation and loneliness • Use validated measures to identify patients at risk • Track risk and progress over time
Respond	• Reinforce the importance of social connection as a protective health factor • Integrate psychosocial support from formal and informal caregivers into the treatment plan • Refer to community resources based on identified needs • Reassess circumstances and needs regularly, and respond accordingly

Source: Adapted from Holt-Lunstad, et al., 2023.[30]

guide intervention,[30] incorporating education on the impact of social connection on health; assessing for loneliness and social isolation and including it in the electronic medical record; and providing support and referral as indicated.

In the Surgeon General's Advisory on loneliness and social isolation, Dr. Vivek Murthy outlined six pillars to advance social connection, as a means to improving the nation's health, safety and prosperity.[1] This strategy is meant not only to improve physical and mental health and well-being for individuals, but to strengthen community health and safety, build resilience against future challenges and advance civic engagement.

The first pillar focuses on strengthening the social infrastructure of communities. The goal is to provide equitable access to a built environment, programs and institutions that promote social interaction. The second pillar acknowledges the role of public policy, encouraging mindfulness across all sectors of society to promote connection and prevent disconnection and cross-departmental leadership to oversee an overarching strategy. The third pillar involves the health sector, due to its role in managing some of the outcomes of social isolation and loneliness. Interventions within health care include training health care providers, assessing and supporting patients and expanding public health surveillance and interventions.

Given the exponential growth of technology, and its major impact on social connection, reform of digital environments is the focus of the fourth pillar of the Surgeon General's strategy. Data transparency will help us understand the impact

TABLE 12.3
Six Pillars to Advance Social Connection

Pillar	Approaches
Strengthen social infrastructure	• Built environment • Community connection programs • Invest in local institutions that bring people together
Public policies	• "Connection-in-all-policies" approach • Policies that minimize harm from disconnection • Cross-departmental leadership at all government levels
Health sector	• Train health care providers • Assess and support patients • Expand public health surveillance/intervention
Digital environment	• Require data transparency • Establish and implement safety standards • Support the development of pro-connection technologies
Knowledge	• National research agenda • Accelerate research funding • Increase public awareness
Culture of connection	• Cultivate values of kindness, respect, service, commitment • Model values in positions of leadership and influence • Expand conversation in schools, workplace, community

Source: From the Surgeon General's Advisory, 2023.[1]

of technology, in order to develop safety standards, and develop and promote technologies that aid in fostering social connection. The fifth pillar speaks to developing and messaging knowledge, through developing, coordinating and funding a national research agenda to understand the causes and consequences of social connection, identify populations at risk and develop effective interventions. This knowledge should be communicated widely, to increase public awareness in order to move policy and create culture change. Last but not least, Dr. Murthy advises cultivating a culture of connection, through discussions throughout our community institutions, and modeling values that promote connection – such as kindness, respect, service and commitment to each other – in positions of leadership and influence.

CONCLUSIONS

There is increasing awareness of the importance of social connection, and the adverse outcomes of social isolation and loneliness – not only to the health of the individual, but to the health of the community. The last several decades have witnessed increasing loneliness and social isolation, and older adults are at high risk, with a significant impact on both morbidity and mortality. Because this issue has become so widespread, it will require both individual and societal approaches to improve outcomes. For optimal results, these efforts should involve not only health care, but public policy, attention to our digital environments and cultivation of a culture of connection.

CLINICAL APPLICATIONS

- Society in general has experienced an increasing prevalence of loneliness and social isolation, and older adults are at high risk of these issues, making screening increasingly important.
- Many tools have been developed to screen for loneliness and social isolation. Two brief validated tools are the UCLA Loneliness Scale and the Berkman–Syme Social Network Index.
- A wide variety of interventions have been developed to address loneliness and social isolation, including social skills development or social cognitive training; social or physical programs; providing support through counseling, therapy or education; internet training; home visits; providing regular contacts, care or companionship; and increasing opportunities for social interaction, such as through online chat rooms, telephone befriending, or a "companion robot" or virtual pet companion.
- Addressing barriers to social connection, such as addressing sensory impairment, improving access to transportation and fostering the use of technology, can improve social connection.
- Due to the individuality of the experience, interventions need to be tailored to suit the needs of the individuals being treated.
- The Surgeon General's advisory on loneliness and social isolation outlined six pillars to advance social connection: community infrastructure, public policy, the health sector, digital technology, research and culture.

REFERENCES

1. U.S. Surgeon General. *Our Epidemic of Loneliness and Isolation: The U.S. Surgeon General's Advisory on the Healing Effects of Social Connection and Community.* US Department of Health and Human Services; 2023:82.
2. Garbarino JT, O'Connor S, Pepin RL, Aitken MS, Flaherty E. Age-friendly health care and the 4Ms in RN-led annual wellness visits. *J Am Geriatr Soc.* May 2024;72 Suppl 2:S13–S20. doi:10.1111/jgs.18671.
3. Buettner D. *The Blue Zones: Lessons for Living Longer from the People Who've Lived the Longest.* National Geographic; 2010:320.
4. American College of Lifestyle Medicine. Accessed October 26, 2024. https://lifestyle-medicine.org/.
5. Rowe JW, Kahn RL. Successful aging. *Gerontologist.* 1997 Aug;37(4):433–440. doi:10.1093/geront/37.4.433.
6. Fakoya OA, McCorry NK, Donnelly M. Loneliness and social isolation interventions for older adults: a scoping review of reviews. *BMC Public Health.* 2020 Feb 14;20(1):129. doi:10.1186/s12889-020-8251-6.
7. Holt-Lunstad J, Robles TF, Sbarra DA. Advancing social connection as a public health priority in the United States. *Am Psychol.* 2017 Sep;72(6):517–530. doi:10.1037/amp0000103.
8. Mulhausen P. Healthy aging: impact of loneliness and social isolation. In: Rippe J, ed. *Lifestyle Medicine.* 4th ed. CRC Press; 2024:1494:chap 109.
9. Bristol City Council. Social isolation and physical and sensory impairment. 2014:1–23. https://www.bristol.gov.uk/files/documents/1417-social-isolation-and-physical-and-sensory-deprivation/file#:~:text=Social%20isolation%2C%20disengagement%2C%20loneliness%2C,of%20social%20support%20may%20result.
10. Wenger GC, Davies R, Shahtahmasebi S, Scott A. Social isolation and loneliness in old age: review and model refinement. *Ageing Soc.* 1996 May;16:333–358. doi:10.1017/S0144686x00003457.
11. Goossens L, van Roekel E, Verhagen M, Cacioppo JT, Cacioppo S, Maes M, Boomsma DI. The genetics of loneliness: linking evolutionary theory to genome-wide genetics, epigenetics, and social science. *Perspect Psychol Sci.* 2015 Mar;10(2):213–226. doi:10.1177/1745691614564878.
12. Matthews T, Danese A, Wertz J, Odgers CL, Ambler A, Moffitt TE, Arseneault L. Social isolation, loneliness and depression in young adulthood: a behavioural genetic analysis. *Soc Psychiatry Psychiatr Epidemiol.* Mar 2016;51(3):339–348. doi:10.1007/s00127-016-1178-7.
13. Putnam RD. *Alone: The Collapse and Revival of American Community.* Simon & Schuster; 2000.
14. Kannan VD, Veazie PJ. US trends in social isolation, social engagement, and companionship – nationally and by age, sex, race/ethnicity, family income, and work hours, 2003–2020. *SSM Popul Health.* Mar 2023;21:101331. doi:10.1016/j.ssmph.2022.101331.
15. Aragao C, Parker K, Greenwood S, Boaronavski C, Mandapat JC. The modern American family: key trends in marriage and family life. *Pew Research Center.* Accessed October 2, 2024. https://www.pewresearch.org/social-trends/2023/09/14/the-modern-american-family/#:~:text=Over%20the%20past%20five%20decades,like%20unmarried%20adults%20raising%20children.
16. Cox DA. *Emerging Trends and Enduring Patterns in American Family Life.* Survey Center of American Life. Accessed October 2, 2024. https://www.americansurveycenter.org/research/emerging-trends-and-enduring-patterns-in-american-family-life/.

17. Dykstra PA, van Tilburg TG, Gierveld JD. Changes in older adult loneliness – results from a seven-year longitudinal study. *Res Aging*. 2005 Nov;27(6):725–747. doi:10.1177/0164027505279712.
18. Wrzus C, Hänel M, Wagner J, Neyer FJ. Social network changes and life events across the life span: a meta-analysis. *Psychol Bull*. 2013 Jan;139(1):53–80. doi:10.1037/a0028601.
19. Nowland R, Necka EA, Cacioppo JT. Loneliness and social internet use: pathways to reconnection in a digital world? *Perspect Psychol Sci*. 2018 Jan;13(1):70–87. doi:10.1177/1745691617713052.
20. Chen YR, Schulz PJ. The effect of information communication technology interventions on reducing social isolation in the elderly: a systematic review. *J Med Internet Res*. 2016 Jan 28;18(1):e18. doi:10.2196/jmir.4596.
21. Cudjoe TKM, Roth DL, Szanton SL, Wolff JL, Boyd CM, Thorpe RJ. The epidemiology of social isolation: National Health and Aging Trends Study. *J Gerontol B Psychol Sci Soc Sci*. 2020 Jan 1;75(1):107–113. doi:10.1093/geronb/gby037.
22. Perissinotto CM, Stijacic Cenzer I, Covinsky KE. Loneliness in older persons: a predictor of functional decline and death. *Arch Intern Med*. 2012 Jul 23;172(14):1078–1083. doi:10.1001/archinternmed.2012.1993.
23. U.S. Centers for Disease Control and Prevention. Health effects of social isolation and loneliness. Accessed October 6, 2024. https://www.cdc.gov/social-connectedness/risk-factors/index.html#:~:text=Certain%20conditions%20or%20experiences%20may,Chronic%20disease%20or%20condition.
24. Wang Q, Zhang SM, Wang Y, Zhao D, Zhou CC. Dual sensory impairment as a predictor of loneliness and isolation in older adults: national cohort study. *Jmir Public Hlth Sur*. 2022 Nov;8(11):e39314. doi:10.2196/39314.
25. National Institute on Aging. Hearing loss: a common problem for older adults. Accessed October 8, 2024. https://www.nia.nih.gov/health/hearing-and-hearing-loss/hearing-loss-common-problem-older-adults#:~:text=About%20one%2Dthird%20of%20older,and%20hearing%20doorbells%20and%20alarms.
26. Killeen OJ, De Lott LB, Zhou Y, et al. Population prevalence of vision impairment in US adults 71 years and older: the National Health and Aging Trends Study. *JAMA Ophthalmol*. 2023Feb 1;141(2):197–204. doi:10.1001/jamaophthalmol.2022.5840.
27. Huang AR, Cudjoe TKM, Rebok GW, Swenor BK, Deal JA. Hearing and vision impairment and social isolation over 8 years in community-dwelling older adults. *BMC Public Health*. 2024 Mar 13;24(1):779. doi:10.1186/s12889-024-17730-8.
28. National Academies of Sciences Engineering and Medicine (U.S.), Board on Health Sciences Policy. Health and Medicine Division, Board on Behavioral Cognitive and Sensory Sciences. Division of Behavioral and Social Sciences and Education. *Social Isolation and Loneliness in Older Adults: Opportunities for the Health Care System*. Consensus study report. National Academies Press; 2020:xvii, 298 pages.
29. Boersma P, Black LI, Ward BW. Prevalence of multiple chronic conditions among US adults, 2018. *Prev Chronic Dis*. 2020 Sep 17;17:E106. doi:10.5888/pcd17.200130.
30. Holt-Lunstad J, Perissinotto C. Social isolation and loneliness as medical issues. *N Engl J Med*. 2023 Jan 19;388(3):193–195. doi:10.1056/NEJMp2208029.
31. Schmidt E. Moving statistics 2024. *Consumer Affairs Journal of Consumer Research*. Accessed October 5, 2024. https://www.consumeraffairs.com/movers/moving-statistics.html.
32. Park J. *Understanding Relocation Patterns of Older Adults*. American Planning Association. Accessed October 6, 2024.

33. Joint Center for Housing Studies of Harvard University. *Housing America's Older Adults 2023*. 2023:1–38. https://www.jchs.harvard.edu/sites/default/files/reports/files/Harvard_JCHS_Housing_Americas_Older_Adults_2023.pdf.
34. Holt-Lunstad J, Smith TB, Layton JB. Social relationships and mortality risk: a meta-analytic review. *PLoS Med*. 2010 Jul;7(7):e1000316. doi:10.1371/journal.pmed.1000316.
35. Rico-Uribe LA, Caballero FF, Martin-Maria N, Cabello M, Ayuso-Mateos JL, Miret M. Association of loneliness with all-cause mortality: a meta-analysis. *PLoS One*. 2018;13(1):e0190033. doi:10.1371/journal.pone.0190033.
36. Pantell M, Rehkopf D, Jutte D, Syme SL, Balmes J, Adler N. Social isolation: a predictor of mortality comparable to traditional clinical risk factors. *Am J Public Health*. 2013 Nov;103(11):2056–2062. doi:10.2105/AJPH.2013.301261.
37. Richard A, Rohrmann S, Vandeleur CL, Schmid M, Barth J, Eichholzer M. Loneliness is adversely associated with physical and mental health and lifestyle factors: results from a Swiss national survey. *PLoS One*. 2017;12(7):e0181442. doi:10.1371/journal.pone.0181442.
38. Hakulinen C, Pulkki-Raback L, Virtanen M, Jokela M, Kivimaki M, Elovainio M. Social isolation and loneliness as risk factors for myocardial infarction, stroke, and mortality: UK Biobank Cohort Study of 479,054 men and women. *Heart*. Sep 2018;104(18):1536–1542. doi:10.1136/heartjnl-2017-312663.
39. Yang YC, Boen C, Gerken K, Li T, Schorpp K, Harris KM. Social relationships and physiological determinants of longevity across the human life span. *Proc Natl Acad Sci U S A*. 2016 Jan 19;113(3):578–583. doi:10.1073/pnas.1511085112.
40. Choi H, Irwin MR, Cho HJ. Impact of social isolation on behavioral health in elderly: systematic review. *World J Psychiatry*. 2015 Dec 22;5(4):432–438. doi:10.5498/wjp.v5.i4.432.
41. Kuiper JS, Zuidersma M, Oude Voshaar RC, Zuidema SU, van den Heuvel ER, Stolk RP, Smidt N. Social relationships and risk of dementia: a systematic review and meta-analysis of longitudinal cohort studies. *Ageing Res Rev*. 2015 Jul;22:39–57. doi:10.1016/j.arr.2015.04.006.
42. Penninkilampi R, Casey AN, Singh MF, Brodaty H. The association between social engagement, loneliness, and risk of dementia: a systematic review and meta-analysis. *J Alzheimers Dis*. 2018;66(4):1619–1633. doi:10.3233/JAD-180439.
43. Gale CR, Westbury L, Cooper C. Social isolation and loneliness as risk factors for the progression of frailty: the English Longitudinal Study of Ageing. *Age Ageing*. 2018 May 1;47(3):392–397. doi:10.1093/ageing/afx188.
44. Uchino BN. Social support and health: a review of physiological processes potentially underlying links to disease outcomes. *J Behav Med*. 2006 Aug;29(4):377–387. doi:10.1007/s10865-006-9056-5.
45. Holt-Lunstad J, Smith TB. Loneliness and social isolation as risk factors for cardiovascular disease: implications for evidence-based patient care and scientific inquiry. *Heart*. 2016 Jul 1;102(13):987–989. doi:10.1136/heartjnl-2015-309242.
46. Stafford M, von Wagner C, Perman S, Taylor J, Kuh D, Sheringham J. Social connectedness and engagement in preventive health services: an analysis of data from a prospective cohort study. *Lancet Public Health*. 2018 Sep;3(9):e438–e446. doi:10.1016/S2468-2667(18)30141-5.
47. Berkman LF, Syme SL. Social networks, host resistance, and mortality: a nine-year follow-up study of Alameda County residents. *Am J Epidemiol*. 1979 Feb;109(2):186–204. doi:10.1093/oxfordjournals.aje.a112674.
48. Lubben JE. Assessing social networks among elderly populations. *Family and Community Health*. 1988;11(3):42–52.

49. Lubben J, Matz-Costa C. Social network index. In: Gu D, Dupre ME, eds. *Encyclopedia of Gerontology and Population Aging*. Springer Nature; 2020:1–3.
50. Cohen S, Mermelstein R, Kamarck T, Hoberman H. Measuring the functional components of social support. In: Sarason IG, Sarason BR, eds. *Social Support: Theory, Research, and Applications*. Martinus Nijhoff; 1985:73–94.
51. Masi CM, Chen HY, Hawkley LC, Cacioppo JT. A meta-analysis of interventions to reduce loneliness. *Pers Soc Psychol Rev*. 2011 Aug;15(3):219–266. doi:10.1177/1088868310377394.
52. Reinemer M, Hood J. Untreated hearing loss linked to depression, social isolation in seniors. *Audiol Today Am Academy of Audiol*. 1999;11(4): 34.
53. Ryerson LM. Innovations in social connectedness. *Public Policy & Aging Report*. 2017;27(4):124–126. doi:10.1093/ppar/prx031.
54. Martire LM, Lustig AP, Schulz R, Miller GE, Helgeson VS. Is it beneficial to involve a family member? A meta-analysis of psychosocial interventions for chronic illness. *Health Psychol*. 2004 Nov;23(6):599–611. doi:10.1037/0278-6133.23.6.599.
55. Smith TB, Workman C, Andrews C, et al. Effects of psychosocial support interventions on survival in inpatient and outpatient healthcare settings: a meta-analysis of 106 randomized controlled trials. *PLoS Med*. 2021 May;18(5):e1003595. doi:10.1371/journal.pmed.1003595.

13 Stress and Its Impact on Older Adults

Meredith Troutman-Jordan and Boyd H. Davis

INTRODUCTION: A FOCUS ON EPIDEMIOLOGY

Stress is a mental reaction to challenging circumstances. A state of worry or mental tension caused by a difficult situation, it is a natural human response that prompts one to address challenges and threats.[1] Though all people experience stress to some degree, an individual's response to stress has a significant impact on overall well-being incorporating physical and mental health. Worldwide, given that 15% of the older adult population experiences mental disorders, it is unsurprising that stress is a specific and major mental health problem affecting a sizeable proportion (10–55%) of this population.[2] The prevalence of stress and anxiety among older adults is increasing and is expected to double in the next decade.[2] In a 2021 poll of 2,023 US adults, 28% of those aged 50–80 years felt depressed or hopeless for several days or more within the past 2 weeks.[3] Even more alarming, 44% reported feeling stressed.

Stress is often associated with various characteristics, some of which are modifiable, and others that are not, such as race, gender and ethnicity. Research literature suggests disparities in exposure to stressors across race/ethnicity, With minority groups reporting a higher stress burden than their White counterparts.[4] In their analysis of *Health and Retirement Study* data from 6,567 adults ages 52 and older, Brown et al.[4] identified significant racial and ethnic differences in both total chronic stress exposure and its appraisal. On average, Black older adults had the highest level of ongoing chronic stress exposure and Whites had the lowest level. Among respondents who reported stress exposure, the average stress appraisal was highest for White older adults and foreign-born Hispanics and lowest for Blacks and US-born Hispanics. The mean appraisal of those reporting stress exposure is approximately the mid-point between *not being upset* and *being somewhat upset*, according to stress appraisal rankings used by Brown et al. (1 = not upsetting, 2 = somewhat upsetting or 3 = very upsetting).

Similar findings have been produced by other researchers; as summarized by Brown et al.[4] (2020), older Black and Hispanic individuals report more chronic stress exposure than Whites and are two to three times as likely to experience financial strain and housing-related stress. Despite experiencing a greater number of stressors, Black and US-born Hispanic older adults are less likely to be upset by exposure to stressors than Whites. US-born Hispanics are particularly less upset by relationship-based stressors, while Black older adults are less upset across all stress domains, and foreign-born Hispanics are only less upset by caregiving strain (Brown et al.).[4]

In their narrative review of epidemiological evidence on how and why the mental health of older adults varies by gender, Kiely, Brady and Byles[5] concluded that throughout the lifecycle women generally have poorer mental health in terms of depression and anxiety symptoms, although gender differences seem to decrease with advancing age. They do note, however, that in many contexts, excess mortality and suicide impacts are greatly elevated for older men. One can infer that poor mental health evaluation is a proxy for poorly managed stress. While race and gender are fixed, other characteristics present are more variable.

Situational factors associated with stress, although somewhat limited, include life events such as managing chronic illness, losing a spouse, being a caregiver or adjusting to changes due to finances, retirement or separation from friends and family.[6] Caregiving responsibilities, loneliness or boredom and any major life changes have also been linked with stress in older adults.[7] One in four older adults experiences issues with their mental health; the most common diagnoses are depression, dementia and anxiety.[8] Of these, depression and dementia are the most common, affecting 5% to 7% of the population over 60. Brennan[8] adds that anxiety – which is clearly a manifestation of stress – follows as a close second, affecting 3.8% of older adults.

Stress and health. It is important to recognize and review the impact of stress not only because of its correlation with mental health diagnoses but also the multitude of associated medical conditions and pathophysiological processes with which it is associated. Chronic medical conditions (particularly chronic obstructive pulmonary disease, cardiovascular disease including arrhythmias and angina, thyroid disease and diabetes), sleep disturbances, side effects of medications (i.e., steroids, antidepressants, stimulants, bronchodilators/inhalers, etc.) and alcohol or prescription medication misuse or abuse are linked with stress and anxiety.[9] Stress can lead to physical symptoms including headaches, GI distress, elevated blood pressure, chest pain and problems sleeping.[10] Research demonstrates that the stress hormone cortisol affects older adults significantly more than younger adults, causing more inflammation.[11] It also impacts physical capacity, weakening muscle signaling; older adults under stress may find it harder to do activities such as climbing stairs. When stress becomes chronic, the brain – dense with cortisol receptors – is repeatedly washed with cortisol surges,[12] which become toxic, increasing the risk of developing dementia.[11] Left untreated, high cortisol levels can result in inflammation, type 2 diabetes and hypertension.[12] Inflammation is linked with more (or worse) health problems, including atherosclerosis, type 2 diabetes, arthritis, dementia and cancer.[7] Thus, chronic stress is a concerning risk factor for numerous serious health conditions.

Perhaps most concerning is the cumulative effect of stress on older adults' cognition, which impacts self-care, quality of life and ability to self-manage all health conditions. Mikneviciute, Ballhausen, Rimmele and Kliegel[13] conducted a systematic review and meta-analysis of research on the effects of acute stress on older adults' cognition, considering the various types of cognition. An analysis of 22 studies suggested that stress in older age impairs verbal fluency. While the effect of stress on episodic memory is unclear, it appears to have no effects on cognitive control, cognitive flexibility and problem-solving/planning in older age. Mikneviciute et al.[13] observed that qualitative evidence suggests potential enhancing effects of stress on response inhibition as well as playing a role in older adults in shifting decision-making concerning more careful strategies. They concluded that stress effects on older adults' memory retention, associative memory, prospective memory, interference control or cognitive flexibility are deeply under-investigated.

In one longitudinal study of 30,239 adults age 45 and older, perceived stress, modeled as a continuous variable in the baseline data set, was associated with 1.08 higher odds of prevalent cognitive impairment, and adjusting for sociodemographic variables, cardiovascular disease risk factors, lifestyle factors and depressive symptoms, there was no appreciable change in the magnitude of this association.[14] In the same study, elevated levels of perceived stress (dichotomized as low stress versus elevated stress) were associated with 1.37 times higher odds of poor cognition after adjusting for sociodemographic variables, CVD risk factors, lifestyle factors and depressive symptoms. Kulshreshtha et al.'s [14] finding suggests that high levels of perceived stress increase the risk of cognitive decline regardless of race. Thus, epidemiological data and research evidence provide compelling reasons for screening, identification and intervention for older adults at risk for or experiencing intense or chronic stress. The wide array of chronic conditions associated with prolonged stress is a compelling reason to optimally manage one's stress, while quality of life is another motivation.

APPROACHES TO ASSESSMENT

It is important to consider screening and assessment for any older adult experiencing psychosocial, health or situational risk factors such as those previously discussed, and interventions should consider age-specific characteristics. A variety of well-established screening tools can be used to help identify stress in older adults. These include the *Perceived Stress Scale*,[15] a 10-item Likert format tool that assesses how different situations affect one's feelings and perceived stress. Items ask about feelings and thoughts during the past month, such as how often they have been upset because something unexpected happened. Perceived Stress Scale scores have been correlated with stress measures, smoking status, self-reported health measures and health behavior measures (Cohen and Williamson, 1988).[15] Possible total scores range from 0 to 56; a higher score indicates greater stress. Perceived Stress Scale norms have been reported for individuals ages 65 and older, as compared to younger age groups.[16] The Perceived Stress Scale has been validated in older adult groups and is a useful tool for evaluating stress in older adults.[17] It is also easily accessible online, free of charge.

Holmes and Rahe's[18] *Stress Inventory* allows self-assessment of the total stress one is experiencing. Comprised of 43 items, it employs a dichotomous response format to assess for experiencing events – ranging from the death of a spouse to taking a vacation – that can contribute to illness. Higher scores indicate a greater risk of health issues; a score of 300 or greater suggests an 80% chance of health breakdown within the next 2 years, according to the Holmes–Rahe statistical prediction model, while 150–300 points indicate a 50% chance of health breakdown in the next 2 years, and 150 points or less implies a relatively low amount of life change and little susceptibility to stress-induced health breakdown.[19]

Perception of stress is important; eustress refers to a positive form of stress having a beneficial effect on health, motivation, performance and emotional well-being. Examples of eustress are a new job or a vacation. Although not all stress is pathological, poor stress management, which can manifest as extreme worry or anxiety, is critical to detect. A limited ability to manage stress as well as chronic stress has harmful physiological and psychological consequences, such as hypertension or depression. The prevalence of anxiety disorders in older adulthood is believed to be underestimated due to the challenges of assessing and diagnosing anxiety in this age group.[20] Various anxiety assessment tools specific to older adults include the Adult Manifest Anxiety Scale,[21] the Worry Scale,[22] the Geriatric Anxiety Scale[23] and the Geriatric Anxiety Inventory.[24]

The Adult Manifest Anxiety Scale is a 50-item self-report measure. Six categories of anxiety are assessed: Somatic Anxiety, Worry and Oversensitivity, Tension and Irritability, Fearfulness and Inhibition, Social Concerns and Cognitive Instability. Items explore different aspects of anxiety, helping professionals gauge an individual's anxious tendencies. The scale has a dichotomous format, with each item being worth 1 point. Scores can range from 0 to 50 with higher scores indicating more severe anxiety.

A second tool is the Worry Scale. With 35 5-point Likert format items, it assesses financial, health and social worries commonly associated with aging. Scores can range from 0 (lower level worry) to 140 (higher level worry). While it could be helpful to determine anxiety characteristics, 50 or even 35 items may not be feasible to assess in clinical practice.

The Geriatric Anxiety Scale might be more suitable in some instances. It has 30 items in a Likert format, that assess somatic, cognitive, and affective symptoms. Responses are rated 0, not at all, to 3 (all of the time), with higher scores indicating greater anxiety. An even shorter tool is the Geriatric Anxiety Inventory, which has just 20 dichotomous items that assess typical common anxiety symptoms. There is a 5-item version of the GAI[22] as well. Each of these tools, while not intended to be diagnostic, is useful for screening and assessment, and has acceptable psychometric properties. Depending upon a patient's literacy and visual acuity, these could be administered during an outpatient clinic visit, and help provide quantifiable data that captures the older adult's subjective experience of anxiety or stress.

Physical signs of stress are also important to assess and can be more difficult to determine. Examples of such symptoms are listed in Table 13.1. The challenge, particularly in the older adult population, is that many of these symptoms correspond with age-related physical changes or common pathophysiologic processes. Thus, a thorough assessment of recent and current symptoms across all systems (e.g., respiratory, cardiovascular) is essential and should be considered as a context for general worries, tensions and of course psychological symptoms. A comprehensive geriatric assessment will help identify both physical and psychological stress and could be a basis for distinguishing between the two.

TABLE 13.1
Common Signs and Symptoms of Stress

- Difficulty breathing/dyspnea
- Panic attacks
- Blurred eyesight or sore eyes
- Sleep difficulties
- Fatigue
- Muscle aches and headaches
- Chest pains and high blood pressure
- Indigestion or heartburn
- Constipation or diarrhea
- Feeling sick, dizzy or fainting
- Sudden weight gain or weight loss
- Developing rashes or pruritis
- Diaphoresis

Depression is more common in people who also have other illnesses or whose function becomes limited.[25] Research demonstrates heightened risk of depression with multiple disease conditions; for example, Yanmin, Ting, Kexin, Xiaoye, Enlai and Jiyan[26] found risk of depression in older adults with cardiovascular diseases was 6.0 times higher than that in those without cardiovascular diseases ($p < 0.001$); and the risk of depression in older patients with peptic ulcer diseases was 4.4 times higher than that in those without peptic ulcer diseases ($p < 0.001$).

In their systematic review on screening and treatment for depression, anxiety disorders and suicide risk in adults, O'Connor, Henninger, Perdue, Coppola, Thomas and Gaynes[27] included one cohort study[28] that found comorbidity patterns of anxiety and depressive disorders in a large cohort study ($N = 1783$); 67% of individuals with a depressive disorder also had a current anxiety disorder, and 75% had a lifetime comorbid anxiety disorder. Thus, it is prudent to rule out depression, as depression (a stressor) often co-occurs with anxiety. Research suggests that there is a higher prevalence of anxiety and somatic symptoms in older adults with depression, and a complete assessment of depression in older adults should include an assessment of anxiety and somatic symptoms.[29]

Older adults with depression are less likely to show affective symptoms such as worthlessness, guilt and dysphoria.[29] Compared to young/middle-aged individuals, depressed older adults more often experience cognitive symptoms such as subjective memory loss and decreased concentration, somatic symptoms, sleep disturbances, fatigue, loss of interest, hopelessness, worry about the future and anxiety.[29] Aside from somatic symptoms of depression common in older adults, many other manifestations of depression in this age group are indicative of mental responses to challenging situations (stress). These include persistent sad, anxious, or "empty" mood; feelings of hopelessness, guilt, worthlessness or helplessness; irritability, restlessness or having trouble sitting still; loss of interest in once pleasurable activities, including sex; decreased energy or fatigue; moving or talking more slowly; difficulty concentrating, remembering or making decisions; difficulty sleeping, waking up too early in the morning or oversleeping; eating more or less than usual, usually with unplanned weight gain or loss; and thoughts of death or suicide, or suicide attempts.[30]

A variety of assessment tools can be used to screen or assess for depression in older adults. The *Geriatric Depression Scale* (GDS) is commonly used and comes in two versions, 30-item[31] and 15-item.[32] Either are dichotomous format scales that detect indicators of depression, such as satisfaction with one's life and dropping of activities and interests. GDS 30 scores of 0–9 are considered normal; 10–19 indicate mild depression; and 20–30, severe depression. For the GDS 15, 0–4 is considered normal; 5–8 suggests mild depression; 9–11, moderate depression; and 12–15 is severe depression.

A second well-known tool for depression screening is the *PHQ9*. This is a 9-item Likert format scale, with items scored 0–3 (not at all, several days, more than half the days, or nearly every day).[33] Major depression is diagnosed if 5 or more of the 9 depressive symptom criteria have been present at least "more than half the days" in the past 2 weeks, and one of the symptoms is depressed mood or anhedonia; other depression is diagnosed if 2, 3 or 4 depressive symptoms have been present at least "more than half the days" in the past 2 weeks, and one of the symptoms is depressed mood or anhedonia.[33] The *PHQ9* can be easily self-administered and also exists in multiple abbreviated forms, the shortest being the *PHQ2*.[34] Like the GDS, the PHQ versions have acceptable reliability and validity.

SCREENING FOR STRESS-RELATED CONDITIONS

With the variety of accessible screening tools to identify stress-related symptomology, the incorporation of screening and assessment into an exam for any older adult can be done with relative ease. A holistic approach to assessing the older adult is aligned with best practice recommendations, many of which entail the identification of stress and impaired coping. The US Preventive Services Task Force (USPSTF) provides recommendations targeting several stress-linked conditions and behaviors. These include smoking, elder abuse, anxiety and depression.

The USPSTF[35] recommends that clinicians ask all adults about tobacco use, advise them to stop using tobacco and provide behavioral interventions and US Food and Drug Administration-approved pharmacotherapy for cessation to nonpregnant adults who use tobacco. Specifically, clinicians should ask about tobacco use and provide behavioral interventions and pharmacotherapy for cessation to those who use tobacco. This recommendation is designated a grade A recommendation; there is high certainty that the net benefit is substantial.

However, the USPSTF[36] offers vague recommendations on elder abuse, concluding that the current evidence is insufficient to assess the balance of benefits and harm of screening for abuse and neglect in all older or vulnerable adults, which are surely stressors. They recognize risk factors for elder abuse include isolation, lack of social support; functional impairment, poor physical health; lower income, and living in a shared living environment with a large number of household members (other than a spouse) as being associated with an increased risk of financial and physical abuse. However, the USPSTF[36] found no valid, reliable screening tools in the primary care setting to identify abuse of older adults without recognizing signs and symptoms of abuse. Moreover, they report limited evidence, which suggests that screening is not commonly occurring in practice. However, there are a host of screening and assessment tools for the detection of elder abuse. The Hartford Institute for Geriatric Nursing[37] identifies the *Elder Assessment Instrument*[38] as one of the best tools for assessing elder abuse. This 41-item Likert format instrument has acceptable reliability and validity and is estimated to take 12–15 minutes to administer.

The USPSTF[39] concludes that the current evidence is insufficient to assess the balance of benefits and harm of screening for anxiety disorders in older adults, noting that few studies reported the accuracy of screening tools in older adults and that the evidence on screening tools in general adults was applicable to older adults. Furthermore, they recommend that health care professionals should use their judgment based on individual patient circumstances when determining whether to screen for anxiety disorders in adults 65 years or older, in the absence of evidence. Additional research evidence may bolster the case for anxiety screening in older adults.

USPSTF[40] recommends depression screening in all adults regardless of risk factors. This recommendation is rated at a level B, indicating high certainty that the net benefit is moderate or there is moderate certainty that the net benefit is moderate to substantial. Depression screening can be included in visits with an older adult, using one of the aforementioned tools. Since depression is a risk for suicide[41] and given the other risk factors in depression often present in older adults, depression screening is essential in older adults, who may not recognize depressive symptoms on their own. For these reasons, clinicians must be mindful of depression risk in this age group; older adults are often misdiagnosed and undertreated. Health care providers may mistake an older adult's depressive symptoms as just a natural reaction to illness or the life changes that may occur with aging, and therefore not see the depression as something to be treated.[25] Older adults themselves often share this belief and do not seek help because they do not understand that they could feel better with appropriate treatment.[25] Despite depression increasing suicide risk, the USPSTF[40] concludes that the current evidence is insufficient to assess the balance of benefits and harm of screening for suicide risk in the adult population, including older adults. The majority of older adults are not depressed; some estimates of major depression in community-dwelling older adults range from less than 1% to about 5% but rise to 13.5% in those who require home-health care and to 11.5% in hospitalized older adults (CDC, 2022a).[25]

LIFESTYLE MEDICINE PILLARS AND THEIR ASSOCIATION WITH STRESS AND STRESS MANAGEMENT

Consideration of the six pillars of lifestyle medicine (nutrition, physical activity, stress management, avoidance of risky substances, restorative sleep and social connections) is essential when working with any older adult.[42] Sleep reduces stress, which allows for the body to repair and replete cellular components necessary for biological functions that become depleted throughout an awake cycle.[43] Exercise and good nutrition improve nearly every aspect of health. All our activities are interconnected and work together to determine our overall health.[44] Caloric management, increased exercise, optimal sleep, stress reduction, avoidance/limited use of harmful substances (e.g., smoking, alcohol) and fostering social connections are recommended[44] for all age groups, but there is heightened importance of the pillars in older adults, who have altered sleep, decreased metabolism and chronic disease-related dietary restrictions (e.g., sodium restriction related to hypertension, etc.) and perhaps reduced social circles, all in the setting of the aging process. Jaqua et al.[42] also point out that the lifestyle management pillars target known modifiable risk factors for major neurocognitive impairment, asserting that simple interventions in the six pillars might prevent, delay and improve neurocognitive impairment. Baban and Morton[45] provide a comprehensive summary of the impact of lifestyle pillars on stress management.

AGE-RELATED SPECIAL CONSIDERATIONS

Dementia and sensory impairment are two potential age-related issues that clinicians should consider when addressing stress in older adults. Both can be identified and treated, and as such, warrant intervention. Anxiety seems to be more common in individuals living with dementia who still have good insight and awareness of their condition, and it can be particularly common in people with vascular or frontotemporal dementia, while it is less common in people with Alzheimer's disease.[46] Alzheimer's disease, the most common form of dementia, results in significant neuropsychiatric symptoms, including apathy, depression, anxiety, agitation, aggression and psychosis.[47] Depression and anxiety disorders are two of the most common neuropsychiatric symptoms in Alzheimer's disease, present in up to 75% of patients with this type of dementia.[48] In addition to feeling anxious persons living with dementia may feel tired, uneasy, irritable, struggle to concentrate and have physical symptoms (such as palpitations, shortness of breath, dizziness, nausea or diarrhea).[46] A person with dementia who has anxiety may also have changes in their behavior, such as restlessness, agitation or hoarding. They may constantly ask for reassurance and not want to be left alone. Or they may closely follow a caregiver or family member around. There are assessment tools and evidence-based interventions, discussed later, to target both anxiety and depression in persons living with dementia (PLWD).

Given the pervasive impact of anxiety on the quality of life in persons living with dementia, it is concerning that anxiety is frequently underdiagnosed and undertreated in this population.[49] The ability to recognize and self-report depressive or anxious symptoms may be impaired in the person living with dementia. Therefore, screening for both anxiety and depression in persons living with dementia is essential.

This can be done through the administration of the *Rating Anxiety in Dementia* (RAID)[50] and *Cornell Scale for Depression in Dementia*. The RAID is an 18-item scale with each item rated according to the person's symptoms and signs of anxiety over the previous 2 weeks. It is reasonably simple to administer and elicit responses from the person living with dementia and their caregiver to determine ratings.

A second useful assessment tool for persons living with dementia is the *Cornell Scale for Depression in Dementia* (CSDD).[51] Specifically developed to assess signs and symptoms of major depression in demented patients, and because some persons living with dementia may give unreliable reports, the CSDD uses a comprehensive interviewing approach that obtains information from the patient and the caregiver informant. Ratings of the CSDD items summed represent the clinician's clinical impression rather than the responses of the informant or the person living with dementia.[51]

Depending upon the severity of cognitive impairment, the person living with dementia may be able to participate in therapy, if assessment findings suggest significant anxiety or depression. *Problem Adaptation Therapy* (PATH) is a home-delivered therapy that aims to improve emotion regulation and reduce the negative impact of behavioral and functional limitations.[52] PATH's strategies aim to help with the regulation of emotions; situation selection, situation modification, attentional deployment, cognitive change and response modulation. To achieve emotion regulation, PATH integrates a problem-solving approach with compensatory strategies, environmental adaptations and caregiver participation.[52]

Outcomes from Kiosses et al.'s[52] 12-week randomized controlled trial with 74 persons living with dementia are promising; PATH participants had a significantly greater reduction in depression than control group participants, and in patients with pharmacotherapy-resistant depression, PATH participants had a significantly greater reduction in depression than control participants.

In a recent systematic review of research on the clinical effectiveness of psychological interventions in reducing depression and anxiety in people with dementia or mild cognitive impairment, Orgeta, et al.[53] appraised 29 randomized controlled trials that compared a psychological intervention for depression or anxiety with treatment as usual or another control condition in people with dementia or mild cognitive impairment. They concluded that cognitive behavioral therapies were probably slightly better than treatment as usual or control conditions for decreasing depressive symptoms, and they may also increase rates of depression remission at the end of treatment. Furthermore, they concluded that cognitive behavioral therapies probably improve patient quality of life and activities of daily living at the end of treatment compared to treatment as usual or active control. However, their meta-analysis revealed that supportive and counseling interventions may have little or no effect on depressive symptoms in people with dementia compared to usual care at the end of treatment. In contrast, Sukhawathanakul et al.'s[54] systematic review of nine studies found support for the effectiveness of psychotherapeutic interventions on improving acceptance and adjustment in older adults with cognitive impairment, particularly with regard to reducing depressive symptoms.

Other therapeutic recommendations include encouraging the person living with dementia (PLWD) to talk about their worries or fears; remaining physically active, including group activities such as dancing or singing; maintaining a healthy diet;[46] and aerobic exercise, meditation and relaxation therapy.[55] Ding et al.[56] conducted a systematic review of 67 studies investigating lifestyle medicine interventions for PLWD. They concluded that because there were only two studies on the effect of mindfulness, and these two studies varied largely in the intervention protocol and participant characteristics, it may not be possible to draw a concrete conclusion about mindfulness for stress management at this point, and that more evidence on lifestyle interventions involving stress management, emotional well-being, and healthy dietary patterns is needed to provide support for the intervention effect on cognitive functions in people with MCI and dementia. Similarly, Forbes et al.'s[57] meta-analysis of seventeen trials with 1,067 participants revealed no evidence of benefit from exercise on cognition, neuropsychiatric symptoms, or depression.

Recommendations for pharmacological intervention for individuals living with dementia are varied. Of utmost concern is the mitigation of troublesome symptoms while avoiding harmful adverse effects. For patients with depression and/or anxiety, Budson[55] advises using low doses of sertraline or escitalopram, both of which he asserts improve depression, anxiety, and often irritability and agitation as well. For patients with depression and apathy, venlafaxine and bupropion can be beneficial in treating both symptoms; however, Budson[55] warns that these stimulating antidepressants can worsen anxiety, so they should be avoided in individuals with anxiety.

The most common treatment for anxiety and agitation is low doses of atypical antipsychotic medications such as risperidone and olanzapine.[57] However, the drugs may increase the risk of strokes, heart attacks and death in older people. Furthermore, anti-anxiety drugs such as diazepam can lead to dizziness and falls in older people. Antidepressants can often help.[58] One clinical trial at Johns Hopkins evaluating the use of the antidepressant citalopram in people with Alzheimer's and anxiety found that it was safer and at least as effective as currently used antipsychotic drugs. Medications such as lorazepam, oxazepam and alprazolam can also help treat anxiety in persons living with dementia.[59] Any psychotropic medication should be used judiciously, and include thorough caregiver education on administration and management as well as side effects.

CONCLUSIONS

This chapter provides an appraisal and recommendations related to the identification and management of stress in older adults. Population projections for this age group and epidemiological trends underscore the criticality of clinician understanding and consideration of psychological and physiological effects and features associated with stress. For adequate problem identification, clinicians should also utilize screening tools designated for this age group, as their manifestation of stress may differ slightly in older adults. Further research is needed to examine ways to inform and educate clinicians about these stress-related issues, suggesting how these factors potentially undermine careful clinical analysis and subsequent treatment and potentially cause reluctance in older persons to seek help.

CLINICAL APPLICATIONS

- Consider administering brief screening tools such as the Perceived Stress Scale to help with the detection of stress in older adults.
- Be cognizant of physical signs and symptoms such as panic attacks and dyspnea; these could be evidence of a pathophysiologic process *or* signs of stress.
- Ask about and assess for stress-related conditions, including tobacco use, elder abuse, anxiety and depression.
- Involve caregivers and utilize dementia-specific screening tools to detect stress and stress-related conditions in persons living with dementia.

REFERENCES

1. World Health Organization. Stress. WHO. Int. 2023. Accessed February 16, 2024. https://www.who.int/news-room/questions-and-answers/item/stress#:~:text=Stress%20can%20be%20defined%20as,experiences%20stress%20to%20some%20degree.
2. World Health Organization. Mental health of older adults. WHO Int. 2017. Accessed February 16, 2024. https://www.who.int/news-room/fact-sheets/detail/mental-health-of-older-adults.
3. Elflein J. Percentage of older adults in the U.S. who felt depressed, stressed, or nervous for several days or more within the past two weeks as of January 2021. *Statista.com*. 2023. Accessed September 4, 2023. https://www.statista.com/statistics/1253613/us-older-adults-feeling-stressed-anxious-or-depressed/.
4. Brown LL, Mitchell UA, Ailshire JA. Disentangling the stress process: race/ethnic differences in the exposure and appraisal of chronic stressors among older adults. *J Gerontol B Psychol Sci Soc Sci*. 2020;75(3):650–660. doi:10.1093/geronb/gby072.
5. Kiely KM, Brady B, Byles J. Gender, mental health and ageing. *Maturitas*. 2019;129:76–84. doi:10.1016/j.maturitas.2019.09.004.
6. Godman H. Stress relief tips for older adults. *Health.Harvard.edu*. 2017. Accessed February 17, 2024. https://www.health.harvard.edu/stress/stress-relief-tips-for-older-adults.
7. National Council on Aging. Stress and how to reduce it: a guide for older adults. *NCOA.org*. 2023. Accessed September 4, 2023. https://www.ncoa.org/article/stress-and-how-to-reduce-it-a-guide-for-older-adults.
8. Brennan D. What to know about mental health in older adults. *WebMD*. 2021. Accessed September 4, 2023. https://www.webmd.com/healthy-aging/mental-health-in-older-adults.
9. Mental Health America. Anxiety in older adults. *mhanational.org*. 2023. Accessed September 4, 2023. https://www.mhanational.org/anxiety-olderadults#:~:text=Anxiety%20in%20older%20adults%20may,Overall%20feelings%20of%20poor%20health.
10. Bhandari S. The effects of stress on your body. *WebMD*. 2021. Accessed September 4, 2023. https://www.webmd.com/balance/stress-management/effects-of-stress-on-your-body#:~:text=Forty%2Dthree%20percent%20of%20all,adverse%20health%20effects%20from%20stress.
11. Broudy O. What stress does to the body after 50. *AARP*. 2023. Accessed September 4, 2023. https://www.aarp.org/health/healthy-living/info-2023/how-stress-affects-your-health-after50.html#:~:text=Stress%20response%20%231%3A%20The%20hormone%20flood%20%EF%BB%BF&text=Studies%20show%20that%20cortisol%20affects,do%20something%20like%20climb%20stairs.

12. Kaiser Permanente Medicine. Stressed out? Too much stress, cortisol can hurt your body. *Mydoctor.kaiserpermanente.org.* 2023. Accessed September 4, 2023. https://mydoctor.kaiserpermanente.org/mas/news/stressed-out-too-much-stress-cortisol-can-hurt-your-body-2218210.
13. Mikneviciute G, Ballhausen N, Rimmele U, Kliegel M. Does older adults' cognition particularly suffer from stress? A systematic review of acute stress effects on cognition in older age. *Neurosci Biobehav Rev.* 2022;132:583–602. doi:10.1016/j.neubiorev.2021.12.009.
14. Kulshreshtha A, Alonso A, McClure LA, Hajjar I, Manly JJ, Judd S. Association of stress with cognitive function among older Black and White US adults. *JAMA Netw Open.* 2023;6(3):e231860. doi:10.1001/jamanetworkopen.2023.1860.
15. Cohen S, Williamson G. Perceived stress in a probability sample of the United States. 1988 In: Spacapan S, Oskamp S, editors, *The Social Psychology of Health.* Sage.
16. Cohen S. Perceived stress scale. *Mindgarden.com.* 1994. Accessed May 6, 2024. https://www.mindgarden.com/documents/PerceivedStressScale.pdf.
17. Ezzati A, Jiang J, Katz MJ, Sliwinski MJ, Zimmerman ME, Lipton RB. Validation of the Perceived Stress Scale in a community sample of older adults. *Int J Geriatr Psychiatry.* 2014;29(6):645–652. doi:10.1002/gps.4049.
18. Holmes TH, Rahe RH. The Social Readjustment Rating Scale. *J Psychosom Res.* 1967;11(2):213–218. doi:10.1016/0022-3999(67)90010-4.
19. American Institute of Stress. The Holmes Rahe Stress Inventory. *Stress.org.* 2023. Accessed September 11, 2023. https://www.stress.org/holmes-rahe-stress-inventory.
20. Mizuno A, Andreescu C. Anxiety in late life. 2019. *Synergies.* Fall 2019. Accessed September 12, 2023. https://www.upmcphysicianresources.com/-/media/physicianresources/pdf-publications/psychiatry/synergies--fall-2019_final.pdf?la=en.
21. Taylor JA. A personality scale of manifest anxiety. *J Abnorm Psychol.* 1953;48(2):285–290. doi:10.1037/h0056264.
22. Balsamo M, Cataldi F, Carlucci L, Fairfield B. Assessment of anxiety in older adults: a review of self-report measures. *Clin Interv Aging.* 2018;13:573–593. Published 2018 Apr 6. doi:10.2147/CIA.S114100.
23. Segal DL, June A, Payne M, Coolidge FL, Yochim B. Development and initial validation of a self-report assessment tool for anxiety among older adults: the Geriatric Anxiety Scale. *J Anxiety Disord.* 2010;24(7):709–714. doi:10.1016/j.janxdis.2010.05.002.
24. Pachana NA, Byrne GJ, Siddle H, Koloski N, Harley E, Arnold E. Development and validation of the Geriatric Anxiety Inventory. *Int Psychogeriatr.* 2007;19(1):103–114. doi:10.1017/S1041610206003504.
25. Centers for Disease Control. Depression is not a normal part of growing older. *CDC.gov.* 2022a. Accessed March 9, 2024. https://www.cdc.gov/aging/depression/index.html#:~:text=Older%20adults%20are%20at%20increased,or%20whose%20function%20becomes%20limited.
26. Ju Y, Liu T, Zhang K, Lin X, Zheng E, Leng J. The relationship between comprehensive geriatric assessment parameters and depression in elderly patients. *Front Aging Neurosci.* 2022;14:936024. doi:10.3389/fnagi.2022.936024.
27. O'Connor E, Henninger M, Perdue LA, et al. *Screening for depression, anxiety, and suicide risk in adults: a systematic evidence review for the U.S. Preventive Services Task Force* [Internet]. Agency for Healthcare Research and Quality (US); 2023 June (Evidence Synthesis, No. 223). https://www.ncbi.nlm.nih.gov/books/NBK592805/.
28. Lamers F, van Oppen P, Comijs HC, et al. Comorbidity patterns of anxiety and depressive disorders in a large cohort study: the Netherlands Study of Depression and Anxiety (NESDA). *J Clin Psychiatry.* 2011;72(3):341–348. doi:10.4088/JCP.10m06176blu.

29. Grover S, Sahoo S, Chakrabarti S, Avasthi A. Anxiety and somatic symptoms among elderly patients with depression. *Am J Psychiatry*. 2019;41:66–72. doi:10.1016/j.ajp.2018.07.009.
30. National Institute on Aging. Depression and older adults. 2021. Accessed December 18, 2023. https://www.nia.nih.gov/health/mental-and-emotional-health/depression-and-older-adults#signs.
31. Yesavage JA, Brink TL, Rose TL, et al. Development and validation of a geriatric depression screening scale: a preliminary report. *J Psychiatr Res*. 1982;17(1):37–49. doi:10.1016/0022-3956(82)90033-4.
32. Sheikh JI, Yesavage JA. Geriatric Depression Scale: recent evidence and development of a shorter version. *Clin Gerontol*. 1986;5:165–173.
33. Kroenke K, Spitzer RL, Williams JB. The PHQ-9: validity of a brief depression severity measure. *J Gen Intern Med*. 2001;16(9):606–613. doi:10.1046/j.1525-1497.2001.016009606.x.
34. American Psychological Association. Patient health questionnaire (PHQ-9 & PHQ-2). *APA.org*. 2022. Accessed December 19, 2023. https://www.apa.org/pi/about/publications/caregivers/practice-settings/assessment/tools/patient-health.
35. U.S. Preventive Services Taskforce. Tobacco smoking cessation in adults, including pregnant persons: interventions. *uspreventiveservicestaskforce.org*. 2021. Accessed December 20, 2023. https://www.uspreventiveservicestaskforce.org/uspstf/recommendation/tobacco-use-in-adults-and-pregnant-women-counseling-and-interventions.
36. U.S. Preventive Services Taskforce. Intimate partner violence, elder abuse, and abuse of vulnerable adults: screening. *uspreventiveservicestaskforce.org*. 2023c. Accessed December 20, 2023. https://www.uspreventiveservicestaskforce.org/uspstf/recommendation/intimate-partner-violence-and-abuse-of-elderly-and-vulnerable-adults-screening.
37. Hartford Institute for Geriatric Nursing. Try this: elder mistreatment assessment. 2019. Accessed December 21, 2023. https://hign.org/consultgeri/try-this-series/elder-mistreatment-assessment.
38. Fulmer TT, Cahill VM. Assessing elder abuse: a study. *J Gerontol Nurs*. 1984;10(12):16–20. doi:10.3928/0098-9134-19841201-06.
39. U.S. Preventive Services Taskforce. Anxiety disorders in adults: screening. *uspreventiveservicestaskforce.org*. 2023a. Accessed February 17, 2024. https://www.uspreventiveservicestaskforce.org/uspstf/recommendation/anxiety-adults-screening.
40. U.S. Preventive Services Taskforce. Depression and suicide risk in adults: screening. *uspreventiveservicestaskforce.org*. 2023b. Accessed December 27, 2023. https://www.uspreventiveservicestaskforce.org/uspstf/recommendation/screening-depression-suicide-risk-adults.
41. Centers for Disease Control. Risk and protective factors. *CDC.gov*. 2022b. Accessed December 21, 2023. https://www.cdc.gov/suicide/factors/index.html.
42. Jaqua E, Biddy E, Moore C, Browne G. The impact of the six pillars of lifestyle medicine on brain health. *Cureus*. 2023;15(2):e34605. doi:10.7759/cureus.34605.
43. Brinkman JE, Reddy V, Sharma S. Physiology of sleep. [Updated 2023 Apr 3]. In: *StatPearls* [Internet]. StatPearls Publishing; 2024 January. https://www.ncbi.nlm.nih.gov/books/NBK482512/.
44. American Institute of Stress. Live better by building on the six pillars of health. *Stress.org*. 2023. Accessed March 7, 2024. https://www.stress.org/live-better-by-building-on-the-six-pillars-of-health.
45. Baban KA, Morton DP. Lifestyle medicine and stress management. *J Fam Pract*. 2022;71(Suppl 1 Lifestyle):S24–S29. doi:10.12788/jfp.0285.

46. Alzheimers Society. Anxiety and dementia. *Alzheimers.org.* 2023. Accessed December 28, 2023. https://www.alzheimers.org.uk/about-dementia/symptoms-and-diagnosis/anxiety-dementia.
47. Mendez MF. The relationship between anxiety and Alzheimer's disease. *J Alzheimers Dis Rep.* 2021;5(1):171–177. doi:10.3233/ADR-210294.
48. Sturm VE, Yokoyama JS, Seeley WW, Kramer JH, Miller BL, Rankin KP. Heightened emotional contagion in mild cognitive impairment and Alzheimer's disease is associated with temporal lobe degeneration. *Proc Natl Acad Sci U S A.* 2013;110(24):9944–9949. doi:10.1073/pnas.1301119110.
49. Goodarzi Z, Samii L, Azeem F, et al. Detection of anxiety symptoms in persons with dementia: a systematic review. *Alzheimers Dement (Amst).* 2019;11:340–347. doi:10.1016/j.dadm.2019.02.005.
50. Shankar KK, Walker M, Frost D, Orrell MW. The development of a valid and reliable scale for rating anxiety in dementia (RAID). *Aging Ment Health.* 1999;3(1):39–49.
51. Alexopoulos GS, Abrams RC, Young RC, Shamoian CA. Cornell Scale for Depression in Dementia. *Biol Psychiatry.* 1988;23(3):271–284. doi:10.1016/0006-3223(88)90038-8.
52. Kiosses DN, Ravdin LD, Gross JJ, Raue P, Kotbi N, Alexopoulos GS. Problem adaptation therapy for older adults with major depression and cognitive impairment: a randomized clinical trial. *JAMA Psychiatry.* 2015;72(1):22–30. doi:10.1001/jamapsychiatry.2014.1305.
53. Orgeta V, Leung P, Del-Pino-Casado R, et al. Psychological treatments for depression and anxiety in dementia and mild cognitive impairment. *Cochrane Database Syst Rev.* 2022;4(4):CD009125. doi:10.1002/14651858.CD009125.pub3.
54. Sukhawathanakul P, Crizzle A, Tuokko H, Naglie G, Rapoport MJ. Psychotherapeutic interventions for dementia: a systematic review. *Can Geriatr J.* 2021;24(3):222–236. doi:10.5770/cgj.24.447.
55. Budson AE. How to treat anxiety and depression in people with dementia. *Psychology Today.* 2019. Accessed December 31, 2023. https://www.psychologytoday.com/us/blog/managing-your-memory/201903/how-treat-anxiety-and-depression-in-people-dementia.
56. Ding Z, Leung PY, Lee TL, Chan AS. Effectiveness of lifestyle medicine on cognitive functions in mild cognitive impairments and dementia: a systematic review on randomized controlled trials. *Ageing Res Rev.* 2023;86:101886. doi:10.1016/j.arr.2023.101886.
57. Forbes D, Forbes SC, Blake CM, Thiessen EJ, Forbes S. Exercise programs for people with dementia. *Cochrane Database of System Rev.* 2015;CD006489. doi:10.1002/14651858.CD006489.pub4. Accessed March 10, 2024.
58. Johns Hopkins Medicine. Beyond memory loss: how to handle the other symptoms of Alzheimer's. *Hopkinsmedicine.org.* 2023. Accessed December 31, 2023. https://www.hopkinsmedicine.org/health/conditions-and-diseases/alzheimers-disease/beyond-memory-loss-how-to-handle-the-other-symptoms-of-alzheimers.
59. Olopaade J, Fletcher J. What are the first-line medications to treat anxiety in those living with dementia? *Medical News Today.* 2022. Accessed January 2, 2024. https://www.medicalnewstoday.com/articles/best-anti-anxiety-medication-for-older-adults--with-dementia.

14 Toxins and Older Adults

Kaku Kuroda

INTRODUCTION

Avoiding harmful toxins is pivotal in enhancing overall well-being and constitutes a crucial aspect of lifestyle medicine. Among the various toxins that significantly impact the quality of life for older adults, this chapter will center on three major ones: alcohol, tobacco and cannabis.

ALCOHOL

Enjoying a glass of beer to relax after a tiring day, savoring a glass of wine during delightful conversations with friends or relishing a cocktail to enhance a meal – when managed prudently, alcohol can color life's experiences. Nonetheless, excessive alcohol intake can result in diverse health issues. These range from immediate concerns, such as experiencing a hangover due to overindulgence, to long-term complications such as liver cirrhosis stemming from prolonged heavy drinking. In this section, we will delve into evidence-based strategies for older adults in managing alcohol consumption.

EPIDEMIOLOGY

The University of Michigan National Poll on Healthy Aging conducted a survey in 2021 among 2,074 adults aged 50–80 who consumed alcohol. It revealed that while the majority drank at low to moderate levels, 27% acknowledged having consumed alcohol at a heavy level on at least one occasion in the past year, with 7% reporting experiencing alcohol-related blackouts.[1] In a separate study involving 1,705 community-dwelling men aged 70 years or older in Sydney, Australia, findings showed a prevalence of 33.7% in daily drinking, 19.2% in heavy/excessive drinking and 14.1% in binge drinking.[2] Although binge drinking is more common in younger age groups compared to older adults, the National Survey on Drug Use and Health in 2021 found that roughly 20% of adults aged 60–64 and approximately 11% of those over 65 reported current binge drinking.[3]

APPROPRIATE AMOUNT OF ALCOHOL CONSUMPTION

How are binge drinking or heavy drinking defined? It is recommended to choose not to drink or limit intake to two drinks or less in a day for men and one drink or less in a day for women when alcohol is consumed, according to the dietary

TABLE 14.1
Amount That Is Equal to One Drink

Type of Beverage	Amount (ounces)
Beer, Ale, Wine Cooler	12
Malt Liquor	8
Wine	5
Distilled Liquor	1.5

guidelines developed by the US Department of Health and Human Services and the US Department of Agriculture.[4]

- For women – one drink or less in a day
- For men – two drinks or less in a day

One drink is equal to the amount shown in Table 14.1.

If an individual consumes wine regularly with dinner, the recommended moderate intake, as per guidelines, is typically considered as no more than two glasses of five ounces of wine for men and one glass for women. This difference is primarily due to how alcohol is metabolized. When a woman and a man of the same weight consume an equal amount of alcohol, the woman's blood alcohol concentration tends to be higher. This occurs because alcohol distributes itself uniformly in body water, and pound for pound, women have proportionally less body water than men.

The patterns below are considered "heavy" drinking,[5,6] which markedly increases the likelihood of alcohol use disorder and other alcohol-related harm:

- For women – 4 or more drinks on any day or 8 or more per week
- For men – 5 or more drinks on any day or 15 or more per week

The risk for alcohol-related harm also depends on a combination of how much, how fast and how often a person drinks. Excessive and rapid alcohol consumption poses significant problems. When a woman consumes four or more drinks, or a man consumes five or more drinks within about 2 hours, this elevation in alcohol intake typically raises the serum alcohol concentration to 0.08% or higher, meeting the criteria for binge drinking.[5] Binge drinking is accountable for more than half of the alcohol-related deaths in the United States, increasing the risk of several adverse outcomes, including but not limited to falls, motor vehicle accidents, memory blackouts, interactions with medications, assaults, drownings and overdose deaths.[7]

THE IMPACT OF ALCOHOL IN OLDER ADULTS: ACUTE AND CHRONIC

The impact of drinking alcohol on the health of the geriatric population, both acute and chronic, is significant. Some of the acute and chronic effects for older adults include the following.

Acute Effects[8,9]
- Increased sensitivity to alcohol leads to a higher risk of falls, motor vehicle accidents and other unintentional injuries.
- Adverse interactions with medications can be dangerous or even deadly when mixed with alcohol. This is more significant in older adults because of age-related physiological changes, such as increased body fat, decreased body water content, decreased liver size and liver blood flow, as well as a higher likelihood of being on multiple medications due to multiple medical conditions.

Chronic Effects[8-11]
- Exacerbation of health problems commonly experienced by older adults, such as diabetes, high blood pressure, congestive heart failure, liver issues, osteoporosis, memory issues and mood disorders
- Increased risk of developing new heart and liver problems, osteoporosis and mood disorders
- For cognitive function, heavy drinking is known as a significant risk factor for dementia.[12] In a cohort study, after excluding past drinkers and individuals with a history of poor health status and diseases, there was an elevated risk of incident dementia in heavy drinkers.[13] This implies that healthier individuals should also exercise caution regarding the potential risk of developing dementia. It suggests that being in better health doesn't necessarily guarantee immunity from the risks associated with alcohol consumption and dementia. Interestingly, within this cohort study, a correlation was found between light-to-moderate alcohol consumption and a reduced risk of dementia. The explanation provided was that individuals who engage in light-to-moderate drinking may have stronger social connections or social bonding, which, in turn, could contribute to a decreased risk of developing dementia.

Other Adverse Neurological Effects[10]
- Orthostasis.
- Myopathy, impaired muscle strength.
- Peripheral neuropathy causing numbness or tingling sensation.
- Cerebellar damage, causing the classically described wide-based ataxic gait.
- Other detrimental effects on gait and balance.

Considerations for Older Adults

Older adults have to be more cautious than young adults about drinking alcohol. This is due to physiological changes, health conditions, medication interactions and impacts of falls and injuries.

- *Physiological changes*: With advancing age, the body undergoes alterations that affect alcohol metabolism. Older adults typically experience a reduced ability to metabolize alcohol due to changes in liver function and decreased body water content. This can lead to higher blood alcohol concentrations and heightened sensitivity to alcohol's effects in older age.

- *Health conditions*: Older adults often have pre-existing health issues such as liver disease, cardiovascular problems and age-related cognitive decline. Alcohol consumption can exacerbate these conditions or interfere with commonly prescribed medications. Thus, it is vital to consider individual health circumstances when contemplating alcohol intake.

- *Medication interactions*: Older adults frequently take several medications for chronic diseases such as high blood pressure, diabetes and arrhythmias. Some medications interact adversely with alcohol, including over-the-counter drugs such as cold and allergy medications, sleep aids and pain relievers. It is advisable to consult a doctor or pharmacist regarding any concerns or inquiries about potential drug interactions.

- *Impact of falls and injuries*: Older adults face a heightened risk of falls and injuries due to factors such as balance issues and decreased bone density. Alcohol further impairs coordination and balance, increasing the likelihood of falls and injuries among this demographic. Falls in older adults can result in severe consequences, such as fractures or head trauma, leading to higher morbidity and mortality rates compared to younger, healthier adults. For instance, a femoral neck fracture in an older adult carries greater health risks than in younger individuals.

ABSTINENCE VERSUS MODERATE ALCOHOL

The longstanding belief that moderate drinking (less than two drinks per day for men, one drink per day for women) might offer certain health benefits has been challenged by newer data. Recent studies indicate that the level of alcohol intake that minimizes the risk of death and disability-adjusted life years is actually **zero** alcohol consumption. Several research studies support this notion, highlighting a shift in the understanding of the potential health effects of alcohol.

In 2017, a significant study examined the link between alcohol consumption and mortality risk in a cohort of 333,247 adults in the United States. The findings suggested that compared to individuals who abstained from alcohol throughout their lives, those who engaged in light or moderate alcohol consumption showed a reduced risk of mortality across all causes, including cardiovascular disease.[14] This contributed to the perception that light or moderate drinking might be superior to abstaining from alcohol, leading some health care providers to recommend moderate alcohol intake.[15] However, subsequent researchers raised concerns regarding this study's methodology. They highlighted that the initial findings might have assumed a higher mortality rate among non-drinkers compared to light drinkers without considering that some individuals might have previously consumed excessive amounts of alcohol and stopped due to health issues rather than merely being lifelong abstainers.[16] Adjusting for this factor in the analysis revealed that abstainers actually exhibited a lower mortality risk. As a result, the recommendation for casual drinking as a means to reduce mortality risk has shifted. Subsequent considerations and analyses have led to the conclusion that abstaining from alcohol might actually confer a lower mortality risk compared to light or moderate drinking. Consequently, the idea of promoting casual alcohol consumption to reduce mortality is no longer supported.[17]

Alcohol metabolism primarily occurs in the liver through two key enzymes that facilitate the breakdown of alcohol. However, certain genetic variations can lead to weaker enzyme activity, notably observed in some Japanese individuals.[18] This results in rapid intoxication, accompanied by symptoms such as nausea and vomiting, as the unprocessed alcohol is converted into a harmful toxin known as acetaldehyde. A global research effort focused on individuals with genetic differences affecting one of these enzymes aimed to investigate whether those with reduced alcohol tolerance due to gene mutations might have a lower risk of cardiovascular diseases such as heart attacks or strokes. The study found that individuals carrying this gene mutation tended to consume less alcohol and displayed lower levels of blood pressure and non-HDL cholesterol.[19] Moreover, they exhibited a reduced risk of experiencing a heart attack compared to individuals without this mutation. These findings suggest a potential link between reduced alcohol consumption, particularly among individuals with genetic variations affecting alcohol metabolism, and improved cardiovascular health. Even for individuals classified as light to moderate drinkers, reducing alcohol intake could potentially benefit cardiovascular health outcomes, as observed in this research study.

Thus, for people who drink alcohol or those who are thinking about starting drinking because they believe an appropriate amount of alcohol provides health benefits, drinking is **not** recommended because there is no health benefit of adding alcohol. Based on current scientific evidence, **zero** alcohol is better than any amount of alcohol consumption for our health. However, we know that occasional alcohol may provide some color in our lives, such as a holiday dinner with precious family or close friends, celebrations for anniversaries or achievements, exploring new beverages while traveling and so on. Assessing risk involves asking a person "what matters the most." If it is health, being abstinent from alcohol would be preferable. If it is a balance between health and leisure, one can consider maintaining an appropriate amount of alcohol intake depending on health conditions.

Is It Too Late to Quit?

Quitting alcohol, even after years of regular consumption, can have significant health benefits for older adults as follows:

- Abstaining from alcohol can significantly reduce the risk of further liver damage and all-cause mortality.[20]

- Ceasing alcohol intake can lead to improvements in blood pressure.[21]
- Quitting alcohol can lower the risk of developing cancer and potentially decrease cancer-related mortality rates.[22,23] In these studies, cancer risk increased 2 years after quitting due to residual effects of past alcohol consumption. But, cancer risk will drop gradually when quitting is sustained.

So, it is never too late to quit drinking to improve health outcomes!

TOBACCO

Tobacco offers no health benefits and is associated with numerous adverse effects. While some may believe that it is too late to quit smoking, it is not. Multiple studies have demonstrated that stopping smoking can bring significant health advantages regardless of age. This section will examine the evidence for how older adults can address smoking.

Epidemiology

In 2021, the percentage of adults aged 65 years and older who were current smokers in the United States stood at 8.3%.[24] Age-adjusted prevalence of current smoking was 14.99% in participants aged 65–74, 7.79% in participants aged 75–84 and 2.78% in participants aged 85 or older.[25] Although the prevalence of smoking is higher in adults under 65 years old compared to older age groups, we cannot simply compare the percentage to think about the impacts on their health because there are many older adults who were heavy smokers and quit for some reason (e.g., severe lung disease).

Negative Effects on Health

While the adverse effects of smoking on health are widely recognized, this summary highlights the extensive range of detrimental health consequences associated with smoking.

- *Lung effects*: Smoking is strongly linked to chronic lung conditions such as chronic obstructive pulmonary disease (COPD), emphysema and chronic bronchitis. These conditions often lead to persistent coughing, excessive sputum production, shortness of breath, dyspnea on exertion and an increased susceptibility to respiratory infections.[26]
- *Heart effects*: Smoking significantly elevates the risk of cardiovascular diseases among older adults, including heart attacks.[27]
- *Vascular diseases, including stroke*: "The more people smoke, the more people stroke," as shown in multiple studies.[28,29] These health issues significantly impact mobility and quality of life in later life.
- *Cancer risks*: Smoking substantially elevates the risk of lung cancer, which stands as the leading cause of smoking-related death among older adults.[30]

Additionally, smoking is responsible for millions of cases of other cancers, including those affecting the mouth, throat, nose, sinuses, esophagus, larynx, stomach, pancreas, liver, kidney, colon, rectum, bladder, cervix and blood-related cancers such as acute myeloid leukemia.[31]
- *Memory issues*: These changes in memory are more likely to occur in older adults.[32] Studies indicate a correlation between smoking and an increased risk of dementia and Alzheimer's disease in older adults.[33] Quitting smoking can aid in preventing these conditions. For individuals already affected by dementia or Alzheimer's disease, ceasing smoking might potentially decelerate the progression of these conditions.[33]
- *Bone health*: Smoking is associated with bone loss[34] and increases the risk of hip fracture.[35,36] If smokers have hip fractures, they are more likely to die than non-smokers.[37]
- *Shortening life expectancy*: Smoking is associated with a reduced life expectancy across all age groups, including older adults.[38]

CHANGES IN RECOMMENDATIONS WITH AGING

Quitting smoking is recommended regardless of age, as numerous studies highlight the significant health benefits associated with smoking cessation at any stage of life.[30,39–42] It is never too late to quit.

Upon quitting smoking, immediate benefits become evident. Within 20 minutes, blood pressure and heart rate fall. Improved lung function ensues over 2 to 3 weeks, facilitated by enhanced blood circulation. By the 1-month mark after quitting, improvements in coughing and shortness of breath become noticeable, accompanied by a reduction in mucus and sputum due to the recovery of lung cilia, which aids in moving mucus out of the lungs.[43]

A comprehensive study conducted in Germany revealed that the risk of experiencing a heart attack significantly decreases within 5 years after quitting smoking.[40] According to this study's findings, a 60-year-old current smoker faces a heart attack risk equivalent to that of a 79-year-old individual who has never smoked, if the smoker continues smoking (based on an estimated risk advancement period of 19.3 years). Moreover, the risk of developing cancers of the mouth, throat and larynx will be halved 5 to 10 years after quitting, while the risk of lung cancer will be approximately half that of an individual who continues to smoke, observed within 10 to 15 years after quitting.[43] These may sound like long timeframes, but the impact is tremendous in the long run to live healthier.

Quitting smoking before the age of 40 substantially diminishes the risk of death linked to persistent smoking by roughly 90%.[38] Even among individuals aged 55–64, ceasing smoking extended life expectancy by up to 4 years.[38] Furthermore, these reductions in risk are influenced by the quantity of smoking, demonstrating a dose-dependent relationship.[39] It is important to note that the risk continues to decline progressively with time following smoking cessation.

Apart from the evident health benefits, individuals who quit smoking stand to save money and time, rid themselves of the smell associated with smoking, experience improved taste and smell sensations and encounter numerous other rewards upon breaking the habit of smoking. The sense of smell diminishes with age without smoking and declines considerably after age 70, so smokers are affected by the dual impacts of aging and tobacco. Quitting smoking is also essential to break the cycle of nicotine addiction, as nicotine elevates dopamine levels in the brain, impacting its reward and pleasure pathways.

AGE-SPECIFIC STRATEGY TO QUIT SMOKING

Generally, older individuals attempting to quit smoking are more likely to succeed in their efforts.[30] This trend may stem from personal insights or self-motivation garnered from firsthand experience of the symptoms or consequences associated with long-term tobacco use. Consequently, health care providers should actively encourage older smokers to quit regardless of age, as it can lead to a positive behavioral change, even after years of continuous smoking.

A study examining 8,332 older adults in the United States revealed that while two-thirds of them received advice from health care providers to quit smoking, just over one-third of those attempting to quit utilized evidence-based tobacco cessation treatments.[44] Additionally, only 1 in 20 individuals managed to quit smoking in the past year successfully. This study highlights the crucial role of health care professionals in supporting smoking cessation efforts by employing evidence-based tobacco cessation methods. These methods encompass various approaches such as one-on-one counseling or cessation clinics, support groups, FDA-approved cessation medications including nicotine replacement therapies (such as patches, gum or lozenges), nicotine nasal spray or inhaler, varenicline and bupropion.

Counseling holds significant importance since older smokers differ from younger smokers and tobacco users in terms of longer duration of use, poor awareness of the adverse effects and poor motivation.[45] Furthermore, the effectiveness of behavioral counseling is directly linked to its intensity, with a higher number of sessions and long-term follow-up correlating with increased success rates. It is essential for current smokers to maintain ongoing discussions with their doctor and persist in efforts to quit. Combining pharmacotherapy treatment with behavioral therapy can significantly enhance a patient's chances of success in quitting smoking.

Nicotine replacement therapy (NRT) stands as the most extensively used and researched pharmacotherapy for addressing nicotine dependence and withdrawal.[46] Various NRT options, including transdermal patches, nasal sprays, gums, lozenges and nicotine inhalers, have demonstrated effectiveness compared to placebos.[47] Varenicline and bupropion are two FDA-approved non-nicotine oral medications used in smoking cessation. Both varenicline and bupropion have shown superior efficacy compared to placebos over one year.[48,49] However, it is worth noting that some studies examining these pharmacotherapies excluded patients aged over 75.

Therefore, individual clinical judgment is crucial for physicians in determining the most suitable intervention strategies for older patients.

Some people may be concerned that smoking cessation may cause unhealthy weight gain. In the study investigating the impact of smoking cessation on blood vessels, it is reported that the function of blood vessels improved in people who quit smoking despite the fact that they gained weight significantly and ended up protecting their hearts and vessels despite weight gain.[50]

FUNCTIONAL AND COGNITIVE STATUS

Smoking can significantly impact physical functional status in various ways. For instance, smokers experiencing lung or heart-related problems that affect breathing may find themselves easily getting out of breath, leading to significant limitations in their range of physical activities. In the event of a stroke, smokers might face enduring paralysis, impacting their mobility and leading to lifelong disability. Furthermore, as smokers accumulate more medical conditions, they may face an increased reliance on daily medications, resulting in a higher pill burden. Managing multiple medications can raise concerns about potential side effects, further affecting overall well-being.

Smokers face an elevated risk of experiencing cognitive decline compared to non-smokers.[33] The risk of developing dementia is directly associated with the quantity of smoking, exhibiting a dose-dependent relationship. Additionally, there appears to be an interaction between high alcohol consumption and smoking, which further escalates the risk of dementia.[13] Moreover, smokers often engage in alcohol consumption, compounding various health risks, as previously discussed. Considering these factors is crucial in determining "what matters the most" for everyone in their later years, emphasizing the significance of addressing smoking and alcohol consumption for better health outcomes in later life.

CANNABIS (MARIJUANA)

In recent years, there has been a noticeable uptick in cannabis use among older adults nationwide. Diverse reasons, including perceived effects on mental and physical health, increased availability, and reduced stigma, drive this rise in usage. Cannabis comprises chemical compounds termed cannabinoids, chiefly THC (tetrahydrocannabinol) and CBD (cannabidiol). These compounds exert multifaceted influences on the brain and body. THC, when consumed, induces the sensation of being "high," altering an individual's cognitive, emotional or perceptual experiences. Conversely, CBD does not produce this high; instead, it is believed to offer calming or relaxing effects. Some individuals turn to CBD for potential health benefits, such as alleviating anxiety or aiding sleep. Cannabis consumption methods vary, encompassing smoking, vaping, ingestion through edibles such as brownies or gummies, or the use of oils or creams derived from cannabis extracts. This section aims to explore the fundamental aspects of cannabis use among older adults, delving into its diverse implications and considerations.

Epidemiology

In recent times, there has been a notable rise in the use of cannabis among older adults.[51] According to one study involving 14,896 respondents aged 65 years and older, the prevalence of past-year cannabis consumption in this age group significantly increased from 2.4% to 4.2% between 2015 and 2018.[51] Several key subgroups have experienced significant increases in cannabis usage, including women, individuals from diverse racial or ethnic backgrounds, those with higher family incomes and individuals dealing with mental health concerns. Notably, there has been a surge in cannabis consumption among older adults who also use alcohol. The risk associated with simultaneous use of both substances exceeds that of using either one alone. A study analyzing trends in alcohol and cannabis co-use following legalization in Washington State revealed marked increases in concurrent consumption of cannabis and alcohol among individuals aged 50 years and older.

Positive Impact of Medical Cannabis and Cannabinoids

There is some scientific evidence for the use of medical cannabis in adults, as follows.

- Both cannabinol (low THC) and THC exhibit moderate to substantial evidence in treating some types of pain.[52] The current evidence suggests that for every 24 patients treated with cannabinol for chronic or neuropathic pain, one patient may experience benefits (i.e., the number needed to treat = 24). Conversely, for every six patients treated with cannabinol, one patient might experience harm, denoted as the "number needed to harm" of six. This suggests that the potential harm from cannabinol treatment may outweigh the benefits. Although these compounds are used for various types of pain, there is no reported evidence supporting their effectiveness specifically for cancer pain.[53]
- Dronabinol, approved by the FDA, has substantial evidence supporting its use as an antiemetic for managing chemotherapy-induced nausea and vomiting.[54]
- Moderate evidence suggests that cannabinoids, particularly nabiximols, are an effective treatment to enhance short-term sleep outcomes in individuals experiencing sleep disturbance linked to obstructive sleep apnea syndrome, fibromyalgia, chronic pain and multiple sclerosis.[54]

Cannabinoid products are frequently utilized for conditions such as anxiety, depression and anorexia; however, the scientific evidence supporting their efficacy for these conditions remains insufficient based on previous studies.[54]

Negative Impact

The rate of cannabis-related emergency department (ED) visits has significantly increased among all age groups, including adults aged 65 and older, in California

TABLE 14.2
Cannabis-Related Disorders Defined in the DSM-5-TR

Disorder Type	Disorder Name
Acute disorder (typically lasting <24 hours)	Cannabis intoxication
Subacute disorders (lasting <1 month)	Cannabis-induced anxiety disorder
	Cannabis-induced psychotic disorder
	Cannabis-induced sleep disorder
	Cannabis-induced delirium
Cannabis withdrawal	
Cannabis use disorder	

between 2005 and 2019.[55] The overall rate escalated from 20.7 per 100,000 ED visits in 2005 to 395.0 per 100,000 ED visits in 2019, signifying an extraordinary 1804% relative increase.

There are cannabis-related disorders defined in the *Diagnostic and Statistical Manual of Mental Disorders*, Fifth Edition, Text Revision (DSM-5-TR) as shown in Table 14.2.

Other potential negative risks include the following:

- *Cognitive Function*: Concerns persist regarding the impact of cannabis on cognitive function in older adults. Studies have yielded conflicting results regarding the effects of long-term cannabis use on cognition and the potential risk of developing or worsening mental health conditions such as anxiety, depression or cognitive decline, particularly in vulnerable older populations.[56]
- *Fall Risk and Mobility Issues*: Cannabis, notably THC, has the potential to influence balance, coordination and reaction time, which might increase the risk of falls among older individuals.[57] Given that falls constitute a significant cause of morbidity in older adults, evaluating the influence of cannabis on fall risk remains crucial.

CAUTIONS WITH AGING

- *Dosing and Administration*: Age-related changes, such as decreased liver size and function, reduced body water and increased fat, may cause older adults to metabolize drugs differently. Establishing appropriate dosing strategies and administration methods for cannabis products in the geriatric population is crucial to minimize potential adverse effects while maximizing therapeutic benefits.
- *Sleep Disorders*: Cannabis is frequently utilized for its sedative effects and potential assistance in managing sleep disorders. However, further investigation is needed to understand the impact of cannabis on sleep architecture, sleep quality and the risk of dependence, especially among older adults.[58]

- *Driving*: Several studies indicate a significant association between marijuana use and motor vehicle accidents across all age groups.[59] Additionally, the enactment of medical cannabis laws in US states appears to be linked with increased instances of driving under the influence of cannabis.[60]

In older adults, current evidence suggests that cannabis use may be associated with higher rates of mental health issues, substance use and increased utilization of acute health care services.[61] Despite the rising trend of cannabis use among older adults, there is limited evidence supporting its use in this population. Additionally, a crucial reminder: *Don't drive under the influence of cannabis.*

CONCLUSIONS

This chapter underscores the importance of addressing harmful toxins, including alcohol, tobacco and cannabis, in enhancing the overall well-being of older adults. It highlights the prevalence of these substances among older populations, with notable findings indicating a significant proportion engaging in heavy alcohol consumption, smoking and a rising trend in cannabis use. Recommendations emphasize abstinence from alcohol and smoking to minimize multiple risks to our health and careful consideration of cannabis use due to potential negative impacts. The fewer toxins in later life, the better the impacts on both physical and cognitive function that affect to quality of life among older adults.

CLINICAL APPLICATIONS

- Both alcohol and tobacco can impact physical and cognitive function in older adults, so it is essential to devote more attention to discussing appropriate usage among older individuals who consume these substances. Health conditions, medication interactions, mobility and cognitive impairment must be carefully assessed.
- Refraining from alcohol consumption leads to better health outcomes than light to moderate use, based on current evidence. Considerations of how much alcohol to drink should be based on individual health conditions and health goals, ensuring a balanced approach.
- For both alcohol and tobacco, it is never too late to consider quitting since cessation can have significant health benefits at any stage of life.
- Cannabis use among older adults might be linked to higher rates of mental health concerns, substance abuse, cognitive decline, increased motor vehicle accidents and escalated utilization of acute health care services. Thus, discussions regarding cannabis use should be approached cautiously and in consultation with a health care professional.

REFERENCES

1. Alcohol Use among Older Adults. National poll on healthy aging. Accessed October 5, 2023. https://www.healthyagingpoll.org/reports-more/report/alcohol-use-among-older-adults
2. Ilomäki J, Gnjidic D, Le Couteur DG, et al. Alcohol consumption and tobacco smoking among community-dwelling older Australian men: the Concord Health and Ageing in Men Project. *Australas J Ageing*. 2014;33(3):185–192. doi:10.1111/ajag.12048
3. Older Adults. Accessed October 5, 2023. https://www.niaaa.nih.gov/alcohols-effects-health/alcohol-topics/older-adults
4. U.S. Department of Agriculture and U.S. Department of Health and Human Services. Dietary Guidelines for Americans, 2020–2025, 9th ed. https://www.dietaryguidelines.gov/sites/default/files/2020-12/Dietary_Guidelines_for_Americans_2020-2025.pdf
5. Drinking Levels Defined. Accessed December 15, 2023. https://www.niaaa.nih.gov/alcohol-health/overview-alcohol-consumption/moderate-binge-drinking
6. CDC. Excessive Alcohol Use. Centers for Disease Control and Prevention. Published February 21, 2023. Accessed December 15, 2023. https://www.cdc.gov/chronicdisease/resources/publications/factsheets/alcohol.htm
7. White AM, Tapert S, Shukla SD. Binge drinking. *Alcohol Res*. 2018;39(1):1–3. https://www.ncbi.nlm.nih.gov/pubmed/30557141
8. Older Adults. Accessed December 15, 2023. https://www.niaaa.nih.gov/alcohols-effects-health/alcohol-topics/older-adults
9. Facts about Aging and Alcohol. National Institute on Aging. Accessed December 15, 2023. https://www.nia.nih.gov/health/alcohol-misuse-or-alcohol-use-disorder/facts-about-aging-and-alcohol
10. Rigler SK. Alcoholism in the elderly. *Am Fam Physician*. 2000;61(6):1710–1716, 1883–1884, 1887–1888 passim. https://www.ncbi.nlm.nih.gov/pubmed/10750878
11. Di Federico S, Filippini T, Whelton PK, et al. Alcohol intake and blood pressure levels: a dose-response meta-analysis of nonexperimental cohort studies. *Hypertension*. 2023;80(10):1961–1969. doi:10.1161/HYPERTENSIONAHA.123.21224
12. Livingston G, Huntley J, Sommerlad A, et al. Dementia prevention, intervention, and care: 2020 report of the Lancet Commission. *Lancet*. 2020;396(10248):413–446. doi:10.1016/S0140-6736(20)30367-6
13. Kawakami S, Yamato R, Kitamura K, et al. Alcohol consumption, smoking, and risk of dementia in community-dwelling Japanese people aged 40–74 years: the Murakami Cohort Study. *Maturitas*. 2023;176:107788. doi:10.1016/j.maturitas.2023.107788
14. Xi B, Veeranki SP, Zhao M, Ma C, Yan Y, Mi J. Relationship of alcohol consumption to all-cause, cardiovascular, and cancer-related mortality in U.S. adults. *J Am Coll Cardiol*. 2017;70(8):913–922. doi:10.1016/j.jacc.2017.06.054
15. Rubin E. To drink or not to drink: that is the question. *Alcohol Clin Exp Res*. 2014;38(12):2889–2892. doi:10.1111/acer.12585
16. Fillmore KM, Stockwell T, Chikritzhs T, Bostrom A, Kerr W. Moderate alcohol use and reduced mortality risk: systematic error in prospective studies and new hypotheses. *Ann Epidemiol*. 2007;17(5 Suppl):S16–S23. doi:10.1016/j.annepidem.2007.01.005
17. Zhao J, Stockwell T, Naimi T, Churchill S, Clay J, Sherk A. Association between daily alcohol intake and risk of all-cause mortality: a systematic review and meta-analyses. *JAMA Netw Open*. 2023;6(3):e236185. doi:10.1001/jamanetworkopen.2023.6185
18. Shibuya A, Yoshida A. Genotypes of alcohol-metabolizing enzymes in Japanese with alcohol liver diseases: a strong association with the usual Caucasian-type aldehyde dehydrogenase gene (ALDH1(2)) with the disease. *Am J Hum Genet*. 1988;43(5):744–748. https://www.ncbi.nlm.nih.gov/pubmed/3189338

19. Holmes MV, Dale CE, Zuccolo L, et al. Association between alcohol and cardiovascular disease: Mendelian randomisation analysis based on individual participant data. *BMJ.* 2014;349:g4164. doi:10.1136/bmj.g4164
20. Hofer BS, Simbrunner B, Hartl L, et al. Alcohol abstinence improves prognosis across all stages of portal hypertension in alcohol-related cirrhosis. *Clin Gastroenterol Hepatol.* 2023;21(9):2308–2317.e7. doi:10.1016/j.cgh.2022.11.033
21. Aguilera MT, de la Sierra A, Coca A, Estruch R, Fernández-Solá J, Urbano-Márquez A. Effect of alcohol abstinence on blood pressure: assessment by 24-hour ambulatory blood pressure monitoring. *Hypertension.* 1999;33(2):653–657. doi:10.1161/01.hyp.33.2.653
22. Rehm J, Patra J, Popova S. Alcohol drinking cessation and its effect on esophageal and head and neck cancers: a pooled analysis. *Int J Cancer.* 2007;121(5):1132–1137. doi:10.1002/ijc.22798
23. Yoo JE, Han K, Shin DW, et al. Association between changes in alcohol consumption and cancer risk. *JAMA Netw Open.* 2022;5(8):e2228544. doi:10.1001/jamanetworkopen.2022.28544
24. CDC. Current Cigarette Smoking among Adults in the United States. Centers for Disease Control and Prevention. Published May 3, 2023. Accessed October 5, 2023. https://www.cdc.gov/tobacco/data_statistics/fact_sheets/adult_data/cig_smoking/index.htm
25. Hunt LJ, Covinsky KE, Cenzer I, et al. The epidemiology of smoking in older adults: a national cohort study. *J Gen Intern Med.* 2023;38(7):1697–1704. doi:10.1007/s11606-022-07980-w
26. CDCTobaccoFree. *2014 SGR: the health consequences of smoking – 50 years of progress.* Centers for Disease Control and Prevention. Published July 27, 2023. Accessed December 30, 2023. https://www.cdc.gov/tobacco/sgr/50th-anniversary/index.htm
27. Ambrose JA, Barua RS. The pathophysiology of cigarette smoking and cardiovascular disease: an update. *J Am Coll Cardiol.* 2004;43(10):1731–1737. doi:10.1016/j.jacc.2003.12.047
28. Shah RS, Cole JW. Smoking and stroke: the more you smoke the more you stroke. *Expert Rev Cardiovasc Ther.* 2010;8(7):917–932. doi:10.1586/erc.10.56
29. Luo J, Tang X, Li F, et al. Cigarette smoking and risk of different pathologic types of stroke: a systematic review and dose-response meta-analysis. *Front Neurol.* 2021;12:772373. doi:10.3389/fneur.2021.772373
30. Burns DM. Cigarette smoking among the elderly: disease consequences and the benefits of cessation. *Am J Health Promot.* 2000;14(6):357–361. doi:10.4278/0890-1171-14.6.357
31. CDCTobaccoFree. Smoking and Cancer. Centers for Disease Control and Prevention. Published November 10, 2023. Accessed December 29, 2023. https://www.cdc.gov/tobacco/campaign/tips/diseases/cancer.html
32. Kleykamp BA, Heishman SJ. The older smoker. *JAMA.* 2011;306(8):876–877. doi:10.1001/jama.2011.1221
33. Peters R, Poulter R, Warner J, Beckett N, Burch L, Bulpitt C. Smoking, dementia and cognitive decline in the elderly: a systematic review. *BMC Geriatr.* 2008;8:36. doi:10.1186/1471-2318-8-36
34. Hollenbach KA, Barrett-Connor E, Edelstein SL, Holbrook T. Cigarette smoking and bone mineral density in older men and women. *Am J Public Health.* 1993;83(9):1265–1270. doi:10.2105/ajph.83.9.1265
35. Baron JA, Farahmand BY, Weiderpass E, et al. Cigarette smoking, alcohol consumption, and risk of hip fracture in women. *Arch Intern Med.* 2001;161(7):983–988. doi:10.1001/archinte.161.7.983

36. Wu ZJ, Zhao P, Liu B, Yuan ZC. Effect of cigarette smoking on risk of hip fracture in men: a meta-analysis of 14 prospective cohort studies. *PLoS One*. 2016;11(12):e0168990. doi:10.1371/journal.pone.0168990
37. Zhang N, Liu YJ, Yang C, et al. Association between cigarette smoking and mortality in patients with hip fracture: a systematic review and meta-analysis. *Tob Induc Dis*. 2022;20:110. doi:10.18332/tid/156030
38. Jha P, Ramasundarahettige C, Landsman V, et al. 21st-century hazards of smoking and benefits of cessation in the United States. *N Engl J Med*. 2013;368(4):341–350. doi:10.1056/NEJMsa1211128
39. Mons U, Müezzinler A, Gellert C, et al. Impact of smoking and smoking cessation on cardiovascular events and mortality among older adults: meta-analysis of individual participant data from prospective cohort studies of the CHANCES consortium. *BMJ*. 2015;350:h1551. doi:10.1136/bmj.h1551
40. Gellert C, Schöttker B, Müller H, Holleczek B, Brenner H. Impact of smoking and quitting on cardiovascular outcomes and risk advancement periods among older adults. *Eur J Epidemiol*. 2013;28(8):649–658. doi:10.1007/s10654-013-9776-0
41. Iso H, Date C, Yamamoto A, et al. Smoking cessation and mortality from cardiovascular disease among Japanese men and women: the JACC Study. *Am J Epidemiol*. 2005;161(2):170–179. doi:10.1093/aje/kwi027
42. Gellert C, Schöttker B, Brenner H. Smoking and all-cause mortality in older people: systematic review and meta-analysis. *Arch Intern Med*. 2012;172(11):837–844. doi:10.1001/archinternmed.2012.1397
43. CDCTobaccoFree. Benefits of quitting. Centers for Disease Control and Prevention. Published November 1, 2023. Accessed December 15, 2023. https://www.cdc.gov/tobacco/quit_smoking/how_to_quit/benefits/index.htm
44. Henley SJ, Asman K, Momin B, et al. Smoking cessation behaviors among older U.S. adults. *Prev Med Rep*. 2019;16:100978. doi:10.1016/j.pmedr.2019.100978
45. Sarkar S, Chawla N, Dayal P. Smoking and tobacco use cessation in the elderly. *J Geriatr Ment Health*. 2020;7:70–77. doi:10.4103/jgmh.jgmh_23_20
46. Henningfield JE, Fant RV, Buchhalter AR, Stitzer ML. Pharmacotherapy for nicotine dependence. *CA Cancer J Clin*. 2005;55(5):281–299; quiz 322–323, 325. doi:10.3322/canjclin.55.5.281
47. West R, Hajek P, Nilsson F, Foulds J, May S, Meadows A. Individual differences in preferences for and responses to four nicotine replacement products. *Psychopharmacology*. 2001;153(2):225–230. doi:10.1007/s002130000577
48. Jorenby DE, Hays JT, Rigotti NA, et al. Efficacy of varenicline, an alpha4beta2 nicotinic acetylcholine receptor partial agonist, vs placebo or sustained-release bupropion for smoking cessation: a randomized controlled trial. *JAMA*. 2006;296(1):56–63. doi:10.1001/jama.296.1.56
49. Gonzales D, Rennard SI, Nides M, et al. Varenicline, an alpha4beta2 nicotinic acetylcholine receptor partial agonist, vs sustained-release bupropion and placebo for smoking cessation: a randomized controlled trial. *JAMA*. 2006;296(1):47–55. doi:10.1001/jama.296.1.47
50. Johnson HM, Gossett LK, Piper ME, et al. Effects of smoking and smoking cessation on endothelial function: 1-year outcomes from a randomized clinical trial. *J Am Coll Cardiol*. 2010;55(18):1988–1995. doi:10.1016/j.jacc.2010.03.002
51. Han BH, Palamar JJ. Trends in Cannabis use among older adults in the United States, 2015–2018. *JAMA Intern Med*. 2020;180(4):609–611. doi:10.1001/jamainternmed.2019.7517

52. Stockings E, Campbell G, Hall WD, et al. Cannabis and cannabinoids for the treatment of people with chronic noncancer pain conditions: a systematic review and meta-analysis of controlled and observational studies. *Pain.* 2018;159(10):1932–1954. doi:10.1097/j.pain.0000000000001293
53. Häuser W, Welsch P, Radbruch L, Fisher E, Bell RF, Moore RA. Cannabis-based medicines and medical cannabis for adults with cancer pain. *Cochrane Database Syst Rev.* 2023;6(6):CD014915. doi:10.1002/14651858.CD014915.pub2
54. National Academies of Sciences, Engineering, and Medicine, Health and Medicine Division, Board on Population Health and Public Health Practice. *The Health Effects of Cannabis and Cannabinoids.* National Academies Press; 2017. doi:10.17226/24625
55. Han BH, Brennan JJ, Orozco MA, Moore AA, Castillo EM. Trends in emergency department visits associated with cannabis use among older adults in California, 2005–2019. *J Am Geriatr Soc.* 2023;71(4):1267–1274. doi:10.1111/jgs.18180
56. Pocuca N, Walter TJ, Minassian A, Young JW, Geyer MA, Perry W. The effects of cannabis use on cognitive function in healthy aging: a systematic scoping review. *Arch Clin Neuropsychol.* 2021;36(5):673–685. doi:10.1093/arclin/acaa105
57. Workman CD, Fietsam AC, Sosnoff J, Rudroff T. Increased likelihood of falling in older Cannabis users vs. Non-Users. *Brain Sci.* 2021;11(2). doi:10.3390/brainsci11020134
58. Wolfe D, Corace K, Rice D, et al. Effects of medical and non-medical cannabis use in older adults: protocol for a scoping review. *BMJ Open.* 2020;10(2):e034301. doi:10.1136/bmjopen-2019-034301
59. Li MC, Brady JE, DiMaggio CJ, Lusardi AR, Tzong KY, Li G. Marijuana use and motor vehicle crashes. *Epidemiol Rev.* 2012;34(1):65–72. doi:10.1093/epirev/mxr017
60. Fink DS, Stohl M, Sarvet AL, Cerda M, Keyes KM, Hasin DS. Medical marijuana laws and driving under the influence of marijuana and alcohol. *Addiction.* 2020;115(10):1944–1953. doi:10.1111/add.15031
61. Wolfe D, Corace K, Butler C, et al. Impacts of medical and non-medical cannabis on the health of older adults: findings from a scoping review of the literature. *PLoS One.* 2023;18(2):e0281826. doi:10.1371/journal.pone.0281826

Section 3

Target Issues

15 Sarcopenia

Aruna Nathan

DEFINITION AND INTRODUCTION

Sarcopenia is a medical condition that primarily affects the geriatric population and is characterized by a progressive loss of skeletal muscle mass and function.[1] Sarcopenia can also be understood as skeletal muscle failure that is progressive and is associated with decreased skeletal muscle performance.[2] This definition has evolved over time (Figure 15.1). The original definition was closer to the literal translation, loss of muscle mass (*sarcopenia* in Greek), and at present, the diagnosis emphasizes muscle strength and functionality. As we move further to the right, the definition is aimed at identifying individuals at risk for mobility disability and other adverse health outcomes.[3–5]

Sarcopenia is primarily associated with aging as observed in several studies. Many physiologic factors such as inflammation and hormonal changes, and lifestyle factors such as immobility and nutrition, play a key role in the progression of sarcopenia. However, it should be noted that the predominant process remains unknown.[2]

The evolving definitions of sarcopenia from various consensus groups with different cutoffs for low muscle mass, strength and physical performance are depicted in Table 15.1.[3–5]

The prevalence of sarcopenia is set to rise globally with the increasing populations of older adults, and though sarcopenia is most commonly present in older individuals, it has been observed in younger populations as well. It can start earlier in certain metabolic conditions such as diabetes and fatty liver disease, certain cancers and in people with chronic kidney and liver diseases. This is of particular concern given the ever-increasing rates of these chronic medical conditions in younger populations, and this will have broad implications for the burden of disease, quality of life and health care costs.[6,7] Sarcopenia is associated with, and often leads to, several adverse health outcomes that include recurrent falls, major injuries such as fractures, worsening functional mobility, lower rates of recovery from illness and, eventually, higher rates of loss of independence with Activities of Daily Living (ADLs), and premature mortality.[8]

Research on sarcopenia is increasing exponentially, as it is a good predictor of health outcomes, and work is being done on therapeutic interventions for sarcopenia in various medical disciplines. However, at present, not much has translated into better patient care and improved outcomes in clinical practice.[1]

In 2016, sarcopenia was recognized as a disease with the International Classification of Diseases, 10th Revision, Clinical Modification (ICD-10) code.

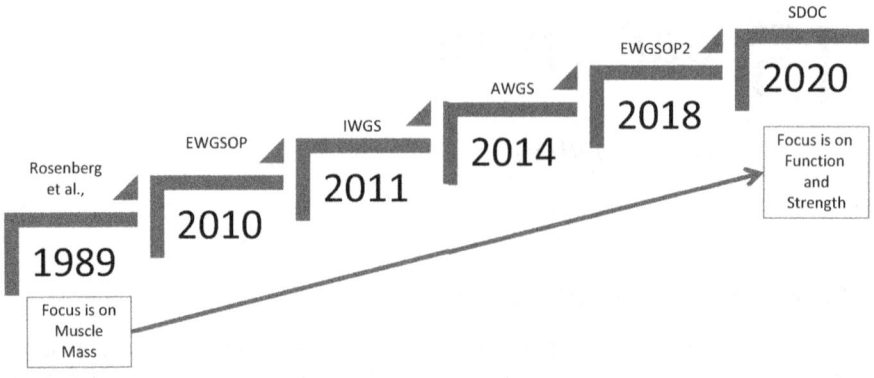

FIGURE 15.1 Evolution of the definition of sarcopenia.

This is a crucial step in addressing sarcopenia as a disease that is treatable. This has allowed clinicians and researchers to work toward better screening, diagnostic and treatment options to address this major public health challenge. A growing consensus in the definition of sarcopenia by various organizations will help in the standardization of diagnostic criteria, making it more practical for everyday clinical application. More work is needed to make this achievable.[8]

PREVALENCE AND EPIDEMIOLOGY

There is a large variation in data on the prevalence of sarcopenia, based on the definition and criteria used in studies to diagnose sarcopenia and the variations in the populations studied. Additionally, studies have used different assessment tools and diagnostic instruments, and there has been no standardization for cutoff points using these tools[7] (as noted in Table 15.1). Diverse settings have been studied, including community-dwelling older adults, people living in long-term facilities, older adults with specific medical conditions and healthier older adults in inpatient and outpatient settings. A few studies have looked at the global prevalence and found variations depending on the definitions used, as well as differences in geographical region, sex, age and medical conditions.[7-11] Taking these issues into consideration, the global prevalence of sarcopenia among community-dwelling older adults ranges from 5 to 27%.[12]

Within the various definitions, the age of the participants and muscle mass cut points were the substantive sources of differences.[8] As the consensus now is to base the definition of sarcopenia on muscle strength and function rather than muscle mass, more research is needed to better study the rates of prevalence using this definition.

As expected, there is a higher prevalence of sarcopenia in patients seen in medical settings. In medical clinics and among people with chronic medical conditions, the prevalence of sarcopenia is much higher compared to the general population. This can range from 18% in patients with diabetes to 66% in patients with unresectable

TABLE 15.1
Sarcopenia Definitions

Working Groups/ Societies Consortium	Definitions	Muscle Mass Cutoff (ASM or ASM/Height^2)	Muscle Strength / Gait Speed Evaluation
EWGSOP	Low Muscle Mass Low Muscle Strength OR Gait Speed	Using BIA: • M < 8.31–10.75 kg/m^2 • W < 6.42–6.75 kg/m^2 Using DXA: • M < 7.23–7.26 kg/m^2 • W < 5.45–5.67 kg/m^2	Grip Strength: • M < 30 kg • W < 20 kg Gait Speed <0.8 m/s M and W
IWGS	Low Muscle Mass Slow Gait Speed	Using BIA: • M < 7.23 kg/m^2 • W < 5.67 kg/m^2 Using DXA: • M < 7.23 kg/m^2 • W < 5.67 kg/m^2	Gait Speed < 1.0 m/s for M and W
AWGS	Low Muscle Mass Low Muscle Strength OR Gait Speed	Using BIA: • M < 7 kg/m^2 • W < 5.7 kg/m^2 Using DXA: • M < 7 kg/m^2 • W < 5.4 kg/m^2	Grip Strength: • M < 26 kg • W < 18 kg Gait Speed < 0.8 m/s for M and W
FNIH	Low Muscle Mass Low Grip Strength	Using DXA: (ASM) • M < 19.75 kg • W < 15.02 kg	Grip Strength: • M < 26 • W < 16 Gait Speed <0.8 for M and W
EWGSOP2	Low Muscle Mass Low Grip Strength	Using DXA: • M < 7 kg/m^2 • W < 5.5 kg/m^2	Grip Strength: • M < 267 kg • W < 16 kg Gait Speed < 0.8 m/s for M and W
SDOC	Low Grip Strength Gait Speed		Grip Strength: • M < 35.5 kg • W < 20 kg Gait Speed < 0.8 m/s for M and W

Abbreviations: ASM, Appendicular Skeletal Mass; AWGS, Asian Working Group for Sarcopenia; BIA, bioelectrical impedance; DXA, dual-energy X-ray absorptiometry; EWGSOP, European Working Group of Sarcopenia in Older People; EWGSOP2, European Working Group of Sarcopenia in Older People2; FNIH, Foundation for National Institute of Health; IWGS, International Working Group of Sarcopenia; SDOC, Sarcopenia Definitions and Outcomes Consortium.

esophageal cancer. Critically ill patients, patients with cirrhosis of the liver, renal transplant patients, patients with cancers and patients on dialysis are some of the patients with the highest prevalence.[7]

RISK FACTORS

As sarcopenia is underrecognized and shows few signs and symptoms until it is severe, knowledge of key associated factors is important. It is especially critical to the early detection, prevention and influence on the trajectory of the illness. Though the number of prospective cohort studies looking at risk factors for sarcopenia are few, and there is always a possibility of reverse causality that can confound data, there is growing evidence of the strong links to various medical conditions.[7]

Some of the risk factors that have been studied are obesity, alcohol consumption, malnutrition, age, sex, smoking, sleep duration, physical inactivity and medical conditions such as diabetes, central obesity, osteoporosis, depression, respiratory diseases, cognitive impairment, peripheral neuropathy, heart disease, osteoarthritis and Parkinson's disease.

AGE

Age is a definitive risk factor for sarcopenia. There is an increase in the inflammatory markers with aging, causing chronic low-grade inflammation. This process dysregulates the acute inflammatory response to illness and infections, and this dysregulation can result in damage to structures like muscle tissue.[13] Aging is associated with accelerated spinal motor neuron apoptosis and distal axon retraction, causing loss of muscle fiber innervated by alpha motor neurons. This is seen as one of the primary causes of sarcopenia. The acceleration of muscle loss starts after age 60 and this accelerates further with more rapid declines in muscle mass and function as one approaches age 75.[14] Aging is also invariably associated with other medical conditions affecting various organ systems, including endocrine, metabolic, liver, kidney, heart, lungs, cognition, brain and an increased incidence of cancers. All of these increase the likelihood of coexisting sarcopenia.[15]

PHYSICAL ACTIVITY

Physical activity protects against sarcopenia. Though this was always common wisdom, it was demonstrated for the first time by a systematic review and meta-analysis by Steffl et al. The review included cross-sectional and cohort studies. The type of physical activity undertaken was not important, as all except one study showed that several different types of physical activity were associated with protection against sarcopenia.[16]

Foong et al. observed that in older adults living in a community, there was a notable positive correlation between physical activity as measured by accelerometers and muscle mass. They discovered that light physical activity (1.5–2.9 METs), moderate activity (3–5.9 METs) and vigorous activity (6 or more METs), all had a significant correlation to the percentage of lean body mass. Notably, the most substantial impact was seen with vigorous physical activity, suggesting a dose-response relationship[17].

In a similar study, Park et al. reported comparable findings within a Japanese population aged 65 to 84 years. However, they only noted significant correlations between muscle mass and physical activity at moderate and vigorous intensity levels.[18]

Studies indicate that older adults tend to engage in sedentary behaviors more frequently than other age groups, and this behavior is linked to increased rates of disease and death. There is evidence that older adults are especially vulnerable to losing muscle quickly during extended periods of inactivity and bed rest, often due to sickness and hospital stays. Research exploring how inactive lifestyles impact muscle mass in healthy older individuals points to a detrimental effect from sedentary habits such as watching TV and sitting for extended periods of time, which is more common in older adults. Foong et al. found that sedentary activities, categorized as less than 1.5 METs, were connected to a reduced percentage of lean body mass in older ages.[19–22]

Decreased muscle mass and physical inactivity directly correlate to decreased energy expenditure that can result in further weight gain, abdominal fat storage and can, in turn, lead to increased proinflammatory cytokines, further negatively impacting muscle mass and strength.[18]

Nutrition

Not consuming the recommended calories per day or low food intake (malnutrition) is often due to physiological and sociological factors associated with aging. This can make it more difficult for older adults to meet the recommended intake of specific nutrients. It is, however, not easy to make direct correlations with specific nutrient intake and sarcopenia.[23,24]

There are several studies looking at protein and a few amino acids that may affect muscle mass and strength. However, current data shows that any gain in muscle strength occurs when nutrient supplementation is implemented alongside physical activity and resistance training. Existing evidence, however, is based on populations differing in age, frailty and nutritional status, making findings inconsistent.[25,26]

Waist Circumference/Obesity

Obesity, waist circumference, and other anthropometric measurements such as waist-to-height ratio and body mass indexes, are linked to sarcopenia in both sexes.[10]

Earlier studies did show some protection from sarcopenia in older adults when middle-aged obesity was present. However, this protective effect is most possibly related to measurements such as BMI and weight that are positively affected by muscle mass.[27,28] Visceral fat and/or waist circumference are better indicators of fat accumulation.[7]

Similar findings were seen in a collaborative study of aging, a survey that was conducted among people aged 65 and older in countries representing a wide geographical variation. A higher percentage of body fat was associated with low muscle mass and a higher presence of sarcopenia.[29]

Another study found a positive association between obesity and late-life sarcopenia, suggesting that obesity might be an important modifiable risk factor related to sarcopenia among men with cardiovascular disease. The participants in this study were 337 men, with a mean age of 56.7 (SD, 6.5) and cardiovascular disease. The participants underwent sarcopenia evaluation 19.9 (SD, 1.0) years after baseline.

The study found sarcopenia among 54.3% of participants with obesity (body mass index [BMI, in kg/m^2] ≥ 30.0), 37.0% of participants who were overweight (25.0 ≤ BMI ≤ 29.9) and 24.8% of participants with normal weight (BMI 18.5 to 24.9). In a comparison of BMI ≥ 25.0 and BMI < 25.0, adjusting for covariates, the odds ratio of having probable sarcopenia was 3.27 (95% CI, 1.68–6.36) and having sarcopenia was 5.31 (95% CI, 2.50–11.27).[30] In this study, probable sarcopenia was defined as low muscle mass or low muscle strength and sarcopenia was defined as low muscle mass and low muscle strength and/or low performance.

The decreased muscle mass and increased fat mass are possibly interdependent, accounting for the correlation between the two factors in older adults with or without other chronic medical conditions.[31] With aging there is some decline in muscle mass, muscle function and muscle endurance, and this can result in lower physical activity. This decreased muscle mass and physical activity can lead to decreased energy expenditure, which, in turn, results in weight gain (fat mass), especially in the abdominal area.[32]

This accumulation of fat, especially in the visceral area, can generate high amounts of proinflammatory cytokines related to macrophages, c-reactive protein and interleukin 6 associated with fats.[33] Obesity-associated inflammation may then have a negative effect on muscle tissue, leading to sarcopenia[34] (Figure 15.2).

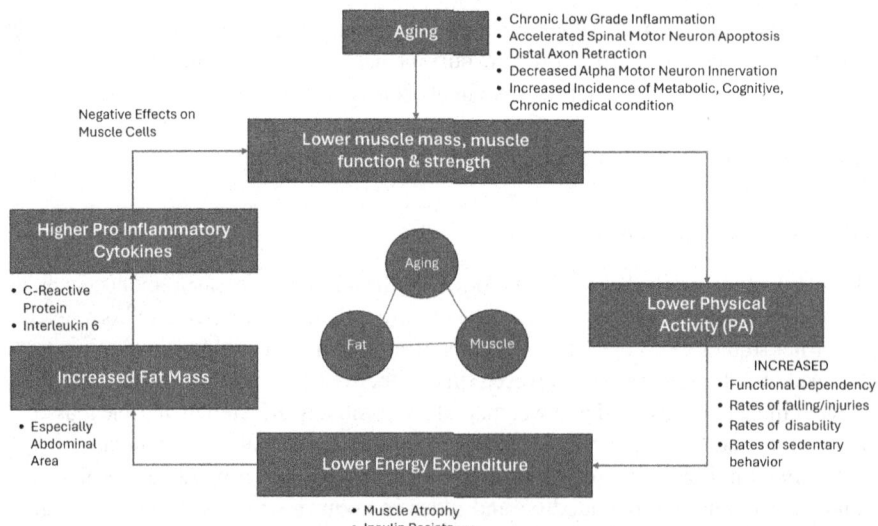

FIGURE 15.2 The sarcopenia cycle.

IMPAIRED FASTING GLUCOSE AND HYPERGLYCEMIA

Hyperglycemia is a risk factor for functional disability and mobility limitations, and several studies have associated type 2 diabetes and sarcopenia. Although ample evidence suggests that older diabetic patients have an increased risk of sarcopenia, so far the underlying mechanism has not been fully clarified. Mitochondrial dysfunction, peripheral neuropathy and microangiopathy have been hypothesized as causes. Observational studies, including one based on the Baltimore Longitudinal Study of Aging data, suggest that treating hyperglycemia early can help mitigate muscle loss.[35]

In a recent study looking for risk factors in community-dwelling adults aged 65 to 74, Hwang et al. found fasting glucose to be a statistically significant variable (p < 0.05) for both men and women[10] cross-sectionally associated with sarcopenia. In the Discussion of this study, the authors made reference to a few previous studies that have found a strong association between sarcopenia and fasting glucose. A study of 157 community-dwelling elderly individuals with sarcopenia demonstrated that the sarcopenic group had a higher incidence of impaired fasting glucose compared to the non-sarcopenic group.[36] Similarly, Ozturk et al. investigated 147 sarcopenia patients at an average age of 70.3 years and found that these patients faced challenges in regulating their blood glucose levels.[37]

SLEEP

Both shorter and longer durations of sleep are positively associated with sarcopenia.[38] More recently, a study that looked at the association between sleep duration and possible sarcopenia and its defining components, based on the China Health and Retirement Longitudinal Study (CHARLS), found short sleep duration to be a risk factor for possible sarcopenia and low handgrip strength.[39]

SMOKING AND ALCOHOL

Smoking is associated with an overall increase in risk for sarcopenia. Shaw et al., in their review titled, "Epidemiology of Sarcopenia: Determinants throughout the Lifecourse," found that research indicates associations between smoking and muscle strength in different age groups:

1. Cross-sectional associations have been observed between smoking and reduced muscle strength in older adults.[40]
2. In a longitudinal study involving healthy younger adults, smoking was inversely associated with knee muscle strength between the ages of 21 and 36, even after adjusting for other lifestyle factors.[41]
3. HALCyon data revealed a strong link between smoking and reduced physical capability in older adults, as measured by grip strength, chair rise speed, TUG/walk speed and balance ability.[40]

Overall smoking was associated with an increased risk of sarcopenia in 29 studies.[28]

Alcohol consumption has not been associated with the risk of sarcopenia in studies as of now.[42] While animal studies have linked alcohol consumption to muscle atrophy, the relationship between alcohol intake and sarcopenia in human studies remains contentious.

Few meta-analyses have explored this association, with only one reported study. In their meta-analysis, Steffl et al. examined data from individuals aged ≥65 years, combining cross-sectional and cohort study data. Surprisingly, they found that alcohol consumption was not a risk factor for sarcopenia within this age group. However, variations in study design and populations across different investigations can impact research outcomes, highlighting a limitation of observational meta-analyses.

Previous studies have explored alcohol's effects on individuals aged 60 years and above. Among older women, high-risk alcohol consumption (as identified by the Alcohol Use Disorders Identification Test) was linked to an increased risk of sarcopenia. Additionally, binge drinkers with weekly or daily alcohol intake faced a higher risk of sarcopenia compared to social drinkers. However, when alcohol consumption was categorized simply as either drinking or non-drinking, it did not emerge as a risk factor for sarcopenia.

In summary, excessive alcohol consumption may contribute to sarcopenia risk, but defining optimal cutoff points or frequencies for this association remains elusive. Furthermore, it is worth noting that alcohol consumption tends to decrease with age, which could partly explain the results observed in the current meta-analysis study where alcohol consumption did not significantly correlate with sarcopenia risk.[43]

CELLULAR AND MOLECULAR CHANGES SEEN IN SARCOPENIA

- *Muscle Fiber Atrophy*: There is a reduction in muscle fiber cross-sectional area, leading to overall muscle shrinkage.
- *Fiber Type Conversion*: There is a shift in muscle fiber types, often with a decrease in the number and size of type II (fast-twitch) fibers.
- *Fat Infiltration*: An increased deposition of fat within muscle tissues, replacing muscle, is seen.
- *Fibrosis*: There is an increase in connective tissue within the muscle, which can cause muscle stiffening and affect muscle adaptability.
- *Mitochondrial Dysfunction*: Changes are seen in muscle metabolism, with a decline in mitochondrial function, leading to reduced/ineffective energy production.
- *Neuromuscular Junction Degeneration*: Deterioration of the neuromuscular junctions, which are critical for muscle contraction, is seen.
- *Satellite Cell Dysfunction*: There is a reduction in the number and regenerative capacity of satellite cells, which are essential for muscle repair and growth.[44,45]

COMMON COEXISTING MEDICAL CONDITIONS

Frailty

Defined as a clinically recognizable state of increased vulnerability resulting from aging-associated decline in reserve and function across multiple physiologic systems such that the ability to cope with everyday or acute stressors is compromised. In the absence of a gold standard, frailty has been operationally defined by Fried et al. as meeting three out of five phenotypic criteria indicating compromised energetics: low grip strength, low energy, slowed walking speed, low physical activity and/or unintentional weight loss.[46]

Multimorbidity

According to the definition of the American Geriatrics Society, multimorbidity in older adults refers to the existence of two or more chronic medical conditions, including common chronic diseases, geriatric syndromes and geriatric problems.[47]

Cachexia

Cachexia is a complicated metabolic syndrome related to underlying illness and characterized by muscle mass loss with or without fat mass loss that is often associated with anorexia, an inflammatory process, insulin resistance and increased protein turnover.[48]

DIAGNOSIS OF SARCOPENIA

Currently, sarcopenia remains underdiagnosed, though it is commonly prevalent in individuals over the age of 60,[7] and the rates of the disease are much higher in patients seen in inpatient and outpatient settings.[49,50] Though every patient over age 60, and younger patients with risk factors,[10] should be screened, this is not always performed in most clinical settings today.

The reason could be multifold, as it is a newer medical condition and there is a general lack of knowledge among clinicians. Consensus on diagnostic criteria is still forming.[51] Additionally, though the diagnosis can be predictive of poor prognosis, it has not found its way into quality assessment metrics for readmission or indicators of worsening prognosis in most health care settings. In current clinical practice, we inquire about the history of falls and it is also part of some screening tools for older patients, and most older patients with falls will also have sarcopenia.[52,53]

Though we don't necessarily look to diagnose sarcopenia in today's clinical practice, we do routinely screen for and treat osteoporosis, seeing patients with fragility fractures (hip, spine and wrists in the setting of bone loss), so we should be alert to the possibility that these patients may also have sarcopenia and, in many cases, frailty as well (another medical diagnosis).[54,55]

Often, in older patients, the diagnoses of frailty and/or cachexia and/or multimorbidity present simultaneously with sarcopenia.[55] On the other hand, among patients aged 60–74, there is an increasing incidence of sarcopenic obesity. This is another condition that needs special attention, which could go unrecognized for a few years before diagnosis.[56] Interventions can be applied to all stages, from identifying people at risk for sarcopenia to the very frail with severe sarcopenia. Multidisciplinary team-based strategies that include preemptive patient education and regular assessments, understanding patient preferences for interventions like exercise and nutrition therapy, and designing a treatment plan with follow-ups can be effective.[57]

Diagnosis of sarcopenia is rarely made in isolation; most people with a diagnosis of sarcopenia will have other comorbid conditions. Sarcopenia is diagnosed both acutely and progressively and can be characterized as both primary and secondary, in combination or alone, based on the causes. Due to the heterogenicity of the presentation of sarcopenia, having a checklist or algorithm will help.[58] The European Working Group on Sarcopenia in Older People (EWGSOP2) has described such an algorithm as follows:

"Find-Assess-Confirm-Severity" or F-A-C-S

F (Find)

Screening tools for sarcopenia help evaluate muscle mass, strength and physical function. There are a few screening tools available today, and we may have more in the future to help simplify identifying patients with sarcopenia. One such screening tool is the SARC-F questionnaire (S = strength, A = assistance walking, R = rising from chair, C = climbing stairs, F = falls). The SARC-F questionnaire is a screening tool that is gaining more acceptance.[58]

The scale is measured from 0–2, from not at all difficult to very difficult. The scale has a total score of 10, with a cutoff point recommended at >= 4.

SARC-F has shown high specificity for the diagnosis of sarcopenia and correlates well with prognosis, though it may have low sensitivity. There are many reports on the usefulness of SARC-F in older adults and in younger people with other underlying diseases.

While taking a history, a clinician should be able to elicit symptoms and look for signs of sarcopenia, such as feeling weaker, walking slower and having more trouble with activities requiring muscle strength and function (based on history, this can range from gardening and yard work to household chores).

Observation includes assessing gait as patients walk in or out of the exam room, and how they sit or get out of a chair. In other words, "eyeball" testing is a good place to start.

A (Assess)

Once the diagnosis of sarcopenia is suspected, muscle strength should be tested. The two standardized tests commonly used are:

- *Handgrip Strength*: Using a Jamar dynamometer, a validated tool to measure grip strength. Handgrip strength correlates with strength in other muscles

Sarcopenia

and therefore serves as a good surrogate. Decreased handgrip strength also serves as a predictor for poor patient outcomes, increased length, functional deficits, and death. The suggested cutoff point for handgrip is <27 kg and <16 kg, for males and females, respectively.[44] Patients should be given the following instructions:

- Stand upright and hold the handgrip dynamometer down by your side, with a slight bend in your elbow. Make sure the dynamometer does not touch your body.
- Squeeze the handgrip dynamometer with as much force as possible.
- Breathe normally and keep the rest of your body still during the test.
- Repeat the procedure twice for your left hand and twice for your right hand, with a rest in between each attempt.
- Record the highest reading displayed on the screen in kilograms (or pounds).
- Add the highest scores from both hands to get your total grip strength.

- *Chair Stand Test*: This test measures the number of times a person can stand and sit from a chair in 30 seconds without using their hands. If a patient cannot do this, it is scored as 0. The suggested cutoff for the chair stand test is >15 seconds for five rises. This test is used as a valid indicator of lower extremity strength.[44,58]

C (Confirm) – Confirming with Body Composition Assessment

Confirming diagnosis and assessing muscle mass can be done with various modalities. MRI and CT are considered gold standards and provide highly accurate muscle mass, but rarely can be done in clinical settings as they require trained professionals, are expensive, lack portability and are time-consuming. DEXA scans are less accurate compared to CT scans and MRIs but are easily available. Bioelectrical Impedance Scans (BIA) are also less accurate but are very portable and can be easily used in a clinical setting.[59]

S (Severity of Sarcopenia)

Measuring physical performance to identify sarcopenia severity.

Once sarcopenia is confirmed through body composition assessment, the severity of the condition is determined by measuring physical performance. Suggested tests and their respective cutoff points for sarcopenia severity as recommended by the EWGSOP2 are listed below.[44]

- *Gait Speed Tests*: These tests are straightforward and predict adverse effects related to sarcopenia. For example, the "four-meter usual walking speed test" assesses sarcopenia severity. During the test, patients walk four meters at their usual pace. A speed of ≤0.8 m/s may indicate severe sarcopenia.
- *Short Physical Performance Battery (SPPB)*: This includes three timed tasks: chair stands, standing balance and walking speed. Scores range from

0 (low performance) to 12 (high performance). A score of ≤8 suggests poor physical performance and greater sarcopenia severity.
- *Timed-Up and Go Test (TUG)*: This measures the time it takes for a patient to rise from a chair, walk three meters away, and return. A time ≥20 seconds indicates physical deficits. Note that this recommendation is based on studies involving older adult female populations.
- *400-Meter Walk Test*: Patients attempt to walk 400 meters (20 laps of 20 meters each) as quickly as possible. Inability to complete or requiring ≥6 minutes suggests significant sarcopenia severity.

MANAGEMENT AND RECOMMENDATIONS

Shared decision-making and a multidisciplinary team approach are essential in any geriatric condition, including sarcopenia. Treatment interventions are based on multiple factors, but nutrition and exercise (resistance/gait and balance, and aerobic) are central.[57]

EXERCISE AND PHYSICAL ACTIVITY RECOMMENDATIONS

Many studies looking at varied physical activity and sarcopenia have been conducted. As mentioned earlier, Steffl et al., in 2017, were the first to perform a systemic review. They found a statistically significant association on the basis of cross-sectional and cohort studies between sarcopenia and decreased physical activity. The researchers also found evidence of the protective role of physical activity against the development of sarcopenia. Data was gained from 40,007 individuals (21,222 males and 18,785 females), with a mean age of 71.6 years (non-sarcopenic males), 74.9 (sarcopenic males), 73.1 (non-sarcopenic females) and 76 (sarcopenic females). Most of the participants lived in a community.

The type of physical activity varied among studies and was mostly gathered through self-reported data. The types of physical activity reported included household work, gardening, doubles tennis, running, climbing, fast cycling, jump rope, singles tennis, etc.

Earlier studies have shown exercise can increase gait speed, balance, and activities of daily living in frail older adults, and improve mobility and physical functioning even among those with mobility problems and physical disability.[17] The 2018 Physical Activity Guidelines incorporating aerobic, resistance, balance and flexibility are most applicable to address sarcopenia. Resistance training or muscle strengthing activities for 2 or more days a week, moderate aerobic physical activity for 150 to 300 minutes (or 75 to 150 minutes of strenuous aerobic activity) and activites or exercises that help with balance and flexibility should be encouraged and prescribed appropriately. Especially for older adults, team-based multimodal exercises incorporating muscle strengthening with balance and aerobic activities should be routine practice. Safety and skill levels should be kept in mind to prevent injuries when making individual recommendations. To implement the guidelines across all demographics, guided programs with exercise physiologists, physical therapists and coaches trained to work with older people should be established.

NUTRITION

Though nutrition is considered important for the health of skeletal muscle, there are many gaps in current evidence to make dietary recommendations for a population. Dietary recommendations for sarcopenia are at present based on consensus with little clinical trial evidence. Most studies focused on individual, isolated macronutrients such as protein, including specific amino acids and other nutrients such as vitamin D and vitamin B; minerals such as magnesium and calcium; and antioxidants such as omega-3 fatty acids. These studies were of shorter duration.

More recently, the focus has been on whole-diet effects over longer periods, and there is growing evidence that links higher quality and a higher nutrient-rich diet to beneficial effects on muscle mass and function. Such diets have a greater range of bioactive nutrients and phytochemicals, as well as favorable acid–base balance and other anti-inflammatory components. Besides nutrients, such quality differences in diet can affect the composition of the gut microbiome, which potentially impacts skeletal muscle mass and function through effects on inflammatory processes and anabolic resistance[60].

Robinson, et al. reported in their 2023 review that a higher quality diet followed habitually across adulthood is linked to better physical performance later in life. Although the authors did state that variations in study designs did limit direct comparisons, the overall data demonstrated a positive correlation between good diet quality across adult life to better muscle function. Many of the dietary pattern studies showed common tenets, such as high consumption of fruits, vegetables and whole grain cereals, and lower amounts of processed foods. Studies with repeated diet assessments are fewer and outcomes do differ between studies, but they do provide some indications of benefits from diet quality.

Diets higher in pro-inflammatory foods at baseline (age 50) did show a decrease in skeletal muscle strength and higher timed up-and-go (TUG) among 522 males who were followed for 15 years.[61] Conversely, the Nurses' Health Study (n = 54,762), using a self-reported functional impairment survey given every 4 years, and comparing this to the cumulative AHEI-2010 scores (Alternative Healthy Eating Index – 2010), showed an association of lower risk for incidental physical impairment with a greater adherence to AHEI-2010.

In the National Survey of Health and Development, United Kingdom (NSHD), diet was assessed longitudinally at ages 36, 43, 53 and 60–64 years of age. Higher diet quality scores at each age were associated with better measurements (chair rise speed, standing balance and TUG). These associations were largely robust to adjustment (age, physical activity, smoking).

Moreover, in the same study, the strongest association was observed with the contemporary diet data in the cross-sectional analysis at ages 60–64 years. This provides evidence that a change in diet to improve quality at this age affects function (chair rise speed, standing balance time). This finding is encouraging and will most likely prompt more studies.

Talegawkar et al. recently published data from a longitudinal study in Baltimore of 1,358 males and females. The Baltimore Longitudinal Study of Aging has many salient components that include repeated assessments of diet, long-term follow-up, comprehensive physical performance measurements and mean MIND scores (Mediterranean–Dietary Approaches to Stop Hypertension Interventions for Neurodegenerative Delay). Higher MIND scores were associated with slower functional decline. They have shown consistent evidence of benefits for measured physical performance and strength, comparable consistent associations in males and females and a significant positive effect, pointing to the importance of this type of diet (more frequent consumption of vegetables (especially greens), berries, nuts and whole grains, and less frequent consumption of red meat and meat products, fast foods, fried foods, pastries and sweets).

Eating a whole food plant-forward diet is a well-understood recommendation when it comes to conditions such as cardiovascular disease, hypertension and diabetes, and most medical societies today recommend this way of eating. However, when it comes to skeletal muscle health, the focus shifts to protein. Though skeletal muscles are the major reservoirs of protein in the body and are made up of mainly proteins, it is important to consider the pathophysiology and causes of sarcopenia when addressing diet. Most adults who are not obtaining the required amount of protein in a day are most likely consuming fewer calories or are on an extremely low nutrient-density diet that is high in processed foods. Also fundamental to muscle health is muscle fiber recruitment, that occurs with all types of physical activity, including both aerobic and resistance training.

Low-Calorie Intake

Irrespective of the underlying and secondary causes and stages of sarcopenia, nutrition plays a role. In the presence of malnutrition, decreased food consumption, that is, low caloric intake over time, results in low body weight as well as low muscle mass. This fall in food intake (calorie intake) is even present in healthy older adults compared to younger adults. Especially in hospital settings, this overlap between sarcopenia and malnutrition may be significant. A recent meta-analysis of pooled data from seven studies shows the odds ratio (OR) for malnutrition among sarcopenic patients to be 4.06 (95% CI).[62]

Providing adequate calorie intake is the treatment for malnutrition that is due to low caloric intake. Macronutrients are the primary building blocks of nutrition, consisting of carbohydrates, fats and proteins. This increased caloric intake needs to be provided and gradually increased as tolerated.

Protein

In 2020, Ganapathy et al. published a comprehensive review on nutrition and sarcopenia, and reviewed protein and amino acids. Several studies show a blunted anabolic response to proteins in older adults.[63] Several cohort studies link sarcopenia to lower protein intake, affecting lean mass and grip strength.[64] Interventional, randomized controlled trials with varying amounts of whey protein supplementation have shown improvements in muscle mass and/or function or strength, but the majority have achieved this only when combined with resistance training of up to 12 weeks duration.[64,65] When protein supplementation was combined with vitamin D, the studies showed mixed results when evaluating improvements in grip strength, gait speed, appendicular skeletal mass and/or skeletal mass index. Another small study with 28 people over the age of 70 used leucine three grams in addition to whey protein. It did not show any improvement in muscle mass or function. All these studies were for a duration of only 12 weeks.[66–69]

In a 2022 Systemic Review of RCTs (18 RTCs and >13,000 people), Hengevald et al. did not find available evidence to make recommendations for increasing protein intake over 0.8 g/kg of body weight for any health benefits. They found a possible beneficial effect on lean body mass in older adults with higher protein intake when combined with physical exercise, but the effects on physical performance were found to be unlikely. This is an important finding, as this study looked at habitual protein intake above the population's reference intake (> = 0.8 grams/kg/day).[68]

A recent review by Hou et al. of 29 studies, including 19 randomized controlled trials, 6 prospective cohort studies and 4 cross-sectional studies and findings, summarized the impact of protein intake and supplementation on sarcopenia in community-dwelling older adults. The study found that in community-dwelling older adults, protein and amino acid supplementation can improve muscle mass in sarcopenia and among pre-frail older adults, with variable effects on muscle strength and physical function. But when supplementation is combined with exercise, muscle mass, strength and physical function improve in the same group compared to either supplementation or exercise alone. The authors also found that with healthy older adults, the results were inconclusive when using protein supplementation with or without exercise on all three criteria of muscle mass, strength and physical function.[70,71]

CLINICAL APPLICATIONS

- Patients seen in a geriatric setting have a very high likelihood of having sarcopenia.
- Routine sarcopenia screenings should be encouraged.
- Much can be accomplished when sarcopenia is diagnosed early, and disease prevention and reversal is a possibility. This will have positive outcome impacts on other chronic medical conditions as well.
- Even older and more frail people, and those with mobility problems and physical disability, can improve with lifestyle interventions. Physical activity and exercise, especially resistance exercise and nutrition, are the pillars that help the most. But in general, any amount of physical activity including aerobic activity can help.
- Most importantly, shared decision-making using motivational interviewing skills, a patient-centered, patient-directed focus and team-based multimodal interventions are needed for the successful implementation of a sarcopenia treatment plan.

REFERENCES

1. Sayer AA, Cruz-Jentoft A. Sarcopenia definition, diagnosis and treatment: consensus is growing. *Age Ageing.* 2022 Oct 6;51(10):afac220. doi:10.1093/ageing/afac220.
2. Coletta G, Phillips SM. An elusive consensus definition of sarcopenia impedes research and clinical treatment: a narrative review. *Aging Res Rev.* 2023 Apr;86:101883. doi:10.1016/j.arr.2023.101883.
3. Carvalho do Nascimento PR, Bilodeau M, Poitras S. How do we define and measure sarcopenia? A meta-analysis of observational studies. *Age Ageing.* 2021 Nov 10;50(6):1906–1913. doi:10.1093/ageing/afab148.
4. Cruz-Jentoft AJ, Bahat G, Bauer J, Boirie Y, Bruyère O, Cederholm T, Cooper C, Landi F, Rolland Y, Sayer AA, Schneider SM, Sieber CC, Topinkova E, Vandewoude M, Visser M, Zamboni M; Writing Group for the European Working Group on Sarcopenia in Older People 2 (EWGSOP2), and the Extended Group for EWGSOP2. Sarcopenia: revised European consensus on definition and diagnosis. *Age Ageing.* 2019 Jan 1;48(1):16–31. doi:10.1093/ageing/afy169. Erratum in: *Age Ageing.* 2019 Jul 1;48(4):601.
5. Bhasin S, Travison TG, Manini TM, Patel S, Pencina KM, Fielding RA, Magaziner JM, Newman AB, Kiel DP, Cooper C, Guralnik JM, Cauley JA, Arai H, Clark BC, Landi F, Schaap LA, Pereira SL, Rooks D, Woo J, Woodhouse LJ, Binder E, Brown T, Shardell M, Xue QL, D'Agostino RB Sr, Orwig D, Gorsicki G, Correa-De-Araujo R, Cawthon PM. Sarcopenia definition: the position statements of the sarcopenia definition and outcomes consortium. *J Am Geriatr Soc.* 2020 Jul;68(7):1410–1418. doi:10.1111/jgs.16372.
6. Watson KB, Carlson SA, Loustalot F, et al. Chronic conditions among adults aged 18–34 years – United States, 2019. *MMWR Morb Mortal Wkly Rep.* 2022;71:964–970. doi:10.15585/mmwr.mm7130a3.
7. Yuan S, Larsson SC. Epidemiology of sarcopenia: prevalence, risk factors, and consequences. *Metabolism.* 2023 Jul;144:155533. doi:10.1016/j.metabol.2023.155533.
8. Mayhew AJ, Amog K, Phillips S, Parise G, McNicholas PD, de Souza RJ, Thabane L, Raina P. The prevalence of sarcopenia in community-dwelling older adults, an exploration of differences between studies and within definitions: a systematic review and meta-analyses. *Age Ageing.* 2019 Jan 1;48(1):48–56. doi:10.1093/ageing/afy106.
9. Therakomen V, Petchlorlian A, Lakananurak N. Prevalence and risk factors of primary sarcopenia in community-dwelling outpatient elderly: a cross-sectional study. *Sci Rep.* 2020 Nov 11;10(1):19551. doi:10.1038/s41598-020-75250-y.
10. Hwang J, Park S. Gender-Specific Risk Factors and Prevalence for Sarcopenia among Community-Dwelling Young-Old Adults. *Int J Environ Res Public Health.* 2022 Jun 13;19(12):7232. doi:10.3390/ijerph19127232.
11. Rodríguez-Rejón AI, Ruiz-López MD, Wanden-Berghe C, Artacho R. Prevalence and diagnosis of sarcopenia in residential facilities: a systematic review. *Adv Nutr.* 2019 Jan 1;10(1):51–58. doi:10.1093/advances/nmy058.
12. Petermann-Rocha F, Balntzi V, Gray SR, Lara J, Ho FK, Pell JP, Celis-Morales C. Global prevalence of sarcopenia and severe sarcopenia: a systematic review and meta-analysis. *J Cachexia Sarcopenia Muscle.* 2022 Feb;13(1):86–99. doi:10.1002/jcsm.12783.
13. Chung HY, Kim DH, Lee EK, Chung KW, Chung S, Lee B, Seo AY, Chung JH, Jung YS, Im E, Lee J, Kim ND, Choi YJ, Im DS, Yu BP. Redefining chronic inflammation in aging and age-related diseases: proposal of the senoinflammation concept. *Aging Dis.* 2019 Apr 1;10(2):367–382. doi:10.14336/AD.2018.0324.
14. Hunter SK, Pereira HM, Keenan KG. The aging neuromuscular system and motor performance. *J Appl Physiol (1985).* 2016 Oct 1;121(4):982–995. doi:10.1152/japplphysiol.00475.2016.

15. Zhang K, Ma Y, Luo Y, Song Y, Xiong G, Ma Y, Sun X, Kan C. Metabolic diseases and healthy aging: identifying environmental and behavioral risk factors and promoting public health. *Front Public Health*. 2023 Oct 13;11:1253506. doi:10.3389/fpubh.2023.1253506.
16. Steffl M, Bohannon RW, Sontakova L, Tufano JJ, Shiells K, Holmerova I. Relationship between sarcopenia and physical activity in older people: a systematic review and meta-analysis. *Clin Interv Aging*. 2017 May 17;12:835–845. doi:10.2147/CIA.S132940.
17. Foong YC, Chherawala N, Aitken D, Scott D, Winzenberg T, Jones G. Accelerometer-determined physical activity, muscle mass, and leg strength in community-dwelling older adults. *J Cachexia Sarcopenia Muscle*. 2016 Jun;7(3):275–283. doi:10.1002/jcsm.12065.
18. Park H, Park S, Shephard RJ, Aoyagi Y. Yearlong physical activity and sarcopenia in older adults: the Nakanojo Study. *Eur J Appl Physiol*. 2010 Jul;109(5):953–961. doi:10.1007/s00421-010-1424-8.
19. Foong YC, Chherawala N, Aitken D, Scott D, Winzenberg T, Jones G. Accelerometer-determined physical activity, muscle mass, and leg strength in community-dwelling older adults. *J Cachexia Sarcopenia Muscle*. 2016 Jun;7(3):275–283. doi:10.1002/jcsm.12065.
20. de Rezende LF, Rey-López JP, Matsudo VK, do Carmo Luiz O. Sedentary behavior and health outcomes among older adults: a systematic review. *BMC Public Health*. 2014 Apr 9;14:333. doi:10.1186/1471-2458-14-333.
21. English KL, Paddon-Jones D. Protecting muscle mass and function in older adults during bedrest. *Curr Opin Clin Nutr Metab Care*. 2010 Jan;13(1):34–39. doi:10.1097/MCO.0b013e328333aa66.
22. Gianoudis J, Bailey CA, Daly RM. Associations between sedentary behaviour and body composition, muscle function and sarcopenia in community-dwelling older adults. *Osteoporos Int*. 2015 Feb;26(2):571–579. doi:10.1007/s00198-014-2895-y.
23. Dennison EM, Sayer AA, Cooper C. Epidemiology of sarcopenia and insight into possible therapeutic targets. *Nat Rev Rheumatol*. 2017 Jun;13(6):340–347. doi:10.1038/nrrheum.2017.60.
24. Robinson S, Cooper C, Aihie Sayer A. Nutrition and sarcopenia: a review of the evidence and implications for preventive strategies. *J Aging Res*. 2012;2012:510801. doi:10.1155/2012/510801.
25. Denison HJ, Cooper C, Sayer AA, Robinson SM. Prevention and optimal management of sarcopenia: a review of combined exercise and nutrition interventions to improve muscle outcomes in older people. *Clin Interv Aging*. 2015 May 11;10:859–869. doi:10.2147/CIA.S55842.
26. Ganapathy A, Nieves JW. Nutrition and sarcopenia – What do we know? *Nutrients*. 2020 Jun 11;12(6):1755. doi:10.3390/nu12061755.
27. Sanada K, Miyachi M, Tanimoto M, Yamamoto K, Murakami H, Okumura S, Gando Y, Suzuki K, Tabata I, Higuchi M. A cross-sectional study of sarcopenia in Japanese men and women: reference values and association with cardiovascular risk factors. *Eur J Appl Physiol*. 2010 Sep;110(1):57–65. doi:10.1007/s00421-010-1473-z.
28. Gao Q, Hu K, Yan C, Zhao B, Mei F, Chen F, Zhao L, Shang Y, Ma Y, Ma B. Associated factors of sarcopenia in community-dwelling older adults: a systematic review and meta-analysis. *Nutrients*. 2021 Nov 27;13(12):4291. doi:10.3390/nu13124291.
29. Tyrovolas S, Koyanagi A, Olaya B, Ayuso-Mateos JL, Miret M, Chatterji S, Tobiasz-Adamczyk B, Koskinen S, Leonardi M, Haro JM. Factors associated with skeletal muscle mass, sarcopenia, and sarcopenic obesity in older adults: a multi-continent study. *J Cachexia Sarcopenia Muscle*. 2016 Jun;7(3):312–321. doi:10.1002/jcsm.12076. Epub 2015 Oct 7.

30. Lutski M, Weinstein G, Tanne D, Goldbourt U. Overweight, obesity, and late-life sarcopenia among men with cardiovascular disease, Israel. *Prev Chronic Dis.* 2020 Dec 24;17:E164. doi:10.5888/pcd17.200167.
31. Zamboni M, Mazzali G, Fantin F, Rossi A, Di Francesco V. Sarcopenic obesity: a new category of obesity in the elderly. *Nutr Metab Cardiovasc Dis.* 2008 Jun;18(5):388–395. doi:10.1016/j.numecd.2007.10.002.
32. Nair KS. Aging muscle. *Am J Clin Nutr.* 2005 May;81(5):953–963. doi:10.1093/ajcn/81.5.953.
33. Tilg H, Moschen AR. Adipocytokines: mediators linking adipose tissue, inflammation, and immunity. *Nat Rev Immunol.* 2006 Oct;6(10):772–783. doi:10.1038/nri1937.
34. Cesari M, Kritchevsky SB, Baumgartner RN, Atkinson HH, Penninx BW, Lenchik L, Palla SL, Ambrosius WT, Tracy RP, Pahor M. Sarcopenia, obesity, and inflammation--results from the trial of angiotensin converting enzyme inhibition and novel cardiovascular risk factors study. *Am J Clin Nutr.* 2005 Aug;82(2):428–434. doi:10.1093/ajcn.82.2.428.
35. Umegaki H. Sarcopenia and diabetes: Hyperglycemia is a risk factor for age-associated muscle mass and functional reduction. *J Diabetes Investig.* 2015 Nov;6(6):623–624. doi:10.1111/jdi.12365.
36. Buscemi C, Ferro Y, Pujia R, Mazza E, Boragina G, Sciacqua A, Piro S, Pujia A, Sesti G, Buscemi S, et al. Sarcopenia and appendicular muscle mass as predictors of impaired fasting glucose/type 2 diabetes in elderly women. *Nutrients.* 2021;13(6):1909. doi:10.3390/nu13061909.
37. Abidin Öztürk ZA, Türkbeyler İH, Demir Z, Bilici M, Kepekçi Y. The effect of blood glucose regulation on sarcopenia parameters in obese and diabetic patients. *Turk J Phys Med Rehabil.* 2017 Nov 14;64(1):72–79. doi:10.5606/tftrd.2018.1068.
38. Chen L, Li Q, Huang X, et al. Association between sleep duration and possible sarcopenia in middle-aged and elderly Chinese individuals: evidence from the China health and retirement longitudinal study. *BMC Geriatr.* 2024;24:594. doi:10.1186/s12877-024-05168-x.
39. Lv X, Peng W, Jia B, et al. Longitudinal association of sleep duration with possible sarcopenia: evidence from CHARLS. *BMJ Open.* 2024;14:e079237. doi:10.1136/bmjopen-2023-079237.
40. Wiener RC, Findley PA, Shen C, Dwibedi N, Sambamoorthi U. Relationship between smoking status and muscle strength in the United States older adults. *Epidemiol Health.* 2020;42:e2020055. doi:10.4178/epih.e2020055.
41. Dennison EM, Sayer AA, Cooper C. Epidemiology of sarcopenia and insight into possible therapeutic targets. *Nat Rev Rheumatol.* 2017 Jun;13(6):340–347. doi:10.1038/nrrheum.2017.60. Epub 2017 May 4.
42. Gao Q, Hu K, Yan C, Zhao B, Mei F, Chen F, Zhao L, Shang Y, Ma Y, Ma B. Associated factors of sarcopenia in community-dwelling older adults: a systematic review and meta-analysis. *Nutrients.* 2021 Nov 27;13(12):4291. doi:10.3390/nu13124291.
43. Hong SH, Bae YJ. Association between alcohol consumption and the risk of sarcopenia: a systematic review and meta-analysis. *Nutrients.* 2022 Aug 10;14(16):3266. doi:10.3390/nu14163266.
44. Ardeljan AD, Hurezeanu R. Sarcopenia. [Updated 2023 Jul 4]. In: StatPearls [Internet]. Treasure Island (FL): StatPearls Publishing; 2024 January. https://www.ncbi.nlm.nih.gov/books/NBK560813/.
45. Siparsky PN, Kirkendall DT, Garrett WE Jr. Muscle changes in aging: understanding sarcopenia. *Sports Health.* 2014 Jan;6(1):36–40. doi:10.1177/1941738113502296.

46. Xue QL. The frailty syndrome: definition and natural history. *Clin Geriatr Med.* 2011 Feb;27(1):1–15. doi:10.1016/j.cger.2010.08.009.
47. Zhou X, Zhang D. Multimorbidity in the elderly: a systematic bibliometric analysis of research output. *Int J Environ Res Public Health.* 2021 Dec 30;19(1):353. doi:10.3390/ijerph19010353.
48. Baker Rogers J, Syed K, Minteer JF. Cachexia. [Updated 2023 Aug 8]. In: *StatPearls* [Internet]. StatPearls Publishing; 2024 January. https://www.ncbi.nlm.nih.gov/books/NBK470208/.
49. Wan SN, Thiam CN, Ang QX, Engkasan J, Ong T. Incident sarcopenia in hospitalized older people: a systematic review. *PLoS One.* 2023 Aug 2;18(8):e0289379. doi:10.1371/journal.pone.0289379.
50. Tan You Mei C, Seah Si Ying S, Yanshan DL, Koh SV, Karthikeyan G, Xia Jiawen O, Low XL, Quek HY, Ong Shuyi A, Low LL, Aw J. Prevalence and factors associated with sarcopenia among older adults in a post-acute hospital in Singapore. *PLoS One.* 2024 Jan 29;19(1):e0291702. doi:10.1371/journal.pone.0291702.
51. Ooi H, Welch C. Obstacles to the early diagnosis and management of sarcopenia: current perspectives. *Clin Interv Aging.* 2024 Feb 20;19:323–332. doi:10.2147/CIA.S438144.
52. Phelan EA, Mahoney JE, Voit JC, Stevens JA. Assessment and management of fall risk in primary care settings. *Med Clin North Am.* 2015 Mar;99(2):281–293. doi:10.1016/j.mcna.2014.11.004.
53. Yeung SSY, Reijnierse EM, Pham VK, Trappenburg MC, Lim WK, Meskers CGM, Maier AB. Sarcopenia and its association with falls and fractures in older adults: a systematic review and meta-analysis. *J Cachexia Sarcopenia Muscle.* 2019 Jun;10(3):485–500. doi:10.1002/jcsm.12411.
54. Reginster JY, Beaudart C, Buckinx F, Bruyère O. Osteoporosis and sarcopenia: two diseases or one? *Curr Opin Clin Nutr Metab Care.* 2016 Jan;19(1):31–36. doi:10.1097/MCO.0000000000000230.
55. Dodds R, Sayer AA. Sarcopenia and frailty: new challenges for clinical practice. *Clin Med (Lond).* 2016 Oct;16(5):455–458. doi:10.7861/clinmedicine.16-5-455.
56. Donini LM, Busetto L, Bischoff SC, Cederholm T, Ballesteros-Pomar MD, Batsis JA, Bauer JM, Boirie Y, Cruz-Jentoft AJ, Dicker D, Frara S, Frühbeck G, Genton L, Gepner Y, Giustina A, Gonzalez MC, Han HS, Heymsfield SB, Higashiguchi T, Laviano A, Lenzi A, Nyulasi I, Parrinello E, Poggiogalle E, Prado CM, Salvador J, Rolland Y, Santini F, Serlie MJ, Shi H, Sieber CC, Siervo M, Vettor R, Villareal DT, Volkert D, Yu J, Zamboni M, Barazzoni R. Definition and diagnostic criteria for sarcopenic obesity: ESPEN and EASO consensus statement. *Obes Facts.* 2022;15(3):321–335. doi:10.1159/000521241.
57. An K, Wu Z, Qiu Y, Pan M, Zhang L, An Z, Li S. Shared decision making in sarcopenia treatment. *Front Public Health.* 2023 Nov 22;11:1296112. doi:10.3389/fpubh.2023.1296112.
58. Cesari M, Kritchevsky SB, Newman AB, Simonsick EM, Harris TB, Penninx BW, Brach JS, Tylavsky FA, Satterfield S, Bauer DC, Rubin SM, Visser M, Pahor M; Health, Aging and Body Composition Study. Added value of physical performance measures in predicting adverse health-related events: results from the Health, Aging and Body Composition Study. *J Am Geriatr Soc.* 2009 Feb;57(2):251–259. doi:10.1111/j.1532-5415.2008.02126.x.
59. Cheng KY, Chow SK, Hung VW, Wong CH, Wong RM, Tsang CS, Kwok T, Cheung WH. Diagnosis of sarcopenia by evaluating skeletal muscle mass by adjusted bioimpedance analysis validated with dual-energy X-ray absorptiometry. *J Cachexia Sarcopenia Muscle.* 2021 Dec;12(6):2163–2173. doi:10.1002/jcsm.12825.

60. Robinson S, Granic A, Cruz-Jentoft AJ, Sayer AA. The role of nutrition in the prevention of sarcopenia. *Am J Clin Nutr.* 2023 Nov;118(5):852–864. doi:10.1016/j.ajcnut.2023.08.015.
61. Davis JA, Mohebbi M, Collier F, Loughman A, Shivappa N, Hébert JR, Pasco JA, Jacka FN. Diet quality and a traditional dietary pattern predict lean mass in Australian women: longitudinal data from the geelong osteoporosis study. *Prev Med Rep.* 2021 Jan 7;21:101316. doi:10.1016/j.pmedr.2021.101316.
62. Ligthart-Melis GC, Luiking YC, Kakourou A, Cederholm T, Maier AB, de van der Schueren MAE. Frailty, sarcopenia, and malnutrition frequently (co-)occur in hospitalized older adults: a systematic review and meta-analysis. *J Am Med Dir Assoc.* 2020 Sep;21(9):1216–1228. doi:10.1016/j.jamda.2020.03.006.
63. Wall BT, Gorissen SH, Pennings B, Koopman R, Groen BB, Verdijk LB, van Loon LJ. Aging is accompanied by a blunted muscle protein synthetic response to protein ingestion. *PLoS One.* 2015 Nov 4;10(11):e0140903. doi:10.1371/journal.pone.0140903.
64. Beasley JM, Wertheim BC, LaCroix AZ, Prentice RL, Neuhouser ML, Tinker LF, Kritchevsky S, Shikany JM, Eaton C, Chen Z, Thomson CA. Biomarker-calibrated protein intake and physical function in the Women's Health Initiative. *J Am Geriatr Soc.* 2013 Nov;61(11):1863–1871. doi:10.1111/jgs.12503. Epub 2013 Oct 28.
65. McLean RR, Mangano KM, Hannan MT, Kiel DP, Sahni S. Dietary protein intake is protective against loss of grip strength among older adults in the Framingham Offspring Cohort. *J Gerontol A Biol Sci Med Sci.* 2016 Mar;71(3):356–361. doi:10.1093/gerona/glv184.
66. Park Y, Choi JE, Hwang HS. Protein supplementation improves muscle mass and physical performance in undernourished prefrail and frail elderly subjects: a randomized, double-blind, placebo-controlled trial. *Am J Clin Nutr.* 2018 Nov 1;108(5):1026–1033. doi:10.1093/ajcn/nqy214.
67. Yamada M, Kimura Y, Ishiyama D, Nishio N, Otobe Y, Tanaka T, Ohji S, Koyama S, Sato A, Suzuki M, Ogawa H, Ichikawa T, Ito D, Arai H. Synergistic effect of bodyweight resistance exercise and protein supplementation on skeletal muscle in sarcopenic or dynapenic older adults. *Geriatr Gerontol Int.* 2019 May;19(5):429–437. doi:10.1111/ggi.13643.
68. Amasene M, Besga A, Echeverria I, Urquiza M, Ruiz JR, Rodriguez-Larrad A, Aldamiz M, Anaut P, Irazusta J, Labayen I. Effects of leucine-enriched whey protein supplementation on physical function in post-hospitalized older adults participating in 12-weeks of resistance training program: a randomized controlled trial. *Nutrients.* 2019 Oct 1;11(10):2337. doi:10.3390/nu11102337.
69. Hengeveld LM, de Goede J, Afman LA, Bakker SJL, Beulens JWJ, Blaak EE, Boersma E, Geleijnse JM, van Goudoever JHB, Hopman MTE, Iestra JA, Kremers SPJ, Mensink RP, de Roos NM, Stehouwer CDA, Verkaik-Kloosterman J, de Vet E, Visser M. Health effects of increasing protein intake above the current population reference intake in older adults: a systematic review of the Health Council of the Netherlands. *Adv Nutr.* 2022 Aug 1;13(4):1083–1117. doi:10.1093/advances/nmab140.
70. Hou V, Madden K. Assessing the effects of dietary protein supplementation on sarcopenia in community-dwelling older adults. *Can Geriatr J.* 2022 Dec 1;25(4):390–403. doi:10.5770/cgj.25.608.
71. Tohyama M, Shirai Y, Kokura Y, Momosaki R. Nutritional care and rehabilitation for frailty, sarcopenia, and malnutrition. *Nutrients.* 2023 Nov 24;15(23):4908. doi:10.3390/nu15234908.

16 Navigating the Landscape of Dementia and Elevating Brain Health in Later Life

Ecler Ercole Jaqua, Mai-Linh N. Tran and Monica Gupta

INTRODUCTION

Globally, an estimated 55 million individuals are currently living with dementia, a number expected to rise significantly to 75 million by 2030 and further escalate to 131 million by 2050.[1] In 2020, the associated care expenses amounted to US$305 billion, and these costs are expected to triple by 2050.[2,3] Given the limitations of existing treatments that cannot reverse cognitive impairment, the evolving field of lifestyle medicine has become a guiding encouragement, emphasizing the profound impact of daily choices on our health.[2,3] The six pillars of lifestyle medicine stand as foundational principles that underscore the complete approach to health care, offering a comprehensive framework for optimizing cognitive function.

As we explore each of these pillars – nutrition, physical activity, sleep, stress management, substance use and social connection – we embark on a journey to understand how these lifestyle choices impact the elaborate workings of the brain.[2,4] A 2020 report from the Lancet Commission identified modifiable risk factors over a lifetime that might prevent or delay up to 40% of dementias. The goal is not merely the absence of disease but also promoting cognitive resilience and longevity.

NOURISHING THE MIND: THE IMPACT OF DIET ON COGNITION AND DEMENTIA PREVENTION

Lifestyle medicine's connection between diet and cognitive health has attracted considerable interest among health care professionals. Researchers and health experts are increasingly recognizing the powerful influence of nutrition on brain function, with particular emphasis on the benefits of a whole food plant-based diet.[2,4] This dietary approach, rich in fruits, vegetables, whole grains and legumes, has shown promising effects in enhancing cognition and reducing the risk of dementia.[2] Additionally, the

MIND (Mediterranean–DASH Diet Intervention for Neurodegenerative Delay) diet, a hybrid of the Mediterranean and DASH (Dietary Approaches to Stop Hypertension) diets, has emerged as a structured dietary plan specifically designed to support brain health. This section will analyze the relationship between a whole food plant-based diet and the MIND diet and their potential roles in improving cognition and preventing dementia.[2,4]

The Whole Food Plant-Based Diet

A whole food plant-based diet centers around the consumption of minimally processed plant foods, emphasizing fruits, vegetables, nuts, seeds, whole grains and legumes while limiting or excluding animal products and refined foods.[4] This dietary pattern is renowned for its rich nutrients, including antioxidants, vitamins, minerals and fiber. Such components play crucial roles in maintaining overall health, and emerging evidence suggests their profound impact on brain function.[1,2]

Whole food plant-based diets are abundant in antioxidants, compounds that combat oxidative stress and inflammation in the body.[2] Oxidative stress is implicated in aging and neurodegenerative diseases, making antioxidants particularly relevant to brain health. Fruits such as berries, rich in polyphenols, have demonstrated neuroprotective effects by scavenging free radicals and reducing inflammation.[1,5]

While a whole food plant-based diet is generally low in saturated fats, it includes essential fatty acids for brain health.[2,4] Omega-3 fatty acids, found in walnuts, flaxseeds and chia seeds, have been associated with improved cognitive performance and a lower risk of dementia. The favorable ratio of omega-3 to omega-6 fatty acids in whole food plant-based diets contributes to a neuroprotective environment, fostering healthy brain aging.[5,6]

The gut microbiome, a complex ecosystem of microorganisms in the digestive tract, has emerged as a key player in brain health.[1,6] Whole food plant-based diets are known to promote the growth of beneficial bacteria in the gut, leading to a more diverse and balanced microbiome. These foods contribute to producing short-chain fatty acids (SCFAs) through microbial fermentation, which can have neuroprotective effects and potentially impact cognitive function.[2,7]

The MIND Diet

The MIND diet, short for the Mediterranean–DASH Diet Intervention for Neurodegenerative Delay, integrates principles from the Mediterranean and DASH (Dietary Approaches to Stop Hypertension) diets. This hybrid dietary pattern specifically targets brain health and has gained attention for its potential to reduce the risk of Alzheimer's disease (AD).[1]

The Mediterranean diet, inspired by the dietary patterns of countries such as Greece and shaped by their connection to the Mediterranean Sea, centers around high consumption of fruits, vegetables, legumes, nuts, cereals and olive oil. It advocates moderate intake of alcohol and dairy while restricting red meat, processed meat, saturated fats and sweets.[8,9] This blend of food groups is believed to supply essential micronutrients and fiber, reducing the risk of neurodegenerative diseases, including AD.[9] A systematic review revealed that randomized controlled trials reported significant improvements in delayed recall, global cognition and working memory, though not in attention, episodic memory, immediate recall, processing speed, paired associates or verbal fluency. Furthermore, studies such as the North Manhattan Study and the Bordeaux Three-City Study found more substantial preservation of white matter microstructure, positive alterations in white matter hyperintensities, and increased total brain matter among individuals compliant with the Mediterranean diet.[8,9] Proposed mechanisms for these findings include the diet's impact on neurovascular health and its role in reducing inflammation and oxidative stress levels.[9]

Similarly emphasizing plant-based foods, the DASH diet limits foods high in saturated fat (such as whole-fat dairy), sugar and sodium. Initially designed to prevent and treat hypertension, longitudinal studies associated the DASH diet with improvements in verbal memory, though not necessarily in visual memory or executive function.[2,4] In multiple studies, higher adherence to the diet correlated with less change in global cognition and episodic memory over time.[4,8] A randomized controlled trial also demonstrated a significant increase in cognitive function and better average cognition when combining the DASH diet with weight management compared to the DASH diet alone.[8]

Combining both Mediterranean and DASH diets, the MIND diet outlines brain-boosting food groups, including vegetables, greens, nuts, berries, beans and whole grains. It limits the consumption of red meats, pastries, sweets, dairy and fast-fried foods.[1,4] By discouraging the intake of these items, the MIND diet aims to minimize factors that may contribute to cognitive decline and neurodegeneration. A longitudinal Australian study revealed a noteworthy 53% reduction in AD risk with high adherence to the MIND diet and a 35% decrease with moderate compliance.[4,10]

While these dietary patterns offer practical applicability for individuals seeking a sustainable dietary pattern, a deeper examination of specific nutritional components underlines the impact of micronutrients in these diets.[4,11] Various studies highlight the importance of vitamin B12, folate, omega-3s and antioxidants. A Swedish longitudinal study, for example, demonstrated that low levels of vitamin B12 and folate doubled the likelihood of developing dementia over 3 years.[11,12]

In a randomized controlled trial involving participants with mild cognitive impairment, taking high folic acid and vitamin B12 and B6 supplements reduced brain atrophy after 2 years of treatment.[2,11] Additional research indicated improved memory, information processing, sensorimotor speed and enhanced response to cholinesterase inhibitors in AD patients. Omega-3 fatty acids, present in the Mediterranean diet through fish consumption, have been individually studied and associated with decreased cognitive decline and amyloid accumulation, increased brain volume and diminished white matter hyperintensities.[11,12]

Antioxidants, such as vitamins A, C and E found in fruits, vegetables, nuts and berries, have demonstrated improved cognition, decreased risk of cerebrovascular events, reduced cognitive impairment and prevention of neurologic dysfunction.[12] Examining these micronutrients within a whole food plant-based diet provides practical insights into why these dietary patterns have proven effective in preventing or slowing cognitive decline.[1,4]

Numerous studies have investigated the impact of these diets on cognitive health in older adults. The results consistently show a potential protective effect against cognitive decline and dementia.[2,4] While fewer studies specifically focus on younger adults, existing research indicates that dietary patterns established earlier in life may influence cognitive outcomes in later years. Adopting brain-healthy diets during youth could contribute to long-term cognitive resilience.[1,2]

The growing field of lifestyle medicine recognizes the profound impact of dietary choices on cognitive health. Both a whole food plant-based diet and the MIND diet offer compelling avenues for individuals seeking to support their minds and potentially mitigate the risk of dementia. By embracing a diverse group of nutrients in a whole food plant-based diet and following a structured dietary plan designed for brain health, individuals can take proactive steps toward maintaining optimal cognitive function throughout their lives. As research in this field continues to unfold, the intersection of nutrition and brain health holds the promise of a brighter and more cognitively resilient future.

UNLOCKING COGNITIVE RESILIENCE: THE TRANSFORMATIVE INFLUENCE OF EXERCISE ON DEMENTIA PREVENTION AND MANAGEMENT

Cognitive impairment evolves as a progressive disease, gradually diminishing cognitive abilities and functional well-being over numerous years. It initiates progressive brain atrophy and memory loss, ultimately culminating in dementia, disability and mortality. The foremost well-established risk factor for dementia is advanced age, with the majority of cases manifesting in individuals aged 65 and older.[13] The intricate process of memory formation relies on the dynamic modulation of synaptic connections in response to changes in neuronal activity.[13,14] In AD-affected brains, toxic proteins such as amyloid-β (Aβ) plaques and tau tangles disrupt synaptic plasticity, impeding effective communication between brain cells. This disruption results in memory loss and various cognitive deficits.[13]

MITIGATING NEURODEGENERATIVE PROCESSES

Physical activity is a cornerstone for promoting holistic health, encompassing physical, social and emotional well-being, particularly for older adults. Recent studies underscore the vital role of regular physical activity in impeding the progression of major neurocognitive disorders, such as AD.[4,13,14] Notably, physical activity fosters the release of brain chemicals and strengthens neuronal connections. These crucial elements decline with the natural aging process.[2,14,15] The relationship between exercise and cognitive function is multifaceted, involving mechanisms such as increased blood flow to the brain, the release of neurotrophic factors and the promotion of synaptic plasticity. Moreover, mobility plays a fundamental role in preventing and improving risk factors associated with neurocognitive impairment, including diabetes mellitus type 2, cardiovascular diseases, hyperlipidemia and metabolic syndrome.[13-15]

IRISIN AND FNDC5: ILLUMINATING PATHS TO COGNITIVE RESILIENCE THROUGH EXERCISE

Recent studies highlight a potential mechanism linking physical activity to preventing neurocognitive decline by elevating Fibronectin Type III Domain-Containing Protein 5 (FNDC5) and irisin in the hippocampus.[15] Irisin, identified as an exercise-induced myokine and a proteolytic product of FNDC5, was first characterized by Bostrom et al. in 2012.[4,15] Extensive research has demonstrated elevated irisin levels in skeletal muscle following prolonged endurance exercise, observed in both human and mice subjects.[15,16] Studies have consistently emphasized the role of exercise in preventing or slowing the progression of AD and related dementias. A plausible mechanism underlying this protective effect is the activation of the FNDC5/irisin pathway by physical activity, which extends into the brain, initiating a signaling cascade that modulates neuronal function.[15-17] Beyond its neuroprotective role, irisin has also been recognized as a myokine capable of inducing the "browning" of white adipose tissue. This process transforms subcutaneous fat into a metabolically active form rich in mitochondria, promoting enhanced fat metabolism, thermogenesis and increased energy expenditure.[4,15,16] FNDC5/irisin also regulates neurogenesis, neurobehavior, neuronal metabolism and memory enhancement.[17,18]

Elevated levels of FNDC5/irisin have been associated with the induction of Brain-Derived Neurotrophic Factor (BDNF) in the hippocampus, a vital process in promoting neuronal cell survival, preserving synaptic integrity and facilitating special memory, key elements for learning development.[16-18]

In the context of AD, studies have revealed diminished levels of FNDC5/irisin in the hippocampus and cerebrospinal fluid of both human subjects and mouse models. Interventions aimed at increasing irisin in the brains of AD mice have demonstrated improvements in synaptic plasticity and memory function.[15,18] Irisin not only diminishes the expression of synapse-related genes induced by Aβ peptides but also reinstates translational suppression associated with Alzheimer's disease in hippocampal neurons.[16-18]

TAILORING EXERCISE INTERVENTIONS

While all forms of exercise contribute to overall health, various studies suggest that aerobic exercise, compared to strength training and multimodal activities, provides more significant advantages in preserving neurocognitive function in patients with Mild Cognitive Impairment (MCI).[2,19] Exercise intensity has also been analyzed, revealing a positive correlation between vigorous physical activity and increased cerebral blood flow, leading to improved executive function, augmented brain size and a reduced risk of neurocognitive decline.[2,19]

Dementia stands as a relentless neurodegenerative condition primarily impacting memory, with no known cure. However, a promising avenue for preventing cognitive decline lies in physical activity, specifically through the elevation of FNDC5/irisin expression in the hippocampus.[16–18] The induction of irisin by exercise serves as a defensive mechanism for the nervous system, promoting neurogenesis and suppressing the accumulation of Aβ.[17,18] Among various lifestyle changes, exercise is shown as a highly effective strategy for reducing the risk of neurocognitive impairment. Embrace regular physical activity to protect against memory loss proactively.

SLEEP AND COGNITIVE HEALTH: UNDERSTANDING PATTERNS, IMPLICATIONS AND STRATEGIES FOR NEUROCOGNITIVE WELL-BEING

The Importance of Quality Sleep

Quality sleep is increasingly recognized as a cornerstone of cognitive health. Adequate and restorative sleep is essential for memory consolidation, emotional regulation and overall cognitive function. Disturbances in sleep patterns have been linked to an increased risk of cognitive decline and dementia.

Sleep plays a crucial role in facilitating the repair and clearance processes necessary for rectifying and preventing neuronal damage while also contributing to learning and synaptic homeostasis.[20] Though we dedicate approximately one-third of our lives to sleep, not all sleep is optimal. To gain insight, we must first grasp the structure of sleep, which is categorized into four stages: N1, N2, N3 (slow sleep) and Rapid Eye Movement (REM), where dreams manifest.[21] The dynamics of sleep shift throughout various life stages, with aging notably influencing these patterns. As individuals age, total sleep time typically decreases from around 14 hours during toddlerhood at 2 years old to approximately 7–9 hours in adults aged 60 years and above.[20,22] Alterations in sleep patterns predominantly manifest before the age of 60.[23] A substantial proportion of American adults, exceeding 50%, self-report experiencing low sleep quality, with a higher prevalence in women over 45 years, reaching parity by the age of 75.[22,23] The total sleep duration has emerged as a potential risk factor for dementia, with the recommended sleep duration for adults falling between 7 and 9 hours.[23,24]

Sleep Architecture throughout the Lifecycle

Age-related hallmark changes in sleep architecture have been well-described. With increased age, there is an increase in daytime napping and nighttime awakenings. There is often an increase in sleep latency (time to fall asleep). There is also an increase in the duration of Stage N1 (transition between awake and asleep) and Stage N2 (throughout sleep). Older adults are more prone to awaken during non-REM sleep. With increased age, there is a decrease in the percent of time spent in REM and a decrease in sleep efficiency (time asleep over time in bed) and total sleep time. There is also a decrease in Stage N3 (slow-wave sleep).[21,25]

It has been suggested that a diminished requirement for sleep in aging individuals may be attributed to the loss of neurons, particularly those linked to rest. This correlation between aging, neuronal loss and reduced sleep is implicated in cognitive decline. Furthermore, the aging process is associated with decreased melatonin secretion, a hormone crucial for regulating the circadian sleep cycle. External factors, such as retirement, altered routines, stressors, caffeine consumption and engaging in exercise before bedtime, also contribute to changes in sleep patterns.[22,25]

SLEEP AND DEMENTIA RISK

Inadequate sleep quality and various sleep disorders, including insomnia, movement disorders and obstructive sleep apnea (OSA), are linked to increased cognitive impairment, type 2 diabetes mellitus, cardiovascular diseases, obesity and depression.[23,25,26] Research supports a direct connection between sleep and an accelerated cognitive decline, manifested through the accumulation of Aβ in Alzheimer's disease and oxidative stress in vascular dementia.[23,26]

Studies have shown that sleep disruption, as often seen in shift workers, affects the release of melatonin in a way that may contribute to cognitive impairment.[2,4] In some studies, male shift workers exhibited diminished cognitive function in a dose-response manner. Those engaged in prolonged periods of shift work experienced greater difficulty with memory, but their cognitive function did improve after discontinuing shift work for at least 4 years.[2] Another investigation revealed that sleep deprivation-induced cellular changes prompted microglia (which typically perform a cleansing function) to phagocytize normal brain tissue.[1,2] Over the long term, this resulted in brain atrophy. One meta-analysis encompassing 7 studies with over 13,000 participants demonstrated that sleep apnea heightened the risk of developing Alzheimer's disease by up to 70%.[2]

Improving sleep quality is an effective strategy for preventing neurocognitive disorders.[26] In non-pharmacological interventions, prioritizing approaches such as cognitive-behavioral therapy for insomnia (CBT-I) and education on sleep hygiene are recommended as the primary therapeutic options, given their superiority over pharmacological treatments.[22] Initiating early screening, diagnosis and treatment for sleep disorders has the potential to reduce the risk of neurocognitive decline and mitigate the onset of other medical conditions.

CHRONIC STRESS AND COGNITIVE HEALTH: UNRAVELING THE IMPACT, LIFESPAN PERSPECTIVES AND STRATEGIES FOR RESILIENCE

CHRONIC STRESS AND THE BRAIN

When assessing a patient vulnerable to dementia, an essential aspect to consider is their stress history. A recent comprehensive review and meta-analysis, encompassing over a thousand studies, revealed a substantial association between elevated perceived stress in adulthood and the development of mild cognitive impairment as well as all-cause dementia.[27,28] The studies underscored the reliability of self-reported stress levels as a metric, indicating the patient's awareness of stress in their life. Addressing stress through interventions such as behavioral health emerged as a valuable strategy for processing and managing the stress experience.[28] Additionally, the same study found that individuals who had encountered more than two significant stressful life events exhibited higher rates of all-cause dementia.[27] In a study by Lupien et al., older participants with increased stress-associated cortisol levels had a 14% reduction in hippocampal volume and impaired memory.[2]

Interestingly, the correlation between a single significantly stressful life event and dementia appears to be insufficient. It suggests a potential interpretation that resilience to stress diminishes with each successive traumatic event. Overall, providing support to patients dealing with stress not only benefits them in the present but may also help mitigate the severity of dementia in the future.

STRESSORS THROUGHOUT THE LIFECYCLE

A substantial body of research has explored the link between the late onset of Alzheimer's disease (AD) and stress. AD, a complex condition influenced by a combination of environmental and genetic factors, results in profound cognitive decline.[28,29] Recent studies propose that this late-age disease might predominantly be instigated by stressors encountered earlier in life, such as insufficient access to food, housing and traumatic experiences.[28] A landmark study has investigated the connection between social factors and late-life AD. Prospective research of women in Gothenburg since 1968 assessed potential dementia risk factors. Women experiencing significant psychosocial stress and a higher frequency of stressful events in midlife exhibited a statistically significant increase in the rate of major neurocognitive impairment three decades later.[29] Psychosocial stressors encompassed widowhood, divorce, limited social connections, receiving support from social security and the presence of mental illness in close relatives.[28,29] Events occurring many years before old age seemed to have enduring effects on the brain, predisposing women to dementia in their later years.

For individuals at risk, it is advisable to conduct thorough history-taking and regular follow-ups to assess stress-related risk factors. Furthermore, incorporating non-pharmacologic interventions can serve as a preventive measure, potentially delaying further brain damage.[28,29]

STRESS MANAGEMENT TECHNIQUES

Stress-reducing activities such as meditation and mindfulness have been linked to lower neural inflammation, decreased atrophy and improved brain function.[30] A study by Harvard University researchers illustrated that individuals with meditation expertise exhibited increased cortical volume and a larger cortex in brain regions associated with attention and sensory processing. Notably, this impact was more pronounced in older individuals, suggesting a heightened effectiveness of meditation on the aging population.[31,32]

MITIGATING SUBSTANCE RISKS FOR COGNITIVE HEALTH

INTRODUCTION

Geriatric substance use poses a significant challenge, demanding careful consideration due to its potential impact on cognitive health and overall well-being in older adults. As the global population ages, grasping the implications of substance use becomes increasingly crucial for health care professionals who serve as primary health care providers for older adults. Substance use in geriatric populations has been on the rise over the last 20 years, according to CDC data showing an increased drug overdose death rate for adults aged 65 years and older, with a higher rate in males compared to females.[33] The importance of geriatric substance use lies not just in its prevalence but also in its potential to exacerbate cognitive decline, contribute to neurodegenerative conditions and complicate the management of common comorbidities in older populations[34,35] (Figure 16.1).

UNIQUE CHALLENGES AND CONSIDERATIONS

Addressing substance use among older adults involves navigating distinct challenges. Unlike their younger counterparts, geriatric individuals often contend with chronic health conditions, polypharmacy and age-related physiological changes that can magnify substance use consequences. Managing substance use in this demographic demands a nuanced approach by recognizing the intricate interplay between physical and mental health, social factors and medication regimens. The stigma surrounding substance use can hinder open communication, requiring health care professionals to foster a trusting and non-judgmental environment. Clinicians must also consider potential substance interactions with medications frequently prescribed to older adults, necessitating a comprehensive and personalized care approach. Understanding the unique challenges of geriatric substance use enables health care

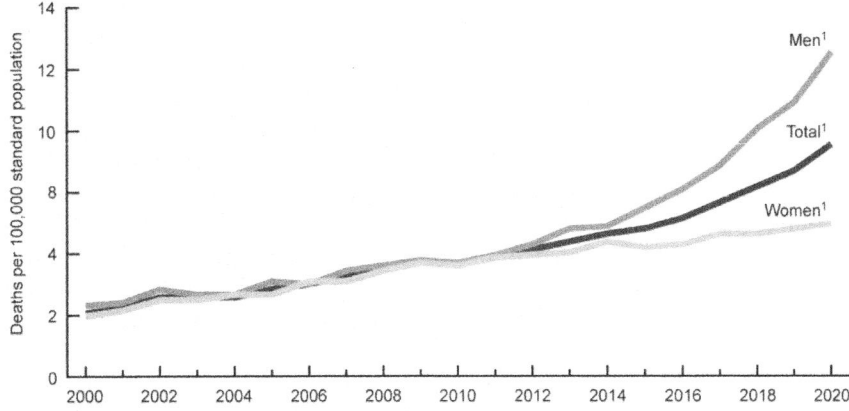

FIGURE 16.1 Age-adjusted drug overdose death rate for adults aged 65 and over, by sex, United States, 2000–2020.

professionals to tailor interventions to the specific needs of their older patients, promoting enhanced brain health and overall quality of life.

Substance Use and Cognitive Health

Cognitive Impact of Substance Use

Exploring the literature on substance use and cognitive health in geriatric patients reveals critical insights. The impact of substance use becomes even more pronounced with age. Older individuals are particularly vulnerable to the adverse effects of risky substances due to changes in metabolism, body composition and cognitive function. Substance use can impair cognitive function, memory and emotional regulation. Alcohol, nicotine, opioids and benzodiazepines are common substances in this demographic and exhibit varying degrees of impact on cognitive function.

Due to physiologic changes, alcohol is metabolized differently in the geriatric population, which leads to increased sensitivity to smaller amounts and increased potential for drug–drug interactions – alcohol on a molecular level functions by increasing GABA activity and blocking N-methyl-D-aspartate (NMDA) receptors. Chronic inhibition of glutamate may cause toxic effects. Not only is alcohol toxic at high levels, but it may also lead to other vitamin deficiencies, such as vitamin B1, vitamin B12 and folate, that contribute to cognitive impairment, mainly affecting memory and executive functions.[36] Even at moderate amounts, chronic alcohol consumption can impair memory, attention and executive function.[36] Chronic alcohol leads to increased cytokines, toll-like receptor activation, prostaglandins, inducible nitric oxide synthase (iNOS) and microglia activation that leads to neurodegeneration and neuronal loss.[37,38] Additional theories linking alcohol to dementia suggest that alcohol is involved in the accumulation of amyloid beta plaques, leading to a continuous cycle of overloaded microglia releasing inflammatory cytokines when consuming the excess plaques to protect brain cells.[38,39] Excessive alcohol use may also lead to liver damage and hepatic encephalopathy.[36] The Lancet Commission 2020 report identified excessive alcohol use along with head injury and air pollution as the three new modifiable risk factors for dementia compared to the 2017 report.[37] This report recommends public health initiatives to minimize detrimental alcohol use that would possibly "reduce young-onset and later-life dementia."[37] Alcohol misuse and drinking more than 21 units weekly increase the risk of dementia.[36] The effects of alcohol are dose-dependent, with light-moderate consumption having cardiovascular protection and increased anti-inflammatory processes.[40] Studies have demonstrated that older patients with a light-moderate amount of alcohol intake can have a decreased risk of cardiovascular disease and dementia.[40] However, the protective effects of alcohol warrant further studies since confounding factors, such as lack of standard definitions and differing methods, may have skewed results.[40]

According to the *Dietary Guidelines for Americans, 2020–2025*, moderate alcohol use guidelines are even more conservative for older adults. Guidelines recommend that men have two drinks or less a day while women have one drink or less a day with no more than seven drinks in a week.[41] A standard drink has 14 grams of alcohol; some examples include 12 ounces of beer, 5 ounces of wine, or 1.5 ounces of spirits.[42] Overall, due to the predominantly adverse effects, the recommendation is to limit alcohol use to promote brain health and overall well-being.

Along with alcohol, nicotine is another substance prevalent in the geriatric population. A cohort study by Hunt et al. demonstrated that smoking prevalence decreased from 15.9% in 1998 to 11.2% in 2028 in older populations, and previous smokers are maintaining cessation.[43] These findings highlight the importance of smoking cessation education. Smokers are at higher risk of dementia compared to non-smokers, though these findings may be biased due to the higher death rate in smokers.[36] Furthermore, smoking has been linked to social isolation, both of which increase the risk for dementia.[36] There are two proposed mechanisms of tobacco use leading to dementia; one involves increased oxidative stress, which in turn increases the formation of neurofibrillary tangles leading to dementia.[44] In another proposed theory, tobacco use causes known cardiovascular effects, including heart disease and strokes, which are correlated to its impacts on the development of dementia on the microvascular scale.[44] Current smoking increases the risk of Alzheimer's disease and other cognitive decline, particularly in those 65 to 75 years old, while smoking cessation of at least 4 years resulted in decreased risk of dementia to that of never-smokers.[44,45] Smoking cessation, even in later years, improves lung function, cardiovascular health and cognitive function.[45] Smoking cessation counseling with the 5 A's framework (Ask, Advise, Assess, Assist, Arrange) and resources are critical for health care professionals to support older individuals in maintaining cognitive health.[46] With these findings, avoiding nicotine use would be ideal. Still, in smokers, smoking cessation counseling should be a primary focus to decrease the risk of dementia and to maintain overall brain health.

Opiates are another detrimental substance that contributes to an increased risk of dementia. Opioid use, often prescribed for pain management, may contribute to cognitive decline, especially with prolonged or inappropriate use. A review study on chronic pain in the older population revealed that geriatric subjects seem to be more susceptible to prolonged pain development due to delayed peripheral nerve injury recovery leading to hyperalgesia and decreased effectiveness of pain inhibitory mechanisms in the brain due to age leading to decreased effectiveness on pain medications acting on the central nervous system.[46] Due to these pathophysiologic changes, specific chronic pain treatment guidelines are needed to treat pain in older adults appropriately.[46] Interestingly, a higher number of chronic pain sites correlated with a future increase in cognitive decline.[47] As such, an interdisciplinary team with clear guidelines on opiate prescriptions would help manage complex chronic opioid use in older patients.[48,49]

Along with alcohol and opiates, the prevalent use of benzodiazepines for anxiety and sleep disorders in older adults poses an additional layer of complexity, with long-term use linked to heightened cognitive impairment. These medications, commonly used as anxiolytics and hypnotics, are increasingly prevalent among women and non-Hispanic White adults, with growing misuse by young adults.[50] The recreational drug market and the internet are witnessing a rise in unregulated psychoactive substances, including designer benzodiazepines.[50] Both benzodiazepines and non-benzodiazepine sedative-hypnotics (Z-drugs) act through GABA-mediated neuronal inhibition, impacting brain reward circuitry and fostering addiction potential.[50] Widespread prescription and misuse of benzodiazepines pose serious risks such as overdose, respiratory depression, memory disturbances, falls and injury, especially when combined with opioids, alcohol or other sedatives.[50] Given age-related hepatic metabolism changes, patients should be counseled about the risks associated with continued benzodiazepine use, irrespective of duration.[50] A retrospective cohort study by Torres-Bondia et al. demonstrated that high doses of short half-lives benzodiazepines and Z-drugs were associated with increased risk of dementia, particularly in women, which shows a dose-response relationship.[51] The increased use of benzodiazepines and Z-hypnotics, coupled with the aging population, raises concerns about their potential contribution to dementia.[52] This cohort study assesses explicitly the risk of developing dementia associated with benzodiazepines and Z-hypnotics, taking into account their respective half-lives and concurrent usage, with results showing an increased dementia risk in participants that took either short or long-acting benzodiazepines for more than 28 days in 3 months.[52] Based on all these findings, avoiding benzodiazepine use, especially in the older population, would be neuroprotective.

As stated at the beginning of this section, illicit drug use has been increasing in the geriatric population over the years, particularly in the baby boomer generation; namely, those born between 1946 and 1965.[53] Substance abuse in people older than 65 years old often goes unnoticed or misdiagnosed since there is a prevalent myth that older people rarely use illicit drugs.[53] With an increased rate of older individuals meeting substance use disorder criteria compared to previous cohorts, this problem is leading to significant adverse effects on both medical and psychiatric conditions.[53] Current management plans need to be revised with collaboration between geriatrics, addiction and psychiatry to establish a comprehensive model that provides specialized interventions and support to address this public health dilemma.[53]

With the increasing prevalence of substance use, having effective screening and diagnosis tools is crucial to elicit a discussion. A screening questionnaire, such as a Drug Screening Questionnaire (DAST), could be a starting point, but this stigmatizing topic can be uncomfortable for patients and clinicians limited by visit time.[54] Admissions data between 2008 and 2018 from substance use treatment facilities showed an increase of admission of adults over 55 years old from 9.04% to 15.64%, with patients mentioning use of these substances: alcohol (66.7%), cocaine (14.8%), cannabis (14.1%), heroin (14.0%), other opioids (8.6%), methamphetamine (5.8%), benzodiazepines (2.4%) and additional (2.7%).[55] Substance use exacerbates age-related cognitive decline, increases the risk of mental health issues, and leads to social isolation.[56]

Understanding potential links between substance use and neurodegenerative conditions is crucial. Emerging research suggests that certain substances may accelerate or exacerbate conditions such as Alzheimer's disease and other dementias in geriatric patients.[56] This underscores the need for holistic assessments that consider substance use and cognitive health simultaneously. With this knowledge and motivational interviewing skills, health care professionals can implement targeted interventions to mitigate potential long-term cognitive consequences. Navigating the nuanced relationship between substance use and cognitive health allows clinicians to enhance the overall well-being of their aging patients with precision and insight.

Polypharmacy and Cognitive Interactions

Effectively managing polypharmacy and its potential interactions with substance use is pivotal in geriatric care. Older adults, often dealing with multiple chronic conditions, frequently find themselves prescribed numerous medications simultaneously – a scenario termed polypharmacy when there is regular use of more than five medications.[57] The challenge intensifies when polypharmacy intersects with substance use, requiring a nuanced approach. The crux of the issue lies in potential interactions between medications and substances, leading to exacerbated cognitive decline in older adults. For instance, combining benzodiazepines or opioids with substances such as alcohol or taking undisclosed over-the-counter medications can heighten sedation and increase the risk of falls, impacting cognitive function.[56] Furthermore, these interactions may compromise the efficacy of prescribed medications, undermining the management of chronic conditions.[57] To make matters more complicated, multiple sub-specialties without primary care physicians to coordinate medications exacerbate adverse consequences of polypharmacy.[57]

Health care professionals must grasp the delicate balance needed to navigate polypharmacy and its intersection with substance use, allowing them to develop tailored interventions. Regular medication reviews by health care professionals with active plans for deprescribing ensure proper dosages and minimize risks of adverse medical outcomes.[57] The five steps to deprescribing include: (1) identifying potentially inappropriate medications, (2) determining if the dosage can be decreased or the medication stopped, (3) creating a tapering plan, (4) monitoring for discontinuation symptoms or need to restart while supporting the patient and (5) documenting outcomes.[56] These steps should be individualized to each case, with each step requiring time, preparation and conversation with patients.[57,58] Clinicians may use the Beers Criteria as an essential reference for medications affecting the older individual that should be deprescribed.[57] By addressing these challenges, clinicians can optimize medication regimens, mitigate cognitive risks and elevate the overall quality of care for their geriatric patients.[57,58]

In conclusion, prioritizing substance avoidance among older adults yields multifaceted benefits. Not only does it contribute to preserved cognitive function, mitigating the risk of neurodegenerative diseases, but it also plays a pivotal role in enhancing physical health by reducing the likelihood of strokes and heart diseases. Additionally, avoiding excessive alcohol helps minimize the occurrence of falls and related injuries, promoting overall safety. Furthermore, substance avoidance supports improved medication management, reducing the risk of adverse drug reactions and ensuring optimal health care outcomes. Embracing a lifestyle that emphasizes the avoidance of risky substances emerges as a comprehensive strategy for fostering cognitive well-being, physical health and overall safety in the aging population.

GERIATRIC SOCIAL CONNECTIONS AND BRAIN HEALTH

In the evolving landscape of geriatric care, the intricate relationship between social connections and brain health is paramount to understanding the multifaceted dynamics of geriatric social connections and exploring their profound impact on cognitive well-being. Recognizing the evolving needs of an aging population, clinicians play a pivotal role in integrating this understanding into their practice to enhance their geriatric patients' overall health and resilience.

Social connections play a crucial role when assessing cognitive concerns in geriatric patients. Social connections are an integral component of brain development and maintaining healthy cognition. This evolutionary aspect suggests that the social brain evolved as a defense mechanism, allowing individuals in complex social groups to engage in more sophisticated computations for cooperation and competition.[59,60]

Recent research suggests a link between increased social relationships and brain preservation. In a randomized control trial involving 250 older adults, scheduled 1-hour group discussion sessions 3 times a week led to a statistically significant increase in brain volume on MRI over 40 weeks and improved neuropsychology testing performance compared to peers without scheduled interaction.[60] The strong connections formed persisted for years beyond the study's conclusion.[60] Another MRI study indicated that patients with more extensive social networks, demonstrating complexity, had larger amygdala volumes.[61] Maintaining such relationships is considered challenging, requiring meaningful cognitive engagement. Some studies utilized 3D "in-degree" depictions of small communities' social networks, revealing that patients with the most connections toward the network's center exhibited high grey matter density in the orbitofrontal cortex and dorsomedial complex on MRI.[62]

Along with social connections being integral to brain development, poor social literacy can be an early sign of cognitive impairment, often manifested as social withdrawal and diminished understanding of cues and situations.[63] Frontotemporal dementia patients struggle with interpreting body language, gestures and facial expressions due to brain atrophy.[64] A prospective cohort study of around 5,800 older women found a two-fold increase in all-cause dementia incidence among those with low social support.[65] Not only does cognitive impairment contribute to decreased socialization but also strong social bonds correlate with lower cognitive impairment risks; this bidirectional relationship underscores the importance of obtaining a comprehensive social history, especially in high-risk older adults.

The geriatric assessment, a multidisciplinary tool, evaluates older individuals' functional ability, physical health, cognition, mental health and socioeconomic factors, which can identify risks for cognitive decline.[66] Physical limitations are assessed using tools such as the Screening Version of the Hearing Handicap Inventory for the Elderly questionnaire.[66] It is crucial to address hearing loss since this is linked to isolation and cognitive dysfunction, even in the absence of dementia.[66] Evaluations for vision loss, balance, fecal and urinary continence and transferring abilities impact social connections due to difficulty leaving home. Early screening for mobility aids reduces stigma and fosters timely access, diminishing mobility-related social isolation.[66] Health care professionals may use these questionnaires for routine assessments to identify social isolation and prevent adverse cognitive outcomes. Assessing social networks and encouraging engagement, intellectual discussions and connecting with younger generations are effective strategies to build social connections. Technology, such as phone or video calls, bridges geographical distances and combats loneliness. Exploring new social opportunities contributes to cognitive reserve, reduces the risk of substance use and promotes mental well-being in geriatric individuals.

This section underscores the importance of recognizing, understanding and addressing the nuanced interplay between geriatric social connections and brain health. By integrating these insights into their practice and obtaining a comprehensive social history, health care professionals can contribute significantly to the holistic well-being of older adults, emphasizing the importance of social connections as a cornerstone of cognitive health in the aging population.

CONCLUSIONS

This chapter emphasizes the vital role of interventions within lifestyle medicine's six pillars in preventing, delaying and improving neurocognitive impairment, particularly in geriatric populations. We recommend that health care professionals offer education and resources on lifestyle changes to middle-aged and older adults at an increased risk of major neurocognitive disorders, with a primary focus on prevention. Empowering individuals to make informed choices and adopt healthier habits optimizes brain function, enhances resilience against neurocognitive challenges and improves the overall quality of life for aging individuals.

CLINICAL APPLICATIONS

- Assess and tailor dietary advice, focusing on elements of a whole food plant-based or MIND diet, considering individual preferences and health status for enhanced adherence and cognitive benefits.
- Integrate brain-healthy dietary interventions into existing treatment plans for those at risk of cognitive decline. Collaborate with nutrition specialists to seamlessly combine dietary recommendations with other therapeutic interventions.
- Tailor exercise recommendations for those at risk of cognitive decline, focusing on aerobic activities. Consider individual health, preferences and adherence for maximum neurocognitive benefits.
- Stress the link between vigorous physical activity and enhanced cognitive function. Encourage activities that boost heart rate and cerebral blood flow, providing a proactive defense against neurocognitive decline, particularly for those with mild cognitive impairment.
- Emphasize the importance of quality sleep for cognitive health. Encourage patients to aim for 7 to 9 hours of sleep per night, addressing factors such as sleep duration, routine and environment.

- Screen for sleep disorders, such as insomnia or sleep apnea, especially in older adults. Early detection and intervention, including non-pharmacological approaches such as cognitive-behavioral therapy for insomnia (CBT-I), can help prevent neurocognitive decline and associated conditions.
- Consider recent and past significant stressful events to inquire about patients' stress history. Understanding a patient's stress experience can provide insights into potential cognitive health risks.
- Advocate for stress management techniques such as meditation and mindfulness. Encourage patients, especially those at risk of dementia, to incorporate these practices into their daily routine as preventive measures for maintaining cognitive resilience.
- Prioritize a substance-free lifestyle for geriatric individuals to promote brain health, preserve cognitive function and enhance overall well-being.
- Health care professionals play a crucial role in offering tailored guidance to help older adults make informed choices about substance use.
- Implement motivational interviewing for more impactful interactions, improved patient outcomes and enhanced overall well-being.
- Understand that positive social connections go beyond companionship, serving as vital elements in promoting brain health and overall well-being in geriatric individuals.

REFERENCES

1. Rippe JM. Lifestyle medicine: the health promoting power of daily habits and practices. *Am J Lifestyle Med.* 2018;12(6):499–512. doi:10.1177/1559827618785554
2. Sherzai D, et al. Lifestyle intervention and Alzheimer disease. *J Fam Pract.* 2022;71(Suppl 1):eS83–eS89. doi:10.12788/jfp.0286
3. Lavretsky H. Lifestyle medicine for prevention of cognitive decline: focus on green tea. *Am J Geriatr Psychiatry.* 2016;24(10):890–892. doi:10.1016/j.jagp.2016.08.002
4. Jaqua E, Biddy E, Moore C, Browne G. The impact of the six pillars of lifestyle medicine on brain health. *Cureus.* 2023;15(2):e34605. doi:10.7759/cureus.34605
5. Abbatecola AM, Russo M, Barbieri M. Dietary patterns and cognition in older persons. *Curr Opin Clin Nutr Metab Care.* 2018;21(1):10–13. doi:10.1097/MCO.0000000000000434
6. Chen X, Maguire B, Brodaty H, O'Leary F. Dietary patterns and cognitive health in older adults: a systematic review. *J Alzheimers Dis.* 2019;67(2):583–619. doi:10.3233/JAD-180468
7. Singh RK, Chang HW, Yan D, et al. Influence of diet on the gut microbiome and implications for human health. *J Transl Med.* 2017;15(1):73. doi:10.1186/s12967-017-1175-y
8. Van den Brink AC, Brouwer-Brolsma EM, Berendsen AAM, van de Rest O. The Mediterranean, dietary approaches to stop hypertension (DASH), and Mediterranean-DASH intervention for neurodegenerative delay (MIND) diets are associated with less cognitive decline and a lower risk of Alzheimer's disease: a review. *Adv Nutr.* 2019;10(6):1040–1065. doi:10.1093/advances/nmz054
9. Loughrey DG, Lavecchia S, Brennan S, Lawlor BA, Kelly ME. The impact of the Mediterranean diet on the cognitive functioning of healthy older adults: a systematic review and meta-analysis. *Adv Nutr.* 2017;8(4):571–586. doi:10.3945/an.117.015495

10. Barnes LL, Dhana K, Liu X, et al. Trial of the MIND diet for prevention of cognitive decline in older persons. *N Engl J Med.* 2023;389(7):602–611. doi:10.1056/NEJMoa2302368
11. Smith PJ, Blumenthal JA. Dietary factors and cognitive decline. *J Prev Alzheimers Dis.* 2016;3(1):53–64. doi:10.14283/jpad.2015.71
12. Harrison FE. A critical review of vitamin C for the prevention of age-related cognitive decline and Alzheimer's disease. *J Alzheimers Dis.* 2012;29(4):711–726. doi:10.3233/JAD-2012-111853
13. Jaqua E, Deschamps J. The FNDC5/irisin pathway correlation with exercise and neurodegenerative disease. *J Gerontol Geriatr Med.* 2021;6:165–166. doi:10.19080/OAJGGM.2021.05.555682
14. Waseem R, Shamsi A, Mohammad T, et al. FNDC5/Irisin: physiology and pathophysiology. *Molecules.* 2022;27(3):1118. doi:10.3390/molecules27031118
15. Wrann CD. FNDC5/irisin – their role in the nervous system and as a mediator for beneficial effects of exercise on the brain. *Brain Plast.* 2015;1(1):55–61. doi:10.3233/BPL-150019
16. Jin Y, Sumsuzzman DM, Choi J, Kang H, Lee SR, Hong Y. Molecular and functional interaction of the myokine irisin with physical exercise and Alzheimer's disease. *Molecules.* 2018;23(12):3229. doi:10.3390/molecules23123229
17. Lourenco MV, Frozza RL, de Freitas GB, et al. Exercise-linked FNDC5/irisin rescues synaptic plasticity and memory defects in Alzheimer's models. *Nat Med.* 2019;25(1):165–175. doi:10.1038/s41591-018-0275-4
18. Pignataro P, Dicarlo M, Zerlotin R, et al. FNDC5/Irisin system in neuroinflammation and neurodegenerative diseases: update and novel perspective. *Int J Mol Sci.* 2021;22(4):1605. doi:10.3390/ijms22041605
19. Falck RS, Davis JC, Liu-Ambrose T. What is the association between sedentary behavior and cognitive function? A systematic review. *Br J Sports Med.* 2017;51(10):800–811. doi:10.1136/bjsports-2015-095551
20. Benca RM, Teodorescu M. Sleep physiology and disorders in aging and dementia. In: *Handbook of Clinical Neurology.* 2019;167:477–493. doi:10.1016/B978-0-12-804766-8.00026-1
21. Alessi CA. *Geriatrics Review Syllabus (GRS 11),* Vol. 11. American Geriatrics Society; 2022. Sleep issues.
22. Sexton CE, et al. Connections between insomnia and cognitive aging. *Neurosci Bull.* 2020;36(1):77–84. doi:10.1007/s12264-019-00401-9
23. Taillard J, et al. Sleep in normal aging, homeostatic and circadian regulation and vulnerability to sleep deprivation. *Brain Sci.* 2021;11(8):1003. doi:10.3390/brainsci11081003
24. Xu W, et al. Sleep problems and risk of all-cause cognitive decline or dementia: an updated systematic review and meta-analysis. *J Neurol Neurosurg Psychiatry.* 2020;91(3):236–244. doi:10.1136/jnnp-2019-321896
25. Suzuki K, et al. Sleep disorders in the elderly: diagnosis and management. *J Gen Fam Med.* 2017;18(2):61–71. doi:10.1002/jgf2.27
26. Kitamura T, et al. Insomnia and obstructive sleep apnea as potential triggers of dementia: is personalized prediction and prevention of the pathological cascade applicable? *EPMA J.* 2020;11(3):355–365. doi:10.1007/s13167-020-00219-w
27. Franks KH, et al. Association of stress with risk of dementia and mild cognitive impairment: a systematic review and meta-analysis. *J Alzheimers Dis.* 2021;82(4):1573–1590. doi:10.3233/JAD-210094
28. Lemche E. Early life stress and epigenetics in late-onset Alzheimer's dementia: a systematic review. *Curr Genomics.* 2018;19(7):522–602. doi:10.2174/1389202919666171229145156

29. Ritchie K, et al. Is late-onset Alzheimer's disease really a disease of midlife? *Alzheimers Dement (N Y)*. 2015;1(2):122–130. doi:10.1016/j.trci.2015.06.004
30. Lardone A, et al. Mindfulness meditation is related to long-lasting changes in hippocampal functional topology during resting state: a magnetoencephalography study. *Neural Plast*. 2018;2018:5340717. doi:10.1155/2018/5340717
31. Kurth F, et al. Reduced age-related degeneration of the hippocampal subiculum in long-term meditators. *Psychiatry Res Neuroimaging*. 2015;232(3):214–218. doi:10.1016/j.pscychresns.2015.03.008
32. Lazar SW, et al. Meditation experience is associated with increased cortical thickness. *Neuroreport*. 2005;16(17):1893–1897. doi:10.1097/01.wnr.0000186598.66243.19
33. Centers for Disease Control and Prevention. Data Brief 455: figure 1. Published 2023. Accessed December 3, 2023. https://www.cdc.gov/nchs/images/databriefs/451-500/db455-fig1.png
34. Kuerbis A, Sacco P, Blazer DG, Moore AA. Substance abuse among older adults. *Clin Geriatr Med*. 2014;30(3):629–654. doi:10.1016/j.cger.2014.04.008
35. Kuerbis A. Substance use among older adults: an update on prevalence, etiology, assessment, and intervention. *Gerontology*. 2020;66(3):249–258. doi:10.1159/000504363
36. Livingston G, Huntley J, Sommerlad A, et al. Dementia prevention, intervention, and care: 2020 report of the Lancet Commission. *Lancet*. 2020;396(10248):413–446. doi:10.1016/S0140-6736(20)30367-6
37. Sinforiani E, Zucchella C, Pasotti C, Casoni F, Bini P, Costa A. The effects of alcohol on cognition in the elderly: from protection to neurodegeneration. *Funct Neurol*. 2011;26(2):103–106.
38. Wiegmann C, Mick I, Brandl EJ, Heinz A, Gutwinski S. Alcohol and dementia—What is the link? A systematic review. *Neuropsychiatr Dis Treat*. 2020;16:87–99. doi:10.2147/NDT.S198772
39. Venkataraman A, Kalk N, Sewell G, Ritchie CW, Lingford-Hughes A. Alcohol and Alzheimer's disease—Does alcohol dependence contribute to beta-amyloid deposition, neuroinflammation, and neurodegeneration in Alzheimer's disease? *Alcohol Alcohol*. 2017;52(2):151–158. doi:10.1093/alcalc/agw092
40. Kim JW, Lee DY, Lee BC, et al. Alcohol and cognition in the elderly: a review. *Psychiatry Investig*. 2012;9(1):8–16. doi:10.4306/pi.2012.9.1.8
41. Dietary Guidelines for Americans. Dietary guidelines for Americans, 2020–2025 and online materials. Published 2020. Accessed December 3, 2023. https://www.dietaryguidelines.gov/resources/2020-2025-dietary-guidelines-online-materials
42. Rigler SK. Alcoholism in the elderly. *Am Fam Physician*. 2000;61(6):.
43. Hunt LJ, Covinsky KE, Cenzer I, et al. The epidemiology of smoking in older adults: a national cohort study. *J Gen Intern Med*. 2023;38(7):1697–1704. doi:10.1007/s11606-022-07980-w
44. Zhong G, Wang Y, Zhang Y, et al. Smoking is associated with an increased risk of dementia: a meta-analysis of prospective cohort studies with investigation of potential effect modifiers. *PLoS One*. 2015;10(3):e0118333. doi:10.1371/journal.pone.0118333
45. Peters R, Poulter R, Warner J, et al. Smoking, dementia, and cognitive decline in the elderly: a systematic review. *BMC Geriatr*. 2008;8:36. doi:10.1186/1471-2318-8-36
46. Centers for Disease Control and Prevention. Clinical tools. Published December 15, 2021. Accessed December 3, 2023. https://www.cdc.gov/tobacco/patient-care/clinical-tools/index.html
47. Tinnirello A, Mazzoleni S, Santi C. Chronic pain in the elderly: mechanisms and distinctive features. *Biomolecules*. 2021;11(8):1256. doi:10.3390/biom11081256
48. Guo X, Hou C, Tang P, Li R. Chronic pain, analgesics, and cognitive status: a comprehensive Mendelian randomization study. *Anesth Analg*. 2023;137(4):896–905. doi:10.1213/ANE.0000000000006514

49. Azubike N, Moseley M, Powers JS. Opioid management in older adults: lessons learned from a geriatric patient-centered medical home. *Fed Pract*. 2021;38(4):168–173. doi:10.12788/fp.0110
50. Peng L, Morford KL, Levander XA. Benzodiazepines and related sedatives. *Med Clin North Am*. 2022;106(1):113–129. doi:10.1016/j.mcna.2021.08.012
51. Torres-Bondia F, Dakterzada F, Galván L, et al. Benzodiazepine and Z-drug use and the risk of developing dementia. *Int J Neuropsychopharmacol*. 2022;25(4):261–268. doi:10.1093/ijnp/pyab073
52. Tseng LY, Huang ST, Peng LN, et al. Benzodiazepines, z-hypnotics, and risk of dementia: special considerations of half-lives and concomitant use. *Neurotherapeutics*. 2020;17(1):156–164. doi:10.1007/s13311-019-00801-9
53. Yarnell S, Li L, MacGrory B, et al. Substance use disorders in later life: a review and synthesis of the literature of an emerging public health concern. *Am J Geriatr Psychiatry*. 2020;28(2):226–236. doi:10.1016/j.jagp.2019.06.005
54. Han BH, Moore AA. Prevention and screening of unhealthy substance use by older adults. *Clin Geriatr Med*. 2018;34(1):117–129. doi:10.1016/j.cger.2017.08.005
55. Weber A, Lynch A, Miskle B, Arndt S, Acion L. Older adult substance use treatment first-time admissions between 2008 and 2018. *Am J Geriatr Psychiatry*. 2022;30(10):1055–1063. doi:10.1016/j.jagp.2022.03.003
56. Lin J, Arnovitz M, Kotbi N, Francois D. Substance use disorders in the geriatric population: a review and synthesis of the literature of a growing problem in a growing population. *Curr Treat Options Psychiatry*. Published online June 5, 2023. doi:10.1007/s40501-023-00291-9
57. Farrell B, Mangin D. Deprescribing is an essential part of good prescribing. *Am Fam Physician*. 2019;99(1):7–9.
58. Sawan M, Reeve E, Turner J, et al. A systems approach to identifying the challenges of implementing deprescribing in older adults across different healthcare settings and countries: a narrative review. *Expert Rev Clin Pharmacol*. 2020;13(3):233–245. doi:10.1080/17512433.2020.1730812
59. Dunbar RI. The social brain hypothesis and its implications for social evolution. *Ann Hum Biol*. 2009;36(5):562–572. doi:10.1080/03014460902960289
60. Mortimer JA, Ding D, Borenstein AR, et al. Changes in brain volume and cognition in a randomized trial of exercise and social interaction in a community-based sample of non-demented Chinese elders. *J Alzheimers Dis*. 2012;30(4):757–766. doi:10.3233/JAD-2012-120079
61. Bickart KC, Wright CI, Dautoff RJ, et al. Amygdala volume and social network size in humans. *Nat Neurosci*. 2011;14(2):163–164. doi:10.1038/nn.2724
62. Kwak S, Joo WT, Youm Y, Chey J. Social brain volume is associated with in-degree social network size among older adults. *Proc Biol Sci*. 2018;285(1871):20172708. doi:10.1098/rspb.2017.2708
63. Saczynski JS, Pfeifer LA, Masaki K, et al. The effect of social engagement on incident dementia: the Honolulu-Asia aging study. *Am J Epidemiol*. 2006;163(5):433–440. doi:10.1093/aje/kwj061
64. Bickart KC, Brickhouse M, Negreira A, et al. Atrophy in distinct corticolimbic networks in frontotemporal dementia relates to social impairments measured using the social impairment rating scale. *J Neurol Neurosurg Psychiatry*. 2014;85(4):438–448. doi:10.1136/jnnp-2012-304656
65. Oh DJ, Yang HW, Kim TH, et al. Association of low emotional and tangible support with risk of dementia among adults 60 years and older in South Korea. *JAMA Netw Open*. 2022;5(8):e2226260. doi:10.1001/jamanetworkopen.2022.26260
66. Elsawy B, Higgins KE. The geriatric assessment. *Am Fam Physician*. 2011;83(1):48–56

17 Depression

Fiona Yan-Yee Ho and Vincent Wing-Hei Wong

INTRODUCTION

While aging is an inherent aspect of the human experience, depression is not an inevitable outcome of the aging process. The global demographic shift toward a larger older adult population is expected to lead to a higher prevalence of geriatric depression, which poses significant challenges for public health infrastructures across the globe. Considering these pressing issues, lifestyle medicine (LM) has emerged as an important strategy for preventing and managing depression among older adults. LM offers a clinically, cost-effective, safe, non-stigmatizing and low-cost approach that empowers individuals through self-management. This chapter aims to provide an overview of the epidemiology of depression among older adults, delve into the underlying pathophysiology and the rationale of LM for depression and review how different pillars of LM, including nutrition and diet, physical activity, sleep management, stress reduction, social connection and substance use, can be leveraged to effectively manage depression in older adults.

EPIDEMIOLOGY OF DEPRESSION IN OLDER ADULTS

The global prevalence of depression among older adults has been extensively studied in the existing literature. A recent meta-analytic review, which aggregated data from 55 epidemiological and cross-sectional studies with 59,851 older adults, indicated an overall global prevalence of depressive symptoms of 35.1%.[1] However, an earlier meta-analysis conducted by Hu et al. indicated that the prevalence rate of depressive symptoms varied depending on the type of screening tool used, with estimates ranging from 15.6% to 31.5%.[2] Regarding major depression, a meta-analysis by Abdoli et al., which focused on 18,953 older adults, revealed a global prevalence rate of 13.3%.[3] Furthermore, Zhang et al. found that approximately 13% of older adults globally exhibited sub-threshold depressive symptoms.[4] Although existing epidemiological research has shown that depression is a prevalent condition among the global older adult population, it is important to note that the reported prevalence rates varied considerably among individual epidemiological studies, ranging from as low as 5% to as high as 81.1%.[1]

The wide range of reported prevalence rates can be partially explained by variations in methodological approaches.[1,2] Studies that solely rely on rating scales for assessing depression tended to report higher prevalence rates in contrast to those utilizing diagnostic interviews.[5] Additionally, smaller-scale studies with fewer than 200 participants tended to report a higher prevalence of depression at 40.5%, whereas studies with 200 or more participants indicated a lower prevalence rate of 27.4%.[2] Sampling methods also appeared to be a significant moderator for the prevalence rates, with cluster random sampling resulting in a prevalence of 54.8%, whereas the stratified random sampling method yielded a rate of 22.9%.[2] In addition to methodological differences, variations in geographic and cultural backgrounds, country income level and sample characteristics also contribute to the observed heterogeneity in prevalence rates. Evidence suggested that prevalence estimates of depression differ by continent, with Africa reporting the highest prevalence at 41.1%, followed by Asia at 29.9%, North and South Americas at 24.2% and Europe at 21.1%.[2] When focusing solely on Major Depressive Disorder (MDD), Australia exhibits the highest prevalence at 20.1%, with rates of 12.9% in Europe, 11% in North and South Americas, and the lowest in Asia at 10%.[3] Country income level also serves as a moderating factor contributing to the observed variability in depression prevalence rates among older adults, with a prevalence of 41.3% in low- and middle-income countries, 24.3% in upper-middle-income countries and 20% in high-income countries.[1]

Additionally, epidemiological studies that sampled from community settings generally found a lower prevalence of depression at 7.9% in older adults, compared to studies that recruited participants from geriatric outpatient clinics, primary care clinics and other medical settings, where the prevalence was significantly higher at 23.8%.[5] Moreover, evidence indicates an age-associated increase in the prevalence of MDD among the geriatric population.[3] Luppa et al. reported that individuals aged between 85 and 89 had a 20% to 25% higher prevalence of depression when compared to their counterparts aged between 75 and 79.[6] Notably, this prevalence rate further escalated by 30% to 50% in individuals aged 90 and above. This upward trend can be partially attributed to a confluence of factors that are more common with advancing age, such as higher incidence of multimorbidity, greater levels of physical and cognitive decline, reduced mobility and independence and lower socioeconomic status.[6]

The growing body of theoretical and empirical evidence has highlighted the role of lifestyle factors in the onset and development of depression among older adults. Wu et al. synthesized data from 25 systematic reviews and meta-analyses with over 1.1 million older adults to evaluate the association strength of 82 factors and the onset of depression.[7] Their findings identified certain lifestyle-related factors, including a healthy dietary pattern, regular physical activity and omega-3 fatty acid intake, as protective factors against depression. However, the strength of evidence varied from weak to suggestive levels. Conversely, the use of aspirin, advanced age (80 years and above), living alone, sleep disturbances, hearing and vision impairments and cardiovascular diseases have been identified as risk factors for depression in older adults. Evidence from cross-sectional studies also suggested a cumulative relationship between unhealthy lifestyles and depression. In a cross-sectional study involving 3,700 Korean older adults, it was found that the presence of three or more lifestyle risk factors was significantly associated with a higher depression risk, with odd ratios of 3.1 in men and 2.8 in women.[8] When examining specific lifestyle behaviors, it was found that being physically active, consuming greater quantities of fruit and vegetables and regularly drinking tea were associated with a reduced risk of depression in older adults.[9,10] Smoking and moderate alcohol use were associated with an increased depression risk. With the increasing recognition of lifestyle risk factors in the onset of depression among older adults, the following section will delve into how various lifestyle pillars contribute to the risk of depression through different biological processes.

PATHOPHYSIOLOGY AND RATIONALE FOR LIFESTYLE MEDICINE PILLARS

Evidence suggests that the pathogenesis and progression of depression in older adults cannot be attributed to a single cause. Instead, it is the result of a complex interplay between various biological (e.g., genetic predispositions, neurochemical imbalances, age-related changes in brain structure and function) and psychosocial factors (e.g., bereavement, retirement, loss of social role and social isolation). More recently, theoretical inquiries have conceptualized depression as a disease of modernity. This perspective suggests that the contemporary lifestyle, characterized by a range of unhealthy lifestyle practices such as physical inactivity, poor diet and nutrition and limited social connectedness, plays a role in the pathogenesis and progression of depression. In response to this proposition, a significant body of empirical research has emerged to explore the associations between various lifestyle practices and depression and to elucidate the underlying biological mechanisms. However, much of the current research has predominantly focused on the younger adult demographic, which may limit its applicability to the geriatric cohort. In the following discussion, the key biological mechanisms that potentially underpin the relationship between the core pillars of LM and depression are presented. These mechanisms include monoamine imbalance, inflammation, altered stress response, oxidative stress and dysfunction of brain-derived neurotrophic factor (BDNF).

Monoamine Imbalance

The theory of monoamine imbalance, which centers on the regulation of monoamine neurotransmitters, has long been influential in understanding the pathophysiology of depression. In older adults, the theory becomes more complex due to age-related neurobiological changes. These changes include natural declines in the production and responsiveness of monoamines such as serotonin, norepinephrine and dopamine. Furthermore, older adults are more prone to experiencing comorbid health conditions such as Parkinson's disease and Alzheimer's disease, which can influence the functioning of neurotransmitter systems.[11] Healthy lifestyles are important in modulating the activity of monoamine neurotransmitters. For instance, exercise has been shown to not only boost the release of neurotransmitters such as dopamine, serotonin and norepinephrine but also to modulate the circulating levels of these mood-regulating chemicals, thus exerting antidepressant effects.[12] Diets rich in tryptophan and tyrosine play a significant role in mood regulation, as these amino acids are precursors for serotonin and dopamine synthesis in the brain, respectively.[13]

Additionally, effective stress management is imperative given that emotional states related to stress can markedly increase inflammatory markers. This, in turn, may reduce monoamine neurotransmission through oxidative stress pathways, thereby heightening susceptibility to depression.[14] Finally, while tobacco use may initially inhibit the action of monoamine oxidase and alcohol use might transiently elevate serotonin in brain regions associated with the reward circuitry (e.g., ventral tegmental area, amygdala, hippocampus), chronic use may lead to neuroadaptations that diminish monoamine function, and ultimately contributing to the development of depression and other mood disorders.[15,16]

INFLAMMATION

Inflammation has emerged as a significant mechanism in the pathophysiology of geriatric depression. Research indicates that chronic low-grade systemic inflammation, characterized by an overproduction of pro-inflammatory markers (e.g., interleukin-6 and tumor necrosis factor-alpha), is frequently observed in the aging population, even in the absence of acute immunological provocations (i.e., inflammaging).[17] Bodai et al. and Vodovotz et al. have described the potential biological processes in which unhealthy lifestyle (i.e., physical inactivity, sedentary behaviors, poor diet and nutrition, limited social connectedness, sleep disturbance, elevated stress and substance use) may exacerbate chronic inflammation, which ultimately contributes to the development of depression.[18,19] Specifically, an unhealthy lifestyle can lead to changes in the gut microbiome that can result in dysbiosis, alteration in gene expression and cellular damage. These changes can individually and collectively precipitate inflammatory responses, leading to further imbalances in the microbiome, the formation of new epigenetic modifications and additional cellular damage. This cyclical mechanism, where inflammation perpetuates itself and becomes chronic, can lead to the manifestation of depressive symptoms.

OXIDATIVE STRESS

Oxidative stress becomes increasingly relevant to depression as individuals age. The natural progression of aging presents a dual challenge: the body tends to produce more reactive oxygen species, while the efficiency of the antioxidant defense systems naturally declines.[20] This imbalance can result in elevated levels of reactive oxygen species, resulting in oxidative stress. Oxidative stress, in turn, can cause neuronal damage and death, neuroinflammation and neurotransmitter imbalance, all of which contribute to the onset of depression. Therefore, bolstering antioxidant defenses through various healthy lifestyle practices becomes an important area of focus for both the prevention and treatment of depression in older adults. For example, research indicates that engaging in regular exercise can result in a range of cellular and systemic neuroimmune changes that contribute to the reduction of oxidative stress.[21] Additionally, maintaining a balanced diet is crucial in managing oxidative stress, as both malnutrition and overnutrition can disrupt the oxidative balance.[22] Moreover, an increased consumption of antioxidant-rich fruits and vegetables has been linked to a reduction in depressive symptoms. Adequate sleep also plays a significant role, as it is associated with a favorable pro-oxidant/antioxidant balance and a decrease in depressive symptoms.[23] Stress reduction is equally important, considering that chronic stress (e.g., loss of loved ones, financial problems, loneliness and social isolation) has been implicated in inducing oxidative stress within brain regions associated with the pathogenesis of depression. Lastly, substance management is important for maintaining oxidative balance, as solid evidence demonstrated that individuals with substance use disorder had significantly higher oxidant markers but lower antioxidant markers when compared to healthy controls.[24]

Hypothalamic–Pituitary–Adrenal Axis

The hypothalamic–pituitary–adrenal (HPA) axis serves as the central stress response system that regulates the release of cortisol to aid the body in coping with everyday stressors. However, the regulation of the HPA axis may become less efficient as the aging process unfolds. A robust body of research has demonstrated that chronic overactivation of the HPA axis is observed in individuals with MDD. This dysregulation carries significant prognostic implications, as it has been identified as a contributing factor for both relapse and suicidal behaviors in affected individuals.[25] Moreover, elevated cortisol induced by stress can lead to increased serotonin uptake and potentially contribute to the atrophy of the hippocampus, which may exacerbate depressive symptoms. The link between maladaptive stress responses and depression underscores the importance of stress management in both the prevention and treatment of depression. Moreover, research indicates that exercise has a modulating effect on the HPA axis, leading to an adaptive response when confronted with stress and resulting in diminished tissue sensitivity to cortisol.[26] This suggests that regular physical activity can help regulate the stress response system. While the relationship between diet and the HPA axis is not yet fully understood, there is evidence that maintaining a healthy dietary pattern can support the proper function of the HPA axis.[27] Furthermore, the HPA axis plays a pivotal role in regulating circadian rhythms, and sleep disturbances have been associated with dysregulation of the HPA axis.[28] This dysregulation can potentially contribute to the onset or exacerbation of depression. Therefore, it is imperative to integrate sleep management as an integral part of LM interventions for depression.

Dysfunction of Brain-Derived Neurotrophic Factor

Brain-derived neurotrophic factor (BDNF) is a neurotrophin essential for neuronal growth, maintenance and survival, and neuroplasticity. With advancing age, there is a natural decline in BDNF levels, which can increase the vulnerability of the aging brain to depression. Evidence from meta-analytic reviews has shown that depressed individuals have reduced levels of BDNF, particularly in brain regions involved in mood regulation and cognitive function, such as the hippocampus and prefrontal cortex.[29] Promoting a range of healthy lifestyle practices can effectively offset the neurobiological and clinical effects of BDNF dysfunction. For example, exercise has been found to stimulate the production of BDNF through the action of the ketone body β-hydroxybutyrate.[30] On the other hand, avoiding Western diets that are typically loaded with glycaemic carbohydrates, sugars, trans and saturated fats and salt can help maintain normal levels of BDNF. In addition, practicing stress and sleep management is important for maintaining optimal BDNF levels, as there is evidence that sleep mediates the relationship between stress and BDNF levels.[31]

RESEARCH ON THE IMPACT OF LIFESTYLE PILLARS ON DEPRESSION IN OLDER ADULTS

NUTRITION AND DIET

Associations between Nutrients/Dietary Patterns and Depression Risk

Numerous research studies have delved into the connections between nutrients/dietary patterns and depression. Certain nutrients have been identified as crucial for managing depression in older adults, such as omega-3 fatty acids and vitamin B.[32,33] For instance, a meta-analysis of six randomized controlled trials (RCTs) demonstrated the effectiveness of omega-3 fatty acids, commonly found in fatty fish, nuts, flaxseed, chia seed and certain plant oils, in treating depression among older individuals, yet the benefits were significant only for those with mild to moderate depression.[32] In addition, a 4-year longitudinal study found that a higher intake of vitamin B6 and B12 was associated with a reduced risk of depression among community-dwelling older adults.[33]

In terms of dietary patterns, a meta-analysis of 41 observational studies (20 longitudinal and 21 cross-sectional) revealed that adhering to healthy diets, such as the Mediterranean diet and avoiding pro-inflammatory diets, was linked to a lower incidence of depression.[34] Similarly, a more recent meta-analysis of 33 studies investigated the longitudinal association between diet and the occurrence of depression in middle-aged and older adults.[35] The findings indicated that higher consumption of pro-inflammatory diets and Western diets was associated with a higher likelihood of developing depression, while consuming higher quantities of fruits and vegetables was associated with a reduced risk of depression. However, this study did not find a significant association between "healthy" and Mediterranean diet and depression risks, which contradicted the findings of a recent meta-analysis.[34] The authors speculated that the absence of significant results may be attributed to the diverse range of methodologies used to define Mediterranean and "healthy" diets across the included studies.

Prevention/Treatment Effect of Nutrients/Dietary Patterns on Depression

A meta-analysis of six RCTs provided evidence supporting the potential benefits of omega-3 fatty acids in the treatment of depression among older adults. However, the effects of omega-3 polyunsaturated fatty acids (n-3 PUFAs) supplementation were found to be significant only in older adults with mild to moderate depression.[36] These findings align with the practice guideline published by the International Society for Nutritional Psychiatry Research, which recommends the use of n-3 PUFAs in treating clinical depression in older adults.[37]

While an RCT demonstrated the effectiveness of a Mediterranean-style dietary intervention supplemented with fish oil in reducing depression symptoms in young and middle-aged adults at 3 months, with sustained benefits observed at 6 months,[38] further large-scale RCTs are needed to confirm the effects of this intervention on older adults with depression. Moreover, more research is necessary to fully understand the mechanisms underlying these associations. Nevertheless, the current evidence suggests that incorporating a healthy and balanced diet that includes specific nutrients and adhering to certain dietary patterns appears to reduce depression risks in geriatric populations.

Physical Activity

Associations between Physical Activity and Depression Risk

Numerous studies examining the relationship between physical activity and the risk of depression among older adults have consistently demonstrated a beneficial effect. A meta-analysis of 49 cohort studies investigated the prospective association between physical activity and the incidence of depression. The findings revealed a significant inverse relationship, indicating that higher levels of physical activity were associated with a lower likelihood of developing depression compared to individuals with lower physical activity levels.[39] Notably, a sensitivity analysis further confirmed the protective effects of engaging in high levels of physical activity against the risk of depression in older adults.

Prevention/Treatment Effect of Physical Activity on Depression

The beneficial effect of exercise interventions for preventing depression was supported by a systematic review that included 8 meta-analyses of 134 RCTs.[40] The findings indicated that exercise interventions as a preventive measure may have a moderate effect in alleviating depressive symptoms across a wide age range, including older adults, in the general population. Additionally, some studies with lower methodological quality suggested that low-intensity exercise may have comparable efficacy in lowering depression severity compared to high-intensity exercise.

Several studies have investigated the impact of different types of exercise on depression. A meta-analysis of 33 RCTs found that resistance exercise training was associated with a significant reduction in depressive symptoms, irrespective of participants' age, suggesting it serves as an alternative or adjunct therapy for depression.[41] In a network meta-analysis of 15 eligible RCTs, the comparative effectiveness of exercise types (aerobic, resistance and mind–body exercise) in treating clinical depression in older adults was explored. The study recommended that older adults self-select their preferred exercise type, and clinicians prescribe exercise alongside conventional treatments.[42] Furthermore, an umbrella review of systematic reviews and meta-analyses, including 12 meta-analyses comprising 97 RCTs, demonstrated a moderate improvement in depression and depressive symptoms among older adults engaging in physical activities. The review further supported the antidepressant effect of various types of physical activity, with aerobic exercises (e.g., walking, running or swimming) showing robust evidence, followed by strength exercises (e.g., weightlifting) and mixed exercises.[43]

Sleep

Associations between Sleep and Depression Risk

The relationship between sleep and depression is intricately connected, and it holds particular relevance among older adults due to the high prevalence of both sleep disturbances and depression in this population. A meta-analysis of nine studies yielded a significant association between sleep and depression.[44] Specifically, older adults who reported poor sleep quality were found to have a higher likelihood of experiencing depressive symptoms. Further evidence comes from a longitudinal study involving 10,794 community-dwelling middle-aged and older adults. The study revealed that individuals with short sleep duration (less than 6 hours) had a higher risk of developing depression and experiencing recurrent episodes compared to those with normal sleep duration (7 to 9 hours).[45] However, long sleep durations (more than 9 hours) did not show a significant effect on depression risks after adjusting for confounding factors. Moreover, a meta-analysis of 23 cohort studies indicated that persistent sleep disturbances were associated with an increased risk of the development, recurrence and exacerbation of depression in older adults.[46]

Prevention/Treatment Effect of Sleep Management on Depression

An RCT was conducted to evaluate the effectiveness of a sleep-focused intervention, specifically cognitive behavioral therapy for insomnia (CBT-I), in preventing and reducing the risk of MDD among 291 older adults who experienced insomnia and resided in the community.[47] Participants were randomly assigned to either a 2-month group-based CBT-I or a sleep education therapy. The findings showed that the intervention group, compared to the active control group (sleep education therapy), achieved a significant reduction of over 50% in both the incidence and recurrence of MDD within the population. This study highlights the significance of sleep management in preventing depression. Another RCT investigated the efficacy of CBT-I for older adults with comorbid insomnia and depression within community mental health services.[48] The participants received 8 weeks of group-based treatment, including one of the following: (1) CBT-I, (2) CBT-I plus positive mood strategies or (3) psychoeducation control. The results demonstrated that both CBT-I and CBT-I plus positive mood strategies were effective in mitigating both insomnia and depressive symptoms. This study supports the implementation of sleep-targeted treatments in community mental health services to address the comorbidity of insomnia and depression in older adults.

Stress Management

Associations between Stress and Depression Risk

Older adults often face unique stressful events which can contribute to the onset or worsening of depression. Retirement, in particular, represents a significant life transition with implications for mental health, both positive and negative. To explore the relationship between retirement and the occurrence of depression among older adults, a meta-analysis of 41 studies was conducted.[49] The findings revealed a protective effect of retirement against the risks of depression, with a reduction of nearly 20%. Additionally, the study emphasized the potential preventive effect of flexible retirement timing in the development of depression. Another meta-analysis of 25 longitudinal studies further supported the longitudinal association between the transition to retirement and depression risks.[50]

The decline in physical health, chronic conditions, functional limitations and cognitive changes that come with aging can also increase the risk of depression among older adults. To investigate the bidirectional relationship between physical health and mental health in later adulthood, a longitudinal study spanning 21 years and involving 16,417 older adults was conducted.[51] The findings revealed a reciprocal relationship, with physical health exerting a larger impact on mental health compared to the reverse influence.

Prevention/Treatment Effect of Stress Management on Depression

Effective stress management can help individuals better cope with life stressors, enhance resilience and protect against the development of mental health problems. A meta-analysis of 12 RCTs and 3 non-RCTs examined the effects of relaxation interventions on depression and anxiety in older adults.[52] The results indicated that older adults who participated in relaxation interventions, such as progressive muscle relaxation, music intervention and yoga, experienced significant improvements in depression compared to both active and inactive control groups. Furthermore, the positive effects of these relaxation techniques persisted for 14 to 24 weeks after the interventions were completed.

Mindfulness-based interventions have also been investigated as a potential approach for addressing depression in geriatric populations. A meta-analysis of 19 primary studies examined the effects of mindfulness meditation interventions on depression among older adults.[53] The findings from the meta-analysis provided evidence that even brief mindfulness meditation interventions, as brief as 4 weeks in duration, can lead to improvements in depressive symptoms among older adults. This suggests that mindfulness-based interventions could be implemented alongside conventional approaches for managing depression.

Social Connection

Associations between Social Connection and Depression Risk

Social isolation is another significant factor that can contribute to depressive symptoms among older adults. To examine the impact of social isolation from family and friends on depressive symptoms, a survey was conducted on a nationally representative sample of 1,439 older adults.[54] The study revealed that feeling subjectively isolated from both family and friends was associated with higher levels of depressive symptoms. Importantly, the findings highlighted that the significant relationship between subjective isolation and psychological stress was specifically observed in cases of isolation from friends.

Furthermore, a systematic review, which included ten longitudinal studies, aimed to explore the relationship between loneliness and depressive symptoms in older adults.[55] The findings of this review demonstrated a significant positive association between loneliness at baseline and depressive symptoms during the follow-up period among older adults. It was observed that older adults who reported higher levels of loneliness were more prone to experiencing an escalation in depressive symptoms, which impeded their recovery from depression. The study also found that loneliness at baseline was associated with an unfavorable clinical course of depression. To gain further insights into the effects of social support and loneliness on depression, a cross-sectional study involving a total of 320 older adults was conducted. The study aimed to explore the influence of loneliness on depression and examine the mediating role of social support.[56] The findings indicated significant associations between loneliness, social support and depression. Moreover, the study revealed that social support partially mediated the relationship between loneliness and depression. These results offer additional evidence supporting the idea that interventions targeting the enhancement of social support networks may be beneficial in reducing loneliness and alleviating depressive symptoms in older adults.

Another systematic review comprising 51 studies aimed to investigate the impact of social relationships on depression outcomes in this population.[57] The findings confirmed the notion that certain factors related to social relationships acted as significant protective factors against depression. These factors included perceived emotional support, which involves having someone available to listen, offer sympathy or provide advice during times of crisis or hardship. Additionally, perceived instrumental support, which involves having someone available to offer physical or financial assistance, was identified as another protective factor. Furthermore, the presence of large and diverse social networks was also associated with a reduced risk of depression.

Treatment Effect of Interpersonal Support and Training on Depression

An RCT with 60 community-dwelling older Chinese immigrants in Canada examined the efficacy of a peer-based intervention in addressing loneliness and social isolation.[58] The participants received an 8-week peer support intervention that covered various topics such as understanding mental health, acquiring knowledge and skills to provide peer support, managing grief and loss, developing self-help skills, stress management, goal setting and building healthy relationships. The results demonstrated that the intervention effectively reduced feelings of loneliness and barriers to social participation, while also enhancing resilience among socially isolated older adults in comparison to the control group. In addition, the intervention group exhibited significant improvements in depressive symptoms, life satisfaction, and happiness, which were not observed in the control group.

SUBSTANCE USE

Associations between Substance Use and Depression Risks

Substance use, which includes the consumption of substances such as alcohol and tobacco, has been a subject of study in relation to its impact on mental health. A study that included a large sample of participants from 19 countries investigated the long-term association between alcohol consumption and the incidence of depressive episodes among older adults over a 10-year period.[59] The findings revealed a differential association between alcohol consumption and the incidence of depressive episodes in older adults. While both heavy drinkers and long-term alcohol abstainers had the highest rates of depressive episodes, moderate drinkers had the lowest risk of developing depressive episodes. Moreover, the authors noted that excessive alcohol use poses significantly greater harm in older ages compared to younger ages.

Another longitudinal study utilized individual-level data from 1992 to 2012 of the Health and Retirement Study.[60] The study aimed to investigate the correlation between smoking, heavy drinking and depression among middle-aged and older adults in the United States. The findings indicated that there was indeed a bidirectional association between smoking and depression, suggesting that smoking predicted future depression and vice versa. The study further revealed that smokers had a 20% higher likelihood of developing depression during the follow-up period compared to non-smokers. Additionally, participants who were initially non-smokers but experienced depression were 41% more likely to start smoking during the follow-up period. In contrast, the study did not find a significant link between heavy drinking and the onset of depression among people who were not depressed at baseline.

CLINICAL CONSIDERATIONS

Existing research indicates that various unhealthy lifestyle factors contribute to the development and progression of depression. Therefore, adopting a multicomponent intervention approach has the potential to maximize the clinical benefits of LM for managing depression. However, simultaneously modifying multiple lifestyle factors requires a considerable level of motivation and effort, which can be particularly challenging for older adults with depression due to symptoms such as low energy and a lack of motivation. To cultivate the motivation necessary for lifestyle modifications, it is important to ensure that older adults understand the tangible benefits that lifestyle changes will bring to their mental health. Additionally, health care providers should assess individual patient needs, readiness to change, preferences, existing health conditions and limitations prior to prescribing lifestyle advice. This personalized approach ensures that lifestyle advice is not only feasible but also aligns closely with each patient's specific medical and psychological conditions, enhancing the likelihood of long-term adherence and success. Moreover, motivation can be substantially enhanced through the strategic implementation of structured action plans and goal-setting methodologies, such as SMART goal setting. Furthermore, providing regular feedback and recognition of progress are also vital for sustaining motivation for lifestyle modifications, as they reinforce the value of the changes, provide a sense of accomplishment and boost patients' confidence in their ability to make and sustain these modifications. Lastly, involving caregivers and family members in the planning and execution of lifestyle modifications is crucial. Their role is fundamental not only for motivating lifestyle changes but also for ensuring adherence, considering that they often provide the daily support needed to implement lifestyle changes, such as meal preparation, physical activity and emotional support and encouragement.

CONCLUSIONS

The ongoing demographic shift toward an older global population presents a dual facet of obstacles and prospects for societies around the world. This shift necessitates a comprehensive reassessment of public policy, health care frameworks and social support systems to effectively respond to the evolving mental health demands of this demographic. LM emerges as a potentially promising approach to offer clinically, cost-effective, safe, non-stigmatizing and easily accessible interventions for depression in older adults. It has the potential to address a wide range of physical and mental health conditions attributed to lifestyle factors within the aging population. Beyond its clinical benefits, the LM approach has the potential to broaden the reach of mental health care on a population-wide scale.

CLINICAL APPLICATIONS

- Adopting a multicomponent approach may maximize the clinical benefits of lifestyle interventions for addressing depression in older adults.
- Take into account the motivation and effort required from older adults with depression to adopt and sustain these lifestyle changes.
- Assess individual patient needs, readiness to change, preferences, existing health conditions and limitations of each individual patient prior to providing lifestyle advice.
- Regular feedback and recognition of progress are vital for sustained motivation for lifestyle modifications.
- Implementing structured action plans, utilizing goal-setting techniques, and involving caregivers and family members are important for initiating and maintaining long-term lifestyle modifications in older adults.

REFERENCES

1. Cai H, Jin Y, Liu R, Zhang Q, Su Z, Ungvari GS, Xiang YT. Global prevalence of depression in older adults: a systematic review and meta-analysis of epidemiological surveys. *Asian J Psychiatry.* 2023;80:103417.
2. Hu T, Zhao X, Wu M, Li Z, Luo L, Yang C, Yang F. Prevalence of depression in older adults: a systematic review and meta-analysis. *Psychiatry Res.* 2022;311:114511.
3. Abdoli N, Salari N, Darvishi N, Jafarpour S, Solaymani M, Mohammadi M, Shohaimi S. The global prevalence of major depressive disorder (MDD) among the elderly: a systematic review and meta-analysis. *Neurosci Biobehav Rev.* 2022;132:1067–1073.
4. Zhang R, Peng X, Song X, Long J, Wang C, Zhang C, Lee TM. The prevalence and risk of developing major depression among individuals with subthreshold depression in the general population. *Psychol Med.* 2023;53(8):3611–3620.
5. Edwards N, Walker S, Paddick SM, Prina AM, Chinnasamy M, Reddy N, Dotchin C. Prevalence of depression and anxiety in older people in low-and middle-income countries in Africa, Asia and South America: a systematic review and meta-analysis. *J Affect Disord.* 2023;325:656–674.

6. Luppa M, Sikorski C, Luck T, Ehreke L, Konnopka A, Wiese B, Riedel-Heller SG. Age-and gender-specific prevalence of depression in latest-life—systematic review and meta-analysis. *J Affect Disord*. 2012;136(3):212–221.
7. Wu Q, Feng J, Pan CW. Risk factors for depression in the elderly: an umbrella review of published meta-analyses and systematic reviews. *J Affect Disord*. 2022;307:37–45.
8. Kim S. The relationship between lifestyle risk factors and depression in Korean older adults: a moderating effect of gender. *BMC Geriatr*. 2022;22:1–10.
9. Cassidy K, Kotynia-English R, Acres J, Flicker L, Lautenschlager NT, Almeida OP, Almeida OP. Association between lifestyle factors and mental health measures among community-dwelling older women. *Aust N Z J Psychiatry*. 2004;38(11–12):940–947.
10. Tsai AC, Chi SH, Wang JY. Cross-sectional and longitudinal associations of lifestyle factors with depressive symptoms in ≥53-year-old Taiwanese – Results of an 8-year cohort study. *Prev Med*. 2013;57(2):92–97.
11. Lee J, Kim HJ. Normal aging induces changes in the brain and neurodegeneration progress: review of the structural, biochemical, metabolic, cellular, and molecular changes. *Front Aging Neurosci*. 2022;14:931536.
12. Marques A, Marconcin P, Werneck AO, Ferrari G, Gouveia ER, Kliegel M, Peralta M, Ihle A. Bidirectional Association between physical activity and dopamine across adulthood-a systematic review. *Brain Sci*. 2021;11(7):829.
13. Reuter M, Zamoscik V, Plieger T, Bravo R, Ugartemendia L, Rodriguez AB, Kirsch P. Tryptophan-rich diet is negatively associated with depression and positively linked to social cognition. *Nutr Res*. 2021;85:14–20.
14. Jiang Y, Zou D, Li Y, Gu S, Dong J, Ma X, Xu S, Wang F, Huang JH. Monoamine neurotransmitters control basic emotions and affect major depressive disorders. *Pharmacol*. 2022;15(10):1203.
15. Quattrocki E, Baird A, Yurgelun-Todd D. Biological aspects of the link between smoking and depression. *Harv Rev Psychiatry*. 2000;8(3):99–110.
16. Ketcherside A, Matthews I, Filbey F. The serotonin link between alcohol use and affective disorders. *J Addict Prev*. 2013;1(2):3.
17. Matison AP, Mather KA, Flood VM, Reppermund S. Associations between nutrition and the incidence of depression in middle-aged and older adults: a systematic review and meta-analysis of prospective observational population-based studies. *Ageing Res Rev*. 2021;70:101403.
18. Bodai BI, Nakata TE, Wong WT, Clark DR, Lawenda S, Tsou C, Liu R, Shiue L, Cooper N, Rehbein M, Ha BP, Mckeirnan A, Misquitta R, Vij P, Klonecke A, Mejia CS, Dionysian E, Hashmi S, Greger M, Stoll S, Campbell TM. Lifestyle medicine: a brief review of its dramatic impact on health and survival. *Perm J*. 2018;22:17–025.
19. Vodovotz Y, Barnard N, Hu FB, Jakicic J, Lianov L, Loveland D, Buysse D, Szigethy E, Finkel T, Sowa G, Verschure P, Williams K, Sanchez E, Dysinger W, Maizes V, Junker C, Phillips E, Katz D, Drant S, Jackson RJ, Parkinson MD. Prioritized research for the prevention, treatment, and reversal of chronic disease: recommendations from the lifestyle medicine research summit. *Front Med*. 2020;7:585744.
20. Maldonado E, Morales-Pison S, Urbina F, Solari A. Aging hallmarks and the role of oxidative stress. *Antioxidants*. 2023;12(3):651.
21. Yatabe K, Muroi R, Kumai T, Kotani T, Somemura S, Yui N, Murofushi Y, Terawaki F, Kobayashi H, Yudoh K, Sakurai H, Miyano H, Fujiya H. Effects of different exercise conditions on antioxidant potential and mental assessment. *Sports*. 2021;9(3):36.
22. Diamanti-Kandarakis E, Papalou O, Kandaraki EA, Kassi G. Mechanisms in endocrinology: nutrition as a mediator of oxidative stress in metabolic and reproductive disorders in women. *Eur J Endocrinol*. 2017;176(2):R79–R99.

23. Darroudi S, Eslamiyeh M, Jaber Al-Fayyadh KK, Zamiri Bidary M, Danesteh S, Hassanzadeh Gouji A, Ferns GA. Prognostic factors associated with sleep duration: serum pro-oxidant/antioxidant balance and superoxide dismutase 1 as oxidative stress markers and anxiety/depression. *Int J Public Health*. 2023;68:1606014.
24. Viola TW, Orso R, Florian LF, Garcia MG, Gomes MGS, Mardini EM, Niederauer JPO, Zaparte A, Grassi-Oliveira R. Effects of substance use disorder on oxidative and antioxidative stress markers: a systematic review and meta-analysis. *Addict Biol*. 2023;28(1):e13254.
25. Mikulska J, Juszczyk G, Gawrońska-Grzywacz M, Herbet M. HPA Axis in the pathomechanism of depression and schizophrenia: new therapeutic strategies based on its participation. *Brain Sci*. 2021;11(10):1298.
26. Duclos M, Tabarin A. Exercise and the hypothalamo-pituitary-adrenal axis. *Front Horm Res*. 2016;47:12–26.
27. Lopresti AL, Hood SD, Drummond PD. A review of lifestyle factors that contribute to important pathways associated with major depression: diet, sleep and exercise. *J Affect Disord*. 2013;148(1):12–27.
28. Chrousos G, Vgontzas AN, Kritikou I. HPA axis and sleep. *Endotext* [Internet]. 2016;18:2000. Available from: https://www.endotext.org.
29. Kishi T, Yoshimura R, Ikuta T, Iwata N. Brain-derived neurotrophic factor and major depressive disorder: evidence from meta-analyses. *Front Psychiatry*. 2018;8:308.
30. Sleiman SF, Henry J, Al-Haddad R, El Hayek L, Abou Haidar E, Stringer T, Ulja D, Karuppagounder SS, Holson EB, Ratan RR, Ninan I, Chao MV. Exercise promotes the expression of brain derived neurotrophic factor (BDNF) through the action of the ketone body β-hydroxybutyrate. *eLife*. 2016;5:e15092.
31. Giese M, Unternaehrer E, Brand S, Calabrese P, Holsboer-Trachsler E, Eckert A. The interplay of stress and sleep impacts BDNF level. *PLoS One*. 2013;8(10):e76050.
32. Bae JH, Kim G. Systematic review and meta-analysis of omega-3 fatty acids in elderly patients with depression. *Nutr Res*. 2018;50:1–9.
33. Gougeon L, Payette H, Morais JA, Gaudreau P, Shatenstein B, Gray-Donald K. Intakes of folate, vitamin B6 and B12 and risk of depression in community-dwelling older adults: the Quebec longitudinal study on nutrition and aging. *Eur J Clin Nutr*. 2016;70(3):380–385.
34. Lassale C, Batty GD, Baghdadli A, Jacka F, Sánchez-Villegas A, Kivimäki M, Akbaraly T. Healthy dietary indices and risk of depressive outcomes: a systematic review and meta-analysis of observational studies. *Mol Psychiatry*. 2019;24(7):965–986.
35. Matison AP, Mather KA, Flood VM, Reppermund S. Associations between nutrition and the incidence of depression in middle-aged and older adults: a systematic review and meta-analysis of prospective observational population-based studies. *Ageing Res Rev*. 2021;70:101403.
36. Bae JH, Kim G. Systematic review and meta-analysis of omega-3 fatty acids in elderly patients with depression. *Nutr Res*. 2018;50:1–9.
37. Guu TW, Mischoulon D, Sarris J, Hibbeln J, McNamara RK, Hamazaki K, Su KP. International society for nutritional psychiatry research practice guidelines for omega-3 fatty acids in the treatment of major depressive disorder. *Psychother Psychosom*. 2019;88(5):263–273.
38. Parletta N, Zarnowiecki D, Cho J, Wilson A, Bogomolova S, Villani A, O'Dea K. A Mediterranean-style dietary intervention supplemented with fish oil improves diet quality and mental health in people with depression: a randomized controlled trial (HELFIMED). *Nutr Neurosci*. 2019;22(7):474–487.

39. Schuch FB, Vancampfort D, Firth J, Rosenbaum S, Ward PB, Silva ES, Stubbs B. Physical activity and incident depression: a meta-analysis of prospective cohort studies. *Am J Psychiatry.* 2018;175(7):631–648.
40. Hu MX, Turner D, Generaal E, Bos D, Ikram MK, Ikram MA, Penninx BW. Exercise interventions for the prevention of depression: a systematic review of meta-analyses. *BMC Public Health.* 2020;20(1):1–11.
41. Gordon BR, McDowell CP, Hallgren M, Meyer JD, Lyons M, Herring MP. Association of efficacy of resistance exercise training with depressive symptoms: meta-analysis and meta-regression analysis of randomized clinical trials. *JAMA Psychiatry.* 2018;75(6):566–576.
42. Miller KJ, Goncalves-Bradley DC, Areerob P, Hennessy D, Mesagno C, Grace F. Comparative effectiveness of three exercise types to treat clinical depression in older adults: a systematic review and network meta-analysis of randomized controlled trials. *Ageing Res Rev.* 2020;58:100999.
43. Bigarella LG, Ballotin VR, Mazurkiewicz LF, Ballardin AC, Rech DL, Bigarella RL, Selistre LDS. Exercise for depression and depressive symptoms in older adults: an umbrella review of systematic reviews and meta-analyses. *Aging Ment Health.* 2022;26(8):1503–1513.
44. Becker NB, Jesus SN, Joao KA, Viseu JN, Martins RI. Depression and sleep quality in older adults: a meta-analysis. *Psychol Health Med.* 2017;22(8):889–895.
45. Sun Y, Shi L, Bao Y, Sun Y, Shi J, Lu L. The bidirectional relationship between sleep duration and depression in community-dwelling middle-aged and elderly individuals: evidence from a longitudinal study. *Sleep Med.* 2018;52:221–229.
46. Bao YP, Han Y, Ma J, Wang RJ, Shi L, Wang TY, Lu L. Cooccurrence and bidirectional prediction of sleep disturbances and depression in older adults: meta-analysis and systematic review. *Neurosci Biobehav Rev.* 2017;75:257–273.
47. Irwin MR, Carrillo C, Sadeghi N, Bjurstrom MF, Breen EC, Olmstead R. Prevention of incident and recurrent major depression in older adults with insomnia: a randomized clinical trial. *JAMA Psychiatry.* 2022;79(1):33–41.
48. Sadler P, McLaren S, Klein B, Harvey J, Jenkins M. Cognitive behavior therapy for older adults with insomnia and depression: a randomized controlled trial in community mental health services. *Sleep.* 2018;41(8):zsy104.
49. Odone A, Gianfredi V, Vigezzi GP, Amerio A, Ardito C, d'Errico A, Costa G. Does retirement trigger depressive symptoms? A systematic review and meta-analysis. *Epidemiol Psychiatr Sci.* 2021;30:e77.
50. Li W, Ye X, Zhu D, He P. The longitudinal association between retirement and depression: a systematic review and meta-analysis. *Am J Epidemiol.* 2021;190(10):2220–2230.
51. Luo MS, Chui EWT, Li LW. The longitudinal associations between physical health and mental health among older adults. *Aging Ment Health.* 2020;24(12):1990–1998.
52. Klainin-Yobas P, Oo WN, Suzanne Yew PY, Lau Y. Effects of relaxation interventions on depression and anxiety among older adults: a systematic review. *Aging Ment Health.* 2015;19(12):1043–1055.
53. Reangsing C, Rittiwong T, Schneider JK. Effects of mindfulness meditation interventions on depression in older adults: a meta-analysis. *Aging Ment Health.* 2021;25(7):1181–1190.
54. Taylor HO, Taylor RJ, Nguyen AW, Chatters L. Social isolation, depression, and psychological distress among older adults. *J Aging Health.* 2018;30(2):229–246.
55. Van As BAL, Imbimbo E, Franceschi A, Menesini E, Nocentini A. The longitudinal association between loneliness and depressive symptoms in the elderly: a systematic review. *Int Psychogeriatr.* 2022;34(7):657–669.

56. Liu L, Gou Z, Zuo J. Social support mediates loneliness and depression in elderly people. *J Health Psychol.* 2016;21(5):750–758.
57. Santini ZI, Koyanagi A, Tyrovolas S, Mason C, Haro JM. The association between social relationships and depression: a systematic review. *J Affect Disord.* 2015;175:53–65.
58. Lai DW, Li J, Ou X, Li CY. Effectiveness of a peer-based intervention on loneliness and social isolation of older Chinese immigrants in Canada: a randomized controlled trial. *BMC Geriatr.* 2020;20:1–12.
59. Keyes KM, Allel K, Staudinger UM, Ornstein KA, Calvo E. Alcohol consumption predicts incidence of depressive episodes across 10 years among older adults in 19 countries. *Int Rev Neurobiol.* 2019;148:1–38.
60. An R, Xiang X. Smoking, heavy drinking, and depression among US middle-aged and older adults. *Prev Med.* 2015;81:295–302.

18 Urinary Incontinence in Older Adults
A Lifestyle Medicine Approach

Cristina H. Davis, Dawn Woods,
Kamal Wagle and Kelly Freeman

EPIDEMIOLOGY

Urinary incontinence (UI) is one of the key health challenges of the geriatric population as it has been associated with loss of independence, reduction in domestic and social participation, significant financial burden, decrease in self-esteem, depressive symptoms, increase in caregiver burden, falls, reduced quality of life and even long-term care admissions.[1-8] UI is also associated with other geriatric syndromes such as gait impairment, cognitive impairment, frequent falls and depression.[6,7,9,10]

It is worth highlighting that UI is not a part of normal aging physiology.[6] In older adults, the prevalence and severity of UI increases with age and affects women more than men.[6,11-14] Among community-dwelling older women, UI prevalence ranges from 17 to 55% with a median of 45% and mean of 34%.[2] For older men the prevalence is 11 to 34% with a median of 17% and a pooled mean of 22%.[2] The same study investigated daily UI prevalence, which was 3–17% for older women (median 14%, pooled mean 12%) and 2–11% for older men (median 4%, pooled mean 5%).[2] In older women, factors that increase the risk of UI include advanced age, low education, history of vaginal deliveries, smoking, impaired activities of daily living and other comorbidities such as obesity, hypertension, diabetes, depression, parkinsonism, stroke, dementia and recurrent urinary tract infections.[2,13-16]

PATHOPHYSIOLOGY

Like many other functions in the human body, the nerve supply to the urinary bladder and how it coordinates with muscles leading to urination is quite sophisticated.[17] Simply put, the urinary bladder functions as a reservoir for urine, and the outlet part of the urinary bladder along with the urethra and urethral sphincter coordinates for the elimination of urine.[17] These functions are only possible due to the coordination of complex neural control in both central and peripheral nervous systems.[17] Some of these functions are involuntary, but voiding, including the function of external sphincter and contraction of pelvic skeletal muscles, is voluntary.[17] Due to this dual complexity, voiding patterns are also influenced by learned behavior.[17]

Regarding neural connection and receptors, the parasympathetic nerves ending in the bladder cause bladder contraction by releasing the neurotransmitter acetylcholine that stimulates muscarinic receptors in the bladder, whereas sympathetic nerves ending in the bladder release noradrenaline that stimulates beta 3 adrenergic receptors to relax bladder smooth muscles.[17] Stimulation of muscarinic and adrenergic receptors will lead to either contraction or relaxation of smooth muscles of the bladder called the detrusor muscle.[17] Of note, the detrusor muscle of the bladder is continuous with the urethral sphincter in the neck of the bladder.[17]

Pelvic floor muscles are key in the pathophysiology of urination.[18] These are skeletal muscles around pelvic bones surrounding the genitourinary system.[18] They consist of a group of muscles called levator ani that includes puborectalis, pubococcygeal and iliococcygeus muscles.[19] When these muscles are well-conditioned and strong, they support the urethra and prevent leaking by suppressing the urgency of urination.[19] Involuntary detrusor contraction can be voluntarily inhibited to some extent by pelvic floor muscle activation.[19] If these muscles become deconditioned due to loss of support to the urethra, there is a higher incidence of UI.[19] In men, enlargement of the prostate can contribute to bladder outlet obstruction and thus to urgency and urge UI.[19]

TYPES OF URINARY INCONTINENCE

UI is defined as any involuntary loss or leakage of urine.[20] Several types of UI impact older adults. Tools to assess for UI can be found in Table 18.1.

TABLE 18.1
Tools to Assess for Incontinence

General assessments to determine if incontinence is present	• 3 Incontinence Questionnaire (3IQ) • Michigan Incontinence Screening Index (M-ISI)[74,75]
Assessments to discriminate type of urinary incontinence	• Questionnaire for Urinary Incontinence (QUID) (Stress versus Urgency)[75] • Urodynamic Testing
Stress incontinence	• Pad Test • Cough Test[76]
Urge incontinence	• Overactive Bladder Symptom Score • International Prostate Symptom Score–Storage Subscore • Urgency Severity Score in Patients with Overactive Bladder and Hypersensitive Bladder
Functional	• Observational/Patient History
Overflow/chronic urinary retention	• Bladder Scan • Bladder Catheterization

Stress Incontinence

Stress urinary incontinence (SUI) occurs when there is a sudden and involuntary leakage of urine following increased pressure on the bladder.[21] Common activities that precipitate SUI by causing increased pressure in the abdomen and bladder include sneezing, exercising, coughing, laughing, jumping, bending over, or straining.[21] This type of UI is most common in younger and middle-aged women.[22] SUI can be caused by various conditions that contribute to loss of support from the pelvic floor muscles and connective tissue, including pregnancy, menopause, constipation, heavy lifting, smoking, obesity, pelvic floor trauma following vaginal delivery, chronic cough and connective tissue disorders.[21]

Urge Incontinence

Urge urinary incontinence (UUI) is the sudden, involuntary loss of urine after experiencing a sudden urge to void.[22] UUI is also referred to as overactive bladder disease (OAB). UUI is commonly caused by irritation of the bladder or loss of control of bladder contractions.[23] OAB is a syndrome of urinary urgency, with or without incontinence.

Functional Incontinence

Functional incontinence is a type of UI that commonly occurs in individuals with normal bladder function but who are unable to make it to the toilet due to underlying medical conditions that make it challenging to get to the restroom, such as arthritis.[22]

Overflow Incontinence/Chronic Urinary Retention

Overflow incontinence is a type of involuntary loss of urine caused by leaking from a full bladder.[22] This type of UI often involves small amounts of urine leaking from a constantly full bladder and has more recently been termed "chronic urinary retention."[22] Chronic urinary retention can sometimes be caused in men by an enlarged prostate blocking the urethra, making it difficult to empty the bladder.[22] Other conditions associated with overflow incontinence include diabetes, spinal cord injuries, constipation and other neurologic conditions that impact the innervation of the bladder as a muscle.[22]

Mixed Incontinence

Mixed incontinence involves both features of stress and urge incontinence.[24] In other words, the involuntary leaking of urine can occur both with the sensation of a sudden urge to void as well as with activities that increase abdominal pressure such as coughing, sneezing, laughing or exercising.[25] It is reported that about 30% of women with UI experience mixed incontinence.[20] It is common for women with mixed urinary incontinence to experience predominantly one type, either stress or urge.[20]

MEDICATIONS COMMONLY ASSOCIATED WITH URINARY INCONTINENCE

There are many commonly prescribed medications in the United States that are associated with UI. The application of lifestyle medicine, which can reduce chronic diseases, can reduce polypharmacy, which in turn may reduce the risk of UI. These medications include alpha-blockers, antipsychotics, antihypertensives, estrogens, opioids, diuretics and antihistamines.[26] A list of these medications is provided in Table 18.2.

Alpha-blockers, also known as alpha-1 adrenergic receptor antagonists, bind to and block type 1 alpha-adrenergic receptors, preventing the contraction of smooth muscle. Their main applications are for symptomatic benign prostatic hypertrophy and hypertension. Their use in the treatment of hypertension is based on the fact that alpha-adrenergic blocking inhibits vascular resistance in arterioles, which raises venous capacitance and lowers blood pressure.[27] Norepinephrine's activation of alpha1-adrenoceptors causes an increase in bladder outlet resistance; these receptors affect smooth muscle of the lower urinary tract directly as well as at the level of the spinal cord ganglia and nerve terminals by mediating somatic, sympathetic and parasympathetic outputs to the bladder, prostate and external urethral sphincter.[27,28] Alpha-blockers, listed in Table 18.2, diminish bladder outlet resistance and result in decreased bladder outlet resistance and, as a result, lead to incontinence.[27] According to one study,[29] using alpha-blockers raised older African American and White women's risk of UI by almost five times.[30] A different investigation[31] revealed that over 40% of female participants on an alpha-blocker reported UI.[31] Many antidepressants and antipsychotics have significant alpha1-adrenoceptor antagonist action as well.[26]

Antipsychotics are useful in the treatment of psychosis and positive symptoms of schizophrenia; however, they are accompanied by a wide range of side effects, many of which are severe.[32] Although the mechanisms of these medications' side effects are not fully understood in relation to UI, numerous explanations have been suggested.[33,34] Antipsychotics can produce incontinence through one or more of the following mechanisms: alpha-adrenergic blockade, dopamine blockade and cholinergic bladder activities.[31] Typical antipsychotics are predominantly dopamine antagonists that cause SUI, whereas atypical antipsychotics are serotonin receptor antagonists.[32] Some individuals suffer UI within hours of starting antipsychotic therapy, while others do not experience UI for weeks. When the antipsychotic is stopped, the UI usually goes away on its own.[26]

There are several types of antidepressants, each with unique pharmacologic features. Proposed mechanisms for antidepressant-induced UI include modulation of bladder sphincter tone, interaction with downstream dopaminergic effects, and potentiation of cholinergic neuromuscular transmission within the detrusor muscle of the bladder through serotonin-induced activation.[35] All antidepressants have been associated with urinary retention and overflow incontinence. Most antidepressants are norepinephrine and/or serotonin uptake inhibitors. At therapeutic concentrations, some operate as antagonists at adrenergic, cholinergic or histaminergic receptors.[26]

Diuretics, which help the kidneys remove salt and water through the urine, can contribute to UI as a result of overfilling the bladder, which in turn increases urine frequency and may result in urinary urgency and UI. In one study, using an alpha-blocker in combination with a loop diuretic nearly doubled the risk of UI compared to using an alpha-blocker alone. However, using thiazide diuretics or potassium-sparing diuretics did not increase risk.[36]

Sedative hypnotics can cause immobility as a result of sedation, which leads to functional incontinence; sedation also causes patients not to wake up when their bladders are full.[30] Because benzodiazepines affect type A receptors for gamma-aminobutyric acid in the central nervous system, they can relax a striated muscle, causing urine retention and UI.[30]

Additionally, antihypertensives such as angiotensin-converting enzyme (ACE) inhibitors, angiotensin receptor blockers (ARBs) and calcium channel blockers (CCBs) contribute to UI. The renin–angiotensin system is found only in the bladder, urethra and kidneys. ACE inhibitors and ARBs diminish both detrusor overactivity and urethral sphincter tone, resulting in less urge incontinence and more SUI.[37] ACE inhibitors may also produce persistent dry cough, which can lead to SUI by raising urethral pressure.[37] CCBs are also used to reduce blood pressure. Calcium causes the heart and arteries to contract more strongly. CCBs prevent calcium from entering cells, allowing blood vessels to open and relax. CCBs also decrease smooth-muscle contractility in the bladder. This causes urinary retention and leads to overflow incontinence.[26]

According to one study, oral and transdermal estrogen, with or without progestin, raised the incidence of UI in elderly women by 45% to 60%.[38] A review of randomized controlled trials found that using oral estrogen raised the risk of UI by 50% to 80%;[39] a 2012 systematic review further concluded that systemic hormone therapy may worsen UI.[40] Combination estrogen–progestin therapy also increased the risk of developing UI in women with a history of cardiovascular disease.[41] The exact mechanism for hormone therapy's impact on UI is unclear; one proposed mechanism relates to the presence of α- and β-estrogen receptors throughout the urogenital tract, including the bladder mucosa, trigone, urethra and vaginal mucosa, in addition to structures that support the pelvic organs such as uterosacral ligaments, levator ani muscles and pubocervical fascia, suggesting that estrogen may have a role in both the structure and function of the UI mechanism.[42] The use of topical vaginal estrogen in the treatment of UI in postmenopausal women has demonstrated inconsistent results thus far. Despite evidence that oral and transdermal estrogen raises the risk of UI, some studies have demonstrated improvement in OAB symptoms with the use of topical estrogen.[40,43] A proposed mechanism for this involves vaginal estrogen increasing vaginal blood flow and reducing the density of vaginal autonomic and sensory nerves.[43] Vaginal estrogen also alters the microbiome of the bladder with noted increased lactobacillus levels in one single-arm study examining OAB symptoms, and this increase was associated with modest improvement in UI symptoms.[43] Further studies are needed to explore the impact of topical estrogen in the prevention and treatment of UI.

TABLE 18.2
Commonly Prescribed Medications Associated with UI

Antipsychotics	1st Generation • Haloperidol • Thorazine • Loxitane • Molindone • Thioridazine • Mesoridazine • Thiothixene	2nd Generation • Clozapine • Risperidone • Ziprasidone • Quetiapine • Paliperidone • Olanzapine • Aripiprazole
Alpha-Blockers	Alpha-Blockers for Hypertension • Doxazosin • Terazosin • Prazosin	Alpha-Blockers for BPH • Alfuzosin • Doxazosin • Silodosin • Tamsulosin • Terazosin
Antidepressants	• Duloxetine • Desvenlafaxine • Vilazodone • Citalopram • Sertraline	• Fluoxetine • Trazodone • Escitalopram • Paroxetine • Venlafaxine
Angiotensin-Converting Enzyme Inhibitors (ACE Inhibitors)	• Benazepril • Enalapril • Captopril • Fosinopril	• Lisinopril • Moexipril • Perindopril • Quinapril
Angiotensin Receptor Blockers (ARBs)	• Azilsartan • Candesartan • Irbesartan • Losartan	• Olmesartan • Telmisartan • Valsartan

TABLE 18.2 (Continued)
Commonly Prescribed Medications Associated with UI

Calcium Channel Blockers	<ul><li>Amlodipine</li><li>Felodipine</li><li>Nicardipine</li><li>Verapamil</li></ul>	<ul><li>Diltiazem</li><li>Isradipine</li><li>Nifedipine</li></ul>	
Diuretics	Thiazide<ul><li>Chlorothiazide</li><li>Chlorthalidone</li><li>Hydrochlorothiazide</li><li>Indapamide</li><li>Metolazone</li></ul>	Potassium-Sparing<ul><li>Spironolactone</li><li>Amiloride</li><li>Eplerenone</li><li>Triamterene</li></ul>	Loop<ul><li>Bumetanide</li><li>Furosemide</li><li>Torsemide</li></ul>
Sedative Hypnotics (Benzodiazepines)	<ul><li>Lorazepam</li><li>Clonazepam</li><li>Alprazolam</li><li>Diazepam</li></ul>	<ul><li>Halazepam</li><li>Oxazepam</li><li>Chlordiazepoxide</li><li>Clorazepate</li></ul>	
Antihistamines	H1 - 1st Generation<ul><li>Diphenhydramine</li><li>Chlorpheniramine</li></ul>	H1 - 2nd Generation<ul><li>Cetirizine</li><li>Levocetirizine</li><li>Fexofenadine</li><li>Loratadine</li></ul>	
Opioids	<ul><li>Hydrocodone</li><li>Morphine</li><li>Oxycodone</li><li>Buprenorphine</li></ul>	<ul><li>Meperidine</li><li>Hydromorphone</li><li>Fentanyl</li></ul>	
Estrogens	<ul><li>Estrogen-containing vaginal tablets</li><li>Combination estrogen + progestin tablets</li><li>Estrogen-containing vaginal rings</li><li>Estrogen-containing vaginal creams</li></ul>		

Opioids interfere with bladder contraction and worsen constipation, potentially leading to retention of urine. They also cause sedation or drowsiness, which causes a lack of urge to use the restroom, difficulty initiating a urine stream, straining to void, weak stream voiding, leaking in between urinations and urinary frequency.[44]

Antihistamines have a significant degree of anticholinergic effects. They relax the bladder, causing it to retain urine which can lead to UI. Pseudoephedrine tightens the urinary sphincter, causing urine to be retained in the bladder.[44,45]

LIFESTYLE MEDICINE PILLARS AND URINARY INCONTINENCE

Therapeutic lifestyle interventions can potentially alleviate or decrease UI symptoms through various mechanisms. Three known causes for potentially reversible UI are excessive alcohol and caffeine intake, medications and stool impaction. While avoidance of alcohol and caffeine intake and modifying fluid intake may be a direct path towards providing relief for UI, many other lifestyle interventions are also beneficial. These lifestyle interventions also may help alleviate the need for medications that can cause UI, such as the medications listed in Table 18.2.

A randomized prospective cohort study of 6,424 women ≥ 40 years old found that there were some potential increased risks of OAB and SUI with certain lifestyle factors. Significant positive correlations were found between smoking, carbonated drink consumption, and obesity with the outcome of OAB/SUI. Negative correlations were found with total vegetable and bread intake. While many online sources recommend avoiding citrus fruit consumption for those with OAB, a study of over 60,000 women did not find a relationship between citrus fruit consumption and developing any type of UI.[46]

Below are the main types of therapeutic lifestyle interventions, known collectively as lifestyle medicine. Research related to interventions known to decrease UI symptoms will be described. It is important to note the bidirectional association between UI and many of the pillars of lifestyle medicine, as UI can impact an individual's ability to focus on certain lifestyle medicine pillars, while utilizing the pillars can also impact an individual's experience with UI.

NUTRITION

A healthy dietary pattern that includes a variety of nutritious, unprocessed foods such as fruits, vegetables, nuts, seeds and legumes appears to have multiple protective factors against UI. More dietary fiber from these foods may decrease the risk of constipation or stool impaction, reducing the risk of incontinence episodes. This dietary pattern also has the potential to improve blood glucose levels. There is a positive association between increased blood glucose levels and incontinence episodes, with women who have diabetes being at 20% higher risk for UUI than those without diabetes. A healthy dietary pattern tends to align with a healthier weight. A modest weight loss of 10 to 20% of body weight in overweight or obese individuals was shown to decrease incontinence episodes.[47,48]

Fluid Intake

Manipulating the type and quantity of fluid to reduce or eliminate OAB symptoms has been studied. The results of a randomized two-group, prospective cross-over trial of increasing or decreasing fluid intake revealed that 83% of the trial participants reported that what they experienced as being most helpful was a 25% decrease in fluid amounts.[49] However, the concerns with this approach may include the risk of dehydration, dry mouth, constipation, concentrated urine or headaches. If this approach is utilized, a baseline level of daily fluid intake should be measured to ensure that the decrease in fluid consumption would put the individual at an acceptable level of fluid loss.

Caffeine can increase urine urgency and frequency, as well as nocturia symptoms. Individuals suffering from OAB may have bladders that are not only hyperactive but also hypersensitive. Caffeine decreases bladder contents, making the bladder more responsive to bladder filling. This finding supports the notion that coffee or caffeine aggravates OAB symptoms and that caffeine limitation may be advantageous. More than two cups of coffee per day (>250 mg caffeine) is connected with worsening symptoms of overactive bladder. The effect is dose-dependent, and drinking more than four cups of coffee per day may result in the development of OAB symptoms in persons who previously had none. Reducing caffeine intake may improve urinary urgency and frequency, but it is not clear if it is effective in reducing UI.[50]

Sleep

One study demonstrated that older adults who experience UI are four times more likely to have trouble sleeping than those without UI.[51] Avoidance of caffeine may have the double benefit of better sleep and decreased risk of incontinence.[52] There appears to be a positive association between obstructive sleep apnea (OSA) and UI, at least in males.[53] Recognizing and treating OSA in patients with UI, including the lifestyle factors that may contribute to OSA, may improve UI symptoms.

Social Connection

Social connectedness for adults who suffer from UI is often impacted due to concerns regarding self-image.[54] Many adults who experience UI also experience increased depressive symptoms and social isolation related to low self-esteem. The presence of UI can also impact an individual's family relationships, especially with family members serving as caregivers.[54] One study suggests that addressing the psychological components of UI including feelings of shame, embarrassment and low self-esteem is as important as addressing the physical components of this condition.[54] Older women with UI report reluctance to leave their homes due to concerns about a potential loss of bladder control while outside of their home.[55]

Individuals with UI are at an increased risk of social isolation, depressive symptoms and loss of pleasure in daily life as a result.[55] Use of incontinence products such as pads or diapers contributes to further social isolation for older women due to concerns regarding discomfort and distortion of the body where others may notice the use of these products.[55] Programs targeted for older adults with UI may promote social engagement which further offers emotional support and prevention of cognitive decline.[55]

STRESS MANAGEMENT

Stress management is another important aspect of preventing and managing UI in older adults.[56] One study of Korean women with UI demonstrated high-stress levels for women in the study who were affected by UI.[56] Women with UI also experience decreased work productivity, which further leads to increased stress levels and depressive symptoms.[56] Management of stress through the implementation of lifestyle medicine interventions can help manage UI in older adults. Many stress management strategies benefit all aspects of health, though not specifically studied in adults with UI, including gratitude, mindfulness and meditation, exercise, building social support systems, progressive muscle relaxation, bright light therapy, deep or diaphragmatic breathing and positive cognitive restructuring.[57] Mindfulness-based stress reduction (MBSR) has been studied primarily in UUI and does demonstrate a decrease in the number of incontinence episodes per day.[58] In a single-arm pilot study of 7 women, implementation of an MBSR program over an 8-week period was studied utilizing a bladder diary to report incontinence episodes; mean incontinence episodes per day decreased from 4.14 to 1.23, indicating improvement in UI with an MBSR program and suggesting that further research with a larger sample size may be helpful to investigate this intervention in practice.[58]

PHYSICAL ACTIVITY

Physical activity is a multifaceted tool for the management and prevention of UI through both the implementation of specifically targeted exercises to strengthen the pelvic floor as well as generally improved physical health which promotes a healthy weight that helps to prevent UI.[59] By promoting physical activity and improving mobility, the incidence of functional incontinence is also reduced. Obesity and low amounts of physical activity are both associated with the risk of developing OAB.[59] A systematic review involving older women and the association between UI and physical activity levels found that women with sedentary lifestyles and who exercised <150 minutes per week are at an overall increased risk of developing UI, though additional studies are recommended to examine this relationship further.[60] In general, a lifestyle prescription for walking at least 30 minutes per day is recommended to prevent the development of UI.[60] It should be noted that while physical activity is associated with a lower risk of developing either mixed UI or UUI, there is not as strong of an association between physical activity and a decreased risk of development of SUI.[61] Increasing physical activity with the goal of decreasing body weight can also be helpful in the prevention of developing UI.

Avoidance of Risky Substances

Alcohol is a diuretic, which causes an increase in urine production, resulting in more trips to the bathroom. Red wine contains more tannins, which gives it a darker hue. Tannins are found in fruit skins and impart bitterness as well as astringency. Unfortunately, these chemical compounds are bladder irritants and cause discomfort in OAB patients.[62] One study found that there was a highly significant negative association between beer consumption and OAB onset for men, suggesting that beer may be protective against new symptoms of OAB. The researchers concluded that this may be due to some properties of the beer besides alcohol.[63] However, the baseline and follow-up studies were only one year apart, which may not have been a long enough exposure period to determine the true effects of beer. Considerations that should discourage providers from recommending beer as a potential preventative behavior for OAB would be the extra calories, poor nutritional value and risk of alcohol consumption sequelae including alcoholism, accidents, liver disease and early death.[63,64]

Cigarette compounds, such as nicotine and tar, can irritate the bladder lining, causing inflammation and increased sensitivity. This inflammation may aggravate the symptoms of overactive bladder. Smoking has been linked to a reduction in bladder capacity, which means the bladder can store less urine before feeling the need to empty. This decreased capacity can increase the frequency and urgency of urination. Cigarette smoking frequently causes persistent coughing, which can place additional strain on the bladder muscles. Coughing and sneezing exert recurrent pressure on the pelvic floor muscles, making it more difficult to regulate urination. Additionally, smoking constricts blood vessels, which lowers blood flow to the bladder. OAB may develop because of an inadequate blood supply, which can also affect bladder function.[65]

Behavioral Approaches to Incontinence Management

Behavioral approaches to the management of UI are the first-line treatment for both UUI and SUI. While medications are useful, the risk of side effects in these medications for older adults often outweigh the potential benefits.[66] Behavioral interventions have been found, both alone and in combination with other interventions, to be more effective than pharmacological therapies alone in managing UI.[66] Some behavioral approaches to UI include bladder training, biofeedback, diet and fluid modification, bladder support (pessaries), weight loss, yoga, heat therapy, pelvic floor muscle training (PFMT), heat therapy, education, vaginal cones, toileting schedules and mindfulness-based stress reduction (MBSR).[66] MBSR is discussed under the stress management pillar more extensively.

PFMT will be the primary focus of the discussion of prevention and reduction of UI symptoms due to strong evidence for it. PFMT is defined by the International Continence Society as exercise that targets and improves pelvic floor muscle strength, endurance, power, relaxation or any combination of these parameters.[67] There are many different types of PFMT including dilation, isometric exercises,

TABLE 18.3
Lifestyle Medicine Prescriptions and Rationale

Intervention Target	Lifestyle Medicine Therapeutic Intervention	Rationale
Fluids	Increase or decrease overall fluid intake[49]	Research has demonstrated that patients respond differently to fluid intake. While some have an improvement in urinary symptoms with an increase in fluid intake, patients more often experience improvement with a 25% decrease in fluid intake. This can be a first-line intervention as it is person-centered, inexpensive, and simple, with minimal or no side effects and almost immediate results.[49]
Fluids	Avoid carbonated beverages	Carbonated beverages are associated with earlier onset of OAB.[59]
Fluids	Avoid caffeinated beverages	Caffeine consumption of 250 mg daily (approximately two cups of coffee) was significantly associated with moderate to severe urinary incontinence in men.[52]
Dietary intake	Increase fiber and fluids	Constipation is associated with urinary incontinence so by increasing fiber and fluid intake, the risk of constipation may be decreased.[49]
Dietary intake	Increase vegetables	Vegetable intake is negatively associated with the onset of OAB.[59]
Dietary intake	Increase fruit	Reduced risk of urinary symptoms have been reported with increased fruit consumption. Citrus fruits do not need to be avoided.[46]
Dietary intake	Avoid red meat	Red meat intake was demonstrated to increase the risk of urinary symptoms.[59]
Weight loss	Increased physical activity, and dietary modification to decrease body weight	Obesity is significantly associated with an increased risk of OAB.[59]
Physical activity	Increase physical activity	Low physical activity is significantly associated with an increased risk of OAB.[59]
Avoidance of risky substances	Smoking cessation	Smoking is significantly associated with an increased risk of OAB.[59]
Stress management	Implement stress-management techniques	MBSR has been studied in UI and has shown improvement in UI symptoms by decreasing the number of incontinence episodes per day.[58]

relaxation, resistance, strength training, stretching and the use of vaginal cones.[67] PFMT with resistance bands has also been proven to be effective in helping men with incontinence regain continence following radical prostatectomy.[68] As noted above, pelvic floor muscles can be strengthened to prevent urinary leakage by temporarily suppressing voiding. PFMT is often recommended as first-line treatment and is widely recommended by multidisciplinary health care team members. In a motivated patient, this has been shown to reduce UI by over 50%.[19] Referral to a pelvic floor specialist is recommended for patients with UI.

Vaginal cones are also utilized to strengthen the pelvic floor in UI; this practice involves inserting cone-shaped weights into the vagina and subsequently contracting the pelvic floor muscles to prevent the weighted cone from slipping out of the vagina.[69] Vaginal cones were reviewed in a systematic review of over 23 studies and found to have similar effectiveness as PFMT in improving UI symptoms and overall to be more effective than no treatment in improving UI symptoms, though larger studies over a longer time frame have been recommended in order to study this further.[69] Many women find cones to be uncomfortable which can be a limitation in utilizing this intervention.[69] Neuromodulation through electrical stimulation of the nerves within the muscles of the pelvic floor has primarily been studied in urgency UI using electroacupuncture, implanted sacral neuromodulation devices, magnetic stimulation and TENS units and is considered a third-line treatment for UI that does show some improvement in UI symptoms when compared with no treatment.[66] Kegel balls, pelvic floor or thigh exercisers and electric probes may also provide some benefits, and these products can be purchased over the counter.[70] There is limited rigorous evaluation of these products in practice and the one study comparing these products utilized a cross-sectional analysis of reviews on the internet; randomized controlled trials related to this are lacking.

While timed voiding, also known as a toileting schedule, and habit retraining have often been recommended to improve UI symptoms, there is limited evidence on whether this impacts UI significantly.[71] The available studies thus far demonstrate little impact on the frequency of incontinence episodes.[71] It is also important to note that there are limited studies that evaluate timed voiding independently of other interventions, which makes it difficult to extrapolate data and draw conclusions regarding its impact on UI.[72] It is often difficult for caregivers to adhere to a timed voiding schedule for patients with UI which additionally limits its impact.[72]

These behavioral approaches encompass several pillars of lifestyle medicine including physical activity, nutrition and stress management. The physical activity pillar relates to behavioral approaches such as yoga and PFMT. While there is limited evidence regarding yoga as a specific intervention to target UI,[73] there is evidence for the use of MBSR for these purposes, highlighting the stress management pillar of lifestyle medicine in managing UI. There is substantial evidence to demonstrate the effectiveness of pelvic floor muscle training (PFMT) on UI, both with and without the addition of biofeedback.[66]

CONCLUSIONS

UI is a common problem for older adults that impacts their quality of life in significant ways including promotion of social isolation, development of skin breakdown and physical discomfort due to briefs/pads. Lifestyle medicine can be utilized to target distressing symptoms of UI and potentially assist in the management of this condition in conjunction with traditional medical and surgical therapies. Avoidance of risky substances is key in the management of UI in both men and women; an association between consumption of alcohol is highly connected with an increase in UI. Support for discontinuation of nicotine products and cigarettes is encouraged as these substances are associated with increased incidence of UI and other health problems; smoking cessation is therefore recommended. Addressing nutrition is also essential in managing UI in older adults; specific recommendations include increasing fruits and vegetables, avoiding red meat, increasing fiber and fluids and avoiding carbonated beverages. Additionally, excessive weight is associated with an increased risk of UI, so patients should be counseled on weight loss, focusing on both dietary modifications and physical activity to achieve this. Older adults impacted by UI tend to experience more depressive symptoms and social isolation, and this should be addressed as part of a multidimensional approach to the prevention and treatment of UI. Physical activity has been proven to prevent and improve symptoms of UI, and a lifestyle medicine prescription for physical activity is recommended. Stress has also been linked to UI, and older adults with UI in particular report increased stress levels. Evidence-based stress management techniques including MBSR should be recommended as part of the treatment of UI in older adults. Additionally, referral to a pelvic floor rehabilitation specialist is critical as there is substantial evidence to highlight the positive impact PFMT has on the impact of UI.

A lifestyle medicine approach to the management of UI can serve as first-line treatment for older adults suffering from this condition, in an attempt to reduce the need for surgical intervention as well as possible side effects from medications commonly utilized in the management of UI. Adopting the outlined lifestyle medicine approaches can help older adults experience decreased morbidity and mortality related to UI while improving perceived quality of life.

CLINICAL APPLICATIONS

- Consider referring patients to health professionals specializing in UI and pelvic floor rehabilitation.
- Engage individuals in lifestyle medicine programming to support improved outcomes.
- Recommend fluid intake adjustments as first-line interventions for incontinence; avoid carbonated and caffeinated beverages. Increase or decrease fluids based on individual response; many patients find improvement with a 25% decrease in fluid intake, although some individuals benefit from an increase in fluid intake.
- Recommend dietary interventions, including increasing fruit, vegetable and fiber intake while avoiding red meat. This helps manage and reduce body weight which further manages and reduces the incidence of OAB.
- Recommend increasing physical activity due to low physical activity being associated with increased risk of OAB.

REFERENCES

1. Hunskaar S, Vinsnes A. The quality of life in women with urinary incontinence as measured by the sickness impact profile. *J Am Geriatr Soc.* 1991;39(4):378–382.
2. Thom D. Variation in estimates of urinary incontinence prevalence in the community: effects of differences in definition, population characteristics, and study type. *J Am Geriatr Soc.* 1998;46(4):473–480.
3. Grimby A, Milsom I, Molander U, Wiklund I, Ekelund P. The influence of urinary incontinence on the quality of life of elderly women. *Age Ageing.* 1993;22(2):82–89.
4. Coward RT, Horne C, Peek CW. Predicting nursing home admissions among incontinent older adults: a comparison of residential differences across six years. *Gerontologist.* 1995;35(6):732–743.
5. Wilson L, Brown JS, Shin GP, Luc KO, Subak LL. Annual direct cost of urinary incontinence. *Obstet Gynecol.* 2001;98(3):398–406.
6. Khandelwal C, Kistler C. Diagnosis of urinary incontinence. *Am Fam Physician.* 2013;87(8):543–550.
7. Brown JS, Vittinghoff E, Wyman JF, et al. Urinary incontinence: does it increase risk for falls and fractures? Study of osteoporotic fractures research group. *J Am Geriatr Soc.* 2000;48(7):721–725.
8. Tran LN, Puckett Y. *Urinary Incontinence.* StatPearls Publishing; 2023.
9. Suskind AM, Cawthon PM, Nakagawa S, et al. Urinary incontinence in older women: the role of body composition and muscle strength: from the health, aging, and body composition study. *J Am Geriatr Soc.* 2017;65(1):42–50.
10. Parker-Autry C, Neiberg RH, Leng I, Colombo L, Kuchel GA, Kritchevsky SB. The geriatric incontinence syndrome: characterizing geriatric incontinence in older women. *J Am Geriatr Soc.* 2021;69(11):3225–3231.
11. Roberts RO, Jacobsen SJ, Rhodes T, et al. Urinary incontinence in a community-based cohort: prevalence and healthcare-seeking. *J Am Geriatr Soc.* 1998;46(4):467–472.
12. Roberts RO, Jacobsen SJ, Reilly WT, Pemberton JH, Lieber MM, Talley NJ. Prevalence of combined fecal and urinary incontinence: a community-based study. *J Am Geriatr Soc.* 1999;47(7):837–841.
13. Wu JM, Matthews CA, Vaughan CP, Markland AD. Urinary, fecal, and dual incontinence in older U.S. Adults. *J Am Geriatr Soc.* 2015;63(5):947–953.
14. Batmani S, Jalali R, Mohammadi M, Bokaee S. Prevalence and factors related to urinary incontinence in older adults women worldwide: a comprehensive systematic review and meta-analysis of observational studies. *BMC Geriatr.* 2021;21(1):212.
15. Brandeis GH, Baumann MM, Hossain M, Morris JN, Resnick NM. The prevalence of potentially remediable urinary incontinence in frail older people: a study using the Minimum Data Set. *J Am Geriatr Soc.* 1997;45(2):179–184.
16. Dugan E, Cohen SJ, Bland DR, et al. The association of depressive symptoms and urinary incontinence among older adults. *J Am Geriatr Soc.* 2000;48(4):413–416.
17. Fowler CJ, Griffiths D, de Groat WC. The neural control of micturition. *Nat Rev Neurosci.* 2008;9(6):453–466.
18. Sam P, Nassereddin A, LaGrange CA. Anatomy, abdomen and pelvis: bladder detrusor muscle. In: *StatPearls.* StatPearls Publishing; 2023. https://www.ncbi.nlm.nih.gov/books/NBK482181/
19. Cho ST, Kim KH. Pelvic floor muscle exercise and training for coping with urinary incontinence. *J Exerc Rehabil.* 2021;17(6):379–387.
20. ICS. ICS. Accessed December 7, 2023. https://www.ics.org/glossary/symptom/urinaryincontinence
21. Lugo T, Riggs J. *Stress Incontinence.* StatPearls Publishing; 2023.

22. Strong N, Salim SZ, Nickels JL, Poduri KR. Urinary incontinence in older adults. In: *Geriatric Rehabilitation*. CRC Press; 2017:157–177. https://www.routledge.com/Geriatric-Rehabilitation-From-Bedside-to-Curbside/Poduri/p/book/9780367868802?srsltid=AfmBOoqX-F7cQEBecBEQgGhlH91qd5SzEJzEIL2CaCNev9YaUMaUB45-Chapter 9
23. Nandy S, Ranganathan S. *Urge Incontinence*. StatPearls Publishing; 2022.
24. Harris S, Riggs J. *Mixed Urinary Incontinence*. StatPearls Publishing; 2023.
25. ICS. ICS. Accessed December 7, 2023. https://www.ics.org/committees/standardisation/terminologydiscussions/femalemixedurinaryincontinencemui
26. Drug-induced urinary incontinence. *Prescrire Int*. 2015;24(162):180–182.
27. Andersson KE, Lepor H, Wyllie MG. Prostatic alpha 1-adrenoceptors and uroselectivity. *Prostate*. 1997;30(3):202–215.
28. Drake MJ, Nixon PM, Crew JP. Drug-induced bladder and urinary disorders. Incidence, prevention and management. *Drug Saf*. 1998;19(1):45–55.
29. Ruby CM, Hanlon JT, Boudreau RM, et al. The effect of medication use on urinary incontinence in community-dwelling elderly women. *J Am Geriatr Soc*. 2010;58(9):1715–1720.
30. Landi F, Cesari M, Russo A, et al. Benzodiazepines and the risk of urinary incontinence in frail older persons living in the community. *Clin Pharmacol Ther*. 2002;72(6):729–734.
31. Marshall HJ, Beevers DG. Alpha-adrenoceptor blocking drugs and female urinary incontinence: prevalence and reversibility. *Br J Clin Pharmacol*. 1996;42(4):507–509.
32. Fuller MA, Borovicka MC, Jaskiw GE, Simon MR, Kwon K, Konicki PE. Clozapine-induced urinary incontinence: incidence and treatment with ephedrine. *J Clin Psychiatry*. 1996;57(11):514–518.
33. Kiruluta HG, Andrews K. Urinary incontinence secondary to drugs. *Urology*. 1983;22(1):88–90.
34. Ambrosini PJ. A pharmacological paradigm for urinary incontinence and enuresis. *J Clin Psychopharmacol*. 1984;4(5):247–253.
35. Tsakiris P, Oelke M, Michel MC. Drug-induced urinary incontinence. *Drugs Aging*. 2008;25(7):541–549.
36. Peron EP, Zheng Y, Perera S, et al. Antihypertensive drug class use and differential risk of urinary incontinence in community-dwelling older women. *J Gerontol A Biol Sci Med Sci*. 2012;67(12):1373–1378.
37. Elliott CS, Comiter CV. The effect of angiotensin inhibition on urinary incontinence: data from the national health and nutrition examination survey (2001–2008). *Neurourol Urodyn*. 2014;33(8):1178–1181.
38. Grodstein F, Lifford K, Resnick NM, Curhan GC. Postmenopausal hormone therapy and risk of developing urinary incontinence. *Obstet Gynecol*. 2004;103(2):254–260.
39. Shamliyan TA, Kane RL, Wyman J, Wilt TJ. Systematic review: randomized, controlled trials of nonsurgical treatments for urinary incontinence in women. *Ann Intern Med*. 2008;148(6):459–473.
40. Cody JD, Jacobs ML, Richardson K, Moehrer B, Hextall A. Oestrogen therapy for urinary incontinence in post-menopausal women. *Cochrane Database Syst Rev*. 2012;10(10):CD001405.
41. Hendrix SL, Cochrane BB, Nygaard IE, et al. Effects of estrogen with and without progestin on urinary incontinence. *JAMA*. 2005;293(8):935–948.
42. Steinauer JE, Waetjen LE, Vittinghoff E, et al. Postmenopausal hormone therapy: does it cause incontinence? *Obstet Gynecol*. 2005;106(5 Pt 1):940–945.
43. Thomas-White K, Taege S, Limeira R, et al. Vaginal estrogen therapy is associated with increased Lactobacillus in the urine of postmenopausal women with overactive bladder symptoms. *Am J Obstet Gynecol*. 2020;223(5):727.e1–e727.e11.

44. Medications that can cause urinary incontinence. Harvard Health. Published August 28, 2019. Accessed January 4, 2024. https://www.health.harvard.edu/bladder-and-bowel/medications-that-can-cause-urinary-incontinence
45. Simons FER, Simons KJ. H1 antihistamines: current status and future directions. *World Allergy Organ J.* 2008;1(9):145–155.
46. Townsend MK, Devore EE, Resnick NM, Grodstein F. Acidic fruit intake in relation to incidence and progression of urinary incontinence. *Int Urogynecol J.* 2013;24(4):605–612.
47. Wing RR, Creasman JM, West DS, et al. Improving urinary incontinence in overweight and obese women through modest weight loss. *Obstet Gynecol.* 2010;116(2 Pt 1):284–292.
48. Danforth KN, Townsend MK, Curhan GC, Resnick NM, Grodstein F. Type 2 diabetes mellitus and risk of stress, urge and mixed urinary incontinence. *J Urol.* 2009;181(1):193–197.
49. Hashim H, Abrams P. How should patients with an overactive bladder manipulate their fluid intake? *BJU Int.* 2008;102(1):62–66.
50. Swithinbank L, Hashim H, Abrams P. The effect of fluid intake on urinary symptoms in women. *J Urol.* 2005;174(1):187–189.
51. Nazaripanah NS, Momtaz YA, Mokhtari F, Sahaf R. Urinary incontinence and sleep complaints in community dwelling older adults. *Sleep Sci.* 2018;11(2):106–111.
52. Davis NJ, Vaughan CP, Johnson TM 2nd, et al. Caffeine intake and its association with urinary incontinence in United States men: results from national health and nutrition examination surveys 2005–2006 and 2007–2008. *J Urol.* 2013;189(6):2170–2174.
53. Kemmer H, Mathes AM, Dilk O, Gröschel A, Grass C, Stöckle M. Obstructive sleep apnea syndrome is associated with overactive bladder and urgency incontinence in men. *Sleep.* 2009;32(2):271–275.
54. Peroni L, Armaingaud D, Yakoubi T, Rothan-Tondeur M. Social representations of urinary incontinence in caregivers and general population: a focus group study. *Int J Environ Res Public Health.* 2022;19(19). doi:10.3390/ijerph191912251
55. Park GR, Park S, Kim J. Urinary incontinence and depressive symptoms: the mediating role of physical activity and social engagement. *J Gerontol B Psychol Sci Soc Sci.* 2022;77(7):1250–1258.
56. Lee HY, Rhee Y, Choi KS. Urinary incontinence and the association with depression, stress, and self-esteem in older Korean women. *Sci Rep.* 2021;11(1):9054.
57. Merlo G, Nikbin A, Ryu H. Emotional wellness and stress resilience. In: *Improving Women's Health Across the Lifespan.* CRC Press; 2021:85–103. https://www.taylorfrancis.com/chapters/edit/10.1201/9781003110682-5/emotional-wellness-stress-resilience-gia-merlo-ariyaneh-nikbin-hanjun-ryu
58. Baker J, Costa D, Nygaard I. Mindfulness-based stress reduction for treatment of urinary urge incontinence: a pilot study. *Female Pelvic Med Reconstr Surg.* 2012;18(1):46–49.
59. Dallosso HM, McGrother CW, Matthews RJ, Donaldson MMK, Leicestershire MRC incontinence study group. The association of diet and other lifestyle factors with overactive bladder and stress incontinence: a longitudinal study in women. *BJU Int.* 2003;92(1):69–77.
60. Faleiro DJA, Menezes EC, Capeletto E, Fank F, Porto RM, Mazo GZ. Association of physical activity with urinary incontinence in older women: a systematic review. *J Aging Phys Act.* 2019;27(4):906–913.
61. Bauer SR, Kenfield SA, Sorensen M, et al. Physical activity, diet, and incident urinary incontinence in postmenopausal women: women's health initiative observational study. *J Gerontol A Biol Sci Med Sci.* 2021;76(9):1600–1607.

62. University of Colorado Urogynecology. Overactive bladder diet drinking tips. Published December 17, 2016. Accessed January 8, 2024. https://urogyn.coloradowomenshealth.com/blog/overactive-bladder-diet.html
63. Dallosso HM, Matthews RJ, McGrother CW, Donaldson MMK, Shaw C, Leicestershire MRC Incontinence Study Group. The association of diet and other lifestyle factors with the onset of overactive bladder: a longitudinal study in men. *Public Health Nutr.* 2004;7(7):885–891.
64. Jani BD, McQueenie R, Nicholl BI, et al. Association between patterns of alcohol consumption (beverage type, frequency and consumption with food) and risk of adverse health outcomes: a prospective cohort study. *BMC Med.* 2021;19(1):8.
65. Kawahara T, Ito H, Yao M, Uemura H. Impact of smoking habit on overactive bladder symptoms and incontinence in women. *Int J Urol.* 2020;27(12):1078–1086.
66. Balk EM, Rofeberg VN, Adam GP, Kimmel HJ, Trikalinos TA, Jeppson PC. Pharmacologic and nonpharmacologic treatments for urinary incontinence in women: a systematic review and network meta-analysis of clinical outcomes. *Ann Intern Med.* 2019;170(7):465–479.
67. Bo K, Frawley HC, Haylen BT, et al. An International Urogynecological Association (IUGA)/International Continence Society (ICS) joint report on the terminology for the conservative and nonpharmacological management of female pelvic floor dysfunction. *Neurourol Urodyn.* 2017;36(2):221–244.
68. Pan LH, Lin MH, Pang ST, Wang J, Shih WM. Improvement of urinary incontinence, life impact, and depression and anxiety with modified pelvic floor muscle training after radical prostatectomy. *Am J Mens Health.* 2019;13(3):1557988319851618.
69. Herbison GP, Dean N. Weighted vaginal cones for urinary incontinence. *Cochrane Database Syst Rev.* 2013;2013(7):CD002114.
70. Thomas HS, Lee AW, Nabavizadeh B, et al. Evaluating the primary use, strengths and weaknesses of pelvic floor muscle training devices available online. *Neurourol Urodyn.* 2021;40(1):310–318.
71. Ostaszkiewicz J, Johnston L, Roe B. Habit retraining for the management of urinary incontinence in adults. *Cochrane Database Syst Rev.* 2004;2004(2):CD002801.
72. Ostaszkiewicz J, Johnston L, Roe B. Timed voiding for the management of urinary incontinence in adults. *Cochrane Database Syst Rev.* 2004;2004(1):CD002802.
73. Susan Wieland L, Shrestha N, Lassi ZS, Panda S, Chiaramonte D, Skoetz N. Yoga for treating urinary incontinence in women. *Cochrane Database Syst Rev.* 2019;(2). doi:10.1002/14651858.CD012668.pub2
74. Khan MJ, Omar MA, Laniado M. Diagnostic agreement of the 3 Incontinence Questionnaire to video-urodynamics findings in women with urinary incontinence: Department of Urology, Frimley Health NHS Foundation Trust Wexham Park Hospital Slough, Berkshire, United Kingdom. *Cent European J Urol.* 2018;71(1):84–91.
75. Suskind AM, Dunn RL, Morgan DM, DeLancey JOL, Rew KT, Wei JT. A screening tool for clinically relevant urinary incontinence. *Neurourol Urodyn.* 2015;34(4):332–335.
76. American Urogynecologic Society and American College of Obstetricians and Gynecologists. Committee opinion: evaluation of uncomplicated stress urinary incontinence in women before surgical treatment. *Female Pelvic Med Reconstr Surg.* 2014;20(5):248–251.

19 Resilience

Halina Kusz and Ali Ahmad

INTRODUCTION

The term resilience was introduced into the English language in the early 17th century from the Latin verb *resilire*, meaning "jump back" or "recoil."[1] Resilience has been defined in numerous ways, and there is no agreed definition of resilience. However, resilience is generally characterized as a system's capability to bounce back, evolve, or withstand disturbances arising from challenges or stressors.[2]

The concept of individual resilience was initially developed by psychologists working on resilience in children, and it is still a relatively new construct in geriatric care. In 2004, Bonnano first defined adult resilience as "the ability that allows older adults to adapt positively when faced with adversity."[3] Since then, research on age-related resilience has been expanding. Following the COVID-19 pandemic, resilience received even more attention from researchers, to further develop new prevention strategies for individuals, communities, and systems.

The concept of resilience has evolved from being viewed as a phenomenon or personality trait to an interactive process and outcome. It is presently conceptualized as a dynamic process of adaptation, which is shaped by both short- and long-term experiences over the lifespan, as well as complex intrinsic and extrinsic factors. While genetics, biological and environmental factors, lifestyle choices, and the aging process contribute significantly to an individual's resilience, it is important to note that diverse cultural and ethnic backgrounds can also elicit different responses to stress. This extends the current understanding of resilience to the bio-psychosocial cultural model.[4]

Resilience and Aging

Older adults are as "resilient" as young adults. The coping skills, experience and wisdom gained over the years seem to protect them, providing stability in times of adversity. The lessons learned from older adults who faced significant changes during the COVID-19 pandemic revealed that they are vulnerable but also demonstrated strengths and great resilience which challenges the stereotypes that portray older adults as "vulnerable and resourceless."[5]

In a previous study comparing psychological resilience between older adults (age > 64) and younger individuals (age < 26), it was found that the older group exhibited higher resilience, particularly in emotional regulation and problem-solving skills.[6] Although there is evidence suggesting that older adults generally have a higher level of well-being than their younger counterparts, they still require support due to physical and cognitive decline. Engaging in resilience practices is beneficial for individuals of all ages, as high resilience has been consistently linked to positive outcomes, such as successful aging, reduced depression and increased longevity.[7] Although the fundamental definition of individual resilience remains unified, common frameworks for practical purposes and resilience studies encompass three closely connected domains: cognitive, physical and psychosocial resilience. These domains are intricately woven together, as stressors in one domain affect the others.[4]

COGNITIVE RESILIENCE

While the symptoms of cognitive aging can be concerning, it is important to understand that some degree of cognitive decline is a natural aspect of the aging process. However, the extent, risk, and progression of cognitive decline varies significantly among individuals. In recent decades, the exploration of cognitive resilience has greatly enhanced our understanding of the individual differences contributing to cognitive advantages in older age.

Cognitive resilience, as outlined in Stern et al.'s framework, comprises three key elements: cognitive reserve, brain maintenance and brain reserve. In this framework, resilience serves as an important term that encapsulates the brain's ability to sustain cognitive function despite the challenges posed by aging and disease. Cognitive reserve refers to the brain's capacity to exhibit cognitive performance beyond expectations, considering life-course-related changes, brain injury or disease. On the other hand, brain maintenance involves the relative absence of alterations in neural resources or neuropathologic changes over time, contributing to preserved cognition in older age. Meanwhile, brain reserve reflects the neurobiological status of the brain, including the numbers of neurons and synapses, at any given point. Although both cognitive reserve and brain maintenance are subject to influences from various genetic and environmental factors throughout the lifespan, brain reserve does not require active adaptation of functional cognitive processes in the presence of injury or disease.[8]

There are several complex and highly interactive factors and mechanisms that lead to cognitive resilience strength. Cognitive resilience is positively impacted by a range of influential factors. These encompass cognitive reserve, intricately linked to one's educational and occupational background; health-promoting lifestyles marked by conscientious choices in diet, exercise and cognitive engagement; as well as positive behaviors such as mindfulness, optimism and self-sufficiency. Genetic influences, specifically through kdm6a and TREM2, play a role in shaping cognitive resilience, alongside the beneficial impact of exposure to greenspace, particularly during early and midlife. Additionally, certain sociodemographic traits, such as younger age and higher income, have been identified as significant contributors to cognitive resilience. Therefore, cognitive resilience is influenced by a multitude of complex factors.[9]

Factors exerting adverse effects on cognitive resilience include vascular risk factors such as hypertension, diabetes, obesity, head injury and lifestyle such as smoking, and alcohol consumption. It is important to note that depression and anxiety also contribute to reduced cognitive resilience. Genetic predispositions, specifically involving MS4A6A and BDNF, further impact cognitive health. Additionally, comorbidities arising from multiple medical conditions, and sociodemographic factors such as low income, advanced age and racial and ethnic disparities may negatively influence cognitive resilience.[9] It is noteworthy that modifiable risk factors contribute significantly, comprising up to 40% of the attributable risk for cognitive decline and Alzheimer's disease and related dementias.[10]

Measuring cognitive resilience is challenging. There is a lack of consensus on how to optimally define and measure cognitive aging and cognitive reserve. The residual approach which uses residuals from regression analysis to quantify cognitive resilience and reserve "better or worse than expected" given a certain level of risk or cerebral damage is commonly used in aging and Alzheimer's disease. While it's important to approach the utilization and interpretation of the residual-based method of cognitive resilience with caution, a thorough review of the literature and meta-analysis affirms the efficacy of residual methods as suitable measures of resilience and resistance. These methods effectively capture clinically meaningful information on aging and Alzheimer's disease.[11]

Alternative indicators of cognitive reserve encompass neuropsychological evaluations of cognitive performance or the Cognitive Reserve Unit Scale (CRUS) which offers a continuous gauge of cognitive reserve, facilitating statistical analyses and comparisons among individuals from various social, racial, ethnic and geographic backgrounds.[9]

COGNITIVE RESILIENCE BIOMARKERS

There are numerous physiological biomarkers of resilience, which include relevant genes, epigenetic changes and protein biomarkers linked to resilient phenotypes. Fluid and neuroimaging biomarkers initially designed for research purposes are now gradually finding application in clinical practice, particularly in dementia. Essential indicators for Alzheimer's disease encompass analyzing amyloid beta (Aβ42), total tau (t-tau) and phosphorylated tau (p-tau) levels in cerebrospinal fluid and blood.[9]

Although biomarkers hold promise in distinguishing individuals with Alzheimer's disease from healthy controls, their ability to predict age-related cognitive decline without dementia remains unclear. Biomarkers such as plasma tau phosphorylated at threonine 181, neurofilament light and fibrillary acidic protein may be valuable in indicating age-related cognitive decline. Furthermore, the efficient clearance of tau phosphorylated at threonine 181 by astrocytes could contribute to cognitive resilience.[12]

Despite advancements in fluid biomarkers, markers that define cognitive resilience are yet to be established. The value of Alzheimer's disease biomarkers in asymptomatic persons is used mainly in research, and its practical implication remains unclear. In addition, it requires interpretation by specialists, making it very limited for practical purposes. Biomarkers for vascular cognitive impairment are currently being studied and are not ready for application in clinical practice.[13]

There are neuroimaging diagnostic tools such as structural neuroimaging (CT, MRI), functional neuroimaging (metabolic PET, SPECT), and biomarker-based (Aβ-PET, tau-PET and fluorodeoxyglucose-PET scan measures). DaT dopamine–transporter single photon emission tomography scan provides quantitative measurements of cortical volume, thickness and surface areas or measurements of amyloid or tau pathology. Although neuroimaging techniques significantly contribute to assessing risks and conducting a differential diagnosis of cognitive decline, there are currently no specific neuroimaging biomarkers identified for cognitive resilience.

GENETIC FACTORS

The genetic factors associated with cognitive resilience are not well understood. There is a suggestion that protective genes could enhance cognitive resilience by lessening the burden of neuropathological accumulation, establishing a higher baseline cognitive reserve, or delaying the onset of clinical diseases. Genome-Wide Association Studies (GWAS), a method that involves comparing the genomes of numerous individuals to identify genetic markers associated with a specific phenotype or disease risk, were conducted. One of these genetic analyses of resilience indicates the presence of a new resilience gene along the bile acid metabolic pathway. Moreover, the genetic structure of resilience seems different from that observed in clinical Alzheimer's disease. This implies that shifting attention to molecular contributors to resilience could unveil new pathways for directed therapy.[14]

In conclusion, despite the substantial progress in cognitive research, a pressing imperative remains for additional investigations into the intricate interplay of genetics, environmental factors and lifelong lifestyle exposures contributing to cognitive resilience in advanced age. The pursuit of interventions geared toward enhancing cognitive resilience emerges as a pivotal strategy in averting cognitive decline and mitigating the susceptibility to Alzheimer's disease and related dementias. These endeavors not only deepen our comprehension of the dynamics of healthy aging but also constitute a crucial contribution to the broader objective of fostering cognitive well-being in older adults.

PHYSICAL RESILIENCE

Older adults are faced with various physical stressors throughout their lives. These may be in the form of an acute illness, chronic disease, personal injury, surgery and hospitalization. Predicting recovery after such stressors is very challenging, even in high-risk patients with multimorbidity and frailty. Patients who manifest resilience in the presence of physical health stressors are more likely to have positive outcomes.

Physical resilience refers to the body's ability to resist functional decline or recover function in response to health stressors.[15] It is an area of growing interest in aging research, at least partially because it is a modifiable target for interventions to optimize function and quality of life in older adults. Physical resilience is influenced by biological, psychological and sociological factors. It is based on physiologic reserve, but also heavily influenced by genetic, environmental and psychosocial factors. Physical resilience can be observed at both the microscopic and macroscopic levels, where an adaptive response is seen in cells, molecules, and bodily organs. At the whole person level, physical resilience involves the restoration of the physiological function of the multiple affected organ systems, for example, circulatory, respiratory, musculoskeletal, neurological and immunological.[15]

Whitson et al. (2016) suggested a framework for understanding physical resilience and its interrelated concepts such as reserve, frailty and robustness. In this perspective, physical resilience is described as an individual's capacity to endure and recover from a decline in functionality following either acute or chronic health stressors. This resilience is observed at a holistic level, influenced by a variety of internal and external factors. The outcome for an individual is shaped by their resilience, in the context of the nature and intensity of the stressor experienced. Physiological reserve refers to the ability of a cell, tissue or organ system to function above its baseline level in response to changes in physiological demands. Frailty can be described as a condition in which there is reduced physiological reserve across biological systems. The reduced physiological reserve, which is in part due to age-related decline in different organ systems, leads to increased vulnerability to health-related stressors.[15]

Physical resilience is not antithetical to frailty. It is important to contrast frailty, physical decline after a stressor, from resilience, and rebounding from functional loss after stressors, as these may be due to different reasons. Both the concepts of physical resilience and frailty are similar in that they involve a physiological decline at the cellular and molecular level in older adults, making some individuals more susceptible to health stressors than others.[16] In addition, differentiation should be drawn between physical resilience and robustness, which is the capacity to withstand deviation from the original state, and resilience, which refers to the ability to recover after such deviation.[17]

Measuring Physical Resilience

Valid and reliable tools have been established to offer quantifiable insights into physical resilience. The Physical Resilience Scale (PRS) is a 17-item questionnaire that assesses physical resilience, as a recovery after a health stressor, and psychological resilience. Recovery in the physical domain is predicted based on psychological attitudes.[18] The Physical Resilience Instrument for Older Adults (PRIFOR) is another 16-item tool that uses self-reported information to assess physical resilience. It has been recognized as a useful tool in identifying factors that protect older adults from poor health outcomes and to test intervention effects on resilience improvement.[19] Differing from the measurement of physical resilience which utilizes surveys, Whitson et al. (2016) have suggested the use of a physical resilience measurement approach that incorporates phenotypes (frail, robust, fatigability), age discrepancy (biological vs. chronological age) and trajectories (prior or after experimental stressors).[15]

To further classify physical resilience in longitudinal data, two alternative methods have been suggested in defining recovery: the recovery phenotype and the expected recovery differential. The "recovery phenotype" applies statistical techniques to characterize the pace and degree of a patient's recovery. The "expected recovery differential" (ERD) assesses the difference between a patient's observed outcome and their anticipated outcome through a population-derived model and individual clinical characteristics during the stressor.[20] Peters et al., in a scoping review identified 22 instruments that can be used to measure physical resilience in older adults. Most of the included articles involved older adults with fractures, cardiac conditions and cancer. Measurement instruments were pooled into four categories: psychological, physiological, motor function and psychosocial scales, for example, measurement instruments for physical resilience in older adults with fractures included psychological measures of depression, psychological resilience measures with the Connor–Davidson Resilience Scale, measures of serum neopterin level, which is an inflammatory biomarker that may predict non-survival after hip fracture, and motor function measures with the Physical Resilience Scale. For older adults with cardiovascular conditions, measurement instruments included psychological resilience measures such as the Connor–Davidson Resilience Scale and combined psychosocial and physical health scores. For older adults with cancer, for example, the 11-item Resilience Scale, and combined psychosocial (e.g., European Organization for Research and Treatment of Cancer Quality of Life Questionnaire [EORTC]) and physical measures were used. However, even among all of these instruments, no single tool incorporates all of the characteristics of physical resilience.[21]

Other potential measurements and biomarkers of physical resilience were identified, and they include: for example, for measuring energy and metabolism: self-perceived fatigue, muscle endurance, malnutrition or nutritional status, body composition and circulating biomarkers of metabolism. To measure neuromuscular function: knee extensor strength, handgrip strength and respiratory muscle strength are used. To measure immune and stress response: circulating biomarkers of inflammation, perceived immune status, oxygen saturation and autonomic function are measured.[22]

The underlying molecular basis of physical resilience is still largely unknown. To identify biomarker associations with better-than-expected recovery (greater ERD) after hip fracture researchers evaluated biomarkers of inflammation, metabolic and mitochondrial function and epigenetic dysregulation. They identified a subset of biomarkers that accounted for 27% of the total variance in the ERD, and therefore could serve for the prediction of physical resilience. This subset of biomarkers included metabolic factors: aspartate, asparagine, C22, C5:1, lactate, glutamate/mine and markers of inflammation: TNFR-I, miR-376a-3p and miR-16-5p.[23]

More research is needed to better understand the molecular underpinning of physical resilience and outcome measures of resilience. The ongoing, prospective cohort study such as the PRIME-Knee (Physical Resilience Indicators and Mechanism in the Elderly), or the Study of Physical Resilience and Aging (SPRING) assessing underlying physical resilience in response to a specific stressor, may contribute more to our better understanding of the physical resilience in older adults.

TABLE 19.1
Characteristics of Resilience Domains in Older Adults

Resilience	Definition	Key Idea	Influences	Measurement	Biomarkers
Cognitive Resilience	Ability to sustain cognitive function despite aging and disease.	• Cognitive reserve • Brain maintenance • Brain reserve	• Education • Occupation • Lifestyle behaviors • Genetics • Social and demographic factors	• Residual approach • Neuropsychological evaluations • Cognitive Reserve Unit Scale[9]	• Aβ42 • t-tau • p-tau • Plasma tau phosphorylated at threonine 181 • neurofilament light • Fibrillary acidic protein
Physical Resilience	Ability to resist functional decline or recover function after health stressors.	• Physiological reserve • Adaptive response is seen in cells, and bodily organs	• Medical comorbidities • Biological factors • Reserve • Frailty • Robustness	• Physical Resilience Scale[18] • Physical Resilience Instrument for Older Adults[19]	• Aspartate • Lactate • Glutamate • TNFR-I • miR-376a-3p • Inflammatory biomarkers
Psychological Resilience	Ability to navigate adversity with a positive adaptive response.	• Positive adaptation • Resisting, bouncing back, and/or growing from stressors	• Emotional regulation • Social support • Environmental influences	• Wagnild and Young's Resilience Scale[26] • Connor–Davidson Resilience Scale[50] • Brief Resilient Coping Scale[27]	• Cortisol • BDNF • Glucose • HbA1c • Catecholamines • Oxytocin • CRP • Interleukins

Abbreviations: Aβ42, amyloid beta; t-tau, total-tau; p-tau, phosphorylated tau; TNFR-I, tumor necrosis factor receptor 1; miR-376a-3p, micro-RNAs; BDNF, brain-derived neurotrophic factor; CRP, C-reactive protein.

PSYCHOLOGICAL RESILIENCE

Psychological resilience, as outlined by the American Psychological Association, is defined as the inherent ability of individuals to navigate adversity, trauma, tragedy, threats or significant stressors with a positive adaptive response. This conceptualization underscores the crucial aspect of individuals' capacity to effectively adjust and thrive in the face of challenging circumstances.[24] Resisting, bouncing back or growing from stressors reflects dominant concepts in resilience. The widely accepted definition of psychological resilience encapsulates the ability to withstand the adverse impacts of stressors, adeptly rebound or "bounce back" from stressors and/or undergo personal growth as a transformative response to stressors. In light of the increasing heterogeneity in research outcomes and measures, some scholars propose a refined approach to better target resilience measures and interventions. Despite controversies in conceptualization and resilience definitions, there is in general agreement that resilience is a complex and dynamic process with "buildable resources." There are environmental and internal factors that promote resilience in an individual.

Measuring Psychological Resilience

Assessment of resilience has been approached in many ways. One commonly used method is psychometric-based and involves the administration of established questionnaires aimed at quantifying resilience. Most resilience scales have been developed in younger populations for which reason validation of these scales in older adults is important. In a systematic review of resilience scales among older adults, Cosco et al. (2016) identified only six studies with psychometric analyses. Among them, three scales demonstrated evidence of psychometric robustness in older adults: Wagnild and Young's Resilience Scale (1993), Connor and Davidson's Connor–Davidson Scale (2003) and Sinclair and Wallston's Brief Resilient Coping Scale (2004). However, it is noteworthy that none of the psychometric evaluations of resilience scales in older adults conducted to date are comprehensive.[25]

The Resilience Scale™ (RS™) developed by Wagnild and Young in 1993, is the original resilience measure considered as the "gold standard" for resilience assessments among researchers around the world. It is a highly valid and reliable 25-item scale that measures resilience in any setting. The original resilience scale was created and validated with a sample of older adults in their fifth to ninth decade of life. Positive results correlate with physical health, morale and life satisfaction, while negative results correlate with depression.[26] The Connor–Davidson Resilience Scale assesses various resilience components, including adaptability to change, stress coping, resilience in the face of failure, and handling emotions such as anger, pain or sadness. Only the CD-RISC-2, CD-RISC-10 and CD-RISC-25 versions are authorized for use. The Brief Resilient Coping Scale (BRCS), a concise four-item measure by Sinclair and Wallston (2004), identifies individuals with potential for enhanced resilient coping skills, making it valuable for targeted interventions.[27]

TABLE 19.2
Examples of Resilience Measurement Scales

Scale	Measurement	Description
Physical Resilience Scale[18]	Developed as a measure of physical resilience and association of resilience to recovery following acute health stressor.	PRS is a 17-item measure that includes characteristics of adaptability, mobilizing one's strengths and social support. • For example, it includes reflections such as "I was determined to recover," "I believe I could recover" and "I accepted the new challenges." • Scores range from 0 to 17 with higher score reflecting greater resilience. • Reliability is good and validity is excellent compared with other general resilience measures. • The PRS does not have license fees.
Resilience Scale[26]	Developed as a general measure of adults' resilience across the lifespan.	The original 25-item RS reflected five interrelated components of resilience, for example, the ability of "mind calmness under the stress"; self-reliance; perseverance; meaning of life and a sense of uniqueness. • It is scored on a 7-item Likert scale with scores ranging between 25 and 175. Higher scores indicate a higher level of resilience. • Responses positively correlate with physical health, morale and life satisfaction; and negatively correlate with depressive symptoms. • It can be used with permission.
Connor–Davidson Resilience Scale[50]	General resilience measure that focuses on coping with stress.	The original CD-RISC is a 25-item self-administered questionnaire that measures e.g., personal competence, positive acceptance of changes, trust in one's instincts, strengthening effect stress, and spiritual influences. • Each item is rated on a 5-point Likert scale, ranging from (0–4) with higher scores indicative of higher levels of resilience. • It is a highly valid and reliable measure of resilience in any setting. • The scale is copyright and not in public domain.

(Continued)

TABLE 19.2 (Continued)

Scale	Measurement	Description
Brief Resilience Scale[51]	Focuses on measuring one's ability to respond to stress and adversity.	BRS is a 6-item self-reported questionnaire in which 3 items are negatively focused and 3 items are positively focused on the ability to recover after stressful experiences, for example, "I tend to bounce back quickly after challenging times." • May provide key insights for individuals facing health-related stressors. • On a 5-point scale response with higher average scores indicate higher levels of perceived resilience. • The BRS does not have license fees.
Brief Resilient Coping Scale[27]	Identify one's ability to cope with stress.	BRCS is a 4-item measure that focuses on adaptive coping, such as using coping strategies to resolve problems despite stressful conditions. • The possible scores range from 4 (low resilience) to 20 (high resilience). • The BRCS is in the public domain.

Abbreviations: PRS, Physical Resilience Scale; RS, Resilience Scale; CD–RISC, Connor–Davidson Resilience Scale; BRS, Brief Resilience Scale; BRCS, Brief Resilient Coping Scale.

PSYCHOLOGICAL RESILIENCE BIOMARKERS

Systems that were found to impact resilience included the Hypothalamic Pituitary Adrenal (HPA) axis, the Autonomic Nervous System (ANS) and associated neuromodulators, the immune system, as well as the endocannabinoid and endorphin (dopamine, serotonin and oxytocin) systems.[28] Potential diagnostic biomarkers of chronic stress included cortisol, ACTH, BDNF, catecholamines, glucose, HbA1c, triglycerides, cholesterol, prolactin, oxytocin, dehydroepiandrosterone sulfate (DHEA-S), CRP and interleukins 6 and 8. Others, including antioxidants and natural killer (NK) cells, require further validation.[29] These physical biomarkers can identify people with low resilience, and therefore at increased risk for neuropsychiatric conditions. It can also help develop therapies that target the physical biomarkers of stress. However, therapies targeting physical biomarkers of resilience are limited in real practice and are still in the research stage.

STRESS AND STRESS-RELATED DISEASES

Chronic stress is intricately connected to many physical and psychological conditions, both positively and negatively impacting health. Existing literature suggests that greater psychological resilience may protect against the onset of diabetes and improve the management of diabetes mellitus (e.g., lower HbA1c levels) in younger people. In a recent analysis of the Look AHEAD Trial, Olson et al. (2023) found that among older individuals with diabetes mellitus, higher levels of psychological resilience were correlated with several positive outcomes. These included reduced hospitalization frequency over the past year, improved physical functioning, lower self-reported disability, enhanced mental quality of life and a diminished likelihood of frailty.[30]

In a cohort of community-dwelling older adults following hip fracture, higher levels of self-reported psychological resilience were associated with greater walking speed and distance.[31] The REGAIN (Regional versus General Anesthesia for Promoting Independence after Hip Fracture) investigators revealed that psychological resilience is associated with better outcomes for older adults after hip fracture surgery. Increasing psychological resilience was associated with lower odds of death or transition to new institutional residence at 60 days after surgery, but among those who do not have postoperative complications. Future interventions may focus on improving psychological resilience preoperatively or providing support to patients with lower psychological resilience.[32]

In older adults, elevated psychological resilience is associated with various health benefits, including enhanced well-being, adoption of healthier lifestyles and a decreased risk of mortality.[33]

INTERVENTIONS TO PROMOTE RESILIENCE

It is important to recognize that the development of resilience interventions follows distinct stages. Researchers first recognize a conceptual framework and specific definitions of resilience. Subsequently, they devise analytical strategies to measure resilience in response to specific stressors. The ongoing work involves identifying biomarkers associated with resilience to better understand underlying mechanisms. The overarching goal is to use evidence-based interventions to promote resilience.

Lifestyle medicine is a new and distinct specialty aiming to prevent, treat and possibly reverse most chronic diseases using the strongest evidence-based approaches available. Lifestyle medicine seeks to address these issues to improve health and well-being at the individual and societal levels. Lifestyle medicine specialists implement interventions to promote resilience and healthy aging. Current evidence demonstrates numerous health benefits by applying six pillars of lifestyle medicine, which include plant-based nutrition, physical activity and exercise, restorative sleep, stress management, avoidance of risky substances and positive social connections.

NUTRITION

Many studies support that adherence to a healthy dietary pattern is associated with slower rates of cognitive and physical decline. Dietary habits are an important modifiable risk factor for neurodegenerative disorders, along with physical inactivity, alcohol and tobacco use.[1] The Study on Nutrition and Cardiovascular Risk in Spain (Seniors–ENRICA Cohort) is a recent study on the association between diet and physical resilience in older adults. The study looks at the Mediterranean diet and other healthy dietary patterns, with physical resilience assessed empirically as a trajectory through exposure to acute and chronic stressors. The study found that in older adults, greater compliance with the Mediterranean diet is associated with increased physical resilience.[34]

There is growing and emerging evidence that diet plays a key role in preventing age-related cognitive decline and Alzheimer's disease. The evidence from epidemiological studies and clinical trials indicates that greater consumption of health-promoting foods and limited intake of unhealthier options, as seen in the Mediterranean diet, the Dietary Approaches to Stop Hypertension (DASH) diet, or the Mediterranean–DASH Interventions for Neurocognitive Delay (MIND) dietary pattern, reduces the risk of neurocognitive disorders, cardiovascular diseases and cancer.[35]

Overall, whole food plant-based diets can support a higher quality of life in older adults, while ultra-processed food is highly associated with cardiometabolic diseases and other non-communicable diseases such as cancer, chronic kidney disease or depression.[36]

The importance of the gut–brain axis in maintaining the body's homeostasis has long been appreciated. However, the research in aging has added to the emergence of microbiota as one of the key regulators of the gut-brain function. A study has implicated gut–brain dysbiosis in neurodegenerative conditions such as Alzheimer's disease and Parkinson's disease, and neuropsychiatric conditions such as anxiety or schizophrenia. Stress, poor nutrition, intestinal inflammation, antibiotics use, environmental factors, host genetics and aging itself can influence gut microbiota composition. More studies are needed to understand the mechanisms underlying the gut–brain axis to develop evidence-based therapeutic strategies to promote healthy aging.[37]

Physical Activity and Exercise

Physical activity and exercise are frequently used interchangeably and are considered potential ways for evaluating and enhancing physical resilience. There is ample evidence supporting a positive correlation between regular physical activity and exercise in preventing diseases and maintaining overall health and longevity. In particular, cardiovascular fitness is a predictor of longer life in older adults, and increasing it can enhance brain function, musculoskeletal health and metabolic status. However, more research is needed to better understand the health benefits related to frequency, intensity and duration of physical activity to determine the optimal dose for older adults.[38] Optimizing physical fitness through activity can improve physical resilience by enhancing physiological responses and reducing reactions to physical stress. Some potential ways to increase physical resilience with aging include engaging in endurance exercises, flexibility and balance activities, resistance training and being outdoors. Tai Chi combines both physical and mental exercises. It is beneficial for preventing falls and enhancing balance in older adults, regardless of whether they are in good health or at a high risk of falling. The effectiveness of Tai Chi is positively associated with the duration and frequency of exercise, with Yang-style Tai Chi demonstrating greater effectiveness than Sun-style Tai Chi.[39]

Current knowledge about how physical activity affects the body at the molecular level indicates that it leads to various changes in metabolism and cells. These changes include alterations in gene activity, epigenetic modifications, increased muscle strength and size and better heart and lung function over time. These molecular and cellular adaptations happen in important parts of the body such as the heart, blood vessels, brain, fat tissue, liver, gut and the immune system. However, there is a poor understanding of how these adaptations occur throughout the entire body due to physical activity, and why the outcomes of physical activity on resilience are inconsistent.[40] The NIH Common Fund's Molecular Transducers of Physical Activity in Humans (MoTrPAC) initiative looks at the benefits of physical exercise at the molecular level. Following completion, it will be the largest research study to examine the link between exercise and its improvement of physical health.

Restorative Sleep

Sleep is a fundamental requirement for both mental and physical well-being. High-quality restorative sleep can enhance the body's ability to resist, adapt and recover from stressors, leading to better health outcomes. There are certain repair processes that occur in the body most effectively during sleep and research findings suggest that the brain has its own "drainage system" that removes toxins during sleep. The CNS glymphatic system, the analog of the lymphatic system in the body, plays a key role in regulating directional interstitial fluid movement, waste clearance, and, potentially, brain immunity.[41] As resilience to brain pathology creates new and promising research directions, and encouraging data are arising from sleep studies that reveal that deep sleep may mitigate Alzheimer's pathology, it is reasonable that sleep could be a modifiable factor in preventing cognitive decline. Recent research shows that in cognitively intact adults with a high beta-amyloid burden, non-REM slow-wave sleep can support cognitive reserve on memory function. On the other hand, adults without significant beta-amyloid pathology burden did not similarly benefit from non-REM slow wave activity.[42] The incorporation of sleep health in resilience research and clinical practice is important for promoting resilience in older adults. Studies supported by the National Institutes of Health (NIH) are investigating sleep as a promoter of molecular, physiological and psychological resilience. These studies explore how sleep contributes to health maintenance, survivorship and protective/preventive pathways.[43]

Researchers are extensively studying non-pharmacological interventions to enhance the quality and amount of sleep in older adults. Methods involving changes in behavior and mind–body exercises have shown the most evidence of improving sleep. Other approaches, including sleep education, relaxation techniques, physical exercise, aromatherapy, massage, psychotherapy and environmental interventions, may also have benefits, although further research is needed.[44]

MANAGING STRESS

Positive attitudes toward aging, social connectedness, improving functioning through healthy diet, physical activity and exercises, restorative sleep and stress management are ways to promote resilience. Mindfulness-based stress reduction (MBSR) techniques and emotional self-management are the most common non-pharmacological stress-related disorders interventions that promote psychological resilience. Developing and practicing stress management techniques, or spiritual practices such as prayer, meditation, mindfulness or yoga, will help to reduce stress and foster psychological resilience. Many classes and workshops on mindfulness and other stress-reduction techniques are organized by communities and the public.

AVOIDING RISKY SUBSTANCES

Avoiding tobacco, alcohol, illicit drugs, but also polypharmacy, will help to foster resilience. Adverse drug interactions and side effects may contribute to declining cognitive health. Data from a UCSF-led study revealed that 58% of seniors with probable or possible dementia had good to excellent health, yet more than half took six or more medications. However, most people with dementia are willing to deprescribe their medications. Deprescribing unnecessary or harmful medications represents an opportunity to improve the quality of life for older adults with dementia.[45]

CULTIVATING POSITIVE PSYCHOLOGY

Positive psychology is the scientific study of optimal human functioning that emphasize on well-being, happiness and personal strengths. Seligman's PERMA model of positive psychology refers to positive emotions, engagement, relationships, meaning and accomplishment. Enjoying life and engaging in social activities that give joy: family, friends, neighborhood, community, volunteering, traveling, studying, gardening, hiking, joining a book club, writing classes, team sports and any other form of socializing helps to promote resilience and healthy aging. Loneliness, social isolation, anxiety and depression have a negative impact on health. Greater social participation in midlife and late life is associated with 30–50% lower subsequent dementia risk.[46] Cultivating positive psychology with optimism, and a positive view of aging may help to foster resilience and healthy aging. Numerous studies have been conducted to examine the longitudinal health effects of subjective aging. Older subjective age is associated with chronic stress and negatively impacts health issues. Younger subjective age produces a lower risk of depression and positively impacts mental health.[47]

There is evidence for the longitudinal relationship of subjective aging with health and longevity. Holding a negative view of one's own aging is associated with a 40% increased risk of heart conditions and a 30% increased risk of stroke.[48] The Successful Aging Evaluation (SAGE) study revealed that younger subjective age compared to chronological age was associated with better mental and physical health and was positively associated with measures of the presence of meaning in life, successful aging, optimism, personal mastery, resilience, curiosity, hope and social support.[49]

Perceived younger age and personal satisfaction with aging have also been demonstrated as a protective mechanism against frailty. Subjective age is a potentially valuable measurement for clinical assessment and intervention, and this possibility should be investigated in future research.

CONCLUSIONS AND PRACTICAL POINTS

The concept of resilience is gaining prominence in geriatric care. Viewing resilience as an individual's capacity to withstand, adapt or recover from health challenges offers a perspective beyond the traditional narrative of aging as a period of losses and declines. Resilience plays a crucial role in optimizing the aging process, promoting health, enhancing well-being and, as a result, contributing to healthy aging. Researchers are actively refining the definition, measurement methods and biomarkers of resilience to develop effective interventions. Concurrently, lifestyle medicine offers evidence-based strategies readily applicable in geriatric practices to enhance resilience among older adults. In clinics dedicated to geriatric well-being and healthy aging, the incorporation of the six pillars of lifestyle medicine is emphasized, covering aspects such as a healthy diet, physical activity, restorative sleep, stress management, avoidance of risky substances and positive psychology. Resilience is also important in discussions of the Geriatric 5Ms: mentation, mobility, multimorbidity, medications and matters most approach.

Routine assessments for healthy aging should include evaluating vital signs and BMI, screening for risky substance use and assessing anxiety and depression using tools such as GAD-2 and PHQ-2 scales. Although there is not enough evidence to screen asymptomatic patients for cognitive decline, any concerns regarding cognitive resilience may be completed using a cognitive assessment.

Adding screening questions regarding patient resilience, such as "What is your resilience level?" by using, for example, the CDR-2, or assessing the ability to manage stress by using the BRCS may provide more insight. It is advisable not to label a patient as "resilient," as this term may be perceived negatively.

Additional questions regarding patients' subjective age may provide insight into their wellness and psychological resilience and help identify patients at risk for future decline.

The use of evidence-based practices, incorporating fundamental blood markers such as CBC, CMP, CRP, TSH and A1c is important in providing insights into physiological reserve.

Tailoring lifestyle medicine recommendations for older adults may differ from those for younger adults, but addressing all aspects remains crucial across ages. For instance, in middle-aged individuals, the emphasis may be on preventing chronic diseases and fortifying reserves for later life through rigorous dietary and exercise regimens, avoiding risky substances and prioritizing stress management. On the other hand, for older adults, the focus may shift toward preserving mobility, prioritizing sleep and incorporating positive psychology principles. Nonetheless, in all cases, an individualized approach proves to be most effective.

Enhancing the health, well-being and resilience of older adults can be achieved by referring them to a certified lifestyle medicine specialist. This specialist provides

TABLE 19.3
Brief Resilient Coping Scale

Instructions: Consider how well the following statements describe your behavior and actions.	Does not describe me at all (1)	Does not describe me (2)	Neutral (3)	Describes me (4)	Describes me very well (5)
I look for creative ways to alter difficult situations.					
Regardless of what happens to me, I believe I can control my reaction to it.					
I believe I can grow in positive ways by dealing with difficult situations.					
I actively look for ways to replace the losses I encounter in life.					

Score	Interpretation
4–13	Low resilient copers
14–16	Medium resilient copers
17–20	High resilient copers

Source: Sinclair, V. G. and Wallston, K.A. (2004). The development and psychometric evaluation of the Brief Resilient Coping Scale. *Assessment, 11 (1)*, 94–101.

counseling, develops non-pharmacological strategies, offers coaching and prescribes evidence-based approaches at a holistic level.

Empathetic interdisciplinary work of geriatricians, lifestyle medicine specialists, nutritionists, physical therapists and psychologists is crucial for "enhancing aging and ending ageism," and promoting healthy aging.

Within the community, it's important to communicate the value of older adults as integral community members. Becoming familiar with available resources, advocating for and directing patients to programs designed for the well-being and physical fitness of older adults – such as Geri-Fit – or encouraging community involvement in meaningful causes and self-expression activities such as art creation, participation in art-based activities or dance classes can contribute significantly to enhancing the resilience of older adults.

Expanding the Age-Friendly Health System with a focus on building health systems that provide high-quality evidence-based health care to older adults will contribute to promoting healthy aging. More research is needed on evidence-based interventions to promote resilience and implement resilience in patient care.

CLINICAL APPLICATIONS

- Resilience in aging empowers individuals to resist, adapt to and overcome health and age-related life adversities, while optimizing personal growth and fulfillment.
- Resilience should be assessed in primary care and healthy aging clinics.
- The Brief Resilience Coping Scale serves as a valuable screening tool.
- Older adults demonstrating low or moderate resilience levels may benefit from further assessment and recommendations.
- Implement the six pillars of lifestyle medicine: nutrition, exercise, sleep, stress management, social connections and avoiding toxins.
- Integrate the "5Ms" of Age-Friendly Health Systems: mentation, mobility, medication, multimorbidity and matters most.
- Incorporate basic blood markers to provide insight into physiological reserve.
- Consider tailored referral to a geriatrician, lifestyle medicine specialist, dietitian, physical therapist, occupational therapist and available community resources.
- Apply positive psychology principles to interactions with older adults.

REFERENCES

1. Merriam-Webster. *Merriam-Webster Dictionary.* Merriam-Webster; 2011.
2. Brown L, Cohen B, Costello R, Brazhnik O, Galis ZS. Next steps: operationalizing resilience research. *Stress Health.* 2023 Sep;39(S1):62–66. doi:10.1002/smi.3256
3. Bonanno GA. Loss, trauma, and human resilience: have we underestimated the human capacity to thrive after extremely aversive events? *Am Psychol.* 2004 Jan;59(1):20–28. doi:10.1037/0003-066X.59.1.20
4. Abadir PM, Bandeen-Roche K, Bergeman C, et al. An overview of the resilience world: proceedings of the American geriatrics society and national institute on aging state of resilience science conference. *J Am Geriatr Soc.* 2023 Aug;71(8):2381–2392. doi:10.1111/jgs.18388
5. Karmann J, Handlovsky I, Lu S, Moullec G, Frohlich KL, Ferlatte O. Resilience among older adults during the COVID-19 pandemic: a photovoice study. *SSM Qual Res Health.* 2023 Jun;3:100256. doi:10.1016/j.ssmqr.2023.100256
6. Gooding PA, Hurst A, Johnson J, Tarrier N. Psychological resilience in young and older adults. *Int J Geriatr Psychiatry.* 2012 Mar;27(3):262–270. doi:10.1002/gps.2712
7. MacLeod S, Musich S, Hawkins K, Alsgaard K, Wicker ER. The impact of resilience among older adults. *Geriatr Nurs.* 2016 Jul–Aug;37(4):266–272. doi:10.1016/j.gerinurse.2016.02.014

8. Stern Y, Albert M, Barnes CA, Cabeza R, Pascual-Leone A, Rapp PR. A framework for concepts of reserve and resilience in aging. *Neurobiol Aging.* 2023 Apr;124:100–103. doi:10.1016/j.neurobiolaging.2022.10.015
9. Joshi MS, Galvin JE. Cognitive resilience in brain health and dementia research. *J Alzheimers Dis.* 2022;90(2):461–473. doi:10.3233/JAD-220755
10. Livingston G, Huntley J, Sommerlad A, et al. Dementia prevention, intervention, and care: 2020 report of the lancet commission. *Lancet.* 2020 Aug 8;396(10248):413–446. doi:10.1016/S0140-6736(20)30367-6
11. Bocancea DI, van Loenhoud AC, Groot C, Barkhof F, van der Flier WM, Ossenkoppele R. Measuring resilience and resistance in aging and alzheimer disease using residual methods: a systematic review and meta-analysis. *Neurology.* 2021 Sep 7;97(10):474–488. doi:10.1212/WNL.0000000000012499
12. Saunders TS, Pozzolo FE, Heslegrave A, et al. Predictive blood biomarkers and brain changes associated with age-related cognitive decline. *Brain Commun.* 2023;5(3):fcad113. doi:10.1093/braincomms/fcad113
13. Dumitrescu L, Mahoney ER, Mukherjee S, et al. Genetic variants and functional pathways associated with resilience to Alzheimer's disease. *Brain.* 2020 Aug 1;143(8):2561–2575. doi:10.1093/brain/awaa209
14. Philip B Gorelick FS. *Practical Aspects of Cognitive Impairment and the Dementias, An Issue of Clinics in Geriatric Medicine.* 1st ed., Vol 39, No 1. Elsevier; 2022.
15. Whitson HE, Duan-Porter W, Schmader KE, Morey MC, Cohen HJ, Colon-Emeric CS. Physical resilience in older adults: systematic review and development of an emerging construct. *J Gerontol A Biol Sci Med Sci.* 2016 Apr;71(4):489–495. doi:10.1093/gerona/glv202
16. Whitson HE, Cohen HJ, Schmader KE, Morey MC, Kuchel G, Colon-Emeric CS. Physical resilience: not simply the opposite of frailty. *J Am Geriatr Soc.* 2018 Aug;66(8):1459–1461. doi:10.1111/jgs.15233
17. Ukraintseva S, Yashin AI, Arbeev KG. Resilience versus robustness in aging. *J Gerontol A Biol Sci Med Sci.* 2016 Nov;71(11):1533–1534. doi:10.1093/gerona/glw083
18. Resnick B, Galik E, Dorsey S, Scheve A, Gutkin S. Reliability and validity testing of the physical resilience measure. *Gerontologist.* 2011 Oct;51(5):643–652. doi:10.1093/geront/gnr016
19. Hu FW, Lin CH, Yueh FR, Lo YT, Lin CY. Development and psychometric evaluation of the physical resilience instrument for older adults (PRIFOR). *BMC Geriatr.* 2022 Mar 21;22(1):229. doi:10.1186/s12877-022-02918-7
20. Colon-Emeric C, Pieper CF, Schmader KE, et al. Two approaches to classifying and quantifying physical resilience in longitudinal data. *J Gerontol A Biol Sci Med Sci.* 2020 Mar 9;75(4):731–738. doi:10.1093/gerona/glz097
21. Peters S, Cosco TD, Mackey DC, Sarohia GS, Leong J, Wister A. Quantifying physical resilience in ageing using measurement instruments: a scoping review. *Physiother Can.* 2022 Nov;74(4):370–378. doi:10.3138/ptc-2020-0134
22. Bautmans I, Knoop V, Amuthavalli Thiyagarajan J, et al. WHO working definition of vitality capacity for healthy longevity monitoring. *Lancet Healthy Longev.* 2022 Nov;3(11):e789–e796. doi:10.1016/S2666-7568(22)00200-8
23. Parker DC, Colomicronn-Emeric C, Huebner JL, et al. Biomarkers associated with physical resilience after hip fracture. *J Gerontol A Biol Sci Med Sci.* 2020 Sep 25;75(10):e166–e172. doi:10.1093/gerona/glaa119
24. Association AP. The road to resilience. Accessed January 11, 2024.
25. Cosco TD, Kok A, Wister A, Howse K. Conceptualising and operationalising resilience in older adults. *Health Psychol Behav Med.* 2019 Mar 28;7(1):90–104. doi:10.1080/21642850.2019.1593845

26. Wagnild GM, Young HM. Development and psychometric evaluation of the resilience scale. *J Nurs Meas*. 1993 Winter;1(2):165–178.
27. Sinclair VG, Wallston KA. *Assessment*. 2004 Mar;11(1):94–101. doi:10.1177/1073 191103258144
28. Ryan M, Ryznar R. The molecular basis of resilience: a narrative review. *Front Psychiatry*. 2022;13:856998. doi:10.3389/fpsyt.2022.856998
29. Noushad S, Ahmed S, Ansari B, Mustafa UH, Saleem Y, Hazrat H. Physiological biomarkers of chronic stress: a systematic review. *Int J Health Sci (Qassim)*. 2021 Sep–Oct;15(5):46–59.
30. Olson KL, Howard M, McCaffery JM, et al. Psychological resilience in older adults with type 2 diabetes from the look AHEAD trial. *J Am Geriatr Soc*. 2023 Jan;71(1):206–213. doi:10.1111/jgs.17986
31. Soliman G, Fortinsky RH, Mangione K, et al. Impact of psychological resilience on walking capacity in older adults following hip fracture. *J Am Geriatr Soc*. 2022 Nov;70(11):3087–3095. doi:10.1111/jgs.17930
32. Investigators R. Preoperative psychological resilience and recovery after hip fracture: secondary analysis of the REGAIN randomized trial. *J Am Geriatr Soc*. 2023 Dec;71(12):3792–3801. doi:10.1111/jgs.18552
33. Resnick B. Resilience in older adults: what it is and how to strengthen it. In: Wister AV, Cosco TD, eds. *Resilience and Aging: Risk, Systems and Decisions*. Springer; 2020: 15–20. https://doi.org/10.1007/978-3-030-57089-7_2 .
34. Sotos-Prieto M, Ortola R, Lopez-Garcia E, Rodriguez-Artalejo F, Garcia-Esquinas E. Adherence to the Mediterranean diet and physical resilience in older adults: the seniors-ENRICA cohort. *J Gerontol A Biol Sci Med Sci*. 2021 Feb 25;76(3):505–512. doi:10.1093/gerona/glaa277
35. Cena H, Calder PC. Defining a healthy diet: evidence for the role of contemporary dietary patterns in health and disease. *Nutrients*. 2020 Jan 27;12(2)doi:10.3390/nu12020334
36. Touvier M, da Costa Louzada ML, Mozaffarian D, Baker P, Juul F, Srour B. Ultra-processed foods and cardiometabolic health: public health policies to reduce consumption cannot wait. *BMJ*. 2023 Oct 9;383:e075294. doi:10.1136/bmj-2023-075294
37. Cryan JF, O'Riordan KJ, Cowan CSM, et al. The microbiota-gut-brain axis. *Physiol Rev*. Oct 1 2019;99(4):1877–2013. doi:10.1152/physrev.00018.2018
38. Andrew Wister TC. *Resilience and Aging: Emerging Science and Future Possibilities*. Springer; 2020.
39. Chen W, Li M, Li H, Lin Y, Feng Z. Tai Chi for fall prevention and balance improvement in older adults: a systematic review and meta-analysis of randomized controlled trials. *Front Public Health*. 2023;11:1236050. doi:10.3389/fpubh.2023.1236050
40. Baumgartner JN, Kowtha B, Riscuta G, Wali A, Gao Y. Molecular underpinnings of physical activity and resilience: a brief overview of the state-of-science and research design needs. *Stress Health*. 2023 Sep;39(S1):14–21. doi:10.1002/smi.3258
41. Hablitz LM, Nedergaard M. The glymphatic system: a novel component of fundamental neurobiology. *J Neurosci*. 2021 Sep 15;41(37):7698–7711. doi:10.1523/JNEUROSCI.0619-21.2021
42. Zavecz Z, Shah VD, Murillo OG, et al. NREM sleep as a novel protective cognitive reserve factor in the face of Alzheimer's disease pathology. *BMC Med*. 2023 May 3;21(1):156. doi:10.1186/s12916-023-02811-z
43. Guida JL, Alfini A, Lee KC, et al. Integrating sleep health into resilience research. *Stress Health*. 2023 Sep;39(S1):22–27. doi:10.1002/smi.3244
44. Carroll JE, Prather AA. Sleep and biological aging: a short review. *Curr Opin Endocr Metab Res*. 2021 Jun;18:159–164. doi:10.1016/j.coemr.2021.03.021

45. Growdon ME, Espejo E, Jing B, et al. Attitudes toward deprescribing among older adults with dementia in the United States. *J Am Geriatr Soc.* 2022 Jun;70(6):1764–1773. doi:10.1111/jgs.17730
46. Sommerlad A, Kivimaki M, Larson EB, Rohr S, Shirai K, Singh-Manoux A, Livingston G. Social participation and risk of developing dementia. *Nat Aging.* 2023 May;3(5):532–545. doi:10.1038/s43587-023-00387-0
47. Mitina M, Young S, Zhavoronkov A. Psychological aging, depression, and well-being. *Aging (Albany NY).* 2020 Sep 18;12(18):18765–18777. doi:10.18632/aging.103880
48. Stephan Y, Sutin AR, Wurm S, Terracciano A. Subjective aging and incident cardiovascular disease. *J Gerontol B Psychol Sci Soc Sci.* 2021 Apr 23;76(5):910–919. doi:10.1093/geronb/gbaa106
49. Atkins D, Best D, Briss PA, et al. Grading quality of evidence and strength of recommendations. *BMJ.* 2004 Jun 19;328(7454):1490. doi:10.1136/bmj.328.7454.1490
50. Connor KM, Davidson JR. Development of a new resilience scale: the Connor-Davidson resilience scale (CD-RISC). *Depress Anxiety.* 2003;18(2):76–82.
51. Smith BW, Dalen J, Wiggins K, Tooley E, Christopher P, Bernard J. The brief resilience scale: assessing the ability to bounce back. *Int J Behav Med.* 2008;15(3):194–200.

20 Palliative Care in Older Adults
A Lifestyle Medicine Approach

Tiffany Jackson and Cristina H. Davis

INTRODUCTION: DEFINING PALLIATIVE CARE

Palliative care is a specialized model of medical care in which individuals with serious illness, or advanced disease that is often terminal, have an opportunity to focus on symptom relief and coping with the stress of their illness with a goal of improved quality of life (QOL).[1] Palliative care is delivered through an interdisciplinary team typically consisting of physicians, nurses, social workers and other specialists who collaborate to provide patients and their families with an extra layer of support as they navigate and experience serious illness; it can be provided alongside curative treatments.[1] This model of care is delivered in community-based settings including patient homes and skilled nursing facilities, inpatient hospital settings and outpatient clinic settings.[1]

Whereas palliative care was once considered end-stage or end-of-life care for patients with advanced disease who were not yet ready to enroll in hospice care, it is now recognized as a fundamental aspect of care for individuals with serious illness at any stage of disease. The World Health Organization (WHO) emphasizes the importance of initiating palliative care as early as possible to promote better outcomes for QOL and reduce the chances of symptoms becoming unmanageable at the end of life.[2] The WHO suggests that symptoms that are not managed early in the disease process may become difficult to manage if not addressed until later.[2] While pain management was once a primary focus of palliative care, it is now recommended to consider the physical, spiritual and emotional needs of patients suffering from serious illness as well as addressing all distressing symptoms of a person's illness, including nausea and vomiting, fatigue, dyspnea, delirium and agitation, anxiety and depression, insomnia, loss of appetite and constipation.[1,2]

EPIDEMIOLOGY: IMPACT AND PREVALENCE OF PALLIATIVE CARE IN THE UNITED STATES/WORLDWIDE

Palliative care is a specialty that is essential for patients with serious illness but is highly underutilized. The WHO reports that 56.8 million people, including 25.7 million in the last year of their life, are in need of palliative care.[3] Globally, only about 14% of people who need palliative care are receiving it.[3] It is clear from current literature that the United States health care systems are not meeting the needs of patients and families that are living with advanced disease or serious illness. This is evidenced by frequent avoidable hospitalizations related to symptom management; poor patient and family satisfaction related to care at the end of life; and lack of focus on symptom management, QOL and advance care planning. While palliative care is not available in many health care systems across the country, the United States has demonstrated continued growth in the overall number of hospital palliative care teams since 2019, with 72% of hospitals with 50 or more beds reporting a palliative care team, an increase from 67% in 2015, 53% in 2008 and 7% in 2001.[4] Organizations such as the Center for Advancing Palliative Care (CAPC) are making significant strides to move palliative care forward from a research, availability, training and policy standpoint. CAPC has implemented a publicly accessible database that tracks state policies on palliative care. The database was collaboratively developed with the Solomon Center for Health Law and Policy at Yale Law School, the Veterans Administration (VA), Indian Health Services (IHS) and other stakeholders. Policy innovation that would reduce health care disparities and support research and development in the field of palliative care is one of the many goals of this database.[5] Growth of both hospital and home-based palliative programs is key. There are advancements needed nationally and worldwide to improve the availability of and increase access to palliative care earlier in the disease process. Early implementation of palliative care is key to managing symptoms and improving QOL for older adults with serious illness.

ADVANCE CARE PLANNING AND GOALS OF CARE

Advance care planning (ACP) and goals of care (GOC) discussions are integral parts of palliative care and are often described as one of the most complex aspects of the specialty from a clinician's standpoint. ACP and GOC conversations directly relate to the "Matters Most" element of the 4M framework to promote patient-centered care. What matters to an older adult with a terminal disease in terms of medical interventions, end-of-life wishes, or what they wish to achieve while they are navigating the disease progression will look very different from younger patients. Examples of advance directives include, but are not limited to: living wills, durable power of attorney for health care, Do Not Resuscitate (DNR) orders, Do Not Intubate (DNI), Do Not Hospitalize (DNH), Physician Orders for Life-Sustaining Treatment (POLST) and Medical Orders for Life-Sustaining Treatment (MOLST) forms. The National Institutes of Health describes ACP as discussions and preparation for future medical decision-making when a person becomes seriously ill or unable to express their own wishes.[6] GOC discussions and ACP can be facilitated by a patient's primary care provider or other specialist, although palliative care is often consulted to initiate this process with the patient and family.[6] Meaningful conversations before a disease becomes advanced or before a medical emergency where decisions have to be made under duress is the preferred time to initiate and revisit these delicate, and often emotional, conversations. When a person is able to make their own medical decision for treatment and end of life, this not only promotes autonomy, but also alleviates the family from that emotional burden. Specific documentation, as well as who can sign or execute the documents, varies from state to state. If there are no advance directives in place, state laws will determine who will make medical decisions if a person is ill and unable to make decisions for themselves. ACP has many benefits such as decreasing life-sustaining treatments, increased and earlier use of hospice and palliative care, and reducing avoidable hospitalizations. Advance care planning interventions increase compliance with patients' documented end-of-life wishes.[7]

COMMON CONDITIONS IN PALLIATIVE CARE AFFECTING OLDER ADULTS

Older adults are impacted by many chronic health conditions that can be progressive in nature and eventually may benefit from the implementation of palliative care including cardiac disorders, neoplasms, pulmonary disorders, neurological disease and other conditions that can be life-limiting. For the purpose of this chapter, three of the primary reasons for palliative care consultation will be discussed, including dementia, advanced cardiac disease and advanced pulmonary disease. Dementia is a generalized term used for a condition whereby a person experiences memory loss, language and speech difficulties and difficulties with problem-solving and other thinking abilities in a way that interferes with their daily life and activities of daily living.[8] Dementia is not recognized as a single disease but rather a collection of symptoms that are often caused by another disease such as Alzheimer's disease (AD). There are several specific types of dementia, the most common of which is AD, accounting for 60–80% of dementia cases, with the second most common type being vascular dementia.[8] The CDC estimates that, as of 2014, over 7 million adults over the age of 65 were diagnosed with dementia, with over half having a diagnosis of AD, and the CDC projects that by 2060, the number of older adults with dementia will grow to over 14 million.[9,10] Dementia symptoms are typically progressive in nature and significantly impact relationships, emotions, behaviors and the ability of a person to care for themselves independently, eventually leading to death.[8] Common symptoms experienced by individuals with dementia include loss of short-term memory, difficulty preparing meals, difficulty paying bills, keeping track of personal items, remembering appointments and traveling outside of their immediate neighborhood.[8] While the pathophysiology of AD is not fully understood, current research indicates that AD involves the development and aggregation of amyloid-β or neuritic/senile plaques, and tau plaques or neurofibrillary tangles.[11] Other important features identified in patients with AD on imaging are brain atrophy and glucose hypometabolism.[11] A leading hypothesis regarding AD pathophysiology involves amyloid-β plaques as the inciting event that precipitates subsequent downstream processes of tau deposition and neurodegeneration which eventually leads to dementia.[11] It is theorized that cerebrovascular disease in combination with protein deposition and aggregation may contribute to the development of AD.[11] Genetically, the apolipoprotein E (APOE) gene has been studied with regard to the development of AD, and the APOE ε4 allele has been identified as a risk factor for development of AD.[11] Lifestyle factors also play a crucial role in the pathogenesis of AD; poor sleep has been highly associated with the development of AD.[11] Individuals who participate in cognitive and physical exercises have lower levels of brain amyloid-β plaques, suggesting a protective nature of these activities.[11] Diet appears to play a key role in the pathogenesis of AD, and a standard Western diet is highly associated with the development of AD while whole food plant-based (WFPB) diets, the Mediterranean diet, and the Mediterranean–DASH Intervention for Neurodegenerative Delay (MIND) diet may be neuroprotective, decreasing the risk of developing AD.[12]

Cardiac Disorders

Cardiac diseases are among the most common diagnoses for a palliative care consultation. Heart failure (HF) is associated with significant symptoms such as dyspnea, chest pain, edema and fatigue. HF is generally a chronic, progressive and eventually terminal condition. Heart failure occurs when the heart cannot pump enough blood to the body due to pumping inefficiently or not being able to fill with enough blood. While there is a growing body of evidence to suggest that lifestyle modifications including implementation of a WFPB diet may promote reversal of this condition through targeting the key pathways and underlying conditions that ultimately contribute to HF, this condition continues to be associated with high morbidity and mortality.[13] HF is responsible for thousands of avoidable hospitalizations related to symptom management each year. Palliative care referrals remain widely underutilized in the management of patients with heart disease. Patients with HF experience frequent hospitalizations related to worsening symptoms secondary to a decrease in cardiac output or fluid retention which further contributes to decreased QOL and worsening symptom burden for patients.[14]

A recent systematic review and meta-analysis[15] of PC for patients with HF suggests that PC interventions are associated with improved patient-centered health outcomes, including QOL and symptom control. Palliative care has also been shown to decrease the cost of care and hospitalizations. Early palliative care involvement not only improves symptom management; it also provides earlier opportunities to introduce goals of care and advance directive conversations. Ideally, this should occur during or after each hospitalization because a person's functional status is likely significantly worse than prior to the hospitalization. Functional status of patients with advanced HF directly impacts morbidity and mortality.[14]

Pulmonary Disorders

Pulmonary disorders, especially COPD, are commonly associated with symptoms prompting palliative care consultation, and palliative care for COPD focuses on the management of symptoms, maintaining QOL and good communication amongst the health care team. Symptoms strongly associated with pulmonary disease include dyspnea, fatigue, weight loss/cachexia, depression and anxiety. COPD, like many other serious illnesses, can impact social interaction, nutrition, QOL, physical activity and many other aspects of a person's life. Dyspnea is the primary symptom burden for people suffering from COPD. Dyspnea at rest indicates that the disease is progressing, possibly into end-stage criteria. Strong symptom management in the person's home setting can reduce avoidable hospitalizations, improve QOL, relieve suffering and reduce morbidity and mortality.

> Despite this burden of disease, the vast majority of patients with advanced COPD are not offered palliative care. The underuse of palliative care was first reported nearly 20 years ago and, since then, national and international guidelines have tried to encourage its adoption.[16]

While lifestyle medicine approaches to COPD management can be helpful, anxiolytics, inhaled bronchodilators and opioids remain a current mainstay of symptom management.

LIFESTYLE MEDICINE APPROACHES TO PALLIATIVE CARE

Prescribing lifestyle medicine interventions for individuals receiving palliative care can help alleviate distressing symptoms of disease, thus improving their overall QOL while also empowering patients to participate in the management of their disease with interventions that promote meaningful improvement in their QOL and symptom burden. Recommendations for lifestyle interventions must be considered through the lens of a patient's specific GOC, as prolongation of life may not be aligned with a patient's goals, and some patients may not be willing or able to consider intensive lifestyle changes in advanced disease due to their frailty.[17]

While lifestyle medicine interventions have the potential to improve QOL, daily function and symptom burden in patients receiving palliative care, more research with high-quality studies is needed to evaluate these interventions in practice. Following are the primary therapeutic lifestyle interventions centered on the six pillars of lifestyle medicine. Research with evidence-based modalities to decrease symptom burden and improve QOL for patients with serious illness will be described.

NUTRITION

Nutrition is an important lifestyle medicine pillar that can be targeted in the palliative care population to assist with patients' overall well-being as well as targeting specific symptoms related to their serious illness. Whole food plant-based (WFPB) diets have been studied in the context of cardiovascular disease and have been shown to reduce all-cause mortality and risk of ischemic heart disease; these diets are also implicated in optimizing blood pressure, lipid and glycemic control which can improve QOL by reducing the need for certain medications and associated side effects.[18] While WFPB diets rich in intake of fruits, vegetables, legumes, nuts and whole grains are known to

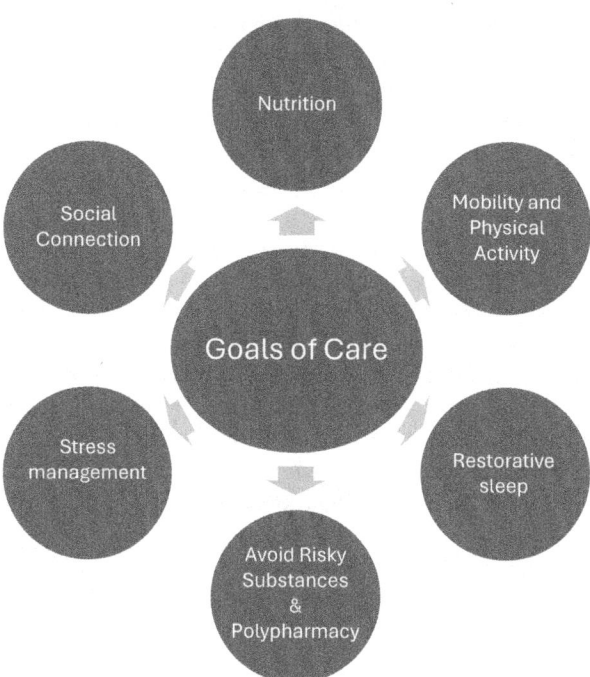

FIGURE 20.1 Goals of care impact how each pillar of lifestyle medicine will be tailored for individuals receiving palliative care.

decrease the risk of developing atherosclerotic cardiovascular disease, there is also strong evidence to support the implementation of these diets to improve symptoms of already existing cardiovascular disease even in patients with advanced disease.[18] The American Heart Association (AHA) now recognizes the importance of nutrition in both the prevention and treatment of cardiac disease and in their most recent recommendations, places an emphasis on a wide variety of fruits and vegetables, whole grains, healthy proteins from mostly plant sources, minimally processed foods, minimal added sugars, foods with little to no salt and limited or preferably no alcohol intake.[19] For patients who are not willing to commit to a WFPB diet, other diets that have been shown to reduce all-cause mortality and major cardiac events for cardiovascular disease include the Mediterranean diet and low-fat diets,[20] although the impact of these diets on symptoms for patients with heart disease has not been extensively studied.

While COPD risk is primarily attributed to smoking tobacco, there is evidence to suggest that individuals adhering to a WFPB diet have a lower risk of developing COPD compared with those not adhering to this diet.[21] A prospective study related to investigating WFPB diets in relation to the primary prevention of COPD has shown that, with tight control for smoking as a factor, individuals with a high plant-based diet index score account for up to a 46% lower risk of developing COPD compared with individuals with a low plant-based diet index score.[21] For individuals who already have COPD, there are few studies examining the impact of a WFPB diet on symptoms; however, one randomized controlled trial (RCT) evaluating 120 patients with COPD found that the intervention group who consumed higher amounts of antioxidant-rich foods including fruits and vegetables experienced improved lung function as measured by predicted forced expiratory lung volume in 1 second compared with the control group, suggesting that dietary interventions may be a future consideration for management of COPD.[22]

Regarding cognition, WFPB diets have been studied with regard to the prevention of cognitive decline and have demonstrated some impact on the risk of developing cognitive impairment and dementia later in life. A 12-year prospective cohort study in Spain examined the role of diet in cognition and found that polyphenol-rich foods, which are primarily found in plant foods, do demonstrate a protective association with regard to the development of cognitive decline.[23] To date, there is limited evidence regarding the implementation of a WFPB diet for patients who have already been diagnosed with dementia, and more high-quality studies are needed to examine their impact. Evidence does suggest that implementation of the Mediterranean diet has been associated with a slower rate of cognitive decline and neurodegeneration, although this has not been specifically studied in high-quality studies for patients who already have dementia and AD.[12]

Physical Activity

A major focus of health and well-being for a person with advanced illness is physical activity. People suffering from advanced serious illness experience significant symptom burden, but also physical and functional debilitation as their disease progresses. Autonomous physical activity is directly related to QOL. While there is often discussion and research on how physical activity is impacted by advanced disease symptoms, it is important to consider the preventative effects of lifestyle medicine. Physical activity can reduce stress, depression and anxiety. It is also directly associated with improvements in pain, appetite and energy.[24] Prescribing suitable exercise programs for patients with advanced disease (specifically cancer) should be a consideration as a holistic approach to their comprehensive individualized treatment program.[24] Physical and occupational therapy consults should be considered when appropriate. Exercise-based cardiac rehabilitation reduced both cardiovascular mortality and hospital admission.[25] Pain, cachexia, weakness, dyspnea, fall risk and other considerations such as safety need to be considered when evaluating the risk versus benefit of physical activity for any patient with advanced serious illness. "A greater exercise rehabilitative focus within palliative care for people with advanced cancer may enable hope and a sense of meaning, while also delaying or improving declines, limiting symptoms, preventing unnecessary hospitalizations and enabling further treatments."[24] Three key interventions have been found to positively impact patient outcomes, including physical activity (PA), nutritional support and palliative symptom management.[26] Validated tools have been used to demonstrate that physical activity, specifically functional status, is directly related to the prognosis for a patient with advanced disease. The Palliative Performance Scale (PPS) is one of the most commonly used prognostication tools used in palliative care. This scale is a modification of the Karnofsky Performance Scale and serves as the gold standard assessment tool for functional capacity and decline in patients receiving palliative care.[27] This scale utilizes percentages from 100% to 0%, declining by increments of 10%; a PPS score of 100% indicates that their medical condition does not affect overall functioning at all whereas a score of 0% represents death.[27] Table 20.1 shows PPS descriptors, as adapted from the Victoria Hospice Society. In current practice, the scale functions in two ways by serving as a reference tool for the assessment of a patient's status and prognosis as well as a tool to assess hospice eligibility across a spectrum of relevant diseases.[28]

SLEEP

Difficulty sleeping is very common for patients with advanced disease and can cause significant decreases in QOL.[29] Good sleep practices are helpful for individuals with or without advanced disease and include behaviors such as exposure to bright light during the day, socialization, optimizing the timing of medications that may impact sleep, avoidance of caffeine and alcohol, performing physical activity, preserving the bed only for sleeping, maintaining a dark and quiet bedroom, providing white noise at night, promotion of a cool body temperature at night, providing a comfortable mattress and maintaining a clean sleeping environment.[30]

Patients with advanced cardiac disease often experience Sleep-Disordered Breathing (SDB) due to a combination of factors including orthopnea, or difficulty lying flat at night due to dyspnea, as well as various types of apnea. Many patients with HF are affected by central sleep apnea or obstructive sleep apnea which can further contribute to poor sleep as their sleep is often disrupted by frequent awakenings due to apneic episodes where the individual ceases to breathe for periods of time, leading to frequent nighttime awakenings.[31,32] For these patients, the primary management tool is optimizing their HF treatment with the use of medications such as diuretics and beta-blockers.[32] The application of the behavioral interventions mentioned above is always considered first-line treatment in SDB for patients with HF to promote sleep without the use of medications with side effects. Additional recommendations specific to this population include avoiding sleeping in supine positions, attempting to lose weight if overweight or obese, and avoiding use of benzodiazepines or alcohol before bed in an effort to decrease the likelihood of airway obstruction during sleep.[32] Treatment of underlying apnea with either mandibular advancement devices or positive airway pressure therapies is also indicated in patients with HF.[32]

Insomnia is present in an estimated one-fourth to one-third of patients with dementia and contributes to caregiver stress, potentially leading to early institutionalization.[30] Insomnia in this population is associated with increased behaviors and agitation which can lead to increased fall risk, stress for caregivers and risk of early institutionalization.[30] Despite limited evidence for improving sleep in older adults and significant side effects, benzodiazepines and sedative-hypnotics are often utilized as a short-term treatment for insomnia.[30] First-line treatment for insomnia in dementia includes promotion of sleep hygiene.[30]

TABLE 20.1
Palliative Performance Scale Descriptors

PPS	Ambulation	Activity and Evidence of Disease	Self-Care	Intake	Level of Consciousness
100%	Full	Normal activity/no evidence of disease	Full	Normal	Full
90%	Full	Normal activity/some evidence of disease	Full	Normal	Full
80%	Full	Normal activity with effort/some evidence of disease	Full	Normal or reduced	Full
70%	Reduced	Unable to do normal work/some evidence of disease	Full	Normal or reduced	Full
60%	Reduced	Unable to do hobbies or housework/significant disease	Occasional assistance necessary	Normal or reduced	Full or confusion
50%	Mainly sit/lie	Unable to do any work/extensive disease	Considerable assistance required	Normal or reduced	Full or confusion
40%	Mainly sit/lie	Unable to do most activities/extensive disease	Mainly assistance	Normal or reduced	Full or drowsy +/− confusion
30%	Totally bed bound	Unable to do any activity/extensive disease	Total care	Reduced	Full or drowsy +/− confusion
20%	Totally bed bound	Unable to do any activity/extensive disease	Total care	Minimal to sips	Full or drowsy +/− confusion
10%	Totally bed bound	Unable to do any activity/extensive disease	Total care	Mouth care only	Drowsy or coma +/− confusion
0%	Death	–	–	–	–

If medications are needed to treat insomnia in these patients, a conversation of risk versus benefits is crucial, and in some cases, the benefits of starting a medication may in fact outweigh the risks.[30] It is also important to consider whether a mood disorder such as anxiety or depression is contributing to insomnia as these are often a prodrome to the development of dementia and are associated with insomnia; treating an underlying mood disorder can be key to managing insomnia and behaviors associated with dementia.[30] Many patients with dementia are on medications which may need to be timed differently in consideration of sleep including antidepressants and acetylcholinesterase inhibitors such as rivastigmine or donepezil, which are known to be wake-promoting medications; conversely, medications that are known to contribute to drowsiness should be adjusted to be administered at night such as muscle relaxers and anxiolytics. Promoting regular activity, social interaction, and regularly timed meals has been shown to help with regulating the circadian rhythm and thus promoting better sleep in this population.[30] Patients with dementia also are often more socially isolated and less engaged in their outside environment, which contributes to less daytime light exposure and can impact sleep; recommendations are for bright light therapy (utilizing a lightbox) for at least 1 hour per day at least 2 hours before bedtime to assist with promotion of sleep at night.[30,33] Melatonin is often utilized to treat insomnia for patients with dementia, and evidence supports improvement in sleep and sundowning behavior with its use.[34]

STRESS MANAGEMENT

High levels of psychological distress often contribute to the development of various medical conditions including cardiac disease. Despite growing evidence to support stress-management techniques in the prevention and treatment of cardiovascular disease, stress-management training has not traditionally been a component of cardiac rehabilitation for patients with cardiovascular disease.[35] When compared with traditional cardiac rehabilitation, an experimental group randomized to cardiac rehabilitation plus stress-management training involving education, cognitive-behavioral therapy (CBT) and group therapy demonstrated greater reductions in global stress scores when compared with the control group.[35] Evidence supports the implementation of a stress-management program as this can impact optimism and HF disease impact in these patients, although this data has not been studied extensively in terms of outcomes related to cardiac events or HF.[36] Management of stress in relation to HF is also linked to other pillars of lifestyle medicine, including social connectedness and physical activity.[36] Individuals with increased social support have perceived lower levels of reported stress and thus tend to experience improved psychological impact of their disease. One study explored the impact of a dual exercise and stress-management program on patients with stable ischemic heart disease and found that the combination of stress management and physical activity improved markers of cardiovascular risk more so than usual medical care.[37] Stress management training involving education regarding their cardiac condition, therapeutic techniques to evaluate their stress levels and thoughts and targeted progressive muscle relaxation and imagery techniques were implemented and, in combination with an aerobic exercise program of 35 minutes 3 times per week, were found to have improved cardiovascular outcomes compared with usual care.[37] Similar positive results related to stress management were demonstrated in the Lifestyle Heart Trial and the subsequent Lifestyle Heart Trial long-term follow-up study through the implementation of stress management techniques that included one hour daily of stress management techniques including stretching, breathing, meditation, progressive relaxation and imagery.[38,39] In combination with other lifestyle interventions including prescribed exercise, adhering to a low-fat vegetarian diet and smoking cessation, patients in the experimental group experienced significant overall regression of coronary atherosclerosis after 1 year of the intervention as well as after 5 years.[38,39]

Stress management is also key in the management of COPD in advanced stages; associations between COPD and psychological distress are thought to be bidirectional in nature as high disease and symptom burden in COPD may contribute to psychological distress while high psychological distress may increase the risk of developing COPD or worsening COPD symptoms, further leading to unhealthy behaviors that may worsen COPD symptoms including smoking and avoiding physical activity.[40] While anxiolytics are often utilized as a palliative measure in end-stage disease to improve QOL for these patients, incorporating lifestyle medicine principles of stress management can help to reduce pill burden and risk of polypharmacy. There is limited research evaluating the use of CBT and other stress management techniques in anxiety management for patients with COPD, although the research on this topic is growing.[40] The strongest evidence to date in improving psychological distress in patients with COPD includes referral for CBT or pulmonary rehabilitation.[40] Psychological distress is underreported and undertreated in this population, and barriers to appropriately addressing this aspect of care include a lack of integration of mental health professionals within pulmonary rehabilitation teams as well as long wait times for patients who have been referred to a mental health professional.[40]

Psychological distress and anxiety are prevalent in patients with dementia and can negatively impact QOL for these individuals as well as their caregivers. Agitation is a behavioral manifestation of anxiety in patients with dementia and is associated with increased falls, fractures, infections and medication use.[41] Psychotropic medications are commonly used to target symptoms of anxiety in older adults with dementia despite a lack of evidence-based guideline recommendations for their use; additionally, the use of psychotropic medications to target anxiety in patients with dementia places them at increased risk for development of adverse effects and polypharmacy.[41] A systematic review of nonpharmacological interventions to target anxiety in this population demonstrated the effectiveness of nonpharmacological interventions in managing anxiety versus usual care; interventions found to be effective include massage, music therapy and those that utilize stimulating cognitive and physical activities such as tailored exercise programs.[41] Conversely, CBT and sensory stimulation were not found to positively impact anxiety in this population.[41] While potential effectiveness has been found in the utilization of medications and supplements such as antipsychotics, antidepressants, probiotics and Ginkgo biloba, safety must be considered and risks versus benefits evaluated since the evidence thus far is limited in support of pharmacologics.[41]

Social Connection

Social connection is an important aspect of health throughout the lifespan but becomes a considerable challenge for adults as they age, particularly for those with serious illnesses. Social isolation is associated with many health risks, including risk for cognitive decline and dementia, increase in death from all-cause mortality, increased risk of heart attack and stroke, and higher rates of depression, anxiety and suicide.[42] Much research related to social connectedness in the palliative care population at present focuses on social isolation, though research in this population is growing with regard to examining social connection as an intervention. Generally, social connection is recommended for prevention but shows promise for those with advanced disease as well.

Social support for patients with cardiac disease is increasingly being implemented as part of overall cardiac care as the benefits are being realized; there is mixed evidence at present regarding the implementation of social connection interventions in this population, despite the well-accepted benefits of social connection in the prevention of cardiac disease. The American Heart Association now recognizes poor social connectedness as a risk factor for death from a heart attack or stroke.[43] One RCT matched 56 patients with cardiac disease undergoing a coronary artery bypass graft for the first time in dyads with an individual who underwent the same surgery previously to form a peer support intervention; anxiety levels were the primary outcome and reported at 24 and 48 hours prior to surgery and again at 5 days and 4 weeks postoperatively, with results indicating that only the experimental group experienced a slight decrease in anxiety levels during hospitalization as well as ongoing decreased anxiety and increased self-efficacy and self-reported physical activity after hospitalization.[44] Another study examining advanced cardiac disease and the impact of social connection on cardiac outcomes focused on a psychosocial approach with counseling as an intervention;[45] this RCT examining interventions of both treating depression and low perceived social support on cardiac events in 2,481 individuals after a myocardial infarction utilized cognitive behavioral therapy (CBT) with counseling sessions aimed at strengthening network ties to be increasingly functional, supportive, and satisfying with some focus on forming new relationships.[45] While this study did demonstrate improvement in depression in this population in the intervention group, there was no statistically significant difference in 4-year survival curves between the intervention and control groups with regard to recurrence of MI or death.[45] Additional research is underway to evaluate the risk of social isolation on the development of HF, though current studies demonstrate a positive association with this.[46] In patients with HF, greater perceived isolation has been associated with increased risk of death and health care use.[47] Research related to this suggests that social isolation may have an impact on prognostication for patients with HF and thus should be assessed by clinicians at every visit.[47] Social connectedness promotes improved medication adherence and therefore improved outcomes in patients with HF in a prospective longitudinal study in this population.[48] Existing research related to cardiac disease and social support primarily evaluates current levels of social support and social isolation, and a 2010 systematic review of peer support intervention trials indicates a need for growing research in this domain to investigate how these interventions support the overall health and cardiac health for patients with known heart disease.[49]

Large-scale research studies implementing social connection interventions in patients with dementia are limited; current research available is primarily qualitative involving small-scale studies which highlight the health benefits of social connectedness in both people living with dementia and their caregivers. One study implemented a community-arts-based intervention involving patients and their caregivers attending art classes and participating in gallery tours at the Frye Art Museum in Seattle, Washington; follow-up telephone surveys with the individuals with dementia indicated a positive trend towards social connectedness through identifying themes of enjoyment, engagement, socialization and personhood.[50] A 2015 systematic review examining the impact of social support groups as an intervention in people living with dementia identified only two studies at the time which may provide psychological benefit through reducing depression and quality of life, though due to limited studies and heterogeneity of available studies, additional multicenter RCTs were recommended.[51]

Patients with COPD experience social isolation as stressors from their disease, embarrassment about symptoms and reduced mobility can disrupt their socialization and increase social isolation.[52] There is a paucity in the literature of high-quality RCTs focusing on a social connection intervention for patients with COPD. Available research indicates a positive association between the existing social network of patients with COPD and their disease severity, self-efficacy for walking, exercise tolerance and breathlessness.[53] A 2020 pilot parallel, single-blind, blocked RCT evaluated the implementation of an intervention called Generating Engagement in Network Support (GENIE) which focused on mapping an individual's current social support, eliciting values and preferences for activities and support resources and linking individuals to their prioritized activities and resources.[54] The intervention group had a noted 55% increase in social interactions and engagement as well as stable COPD symptom burden whereas the control group did not demonstrate any change in their social interactions and had an increased symptom burden related to COPD, though not statistically significant.[54] Another RCT found improved physical and psychological benefits with pulmonary rehabilitation referral for patients with regard to their lung disease, suggesting that referral to pulmonary rehabilitation may improve social connection by providing a larger support network.[53] Additional research in this population is needed with a focus on RCTs.

Avoidance of Risky Substances

Cigarette smoking leads to a variety of health problems, harming almost every organ in the body.[55] While avoiding smoking is important in preventing coronary heart disease, various cancers including lung and oral cancers and stroke, among other diseases, reducing or quitting tobacco use for those with serious illnesses can have a positive impact on QOL although can be difficult to accomplish.[55]

In patients with COPD, smoking cessation is indicated for slowing the progression of the disease, although no research to date exists to demonstrate the reversal of COPD through smoking cessation. Smoking cessation in the early stages of COPD has been associated with decreased all-cause mortality.[56] Patients with COPD who continue to smoke cigarettes experience a rapid decline in lung function and worsening symptoms of their disease.[56]

Smoking cessation in patients with cardiovascular disease has also demonstrated a decreased risk of all-cause mortality, a reduction in risk of death from cardiac causes and sudden death, and a reduction in the risk of new and recurrent cardiac events.[57] It is important to note that the benefit of smoking cessation is not realized immediately with regard to cardiovascular disease but has been demonstrated to be realized over the course of several years when compared with current smokers,[58] and as such, assisting patients to quit smoking early in their diagnosis is most helpful with regard to long-term cardiovascular risk reduction. Screening for smoking and assessing patients for readiness to quit is an important aspect of palliative care interventions for patients with serious illness but also should be considered in light of the patient's GOC and prognosis.

Avoiding alcohol is important for patients receiving palliative care, but it is also a method of primary prevention of serious illness, specifically cancers. The American Cancer Society (ACS) labels alcohol and tobacco as two of the most significant preventable cancer risk factors. Alcohol use accounts for about 6% of all cancers and 4% of all cancer deaths in the United States.[59] Clinicians can use SMART goals to help patients reduce alcohol intake by using individual approaches, patience and support. With the correct approach and follow-up, avoiding alcohol will decrease the risk of chronic disease and death. The 2020–2025 Dietary Guidelines for Americans recommends that adults of legal drinking age can choose not to drink, or to drink in moderation by limiting intake to two drinks or less in a day for men or one drink or less in a day for women, on days when alcohol is consumed.[60] Patients receiving palliative care can participate in counseling to reduce and avoid alcohol as their disease progresses. If a person is suffering from alcohol use disorder, proper referral to a specialist would be recommended due to the risk of adverse events from alcohol withdrawal such as seizures and death.

While pharmaceutical medications do not classically qualify as risky substances, it is important to note that for older adults who experience multimorbidity and use a large number of medications to treat chronic diseases, medications can impact QOL due to numerous adverse effects and drug–drug interactions. Older adults are at an increased risk of polypharmacy and cumulative adverse effects from medications, and it is often indicated for a palliative care provider to work in collaboration with a patient's medical team to consider deprescribing medications that may have bothersome side effects and impact QOL.

CONCLUSIONS

Early palliative care consultation and prescribing lifestyle medicine interventions for patients diagnosed with a progressive serious illness improve overall QOL and health. The additional social support and connection, symptom management and advance care planning, should be considered an integral part of their comprehensive treatment plan. The interdisciplinary palliative care team promotes physical and emotional well-being in addition to alleviating physical and emotional suffering.[61] Every pillar of lifestyle medicine is directly related to palliative care in every aspect to promote the best possible outcomes for seriously ill patients. Aligning palliative care with lifestyle medicine promotes both an individual and holistic care model and patient-centered care.

CLINICAL APPLICATIONS

- Consider referral to palliative care for patients with advanced or terminal disease to help establish individual goals of care to tailor lifestyle medicine interventions.
- While lifestyle interventions can be applied throughout the course of illness for most patients, consideration of a patient's goals and medical frailty is essential when providing recommendations and lifestyle medicine prescriptions.

REFERENCES

1. About Palliative Care. CAPC. Accessed December 7, 2023. https://www.capc.org/about/palliative-care/
2. Sepúlveda C, Marlin A, Yoshida T, Ullrich A. Palliative care: the world health organization's global perspective. *J Pain Symptom Manage*. 2002;24(2):91–96.
3. Palliative care. Accessed January 7, 2024. https://www.who.int/news-room/fact-sheets/detail/palliative-care
4. Palliative Care, Report Card. Published August 18, 2015. Accessed January 7, 2024. https://reportcard.capc.org/
5. Vossel H. CAPC rolls out database on public palliative care policy. *Hospice News*. Published September 15, 2021. Accessed January 7, 2024. https://hospicenews.com/2021/09/15/capc-rolls-out-database-on-public-palliative-care-policy/
6. Advance Care Planning: Advance Directives for Health Care h. National Institute on Aging. Accessed January 7, 2024. tps://www.nia.nih.gov/health/advance-care-planning/advance-care-planning-advance-directives-health-care
7. Brinkman-Stoppelenburg A, Rietjens JAC, van der Heide A. The effects of advance care planning on end-of-life care: a systematic review. *Palliat Med*. 2014;28(8):1000–1025.
8. What is dementia? Alzheimer's Association. Accessed December 7, 2023. https://www.alz.org/alzheimers-dementia/what-is-dementia?utm_source=google&utm_medium=paidsearch&utm_campaign=google_grants&utm_content=dementia&gad_source=1&gclid=Cj0KCQiAm4WsBhCiARIsAEJIEzXCqPzsTiFA04DIyXYrSr9Fn1MZKU9JOMmjtTx5vqa-UL6pTc21Gq8aAvq8EALw_wcB
9. About dementia. Published July 13, 2023. Accessed January 11, 2024. https://www.cdc.gov/aging/alzheimers-disease-dementia/about-dementia.html
10. About Alzheimer's disease. Published July 13, 2023. Accessed January 11, 2024. https://www.cdc.gov/aging/alzheimers-disease-dementia/about-alzheimers.html

11. Jagust W. Imaging the evolution and pathophysiology of Alzheimer disease. *Nat Rev Neurosci.* 2018;19(11):687–700.
12. Arora S, Santiago JA, Bernstein M. Diet and lifestyle impact the development and progression of Alzheimer's dementia. *Frontiers in.* Published online 2023. https://www.ncbi.nlm.nih.gov/pmc/articles/PMC10344607/
13. Choi EY, Allen K, McDonnough M, Massera D, Ostfeld RJ. A plant-based diet and heart failure: case report and literature review. *J Geriatr Cardiol.* 2017;14(5):375.
14. von Schwarz ER, He M, Bharadwaj P. Palliative care issues for patients with heart failure. *JAMA Netw Open.* 2020;3(2):e200011.
15. Diop MS, Rudolph JL, Zimmerman KM, Richter MA, Skarf LM. Palliative care interventions for patients with heart failure: a systematic review and meta-analysis. *J Palliat Med.* 2017;20(1):84–92.
16. Halpin DMG. Palliative care for people with COPD: effective but underused. *Eur Respir J.* 2018;51(2). doi:10.1183/13993003.02645-2017
17. Anandarajah G, Mennillo HA, Rachu G, Harder T, Ghosh J. Lifestyle medicine interventions in patients with advanced disease receiving palliative or hospice care. *Am J Lifestyle Med.* 2020;14(3):243–257.
18. Salehin S, Rasmussen P, Mai S, et al. Plant based diet and its effect on cardiovascular disease. *Int J Environ Res Public Health.* 2023;20(4). doi:10.3390/ijerph20043337
19. The American Heart Association diet and lifestyle recommendations. www.heart.org. Accessed December 19, 2023. https://www.heart.org/en/healthy-living/healthy-eating/eat-smart/nutrition-basics/aha-diet-and-lifestyle-recommendations
20. Karam G, Agarwal A, Sadeghirad B, et al. Comparison of seven popular structured dietary programmes and risk of mortality and major cardiovascular events in patients at increased cardiovascular risk: systematic review and network meta-analysis. *BMJ.* 2023;380:e072003.
21. Varraso R, Dumas O, Tabung FK, et al. Healthful and unhealthful plant-based diets and chronic obstructive pulmonary disease in U.S. adults: prospective study. *Nutrients.* 2023;15(3). doi:10.3390/nu15030765
22. Keranis E, Makris D, Rodopoulou P, et al. Impact of dietary shift to higher-antioxidant foods in COPD: a randomised trial. *Eur Respir J.* 2010;36(4):774–780.
23. González-Domínguez R, Castellano-Escuder P, Carmona F, et al. Food and microbiota metabolites associate with cognitive decline in older subjects: a 12-year prospective study. *Mol Nutr Food Res.* 2021;65(23):e2100606.
24. Myrcik D, Statowski W, Trzepizur M, Paladini A, Corli O, Varrassi G. Influence of physical activity on pain, depression and quality of life of patients in palliative care: a proof-of-concept study. *J Clin Med Res.* 2021;10(5). doi:10.3390/jcm10051012
25. Anderson L, Oldridge N, Thompson DR, et al. Exercise-based cardiac rehabilitation for coronary heart disease: cochrane systematic review and meta-analysis. *J Am Coll Cardiol.* 2016;67(1):1–12.
26. Ester M, Culos-Reed SN, Abdul-Razzak A, et al. Feasibility of a multimodal exercise, nutrition, and palliative care intervention in advanced lung cancer. *BMC Cancer.* 2021;21(1):159.
27. Anderson F, Downing GM, Hill J, Casorso L, Lerch N. Palliative performance scale (PPS): a new tool. *J Palliat Care.* 1996;12(1):5–11.
28. Nasr A. Palliative performance scale as a prognostic tool for pool for patients with dementia in hospice. Published online 2021.
29. Davies A. Sleep problems in advanced disease. *Clin Med.* 2019;19(4):302–305.
30. Molano J, Vaughn BV. Approach to insomnia in patients with dementia. *Neurol Clin Pract.* 2014;4(1):7–15.

31. Sands SA, Owens RL. Congestive heart failure and central sleep apnea. *Crit Care Clin.* 2015;31(3):473–495.
32. Sharma B, Owens R, Malhotra A. Sleep in congestive heart failure. *Med Clin North Am.* 2010;94(3):447–464.
33. McCurry SM, Pike KC, Vitiello MV, Logsdon RG, Larson EB, Teri L. Increasing walking and bright light exposure to improve sleep in community-dwelling persons with Alzheimer's disease: results of a randomized, controlled trial. *J Am Geriatr Soc.* 2011;59(8):1393–1402.
34. de Jonghe A, Korevaar JC, van Munster BC, de Rooij SE. Effectiveness of melatonin treatment on circadian rhythm disturbances in dementia. Are there implications for delirium? A systematic review. *Int J Geriatr Psychiatry.* 2010;25(12):1201–1208.
35. Blumenthal JA, Sherwood A, Smith PJ, et al. Enhancing cardiac rehabilitation with stress management training: a randomized, clinical efficacy trial. *Circulation.* 2016;133(14):1341–1350.
36. Luskin F, Reitz M, Newell K, Quinn TG, Haskell W. A controlled pilot study of stress management training of elderly patients with congestive heart failure. *Prev Cardiol.* 2002;5(4):168–172.
37. Blumenthal JA, Sherwood A, Babyak MA, et al. Effects of exercise and stress management training on markers of cardiovascular risk in patients with ischemic heart disease: a randomized controlled trial. *JAMA.* 2005;293(13):1626–1634.
38. Ornish D, Brown SE, Scherwitz LW, et al. Can lifestyle changes reverse coronary heart disease? The lifestyle heart trial. *Lancet.* 1990;336(8708):129–133.
39. Ornish D, Scherwitz LW, Billings JH, et al. Intensive lifestyle changes for reversal of coronary heart disease. *JAMA.* 1998;280(23):2001–2007.
40. Volpato E, Farver-Vestergaard I, Brighton LJ, et al. Nonpharmacological management of psychological distress in people with COPD. *Eur Respir Rev.* 2023;32(167). doi:10.1183/16000617.0170-2022
41. Fillit H, Aigbogun MS, Gagnon-Sanschagrin P, et al. Impact of agitation in long-term care residents with dementia in the United States. *Int J Geriatr Psychiatry.* 2021;36(12):1959–1969.
42. National Academies of Sciences, Engineering, and Medicine; Division of Behavioral and Social Sciences and Education; Health and Medicine Division; Board on Behavioral, Cognitive, and Sensory Sciences; Board on Health Sciences Policy; Committee on the Health and Medical Dimensions of Social Isolation and Loneliness in Older Adults. *Social Isolation and Loneliness in Older Adults: Opportunities for the Health Care System.* National Academies Press; 2020.
43. Social isolation and loneliness increase the risk of death from heart attack, stroke. American Heart Association. Accessed April 5, 2024. https://newsroom.heart.org/news/social-isolation-and-loneliness-increase-the-risk-of-death-from-heart-attack-stroke
44. Parent N, Fortin F. A randomized, controlled trial of vicarious experience through peer support for male first-time cardiac surgery patients: impact on anxiety, self-efficacy expectation, and self-reported activity. *Heart Lung.* 2000;29(6):389–400.
45. Berkman LF, Blumenthal J, Burg M, et al. Effects of treating depression and low perceived social support on clinical events after myocardial infarction: the Enhancing Recovery in Coronary Heart Disease Patients (ENRICHD) Randomized Trial. *JAMA.* 2003;289(23):3106–3116.
46. Goodlin SJ, Gottlieb SH. Social isolation and loneliness in heart failure: integrating social care into cardiac care. *JACC Heart Fail.* 2023;11(3):345–346.

47. Manemann SM, Chamberlain AM, Roger VL, et al. Perceived social isolation and outcomes in patients with heart failure. *J Am Heart Assoc.* 2018;7(11). doi:10.1161/JAHA.117.008069
48. Wu JR, Frazier SK, Rayens MK, Lennie TA, Chung ML, Moser DK. Medication adherence, social support, and event-free survival in patients with heart failure. *Health Psychol.* 2013;32(6):637–646.
49. Parry M, Watt-Watson J. Peer support intervention trials for individuals with heart disease: a systematic review. *Eur J Cardiovasc Nurs.* 2010;9(1):57–67.
50. Burnside LD, Knecht MJ, Hopley EK, Logsdon RG. here:now - Conceptual model of the impact of an experiential arts program on persons with dementia and their care partners. *Dementia.* 2017;16(1):29–45.
51. Leung P, Orrell M, Orgeta V. Social support group interventions in people with dementia and mild cognitive impairment: a systematic review of the literature. *Int J Geriatr Psychiatry.* 2015;30(1):1–9.
52. Lenferink A, van der Palen J, Effing T. The role of social support in improving chronic obstructive pulmonary disease self-management. *Expert Rev Respir Med.* Published online 2018. https://www.tandfonline.com/doi/full/10.1080/17476348.2018.1489723
53. Grodner S, Prewitt LM, Jaworsk BA, Myers R, Kaplan RM, Ries AL. The impact of social support in pulmonary rehabilitation of patients with chronic obstructive pulmonary disease. *Ann Behav Med.* 1996;18(3):139–145.
54. Welch L, Orlando R, Lin SX, Vassilev I, Rogers A. Findings from a pilot randomised trial of a social network self-management intervention in COPD. *BMC Pulm Med.* 2020;20(1):162.
55. CDCTobaccoFree. Health effects. Centers for Disease Control and Prevention. Published July 21, 2022. Accessed January 7, 2024. https://www.cdc.gov/tobacco/basic_information/health_effects/index.htm
56. Doo JH, Kim SM, Park YJ, et al. Smoking cessation after diagnosis of COPD is associated with lower all-cause and cause-specific mortality: a nationwide population-based cohort study of South Korean men. *BMC Pulm Med.* 2023;23(1):237.
57. CDCTobaccoFree. *Cardiovascular Care Settings and Smoking Cessation.* Centers for Disease Control and Prevention. Published October 26, 2022. Accessed January 7, 2024. https://www.cdc.gov/tobacco/patient-care/care-settings/cardiovascular/index.htm
58. Okorare O, Evbayekha EO, Adabale OK, et al. Smoking cessation and benefits to cardiovascular health: a review of literature. *Cureus.* 2023;15(3):e35966.
59. Alcohol use and cancer. Accessed January 7, 2024. https://www.cancer.org/cancer/risk-prevention/diet-physical-activity/alcohol-use-and-cancer.html
60. Facts about moderate drinking. Published July 25, 2022. Accessed January 7, 2024. https://www.cdc.gov/alcohol/fact-sheets/moderate-drinking.htm
61. Duncan AJ, Holkup LM, Sang HI, Sahr SM. Benefits of early utilization of palliative care consultation in trauma patients. *Crit Care Explor.* 2023;5(9):e0963.

21 Polypharmacy and Deprescribing

Fatoumata Jallow, Patti A. Parker and Kathryn M. Daniel

POLYPHARMACY AND DEPRESCRIBING IN OLDER ADULTS FROM A LIFESTYLE MEDICINE PERSPECTIVE

Polypharmacy in older adults is the concurrent use of five or more prescribed medications daily.[1] Taking multiple medications can lead to significant negative effects on both the patient's health and the overall cost of health care. Aging increases the risk of chronic conditions leading to polypharmacy. As people age and take more medications, their risk of hospitalization due to adverse drug events (ADEs) increases.[2] Adverse drug events account for over 700,000 hospital visits annually in the United States.[3] The percentage of adults with polypharmacy in the United States has increased from 8.2% to 17.1% in recent years.[4] Polypharmacy was significantly more common in older adults, those with heart disease and individuals with diabetes. Men, Mexican Americans and non-Hispanic Blacks showed a more significant increase in polypharmacy than in other race groups.[4]

As the prevalence increases, the adverse effects of polypharmacy increase such as falls, fractures, frailty and increased mortality.[5] The Health, Aging, and Body Composition study investigated the relationship between persistent polypharmacy and the risk of treated fall injury in 1,764 older adults.[6] The researchers found that the combination of persistent polypharmacy and the use of Fall Risk-Increasing Drugs (FRIDs) is linked with a nearly 50% higher risk of treated fall injury in older adults.[6] FRIDs in this study were antiepileptic drugs, hypnotics/sedatives drugs, antipsychotics, antidepressants, benzodiazepines and opioids.[6] Consequences of the use of FRIDs such as falls often lead to a cascade of events and eventually an increase in prescribed medication.[7] Some of the effects of polypharmacy such as falls, and confusion have been mistaken for symptoms of chronic illness or simply deemed a normal part of aging leading to a prescribing cascade, with more drugs being prescribed.[8] Therefore, the prevalence of polypharmacy may be underreported.

There have been several measures put in place to mitigate the risks associated with polypharmacy. The two most widely used tools to detect Potentially Inappropriate Medications (PIMs) in older adults are the American Geriatric Society (AGS) Beers Criteria[9] and the Screening Tool of Older Persons' Prescriptions (STOPP).[10] In spite of the existence of these tools, adverse effects related to polypharmacy continue to rise. Research overwhelmingly shows that older adults are at a higher risk of hospitalization due to adverse effects when they take multiple medications daily.[5] As a result, health care providers must continuously evaluate older adults for PIMs. Providers can use deprescribing to reduce inappropriate medication doses for older adults. This process involves either reducing dosages or stopping certain medications altogether. Deprescribing could result in fewer medications being consumed, reduced side effects and improve health outcomes if done periodically.[11] The challenges of polypharmacy, including drug interactions, side effects and complexities of medication regimen, could undermine medication adherence.

LIFESTYLE PILLARS CONTRIBUTION TO OPPORTUNITIES FOR DEPRESCRIBING AND REDUCING POLYPHARMACY

According to the American College of Preventive Medicine (ACPM), lifestyle medicine (LM) is a medical specialty that uses behavioral interventions to prevent and treat chronic conditions such as diabetes, hypertension and obesity.[12] Clinicians certified in lifestyle medicine use evidence-based research to effectively coach patients on the six pillars of healthy living, resulting in improved health outcomes through intensive intervention. The six pillars of LM are:

1. Physical activity
2. Whole food plant-based nutrition
3. Restorative sleep
4. Stress management
5. Positive social connections
6. Avoidance of risky substances[12]

These lifestyle pillars when applied can help in the prevention, treatment and reversal of chronic illnesses such as cardiovascular disease, diabetes and chronic respiratory illness which account for more than 80% of non-communicable deaths worldwide.[13] In a randomized controlled trial conducted on 48 patients with coronary artery disease, researchers examined the impact of intensive lifestyle changes on their health.[14] The participants were advised to adopt a plant-based diet, enroll in a stress management program, quit smoking and follow aerobic exercise recommendations. After 5 years, the group practicing intensive lifestyle changes experienced less coronary atherosclerosis.[14] In contrast, the control group experienced more progression of coronary atherosclerosis and cardiac events. This suggests adopting healthy lifestyles could reduce chronic illnesses and the need for multiple medications.

PHYSICAL ACTIVITY

Physical activity in older adults is an essential aspect of a healthy lifestyle that offers numerous health benefits, including the prevention of cardiovascular diseases.

Engaging in moderate-intensity aerobic physical activity at least 150 minutes per week can improve overall cardiovascular health.[15] Researchers found that adults who engage in the recommended guidelines of aerobic and muscle-strengthening activities significantly reduce the risk of all-cause mortality.[16] Regular physical activity can effectively control blood glucose levels. Exercise boosts insulin sensitivity, which enables the body to regulate blood sugar levels more effectively, thus reducing the risk of acquiring type 2 diabetes. Resistance training, a more tolerable modality for older adults than intense training, at moderate intensity can improve HbA1c levels in older adults with type 2 diabetes.[17] Furthermore, regular physical activity can help manage weight and prevent obesity, a major factor in chronic diseases such as heart disease, diabetes and some cancers.

Walking, running and weightlifting can preserve bone density, reduce the risk of osteoporosis and strengthen the skeleton.[18] Maintaining healthy bones becomes especially important as we age, as it helps counteract the natural decline in bone density and decreases the likelihood of fractures. Older adults who exercise regularly have greater endurance, improved functional skills and perform daily activities with less difficulty.[19] Physical activity can reduce stress, depression and promote well-being in older adults.[20] Physical inactivity can lead to chronic health issues and contribute to the frailty syndrome.[21] Reduced mobility and muscle strength are criteria for frailty identification models.[21] Older adults should continue to engage in physical activity to prevent the progression of frailty and promote healthy aging.

WHOLE-FOOD PLANT-BASED NUTRITION

Researchers substantiate the efficacy of adopting a holistic dietary approach, primarily centered around plant-based whole foods, as a crucial intervention in mitigating, managing and reversing chronic conditions. To achieve optimal nutrition, one should incorporate a variety of minimally processed vegetables, fruits, whole grains, legumes, nuts and seeds, rich in dietary fiber, antioxidants and essential nutrients.[12] Millions of Americans are currently affected by type 2 diabetes, primarily caused by insulin resistance.[22] Consequently, individuals with this chronic condition often require multiple medications as part of their treatment regimen. It is important to note that obesity and an unhealthy diet are significant factors contributing to insulin resistance. According to a study, patients diagnosed with cardiovascular disease (CVD) who followed a plant-based diet for an average of 3.7 years had significantly lower chances of experiencing further cardiac events.[23] These findings suggest that plant-based nutrition can be a powerful tool in reducing the widespread prevalence of CVD. Consuming more than four servings of ultra-processed foods per day is independently associated with a 62% higher risk of all-cause mortality.[24] Using a Food Frequency Questionnaire (FFQ), researchers found that with each additional serving of ultra-processed food, there is an 18% increase in the risk of all-cause mortality.[24] In a recent study, a plant-based diet was linked to a 58% reduction in polypharmacy in older adults.[25] Therefore, it is desirable to limit the daily consumption of ultra-processed foods to reduce chronic conditions and the risk of all-cause mortality.[26]

Restorative Sleep

Getting enough sleep is crucial for our overall well-being. Lack of sleep can have many adverse effects on our health, such as reduced attention span, depressed mood, poor metabolism, insulin resistance and impaired performance. Therefore, it is recommended that we aim for a minimum of 7 hours of sleep per night to ensure optimal health.[27] Not getting enough sleep, or having too much and irregular sleep patterns can raise the risk of developing cardiovascular disease.[28,29] So, it is important to maintain a regular sleep pattern to improve overall health.

Sleep disorders can have detrimental effects on bone health. Research has shown that individuals with lower bone mineral density are at a higher risk of osteoporosis and fractures.[30] Sleep deprivation can disrupt the hormonal balance in the body, leading to increased inflammation and oxidative stress, both of which can contribute to bone loss and impaired bone healing.[31] Chronic sleep deprivation can also impair the body's ability to regulate insulin and glucose levels, negatively impacting bone health.[31] Additionally, a descriptive, cross-sectional study investigated the relationship between sleep quality, inappropriate medication use and frailty.[32] The researchers found that taking Potentially Inappropriate Medications (PIMs) was linked to lower subjective sleep efficiency.[32] Sleep efficiency is the measure of actual sleep time to the total time spent in bed.[32] The participants who took more PIMs had less efficient sleep. The average number of Potentially Inappropriate Prescriptions (PIPs) was also associated with poor sleep quality among older adults.[32] Chronic sleep deprivation has also been linked to an increased risk of Alzheimer's disease (AD) in later years.[33] During sleep, the brain eliminates toxic proteins such as beta-amyloid, which can accumulate and cause damage over time. Sufficient and high-quality sleep can help reduce the likelihood of developing AD and potentially eliminate the need for medications.

Stress Management

The body responds to stressful situations by producing stress hormones. In moderate amounts, stress motivates us to do our best and helps us accomplish complex tasks. However, excessive or chronic stress can harm our physical and mental well-being. Stress can negatively impact health, including damage to the hippocampus – a critical brain area that plays a crucial role in learning and memory. The hippocampus is sensitive to stress hormones such as cortisol, which is released during chronic stress. High cortisol levels can shrink the hippocampus and impair its functioning, which is critical for older adults.[34] Brain structural changes increase the risk of cognitive impairment, depression, anxiety and Alzheimer's disease (AD) in older adults.[35]

Adopting healthy lifestyle habits, such as getting enough sleep, eating a balanced diet and practicing time management, can also contribute to stress management and protect the hippocampus from long-term damage. For instance, yoga training may prevent cognitive decline.[36] Studies suggest that yoga training is more neuroprotective than memory enhancement training, even over short periods.[36]

Positive Social Connections

Loneliness and lack of social connection are significant concerns among older adults, as they can have detrimental effects on overall health and well-being. Researchers have also focused on the impact of social ties on health outcomes. Study findings show that individuals with cardiovascular disease who experience social isolation have a higher mortality risk than those with robust social ties.[37] Social isolation and loneliness have been linked to unhealthy behaviors such as smoking, poor diet and physical inactivity, all of which contribute significantly to the development of cardiovascular disease.[38] Other researchers have also found a significant association between social connection and cancer outcomes. For instance, women with breast cancer who have stronger social ties have a lower risk of death.[39] In another study, middle-aged men with low social connections have been found to have a higher risk of developing cancer.[40] Being single was also found to be associated with worse cancer outcomes.[40] Strong social ties can influence cancer outcomes through various pathways, including the modulation of immune response, promotion of health-promoting behaviors and buffering against the adverse effects of stress.[41]

The association between polypharmacy and psychosocial factors has gained attention recently. Among older adults, the occurrence of loneliness and social isolation has been found to be associated with polypharmacy.[42] Participants with polypharmacy were more likely to experience social isolation than those without polypharmacy.[42] The relationship between social isolation and polypharmacy may be due to various factors. For instance, side effects associated with the use of FRIDs can prohibit individuals from participating in social activities. Additionally, medication side effects may cause physical discomfort and decreased mobility, which can further limit opportunities for social interaction. The complexity of managing multiple medications can be overwhelming for older adults, also leading to decreased engagement in social activities and reduced social interactions. In a survey of community-dwelling older adults who self-administered daily medications, while occasional use of opioids, benzodiazepines or non-opioid analgesics was not linked to loneliness, polypharmacy was associated with loneliness.[43] Though polypharmacy can lead to decreased socialization, the reverse is also true. Loneliness was found to be a strong predictor of the use of medications used to treat psychosomatic symptoms among older adults in a nationally representative cohort.[44] Additionally, loneliness was significantly associated with pain, insomnia, depression, anxiety and multimorbidity.[44] When depression or anxiety leads to feelings of loneliness, it can worsen these psychological symptoms and trigger a prescription cascade.

Avoidance of Risky Substances

According to a Substance Abuse and Mental Health Services Administration (SAMHSA) report, substance use disorder affects almost 1 million adults aged 65 and above.[45] Substance use among older adults can be harmful to their health and well-being, leading to memory impairment, increased risk of falls and depression. Some common substances older adults misuse are alcohol, cannabis, benzodiazepines and cocaine.[46] Aging can increase sensitivity to alcohol and drugs due to changes in the central nervous system. The blood–brain barrier becomes more permeable, and neuronal receptor sensitivity is heightened, making older adults more susceptible to the effects of alcohol and other substances.[46] Consequences of substance abuse, such as cognitive impairment and depression, can further complicate an individual's medication regimen, as antidepressant medications may need to be added to their existing medication regimen. This increase in the number of medications can compound the challenges of polypharmacy, potentially leading to drug interactions, side effects and difficulties with medication adherence.

CLINICAL APPLICATIONS

- Clinicians should stress the importance of avoiding risky substances among older adults, as this could interfere with medication management.
- Emphasizing exercise can improve overall health, reduce the risk of chronic diseases and decrease the need for medications.
- Encouraging a plant-based diet can reduce the need for multiple medications.
- Limiting the consumption of ultra-processed foods can lower the risk of chronic diseases, mortality and medication burden.

REFERENCES

1. World Health Organization (WHO). *Medication Safety in Polypharmacy*. WHO; 2019. (WHO/UHC/SDS/2019.11). Licence: CC BY-NC-SA 3.0 IGO.
2. Nymoen LD, Björk M, Flatebø TE, et al. Drug-related emergency department visits: prevalence and risk factors. *Intern Emerg Med*. 2022 Aug;17(5):1453–1462. doi: 10.1007/s11739-022-02935-9.
3. Shehab N, Lovegrove MC, Geller AI, Rose KO, Weidle NJ, Budnitz DS. US emergency department visits for outpatient adverse drug events, 2013–2014. *JAMA*. 2016 Nov 22;316(20):2115–2125. doi: 10.1001/jama.2016.16201.
4. Wang X, Liu K, Shirai K, et al. Prevalence and trends of polypharmacy in U.S. adults, 1999–2018. *Glob Health Res Policy*. 2023 Jul 12;8(1):25. doi: 10.1186/s41256-023-00311-4.
5. Li Y, Zhang X, Yang L, et al. Association between polypharmacy and mortality in older adults: a systematic review and meta-analysis. *Arch Gerontol Geriatr*. 2022;100:104630. doi: 10.1016/j.archger.2022.104630.
6. Xue L, Boudreau RM, Donohue JM, et al. Persistent polypharmacy and fall injury risk: the Health, Aging and Body Composition Study. *BMC Geriatr*. 2021 Dec 15;21(1):710. doi: 10.1186/s12877-021-02695-9.
7. Dagli RJ, Sharma A. Polypharmacy: a global risk factor for elderly people. *J Int Oral Health*. 2014;6(6):i-ii.
8. Varghese D, Ishida C, Haseer Koya H. *Polypharmacy*. StatPearls; 2023.
9. American Geriatrics Society (AGS) Beers Criteria® Panel. American Geriatrics Society 2023 updated AGS Beers Criteria® for potentially inappropriate medication use in older adults. *J Am Geriatr Soc*. 2023;71(7):2052–2081. doi: 10.1111/jgs.18372.

10. Gallagher P, Ryan C, Byrne S, Kennedy J, O'Mahony D. STOPP (Screening Tool of Older Person's Prescriptions) and START (Screening Tool to Alert doctors to Right Treatment). Consensus validation. *Int J Clin Pharmacol Ther.* 2008 Feb;46(2):72–83. doi: 10.5414/cpp46072.
11. Elbeddini A, Sawhney M, Tayefehchamani Y, et al. Deprescribing for all: a narrative review identifying inappropriate polypharmacy for all ages in hospital settings. *BMJ Open Qual.* 2021 Jul;10(3):e001509. doi: 10.1136/bmjoq-2021-001509.
12. American College of Lifestyle Medicine (ACLM). Definition of Lifestyle Medicine. Accessed October 2, 2023. https://lifestylemedicine.org/overview/.
13. World Health Organization (WHO). Noncommunicable diseases. https://www.who.int/news-room/fact-sheets/detail/noncommunicable-diseases.
14. Ornish D, Scherwitz LW, Billings JH, et al. Intensive lifestyle changes for reversal of coronary heart disease. *JAMA.* 1998 Dec 16;280(23):2001–2007. doi: 10.1001/jama.280.23.2001.
15. American Heart Association (AHA). American Heart Association Recommendations for Physical Activity in Adults and Kids. https://www.heart.org/en/healthy-living/fitness/fitness-basics/aha-recs-for-physical-activity-in-adults.
16. Zhao M, Veeranki SP, Magnussen CG, Xi B. Recommended physical activity and all-cause and cause-specific mortality in US adults: prospective cohort study. *BMJ.* 2020 Jul 1;370:m2031. doi: 10.1136/bmj.m2031.
17. Jiahao L, Jiajin L, Yifan L. Effects of resistance training on insulin sensitivity in the elderly: a meta-analysis of randomized controlled trials. *J Exerc Sci Fit.* 2021 Oct;19(4):241–251. doi: 10.1016/j.jesf.2021.08.002.
18. Centers for Disease Control and Prevention (CDC). Benefits of Physical Activity. 2023.
19. Parra-Rizo MA, Sanchis-Soler G. Satisfaction with life, subjective well-being, and functional skills in active older adults based on their level of physical activity practice. *Int J Environ Res Public Health.* 2020 Feb 18;17(4). doi: 10.3390/ijerph17041299.
20. Callow DD, Arnold-Nedimala NA, Jordan LS, et al. The mental health benefits of physical activity in older adults survive the COVID-19 pandemic. *Am J Geriatr Psychiatry.* 2020 Oct;28(10):1046–1057. doi: 10.1016/j.jagp.2020.06.024.
21. Woolford SJ, Sohan O, Dennison EM, Cooper C, Patel HP. Approaches to the diagnosis and prevention of frailty. *Aging Clin Exp Res.* 2020 Sep;32(9):1629–1637. doi: 10.1007/s40520-020-01559-3.
22. Centers for Disease Control and Prevention (CDC). Type 2 diabetes. https://www.cdc.gov/diabetes/basics/type2.html#:~:text=More%20than%2037%20million%20Americans,adults%20are%20also%20developing%20it.
23. Esselstyn CB, Gendy G, Doyle J, Golubic M, Roizen MF. A way to reverse CAD? *J Fam Pract.* 2014 Jul;63(7):356–364b.
24. Rico-Campà A, Martínez-González MA, Alvarez-Alvarez I, et al. Association between consumption of ultra-processed foods and all-cause mortality: SUN prospective cohort study. *BMJ.* 2019 May 29;365:l1949. doi: 10.1136/bmj.l1949.
25. Dos Santos H, Gaio J, Durisic A, Beeson WL, Alabadi A. The polypharma study: association between diet and amount of prescription drugs among seniors. *Am J Lifestyle Med.* 2021:15598276211048812. doi: 10.1177/15598276211048812.
26. Shan Z, Wang F, Li Y, et al. Healthy eating patterns and risk of total and cause-specific mortality. *JAMA Intern Med.* 2023 Feb 1;183(2):142–153. doi: 10.1001/jamainternmed.2022.6117.
27. National Institutes of Health (NIH). How much sleep is enough? https://www.nhlbi.nih.gov/health/sleep/how-much-sleep#:~:text=Experts%20recommend%20that%20adults%20sleep,or%20more%20hours%20a%20night.
28. Wang Z, Yang W, Li X, Qi X, Pan KY, Xu W. Association of sleep duration, napping, and sleep patterns with risk of cardiovascular diseases: a nationwide twin study. *J Am Heart Assoc.* 2022 Aug 2;11(15):e025969. doi: 10.1161/JAHA.122.025969.

29. Wang L, Wang K, Liu LJ, et al. Associations of daytime napping with incident cardiovascular diseases and hypertension in Chinese adults: a nationwide cohort study. *Biomed Environ Sci.* 2022 Jan 20;35(1):22–34. doi: 10.3967/bes2022.004.
30. Specker BL, Binkley T, Vukovich M, Beare T. Volumetric bone mineral density and bone size in sleep-deprived individuals. *Osteoporos Int.* 2007 Jan;18(1):93–99. doi: 10.1007/s00198-006-0207-x.
31. Singh T, Ahmed TH, Mohamed N, et al. Does insufficient sleep increase the risk of developing insulin resistance: a systematic review. *Cureus.* 2022 Mar;14(3):e23501. doi: 10.7759/cureus.23501.
32. Kumar S, Wong PS, Hasan SS, Kairuz T. The relationship between sleep quality, inappropriate medication use, and frailty among older adults in aged care homes in Malaysia. *PLoS One.* 2019;14(10):e0224122. doi: 10.1371/journal.pone.0224122.
33. Spira AP, Gamaldo AA, An Y, et al. Self-reported sleep and β-amyloid deposition in community-dwelling older adults. *JAMA Neurol.* 2013 Dec;70(12):1537–1543. doi: 10.1001/jamaneurol.2013.4258.
34. Dronse J, Ohndorf A, Richter N, et al. Serum cortisol is negatively related to hippocampal volume, brain structure, and memory performance in healthy aging and Alzheimer's disease. *Front Aging Neurosci.* 2023;15:1154112. doi: 10.3389/fnagi.2023.1154112.
35. Touron E, Moulinet I, Kuhn E, et al. Depressive symptoms in cognitively unimpaired older adults are associated with lower structural and functional integrity in a frontolimbic network. *Mol Psychiatry.* 2022 Dec;27(12):5086–5095. doi: 10.1038/s41380-022-01772-8.
36. Krause-Sorio B, Siddarth P, Kilpatrick L, et al. Yoga prevents gray matter atrophy in women at risk for Alzheimer's disease: a randomized controlled trial. *J Alzheimers Dis.* 2022;87(2):569–581. doi: 10.3233/JAD-215563.
37. Yu B, Steptoe A, Chen LJ, Chen YH, Lin CH, Ku PW. Social isolation, loneliness, and all-cause mortality in patients with cardiovascular disease: a 10-year follow-up study. *Psychosom Med.* 2020;82(2):208–214. doi: 10.1097/PSY.0000000000000777.
38. Kobayashi LC, Steptoe A. Social isolation, loneliness, and health behaviors at older ages: longitudinal cohort study. *Ann Behav Med.* 2018 May 31;52(7):582–593. doi: 10.1093/abm/kax033.
39. Kroenke CH, Michael YL, Poole EM, et al. Postdiagnosis social networks and breast cancer mortality in the After Breast Cancer Pooling Project. *Cancer.* 2017 Apr 1;123(7):1228–1237. doi: 10.1002/cncr.30440.
40. Kraav SL, Lehto SM, Kauhanen J, Hantunen S, Tolmunen T. Loneliness and social isolation increase cancer incidence in a cohort of Finnish middle-aged men: a longitudinal study. *Psychiatry Res.* 2021 May;299:113868. doi: 10.1016/j.psychres.2021.113868.
41. Roy V, Ruel S, Ivers H, et al. Stress-buffering effect of social support on immunity and infectious risk during chemotherapy for breast cancer. *Brain Behav Immun Health.* 2021 Jan;10:100186. doi: 10.1016/j.bbih.2020.100186.
42. Svensson M, Ekström H, Elmståhl S, Rosso A. Association of polypharmacy with occurrence of loneliness and social isolation among older adults. *Arch Gerontol Geriatr.* 2023 Aug 14;116:105158. doi: 10.1016/j.archger.2023.105158.
43. Vyas MV, Watt JA, Yu AYX, Straus SE, Kapral MK. The association between loneliness and medication use in older adults. *Age Ageing.* 2021 Feb 26;50(2):587–591. doi: 10.1093/ageing/afaa177.
44. Kotwal AA, Steinman MA, Cenzer I, Smith AK. Use of high-risk medications among lonely older adults: results from a nationally representative sample. *JAMA Intern Med.* 2021 Nov 1;181(11):1528–1530. doi: 10.1001/jamainternmed.2021.3775.
45. Substance Abuse and Mental Health Services Administration (SAMHSA). *Results from the 2018 National Survey on Drug Use and Health: Detailed Tables.* Center for Behavioral Health Statistics and Quality, SAMHSA. https://www.samhsa.gov/data/.
46. Coggins M. Substance use disorder in older adults. *Today's Geriatric Medicine.* 2023;18.

22 Caregiver Health

Paul Mulhausen

INTRODUCTION

Every day, millions of informal caregivers place their own health and well-being at risk to support the health and well-being of older adults who depend on them to improve and maintain their quality of life. These caregivers reflect the rich diversity of our society and may be a relative, spouse, partner, friend or neighbor who supports the broad range of needs to the care recipient, typically assisting with activities of daily living or instrumental activities of daily living, and providing emotional support for someone who can no longer care for himself or herself due to illness, injury or disability. Family members are the primary source of support for older adults with chronic illness and disability, playing an essential role in the health care and care management of the community-dwelling, frail elderly. While informal caregiving can be rewarding and personally satisfying, it often comes at a personal cost, with caregivers experiencing higher rates of depression, anxiety and other chronic health conditions.[1] Lifestyle medicine, with its focus on the fundamental pillars of nutrition, physical activity, stress management, sleep optimization and social connections, offers a comprehensive and sustainable approach to improve the overall health of caregivers, reduce their caregiving-related stress and enhance the quality of their life.

EPIDEMIOLOGY

The 2020 survey performed by AARP and the National Alliance for Caregiving reports that about 53 million people in the United States provide informal, and usually unpaid, care and support to older adults and disabled people of all ages.[2] The majority of caregivers are older spouses and middle-aged adult children who care for a parent or a spouse with functional limitations. About 61% of caregivers are women. Their average age is 49. Older adults are not the only care recipients, but about half of caregivers of adults are caring for someone aged 75 or older (46%), with 40% caring for someone aged 50 to 74. The diversity of caregivers reflects the diversity of the population. Caregiving is an activity that crosses all generations, racial and ethnic groups, family types, gender identities and sexual orientation. Sixty-one percent of caregivers are non-Hispanic White, 17% are Hispanic or Latina, 14% are non-Hispanic African American or Black, 5% Asian American and Pacific Islander and 3% some other race/ethnicity, including multiracial. The economic value of this informal caregiving is substantial and surpasses the spending for formal home health care and nursing home care.[3]

CAREGIVING AND ITS IMPACT ON HEALTH AND WELL-BEING

The caregiving role involves multiple domains, including assistance with household tasks, self-care tasks and mobility; provision of emotional support; maintaining social connections; health and medical care; advocacy and care coordination; and surrogacy. Within these domains there are multiple tasks and activities that make up the caregiving experience. Caregiving can be highly variable, especially in terms of its onset, duration and evolution over time. The needs of care recipients, duration of the period of dependency and progression over time depend on the type and precipitating cause of the disability. Despite this considerable variability, a prototypical longitudinal trajectory for older adult caregivers has been described. The trajectory typically includes shared phases of caregiving that include: (1) initial adjustment; (2) stabilization; (3) challenges and strains; (4) long-term adaptation; and (5) the end of caregiving. It is clear, however, that the trajectory of caregiving is not fixed or linear and the transitions between these phases are significantly influenced by personal circumstances and external factors.[4]

Today's caregivers provide, on average, about 24 hours of care each week, with a median of 10 hours. The average duration of caregiving is 4.5 years, with three out of ten caregivers reporting 5 years or more as a caregiver. Caregivers report that they provide support for both physical activities of daily living and the instrumental activities of daily living. Forty-five percent of caregivers report that they help with dressing and 44% provide help with mobility. Thirty-six percent report assisting with eating. At least half of caregivers report that they help their care recipient daily with instrumental activities of daily living, ranging from meal preparation (74%) to helping with finances (50%).[5] More than half of caregivers report that they had no choice

TABLE 22.1
The Caregiving Trajectory

Initial Adjustment	The transition into the caregiving role. Caregivers may experience stress and adjustment challenges as they adapt to caregiving responsibilities.
Stabilization	The caregiver establishes routines and coping mechanisms to manage caregiving duties. They may seek support from personal social networks or community resources to ease caregiver burden.
Challenges and Strains	Over time, caregivers may encounter increased stress, and potential strain on their own health and well-being. The caregiver may experience physical, emotional or financial challenges due to the ongoing demands of caregiving.
Long-Term Adaptation	Some individuals adapt to the demands and develop resilience. They may find ways to balance caregiving with self-care and manage their roles effectively.
Transition or End of Caregiving	The caregiving role may come to an end because the care recipient's health improved, the care recipient was placed under formal care services such as a nursing facility, or due to the passing of the care recipient. This transition phase may bring the caregiver relief, but also has its own potential stressors, including guilt, grief or a loss of purpose.

in taking on the responsibility to provide care for their care recipient and those who report having no choice were found to often face increased stress and strain.[6]

Though there is much yet to know about the impacts of informal caregiving, for many individuals, caring for a care recipient with a disabling chronic illness is a major life stressor. The role generates physical and emotional strain and has the capacity to generate secondary stressors in multiple areas of life. Though caregivers are deeply committed to their caregiving and can find the experience both rewarding and personally satisfying, the research shows that informal caregivers suffer from higher rates of depression than age-matched non-caregivers and they suffer a mortality rate that is 63% higher than non-caregivers.[7]

PATHOPHYSIOLOGY

Caregiver burden describes the stress that caregivers experience in the management of care-related tasks.[8] Most caregivers report that they have less time for family and friends; have increased emotional stress and neglect self-care: healthy sleep, physical activity and healthy dietary habits.[9] Caregivers have higher rates of insomnia and depression, are at risk of serious illness, and are less likely to engage in preventive health measures. Half of all caregivers have at least one chronic health condition.[10] Spousal caregivers who report elevated levels of caregiver strain have a 23% higher Framingham Stroke Risk than their non-caregiver counterparts. One in five caregivers describes their health as fair or poor, and 17% believe that their health has deteriorated because of their work providing care.[11] Barriers to self-care include gender roles, self-sacrificing, minority ethnicity and the physical demands of caregiving, including a lack of time and energy.[12] How much burden an individual caregiver may experience varies considerably.[13] The adverse impacts of caregiving appear to originate in a complex interaction of factors that create stress and burden. Stressors that have been implicated as root causes of caregiver burden include the following: the care needs of the care recipient; the caregiver's resilience – tolerance in the face of those needs; the interaction between care demands and the caregiver's sense of commitment; the caregiver's health status; and the caregiver's self-perceived competence.[14] A majority of caregivers (81%) feel inadequately trained for the skills that they perform, having never received any formal education in caregiving.[15]

The factors that influence caregiver depression have also been investigated. These also appear to interact in an array of determinative factors: characteristics of the care recipient and the caregiver, cultural factors and caregiving demands. Attributes associated with higher rates of depression include the caregiver's relationship to the recipient (highest for wife), hours per week spent caregiving, and poor caregiver physical function.[16]

Social isolation is a frequently reported source of stress among informal caregivers. Caregiving requires time and effort, resulting in diminished social networks. Social isolation has been related to the intensity of the care recipient's care needs and lack of social supports.[17] Despite this well-recognized relationship, most caregivers receive very little informal or formal supports.[18]

TABLE 22.2
Factors in Caregiver Burden

Time Demands	Time demands disrupt caregiver's personal life, social activities and leisure time. Time demands compete with self-care and contribute to exhaustion.
Lack of Social Support	Many caregivers experience diminished social supports and describe concomitant social isolation and loneliness because of their caregiving role.
Neglected Self-Care	Lack of time for self-care is a key barrier to caregiver health. Caregivers may sacrifice their own health and wellness to the demands of the caregiving role.
Disrupted Sleep	Sleep disturbance is a common problem among caregivers. Caregivers report increased rates of sleep disruption and fewer hours of sleep per night.
Physical Demands	The physical tasks involved in caregiving, such as lifting, bathing and assisting with mobility can be physically taxing. Half of all caregivers report at least one chronic health condition.
Care Complexity	Emotional stress has been found to increase with increasing care complexity. Caregivers report a need for information and support to help them master and adjust to the caregiving role.

Sleep disturbances are commonly reported by caregivers and affect physical and mental health. The subjective experience of stress with the caregiving role is associated with sleep disturbances.[19] Wandering behaviors and nighttime urinary incontinence by care recipients are especially disruptive to the sleep of their informal caregivers.[20]

The most important lesson to learn from the research on caregiver burden and the adverse impacts of caregiving on the caregiver is that these experiences need to be viewed from a broad context and social framework. They can only be effectively addressed through multicomponent interventions that encourage social engagement, address emotional well-being, teach stress management techniques and support health-promoting behaviors.[21] These approaches are encompassed in the pillars of lifestyle medicine.

LIFESTYLE MEDICINE AND CAREGIVER HEALTH

Lifestyle medicine builds on the scope of preventative medicine by focusing on the promotion of healthy lifestyles to prevent, treat and reverse chronic diseases caused by behaviors and environmental factors. It focuses on six pillars – healthy eating patterns (especially unprocessed or minimally processed plant-based foods), physical activity, restorative sleep, stress management, positive social connections and avoidance of risky substances.[22] Its focus on "whole person health" presents a multimodal approach to address the many factors that contribute to caregiver burden, stress and burnout.

The actions taken by caregivers to improve their health, maintain good functioning, and increase their well-being are health-promoting self-care behaviors. Much of the health-related research on informal caregivers is about the negative experiences or problems that arise from their caregiving roles and is based on stress-coping frameworks. Though the evidence for successful approaches to improve the overall quality of life for caregivers is limited, there is evidence that multicomponent interventions can have a positive impact on caregiver quality of life. These studies indicate that efforts to support healthy behaviors based on caregiving mastery, self-care promotion, physical activity, nutrition, spiritual growth, interpersonal relationships and stress management reduce measures of caregiver burden and enhance adherence to health-promoting behaviors.[23] In addition, measures to encourage social engagement, address emotional well-being, teach stress management techniques and promote healthy behaviors may lead to improved quality of life.[24]

CAREGIVER ENGAGEMENT

Caregivers and their care recipients highly value the inclusion of the caregiver in discussions about the care recipient's health management.[25] Care plans are often developed for individuals that require caregivers to perform certain tasks, such as medical tasks, personal care tasks, or transportation, without input from the caregiver. Caregivers should be better recognized as integral to the health care of the care recipient and viewed as partners by health care providers. Caregivers often describe feeling invisible when providers working with their care recipient do not consider their own input into the treatment plan or how their own needs impact the plan of care. Fewer than three in ten say a health care provider, such as a doctor, nurse or social worker, has asked about what was needed to care for their care recipient. Just 13% say a health care provider has asked about what they need to care for themselves.[26] The attitudes and behaviors of medical providers, including physicians, affect caregiver well-being. Medical providers should acknowledge and support caregivers in their caregiving role. Caregivers place high value on respectful and open relationships with their medical providers and welcome education about the care recipient's illness and specific care needs.[27] Encourage the caregiver to function as a member of the care team. Care that includes a focus on the caregiver improves self-care behaviors, including prevention measures.[28]

Take the time to perform a systematic process of information gathering to identify the needs, strengths and resources for the caregiver. This can be done by the physician or other members of the health care team. The caregiver evaluation should also include perception of their own well-being, perceived challenges and benefits of caregiving, confidence in their abilities and the need for additional support systems. Caregiver burden should be assessed with inquiry into the extent to which caregivers perceive that care giving has had an adverse effect on their emotional, social, financial, physical and spiritual functioning.[29] The Short Form of the Zarit Burden Interview is one well-validated and readily available tool to measure a caregiver's subjective perceptions of burden.[30]

The degree to which family caregivers feel supported by the physician may influence the caregivers' burden, attitude and emotional health status. In turn, their ability to provide care affects patients' health, rates of hospitalization, and long-term

TABLE 22.3
Short Form Zarit Burden Interview

Do you feel...?	"Never" (0)	"Rarely" (1)	"Sometimes" (2)	"Quite frequently" (3)	"Nearly always" (4)
That because of the time you spend with your relative that you don't have enough time for yourself?					
Stressed between caring for your relative and trying to meet other responsibilities (work/family)?					
Angry when you are around your relative?					
That your relative currently affects your relationship with family members or friends in a negative way?					
Strained when you are around your relative?					
That your health has suffered because of your involvement with your relative?					
That you don't have as much privacy as you would like because of your relative?					
That your social life has suffered because you are caring for your relative?					
That you have lost control of your life since your relative's illness?					
Uncertain about what to do about your relative?					
You should be doing more for your relative?					
You could do a better job in caring for your relative?					

- Total Score is the summation of the 12 items (0 to 4 points per item, total score range 0 to 48).
- Guidelines for Scoring: 0–10 no or mild burden; 10–20 mild to moderate burden; >20 high burden.

Note: Copyrighted, but available for free use by clinicians and for non-funded academic research.

care admission. Caregivers experience significantly less depression when the physician listens to their needs and concerns and validates the importance of the caregiving role.[31]

PHYSICAL ACTIVITY

The health benefits of physical activity for the general population, as well as people with chronic illnesses, are well established. Because of the physical and emotional challenges of caregiving, caregivers may particularly benefit from the health promoting effects of physical activity. Higher levels of physical activity among caregivers are associated with higher levels of physical and mental health quality of life for the caregiver[32] and individualized physical activity programs for caregivers have been associated with increases in physical activity and improved overall affect.[33] Although the evidence base for interventions to increase levels of physical activity among caregivers is not strong, one systematic review concluded that physical activity interventions decrease caregiver distress and increase caregiver well-being, quality of life, sleep quality, levels of physical activity, self-efficacy for caregiving and readiness for exercise.[34] Physical activity may also be viewed as a behavioral and rehabilitation strategy for improving health-related quality of life in the caregiver–care recipient dyad. The Mobility and Vitality Lifestyle Program (MOVE UP) was a pre-post, community-based, 13-month lifestyle intervention study to help older adults improve physical function performance and lose weight. This multimodal intervention improved lower extremity function, weight loss and self-efficacy in caregiver participants. Caregiver participants were as likely to benefit from the MOVE UP intervention as non-caregivers.[35] Activity programs for patients that target the caregiver–care recipient dyad can result in improved caregiver well-being and improved caregiver confidence.[36]

Many barriers exist to lifestyle physical activity among caregivers, including heavy caregiving responsibilities, non-caregiver demands and obligations, resistance to change, depressed mood and fatigue. Because the evidence base for a best-practice intervention is limited, experts in the field recommend a focus on identifying optimal and feasible physical activity regimens for caregivers and ways to integrate physical activity into multicomponent caregiver interventions.[37] Focus groups with caregivers have highlighted the importance of providing high-quality information about

TABLE 22.4

Health Benefits of Physical Activity for Caregivers

Improved Affect
Diminished Stress
Reduced Subjective Burden
Improved Well-Being
Improved Sleep Quality
Increased Caregiving Self-Efficacy

the safety of physical activity and strategies for maintaining ongoing motivation.[38] For caregivers to fully benefit from these interventions, they may require continuing social supports such as ongoing physical activity classes or frequent contact with health educators.[39] Novel approaches to physical activity programs such as home-based program delivery or group-based videoconferencing may help to address barriers related to caregiving time demands and other non-caregiving obligations.[40]

Restorative Sleep

Sleep disturbance is a commonly reported problem among caregivers. Most surveys find between 32% to 74% of informal caregivers report various types of sleep disturbance.[41] Although caregivers do not uniformly endorse sleep as an important self-care need, they are at high risk for low sleep efficiency and caregiver depression has been linked to poor sleep.[42] Studies of caregivers of people with dementia find that poor self-rated sleep quality and more frequent sleep disturbances were related to the care recipients' neuropsychiatric symptoms and nocturnal disruptions.[43] Lower sleep quality is associated with higher frequency of nocturnal disruptions by the care recipient, the care recipient needing to use the bathroom and wandering. Caregivers who experience low sleep quality report higher caregiver depressive symptoms, and higher levels of caregiver role burden.[44] Medical providers should evaluate caregiver sleep patterns and the predisposing and precipitating factors, focusing on modifiable factors to enable intervention and promotion of restorative sleep.[45]

Social Connectedness

Many caregivers associate the caregiving role with positive emotions, including a sense of purpose. These positive emotions, however, may coexist with feelings of stress and strain. Caregiving is often time-intensive and can leave caregivers isolated from friends, family, colleagues and support systems. Caregivers report feeling isolated and alone, finding it difficult to maintain social relationships and expressing a need for social support. Many express feelings of abandonment and struggle to find the resources to support their caregiving.[46]

Social engagement is both a self-care need and a self-care behavior. Social engagement has been shown to promote the health and well-being of caregivers. Support networks are important for sharing the responsibilities and duties of caregiving, promoting self-care advocacy and helping to manage caregiver stress. Social supports lead to more engagement with self-care activities, more positive perceptions of caregiving, reduced psychological distress and less caregiver burden.[47] As with the other approaches to health-promoting caregiver self-care, there is limited evidence to inform best practices for interventions to improve social engagement and social supports for informal caregivers. Most caregiver interventions are best described as multicomponent psychosocial interventions. These include informational or educational components that incorporate measures to educate the caregiver about sources of support.[48] Some caregivers report that they find strength and emotional support from engagement with spiritual and religious activities, such as prayer and church attendance.[49]

TABLE 22.5
Online Support Resources

AARP Resources for Caregivers and Their Families	https://www.aarp.org/caregiving/	Information for caregivers, including planning resources and links to other online materials and tools.
Alzheimer's Association Online Tools	https://www.alz.org/help-support/resources/online-tools	Online tools for caregivers, many of which are useful regardless of disease or condition.
Family Caregiver Alliance	https://www.caregiver.org/	Programs and services designed with caregivers' needs in mind.
Health in Aging Foundation	https://www.healthinaging.org/	Education materials for older adults and caregivers to help older adults and caregivers maintain health, independence and quality of life.
National Alliance for Caregiving	https://www.caregiving.org/resources/	Informational resources for caregivers with many links to a wide variety of available online sources of information and support.
Rosalynn Carter Institute for Caregivers	https://rosalynncarter.org/	Resources for caregiver support and advocacy.
SAGE National Resource Center Caregiving Resource Page	https://www.lgbtagingcenter.org/	A resource center focused on improving the quality of services and supports offered to lesbian, gay, bisexual, and/or transgender older adults, families and caregivers.

Multicomponent interventions that encourage social engagement as part of their integrated approach to promoting caregiver health have demonstrated enhanced adherence to health-promoting behaviors and a reduction in caregiver burden.

STRESS MANAGEMENT

About 40% of caregivers consider their caregiving situation to be highly stressful, while an additional 28% report moderate emotional stress. Twenty-six percent want more information about managing their stress.[50] One of the top unmet needs of informal caregivers is the management of emotional stress.[51] Counseling about caregiver stress, its consequences and ways to manage and reduce stress can reduce burden among caregivers.[52] Psychosocial interventions, including support groups and psychoeducational interventions have shown modest efficacy in mitigating caregiver distress, even if overall burden is minimally impacted.[53] Caregivers are frequently satisfied or very satisfied with these psychosocial interventions; they appraised their own coping skills as improved, reported that their relationship with the patient had improved, identified helpful training elements and most (71%) reported that they would use training again.[54] Individualized stress management techniques used as elements of multi-component interventions have been shown to modestly improve caregiver well-being. Cognitive reframing, a technique used in cognitive behavioral therapy, reduces caregiver psychological morbidity and subjective stress.[55] Mindfulness-based stress reduction may reduce depressive symptoms and anxiety in caregivers caring for people with dementia.[56] Encouraging caregivers to access and use respite services is a key strategy to reduce stress and provide enough relief for caregivers to engage in health-promoting behaviors and improve quality of life.[57] The identification of respite needs and earlier exposure to respite is an approach endorsed by most experts in the field.[58] Under extreme circumstances, it may be appropriate to relieve a vulnerable older person from caregiving responsibilities permanently by finding an alternative caregiver or institutionalizing the care recipient.[59]

CONCLUSIONS

Working with caregivers is a core feature of geriatric care. Either as patients or caregivers to patients, the caregiver is at risk for a variety of poor health outcomes that can be addressed and mitigated with the pillars of lifestyle medicine. Engaging caregivers actively in plans of care, acknowledging the challenges of caregiving and supporting their caregiver efforts is of immense value to caregivers and their work with medical providers. Self-care deficits and caregiving-related emotional distress are a frequent experience for caregivers and can lead to caregiver burden and burnout. Addressing social support and social connectedness can mitigate burden, burnout and emotional distress. The promotion of self-care to increase physical activity has been shown to be feasible and effective at improving physical and emotional well-being. Sleep concerns and sleep deficits are common among informal caregivers and efforts to increase restorative sleep may mitigate emotional distress and fatigue. The stress of caregiving is well-documented and stress management strategies have been shown to reduce depressive symptoms, emotional distress and caregiver quality of life. And, most importantly, the application of the lifestyle medicine pillars presents a multi-component and proactive approach to caregiver well-being with great opportunity to improve their quality of life and reduce their caregiver stress and burden.

CLINICAL APPLICATIONS

- Lifestyle medicine's focus on whole person health presents a multimodal approach to reduce caregiver burden, stress and burnout.
- Acknowledge and support the important role that caregivers have in promoting the health of care recipients.
- Engage caregivers in plans of care. Ask what they need to support the treatment plan and to master their caregiving role.
- Assess caregiver burden, preferably with a valid, standardized tool, such as the Zarit Burden Interview.

- Systematically assess caregiver needs, social supports and the resources available to them.
- Support caregivers in efforts to identify and engage with opportunities to promote social connectedness.
- Be aware of available respite options and encourage use of respite services to support caregiver well-being.
- Support healthy behaviors to reduce caregiver burden and enhance adherence to health-promoting behaviors.
- Educate caregivers about emotional stress, its consequences and ways to manage and reduce stress.

REFERENCES

1. Physicians and Family Caregivers. A model for partnership. Council on Scientific Affairs, American Medical Association. *JAMA*. 1993;269(10):1282-4.
2. AARP and National Alliance for Caregiving. *Caregiving in the United States 2020*. Washington, DC: AARP; May 2020. Accessed November 7, 2023. https://www.aarp.org/ppi/info-2020/caregiving-in-the-united-states.html.
3. Collins LG, Swartz K. Caregiver care. *Am Fam Physician*. 2011;83(11):1309-17.
4. Schulz R, Beach SR, Czaja SJ, et al. Family caregiving for older adults. *Annu Rev Psychol*. 2020;71:635-659.
5. AARP and National Alliance for Caregiving. *Caregiving in the United States 2020*. Washington, DC: AARP; May 2020. Accessed November 7, 2023. https://www.aarp.org/ppi/info-2020/caregiving-in-the-united-states.html.
6. Jacops R, Hopkins CS, Fasolino T. Patient-caregiver dyad: a systematic review informing a concept analysis. *Int J Nurs Health Care Res*. 2022;5:1298.
7. Schulz R, Beach SR. Caregiving as a risk factor for mortality: the Caregiver Health Effects Study. *JAMA*. 1999;282(23):2215-2219.
8. Zarit SH, Todd PA, Zarit JM. Subjective burden of husbands and wives as caregivers: a longitudinal study. *Gerontologist*. 1986;26(3):260-266.
9. Waligora KJ, Bahouth MN, Han HR. The self-care needs and behaviors of dementia informal caregivers: a systematic review. *Gerontologist*. 2019;59(5):e565-e583.
10. Collins LG, Swartz K. Caregiver care. *Am Fam Physician*. 2011;83(11):1309-17.
11. Oliveira D, Sousa L, Orrell M. Improving health-promoting self-care in family carers of people with dementia: a review of interventions. *Clin Interv Aging*. 2019;14:515-523.
12. Waligora KJ, Bahouth MN, Han HR. The self-care needs and behaviors of dementia informal caregivers: a systematic review. *Gerontologist*. 2019;59(5):e565-e583.
13. Liang J, Aranda MP, Lloyd DA. Association between role overload and sleep disturbance among dementia caregivers: the impact of social support and social engagement. *J Aging Health*. 2020;32(10):1345-1354.
14. Physicians and family caregivers. A model for partnership. Council on Scientific Affairs, American Medical Association. *JAMA*. 1993;269(10):1282-1284.
15. Collins LG, Swartz K. Caregiver care. *Am Fam Physician*. 2011;83(11):1309-1317.
16. Covinsky KE, Newcomer R, Fox P, et al. Patient and caregiver characteristics associated with depression in caregivers of patients with dementia. *J Gen Intern Med*. 2003;18(12):1006-1014.
17. Lee J, Baik S, Becker TD, Cheon JH. Themes describing social isolation in family caregivers of people living with dementia: a scoping review. *Dementia (London)*. 2022;21(2):701-721.

18. Oliveira D, Sousa L, Orrell M. Improving health-promoting self-care in family carers of people with dementia: a review of interventions. *Clin Interv Aging.* 2019;14:515–523.
19. Liang J, Aranda MP, Lloyd DA. Association between role overload and sleep disturbance among dementia caregivers: the impact of social support and social engagement. *J Aging Health.* 2020;32(10):1345–1354.
20. Peng LM, Chiu YC, Liang J, Chang TH. Risky wandering behaviors of persons with dementia predict family caregivers' health outcomes. *Aging Ment Health.* 2018;22(12):1650–1657.
21. Belle SH, Burgio L, Burns R, et al. Resources for Enhancing Alzheimer's Caregiver Health (REACH) II Investigators. Enhancing the quality of life of dementia caregivers from different ethnic or racial groups: a randomized, controlled trial. *Ann Intern Med.* 2006;145(10):727–738.
22. Parkinson MD, Stout R, Dysinger W. Lifestyle medicine: prevention, treatment, and reversal of disease. *Med Clin North Am.* 2023;107(6):1109–1120.
23. Homayouni A, Vasli P, Estebsari F, Nasiri M. Reducing care burden and improving adherence to health-promoting behaviors among family caregivers of patients with multiple sclerosis through a healthy lifestyle empowerment program. *BMC Nurs.* 2022;21(1):229.
24. Belle SH, Burgio L, Burns R, et al. Resources for Enhancing Alzheimer's Caregiver Health (REACH) II Investigators. Enhancing the quality of life of dementia caregivers from different ethnic or racial groups: a randomized, controlled trial. *Ann Intern Med.* 2006;145(10):727–738.
25. Kuluski K, Peckham A, Gill A, et al. What is important to older people with multimorbidity and their caregivers? Identifying attributes of person-centered care from the user perspective. *Int J Integr Care.* 2019;19(3):4,1–15.
26. AARP and National Alliance for Caregiving. *Caregiving in the United States 2020.* AARP; May 2020. Accessed November 7, 2023. https://www.aarp.org/ppi/info-2020/caregiving-in-the-united-states.html.
27. Wolff JL, Roter DL. Family presence in routine medical visits: a meta-analytical review. *Soc Sci Med.* 2011;72(6):823–831.
28. Nakayama G, Masumoto S, Haruta J, Maeno T. Family caregivers' experience with healthcare and social care professionals and their participation in health checkups: a cross-sectional study in Japan. *J Gen Fam Med.* 2022;24(2):110–118.
29. Collins LG, Swartz K. Caregiver care. *Am Fam Physician.* 2011;83(11):1309–1317.
30. Bédard M, Molloy DW, Squire L, et al. The Zarit Burden Interview: a new short version and screening version. *Gerontologist.* 2001;41(5):652–657.
31. Mitnick S, Leffler C, Hood VL; American College of Physicians Ethics, Professionalism and Human Rights Committee. Family caregivers, patients, and physicians: ethical guidance to optimize relationships. *J Gen Intern Med.* 2010;25(3):255–260.
32. Fakolade A, Cameron J, McKenna O, et al. Physical activity together for people with multiple sclerosis and their care partners: protocol for a feasibility randomized controlled trial of a dyadic intervention. *JMIR Res Protoc.* 2021;10(6):e18410. doi:10.2196/18410.
33. Farran CJ, Paun O, Cothran F, et al. Impact of an individualized physical activity intervention on improving mental health outcomes in family caregivers of persons with dementia: a randomized controlled trial. *AIMS Med Sci.* 2016;3(1):15–31.
34. Lambert SD, Duncan LR, Kapellas S, et al. A descriptive systematic review of physical activity interventions for caregivers: effects on caregivers' and care recipients' psychosocial outcomes, physical activity levels, and physical health. *Ann Behav Med.* 2016;50(6):907–919.

35. Liu X, King J, Boak B, et al. Effectiveness of a behavioral lifestyle intervention on weight management and mobility improvement in older informal caregivers: a secondary data analysis. *BMC Geriatr.* 2022;22(1):626. doi:10.1186/s12877-022-03315-w.
36. Ng SM, Fung MHY, Chan JSM, et al. Physical activity, confidence, and quality of life among cancer patient-carer dyads. *Sports Med Open.* 2021;7(1):46. doi:10.1186/s40798-021-00333-7.
37. Farran CJ, Staffileno BA, Gilley DW, et al. A lifestyle physical activity intervention for caregivers of persons with Alzheimer's disease. *Am J Alzheimers Dis Other Demen.* 2008;23(2):132–142.
38. Fakolade A, McKenna O, Kamel R, et al. Prioritizing components of a dyadic physical activity intervention for people with moderate to severe multiple sclerosis and their care partners: a modified e-Delphi study. *Int J MS Care.* 2023;25(1):8–14.
39. Handlery R, Regan E, Lewis AF, et al. Active participation of care partners in a physical activity intervention alongside people with stroke: a feasibility study. *Physiother Can.* 2022;74(1):97–110.
40. Castro CM, Wilcox S, O'Sullivan P, et al. An exercise program for women who are caring for relatives with dementia. *Psychosom Med.* 2002;64(3):458–468.
41. Peng HL, Chang YP. Sleep disturbance in family caregivers of individuals with dementia: a review of the literature. *Perspect Psychiatr Care.* 2013;49(2):135–146.
42. Ahn S, Lobo JM, Davis EM, et al. Characterization of sleep efficiency transitions in family caregivers. *J Behav Med.* 2023. doi:10.1007/s10865-023-00461-3.
43. Chiu YC, Lee YN, Wang PC, et al. Family caregivers' sleep disturbance and its associations with multilevel stressors when caring for patients with dementia. *Aging Ment Health.* 2014;18(1):92-101.
44. Creese J, Bédard M, Brazil K, et al. Sleep disturbances in spousal caregivers of individuals with Alzheimer's disease. *Int Psychogeriatr.* 2008;20(1):149–161.
45. Brewster GS, Wang D, McPhillips MV, et al. Correlates of sleep disturbance experienced by informal caregivers of persons living with dementia: a systematic review. *Clin Gerontol.* 2022. doi:10.1080/07317115.2022.2135102.
46. Lilly MB, Robinson CA, Holtzman S, et al. Can we move beyond burden and burnout to support the health and wellness of family caregivers to persons with dementia? Evidence from British Columbia, Canada. *Health Soc Care Community.* 2012;20(1):103–112.
47. Lin X, Moxley JH, Czaja SJ. Caring for dementia caregivers: psychosocial factors related to engagement in self-care activities. *Behav Sci (Basel).* 2023;13(10):851.
48. Schulz R, Beach SR, Czaja SJ, Martire LM, Monin JK. Family caregiving for older adults. *Annu Rev Psychol.* 2020;71:635–659.
49. Waligora KJ, Bahouth MN, Han HR. The self-care needs and behaviors of dementia informal caregivers: a systematic review. *Gerontologist.* 2019;59(5):e565–e583.
50. AARP and National Alliance for Caregiving. *Caregiving in the United States 2020.* AARP; May 2020. Accessed November 7, 2023. https://www.aarp.org/ppi/info-2020/caregiving-in-theunited-states.html.
51. Collins LG, Swartz K. Caregiver care. *Am Fam Physician.* 2011;83(11):1309–1317.
52. Griffin JM, Meis L, Greer N, Jensen A, MacDonald R, Rutks I, Carlyle M, Wilt TJ. *Effectiveness of Family and Caregiver Interventions on Patient Outcomes Among Adults With Cancer or Memory-Related Disorders: A Systematic Review.* Department of Veterans Affairs; April 2013. Accessed March 29, 2023. https://www.hsrd.research.va.gov/publications/esp/caregiver-interventions.pdf.
53. Adelman RD, Tmanova LL, Delgado D, Dion S, Lachs MS. Caregiver burden: a clinical review. *JAMA.* 2014;311(10):1052–1060.
54. Brodaty H, Green A, Koschera A. Meta-analysis of psychosocial interventions for caregivers of people with dementia. *J Am Geriatr Soc.* 2003;51(5):657–664.

55. Vernooij-Dassen M, Draskovic I, McCleery J, Downs M. Cognitive reframing for carers of people with dementia. *Cochrane Database Syst Rev.* 2011;11:CD005318. doi:10.1002/14651858.CD005318.pub2.
56. Liu Z, Sun YY, Zhong BL. Mindfulness-based stress reduction for family carers of people with dementia. *Cochrane Database Syst Rev.* 2018;8:CD012791. doi:10.1002/14651858.CD012791.pub2.
57. Adelman RD, Tmanova LL, Delgado D, Dion S, Lachs MS. Caregiver burden: a clinical review. *JAMA.* 2014;311(10):1052–1060.
58. Oliveira D, Sousa L, Orrell M. Improving health-promoting self-care in family carers of people with dementia: a review of interventions. *Clin Interv Aging.* 2019;14:515–523.
59. Griffin JM, Meis L, Greer N, Jensen A, MacDonald R, Rutks I, Carlyle M, Wilt TJ. *Effectiveness of Family and Caregiver Interventions on Patient Outcomes Among Adults With Cancer or Memory-Related Disorders: A Systematic Review.* Department of Veterans Affairs; April 2013. Accessed March 29, 2023. https://www.hsrd.research.va.gov/publications/esp/caregiver-interventions.pdf.

23 Reducing Fall Risk with Lifestyle Changes

Crystal Arrendell

Falls are the leading cause of injury for adults ages 65 and older. In 2020, 14 million older adults in the United States reported falling.[1] Falls are a serious threat to the health and well-being of older adults due to their high prevalence and potentially severe consequences, including increased morbidity, mortality, reduced quality of life and substantial strain on health care services and costs. Various assessments can be administered in clinical settings to estimate fall risk. STEADI, developed by the CDC, is an algorithm for fall risk screening, assessment and intervention. STEADI recommends yearly screening for fall risk and assessing modifiable risk factors and fall history for at-risk patients. Things that can potentially increase fall risk include gait abnormalities, certain medications, home hazards, blood pressure abnormalities, vision trouble, inappropriate footwear and uncontrolled medical problems. At the same time, many falls occur among older adults with no traditional risk factors.

A person's lifestyle independently affects fall risk.[2] Lifestyle medicine is a medical specialty that focuses on six pillars that can improve health and well-being. These pillars of lifestyle medicine – physical activity, nutrition, restorative sleep, stress management, avoidance of harmful substances and social connection – can also potentially reduce fall risk. Increasing physical activity with attention to strength, balance, flexibility and endurance training has been shown to reduce fall risk. A whole food plant-based diet may reduce comorbidities and polypharmacy, reducing a person's fall risk. Stressful life events have also been shown to increase the risk of falls. Conversely, focusing on stress management and improved mood has been shown to have the opposite effect. Restorative sleep can reduce fall risk by improving physical and cognitive function and mood. Consumption of harmful substances can cause falls by affecting balance, coordination and reaction time while also increasing the potential for risky behavior. Finally, social isolation can contribute to an increased risk of falls. Emphasizing social connection and engagement in life improves physical activity, reduces stress and reduces fall risk.

A person's environment and socioeconomic status, while not typically listed as a pillar of lifestyle medicine, are essential to consider as they can impact the likelihood of a fall. For example, environmental hazards at home can cause a person to fall. Additionally, having a low income is linked to having limited access to health care and an increased risk of falling. The remainder of this chapter will examine how personal lifestyle adjustments can reduce the risk of falls.

EXERCISE

The concept of exercise leading to fall prevention may seem like an obvious statement to many people. However, "exercise" is extremely general and encompasses a wide range of physical activity. Asking five individuals to describe exercise will likely lead to five completely different answers. While exercise is crucial for fall prevention, evidence has identified that exercise programs that focus on specific areas of training are the most effective. It is also important for exercise to be progressively challenging and sustained over time to maximize its effectiveness in reducing falls.[3] Various training areas of focus, including strength, balance, flexibility and endurance training, have been studied and shown effectiveness in reducing fall risk.

Strength training, also known as resistance training, is an exercise that causes muscles to contract against outside resistance. It can help build strength, size, power and muscle endurance. It is also a form of balance training as it can strengthen the muscles that maintain posture and improve stability. Strength training plays a key role in preventing falls as it limits the loss of bone and muscle mass and strength, along with stimulating postural control. Strength training can be done using body weight, such as push-ups, squats and lunges. Weights or resistance bands can also be added to increase the intensity of the exercise.

Pilates is a low-impact exercise method focusing on core strength and using controlled movements. It is a form of strength training that can also improve flexibility and balance and has been shown to have a positive influence on fall prevention.[4] Because Pilates is a low-impact exercise, it is routinely recommended for older adults who are seeking to add strength training to their exercise routine. It is also ideal for those at the beginning stages of their exercise journey.

Flexibility training involves exercises that stretch muscles, ligaments and tendons to improve range of motion. It can help decrease the risk of injuries, increase freedom of movement and help with balance. It is often used in yoga and Pilates routines. Yoga is an ancient system originating from India that focuses on harmonizing the body with the mind and breath. The Successful Ageing (SAGE) yoga trial found that a consistent yoga program can yield several positive outcomes, including improved balance and flexibility along with improved physical and mental health.[5]

Endurance training, also called aerobic exercise, includes activities that increase breathing and heart rate, such as swift walking, jogging, biking or swimming. There are many cardiovascular benefits to endurance training, as it can maintain the health of the heart, lungs and circulatory system while enhancing overall fitness. Consistent aerobic exercise can lead to improved and better-managed comorbidities. There is an association between falls in older adults and the number of chronic diseases an individual has.[6]

Tai Chi is a mind–body exercise that originated in China as a martial art. It combines slow, deliberate movements, meditation and deep breathing. It is a gentle and low-impact activity that can help maintain strength, flexibility and balance. It is also an exercise that can be easily tailored to suit everyone, from those who are highly fit to those who are wheelchair-bound or recovering from surgery. Many studies have shown that Tai Chi has value in treating or preventing many health problems. A systemic review and meta-analysis of randomized controlled trials related to Tai Chi, falls and balance ability concluded that Tai Chi is an effective exercise for preventing falls and improving balance ability in older adults.[7] This study showed improvement in falls risk regardless of risk level. It is important to note that the effectiveness of Tai Chi increases with exercise time and consistency.

Older adults have many exercise options that may reduce fall risk. Focusing on various facets of exercise such as strength training, endurance training, balance and flexibility can improve mobility and function. Low-impact exercises such as Pilates, yoga and Tai Chi are easier on joints and usually well tolerated, even for beginner exercisers. Tai Chi is an ideal activity for older adults who want to improve many aspects of life including health and mobility. Tai Chi classes are often offered at local senior centers or retirement communities.

NUTRITION

Ensuring proper nutritional intake is important for maintaining health. Nutrients provide essential building blocks to maintain all body functions, including energy production, tissue repair and immune system support. Focusing on daily total calories, protein, vitamin D and calcium intake supports the overall health of muscles and bones.

Eating the right amount of calories daily is crucial to maintaining a healthy weight. Being overweight or underweight increases fall risk. The number of daily calories will change depending on the goal. If the goal is losing weight, eating fewer daily calories along with regular aerobic exercise may be beneficial. If the goal is to gain weight, eating small, frequent, calorie-dense meals, along with regular exercise focused on strength training may help.

Dietary protein helps to build and repair muscle and body tissue. The FDA recommends an intake of 50 g of protein per day based on a 2,000-calorie daily diet. Daily protein requirement will vary based on daily calorie needs, as well as activity level.

Dietary vitamin D and calcium intake are important for muscle and bone health. Calcium-rich foods include dairy products, green leafy vegetables and grains. The daily recommendation of vitamin D varies based on the individual. Older adults should see their primary care doctor to assess whether vitamin D supplementation is recommended for them. vitamin D–rich foods include fatty fish such as salmon or tuna, egg yolks and fortified orange juice. Sun exposure leads to the conversion and activation of vitamin D, although this process is less efficient in older adults and individuals with darker skin tones.

Daily water intake is an often-overlooked part of daily intake that can have an impact on health. The total amount of water a person should drink depends on many factors, but a generally recommended daily intake of water ranges from about 11 cups in women to 15 cups in men. Throughout the day, water is ingested through many sources such as coffee, tea, juice, fruits and vegetables. This means that the average person may only need to drink four to six cups of plain water to meet their daily goal. Inadequate hydration increases the risk of dehydration. A retrospective cohort study from the University of Wisconsin showed an association between dehydration and a higher risk of falls.[8]

The lack of adequate dietary intake and hydration can lead to malnutrition. However, the diagnosis of malnutrition is sometimes difficult to make due to inconsistent definitions, varying measurement tools and no clearly established guidelines for diagnosis. A Vermont-based study looked at older adults who were at risk for having poor nutrition and found an association between fall risk and nutrition risk.[9]

A healthy weight and diet can help to manage or resolve medical problems such as high blood pressure, diabetes and obstructive sleep apnea. The management and control of these chronic medical problems with dietary adjustments can lead to reduced polypharmacy as health improves and medications are discontinued. This reduction in polypharmacy can, in turn, reduce fall risk. Several studies have suggested an association between health status and falls in older adults. One study explored the relationship between falls and chronic disease and showed that the higher the number of chronic diseases, the higher the probability of falling.[6]

RESTORATIVE SLEEP

Inadequate sleep is an important yet understudied risk factor for falls. Sleep disturbances have the potential to occur due to many reasons and are often multi-factorial. Some examples of sleep disturbances include long or short sleep duration, fragmented sleep overnight and disordered breathing while sleeping. Most of the research available suggests that 7 to 8 hours of sleep per night is ideal to avoid adverse physiological effects. An average sleep duration in the past month of less than 5 hours has been associated with more frequent falls.[10] In addition, individuals who report unrestful sleep are more likely to have a fall.[11] Sleep may represent a modifiable risk factor to target for reducing the risk of falls in older adults.

Medication has historically been a widely used treatment for insomnia or other sleep disturbances. However, many of the medications used for insomnia-related disorders have extensive side effect profiles and risks. Zolpidem, also known as Ambien, is one of the most prescribed hypnotic drugs in the United States. It is a strong, independent risk factor for falls and can make individuals four times more likely to fall.[12] Diphenhydramine is an over-the-counter medication commonly used for insomnia but can have multiple side effects, especially in older adults. The use of diphenhydramine has been associated with an increased risk of falls with injury.[13]

Cognitive behavioral therapy (CBT) is a non-pharmacological option for the treatment of various sleep disorders. It is widely recognized to be the preferred first-line treatment for insomnia. CBT helps identify the thoughts and behaviors that contribute to or worsen sleep problems. It is a form of therapy that teaches how to replace these thoughts and behaviors with habits that promote healthy, restful sleep.[14] Unlike sleeping pills, CBT addresses the root causes of sleep issues.

There can be challenges with the implementation of CBT as a treatment for insomnia. It is often difficult to locate a treatment center that performs CBT for sleep disturbances, and it can also be difficult to schedule due to a lack of open appointments.

STRESS MANAGEMENT

Living a stressful life can contribute to anxiety, depression, obesity, immune system dysfunction and other health issues. American culture often glamorizes stress and high conflict. In addition, US citizens are thought to live a more stressful life compared to life in other parts of the world. Focusing on stress reduction and management will contribute to overall well-being and can lower the risk of developing various medical problems.

Many studies have investigated the potential repercussions of unmanaged stress. Anxiety disorders and clinically significant levels of anxiety symptoms are common in adults. Unfortunately, elevated levels of anxiety are associated with a 53% increased likelihood of falls, and older age is predictive of a stronger association.[15] Not only has anxiety been linked to increased falls. Falls themselves have been associated with an increased risk of developing anxiety and depression among adults aged greater than 50.[16]

While many things may help an individual reduce stress and anxiety, individuals often do not practice consistent stress reduction practices, as it is not yet common in US culture. Some common stress reduction techniques include participation in an exercise program, meditation, psychotherapy or spending time outdoors. Improving mood with a conservative stress management routine may reduce the need for medications such as antidepressants or anxiolytics, which increase the risk of falls.

Reducing the fear of falling has also been shown to reduce falls.[17] Experiencing a fall in older age can have devastating health outcomes and even lead to death. Fear of falling is a common emotional concern experienced by older adults. It can be described as an individual's anxiety towards normal walking with a perception that they will fall. An exercise program can be beneficial in this situation as building muscle and balance can help someone become more stable and comfortable with ambulation and, thus, less worried about falling.

Not only has chronic stress and anxiety been associated with a greater risk of falls. Individual stressful life events have been shown to significantly increase the risk of falls in older men.[18] Some common stressful life events experienced by older adults are the loss of a spouse, job loss, change in residency and debilitating medical or hospital experiences.

In recent years, the concept of stress management has been more often discussed in American society. It is something that is especially important for older adults as unmanaged stress may lead to falls, which can negatively alter the course of an older person's health and life.

AVOIDANCE OF HARMFUL SUBSTANCES

Some substances are frequently used in the United States and have been shown to cause harm in various ways. That potential for harm increases as a person ages due to physiological changes in how one's body processes and metabolizes these substances. These substances include the ingestion of alcohol, tobacco and polypharmacy (i.e., the use of multiple prescription drugs by a single person).

Reducing Fall Risk with Lifestyle Changes

Alcohol consumption is common in the United States. Celebratory occasions can be defined by multiple toasts throughout the event and easy access to alcoholic beverages. According to the 2023 National Survey on Drug Use and Health, 134.7 million adults reported that they drank alcohol in the past month. It is not a stretch to assume that binge drinking leads to increased falls; however, studies have shown that fall risk also increases with moderate drinking, suggesting that any alcohol consumption may increase the risk for falls.[19]

The number of falls in older adults that are associated with alcohol consumption appears to be increasing. The annual rate of emergency department visits for alcohol-associated falls in adults aged greater than 65 increased annually from 2011–2019.[20] This highlights the importance of screening older adults for alcohol consumption and advising that even minimal alcohol consumption can increase the risk of falls.

Tobacco is a commonly inhaled substance that has been repeatedly shown to be associated with numerous adverse health conditions. It is not uncommon for an individual to use alcohol and tobacco simultaneously. In addition to the association of tobacco with adverse health conditions, tobacco use has also been linked with increased frailty.[21] Older adults may be seen as frail if they have three or more of the following symptoms: weight loss, exhaustion, low physical activity, slowness and weakness.[22] Frailty is a geriatric syndrome that is characterized by decreased physiological reserves and increased vulnerability to adverse health outcomes. Numerous studies have shown that frail older adults have a higher risk of falling compared to more robust older adults.[23] These findings underline the importance of smoking cessation in older adults, as tobacco use may not only worsen health conditions but also increase frailty and the risk of falls.

The ingestion of multiple prescription medications, known as polypharmacy, can also be harmful to health. Polypharmacy is a well-known problem among geriatricians who often see patients who have been on medications for years and continue to be prescribed different medications by various providers. This leads to an extensive medication list with medications that may interact with each other or cause side effects. One of these potential side effects is the increased risk of falls.

Nine unique medication classes were identified as having a side effect of increased fall risk. These include antihypertensive agents, diuretics, beta-blockers, sedatives and hypnotics, neuroleptics and antipsychotics, antidepressants, benzodiazepines, narcotics and nonsteroidal anti-inflammatory drugs.[24] All of these medication classes are very commonly prescribed, and often, patients are taking medications from multiple categories listed. With every addition of one of these medications, fall risk increases.

Polypharmacy is not commonly seen as a "harmful substance," and providers are often hesitant to discontinue medications, especially if a patient has been taking these medications long term. More emphasis should be placed on potential adverse events related to taking multiple medications, which increase as a patient's age increases. Patients are encouraged to meet with their providers for specific office visits to look for polypharmacy and work with their providers to determine the necessity of each medication. As a patient ages, it may improve health outcomes to discontinue medications that have more potential risks than benefits.

SOCIAL CONNECTION

There are certain geographical regions around the world where people are reported to live longer and healthier lives. They are known as "Blue Zones," a term that was coined in 2004 by Dan Buettner, a journalist and National Geographic explorer. The first five Blue Zones identified were Sardinia, Italy; Okinawa, Japan; Nicoya, Costa Rica; Ikaria, Greece; and Loma Linda, California. As researchers looked more closely at these locations, they identified that residents of these areas shared certain characteristic lifestyles that may contribute to their propensity to live longer and healthier.

One of these characteristic lifestyles was that the residents were noted to have "the right tribe," that is, specific social circles that supported healthy behaviors. A prominent example of this can be seen in Okinawa, Japan, where they have a concept of "Moais." Moais are social support groups that start in childhood and last throughout each person's entire life. It is a cultural tradition for built-in companionship.

Social connection is also one of the six pillars of lifestyle medicine and has been linked to preventing certain medical conditions. In contrast, social isolation and loneliness have been linked to adverse health outcomes, one of which is the increased risk of falls.[25,26] Loneliness is not the same as being alone or isolated. People can be alone but not lonely and, conversely, feel lonely around others. Loneliness is an unpleasant, sad and sometimes distressing emotion that comes from being alone or feeling like one is alone.

It is important to establish connections and maintain relationships throughout our lives, especially as we age. A sense of community can improve health outcomes and prevent adverse health events. It is an under appreciated goal of aging that can improve people's lives considerably.

ENVIRONMENTAL CONSIDERATIONS

When discussing falls, it is prudent to consider environmental hazards that may lead to increased falls. The living environment of an individual can be a strong indicator of their likelihood of falling. Common items in hazardous homes include loose rugs, poor lighting, narrow or cluttered hallways, lack of supportive handrails, etc. Additionally, a person's home setup can lead to a reduction in physical activity. For example, a person who lives in a cluttered home with no open spaces may become more sedentary, as moving around the home is more difficult. The need to use an assistive device would further complicate the ability to move about the house.

A home safety evaluation can be performed by an occupational therapist and may be helpful in determining how safe a home situation is. Many times, people are unaware of how their home setup may predispose them to fall. A professional assessment can be both enlightening and prevent a potentially devastating event such as a hard fall.

SOCIOECONOMIC DISPARITIES

In the previous sections, we discussed lifestyle practices that can increase the risk of falls. We have also covered interventions that may reduce an individual's risk. It is also crucial to consider another aspect of a person's life that can greatly affect their overall health and well-being. Socioeconomic status is a term that deals with how well a person can support themselves based on their social class, social standing or economic circumstances. It is measured by education, occupation and income. Lower education levels and occupational positions have been associated with higher fall rates.[27] A higher fall rate can be especially devastating when considering that health care utilization and outcomes often favor those with higher socioeconomic status. Health care utilization can vary in appropriateness, quality and cost. Access to health care is closely linked to the affordability of health insurance. Often, those with a lower income are not able to afford to be seen for preventative visits and may rely on emergency department visits when an acute medical concern arises. Those with greater financial means may be able to prevent adverse health outcomes and falls with the previously mentioned lifestyle changes. Lower financial status may lead to exacerbation of chronic conditions and an increased risk of falls. It is important to consider the socioeconomic status of an individual as it can play a key role in health outcomes and fall risk.

CONCLUSIONS

Falls and fall-related injuries are common among older adults and can have serious consequences. About a third of people over 65 years of age fall each year, and the rate of injuries increases with age.[28] Most falls are minor with injuries such as bruising or sprains, but they are still associated with pain and reduced function and can negatively affect quality of life.

Research regarding falls and fall risk has become increasingly more prevalent over recent years. Falls in older age can be devastating and lead to worsening function, disability or even death. It is encouraging that a focus on lifestyle adjustments can reduce falls as we age and promote living longer with limited medical comorbidities. This chapter provided an overview of lifestyle adjustments that can be made to reduce the risk of falls.

CLINICAL APPLICATIONS

- Physical inactivity increases fall risk, while regular activity can reduce falls. Falls may be avoided by focusing on strength, balance, flexibility and endurance training while exercising. Tai Chi, Pilates and yoga are effective and low-impact exercises that are ideal for older adults.
- An adjustment in diet to consist mostly of whole plant-based foods can improve fall risk by improving medical comorbidities and reducing polypharmacy. Adequate hydration is also important for health, and dehydration may lead to falls.

- A lack of restorative sleep can lead to decreased mobility and physical activity. Adequate sleep can improve mood along with physical and cognitive function. Notably, a long sleep duration of >10 hours is associated with adverse medical outcomes. Although prescriptions for sleep medications are common in the United States, these medications have many side effects that increase the risk of falls.
- Stress management is a focus of lifestyle medicine that is not yet common practice in the United States. Yet stress, depression and anxiety are associated with increased falls. Improved mood with stress-reducing techniques may reduce the need for medications such as antidepressants that increase fall risk.
- There are many harmful substances that should be avoided in older adults to limit fall risk. These include alcohol, tobacco, and the ingestion of multiple prescribed medications. Even moderate use of alcohol is linked to more falls.
- Many older adults suffer from polypharmacy, which can lead to adverse side effects and falls. Patients are encouraged to visit their primary care provider to discuss their medication regimen and potentially discontinue any drugs that are at high risk for adverse outcomes or falls.
- Developing a strong social circle and having social connections can contribute to better health. Social isolation and loneliness have been linked to increased falls and adverse medical outcomes.
- A safe home environment is another important consideration when thinking about fall risk. Simple adjustments in the home may be enough to lead to fewer falls. However, the socioeconomic status of an individual also plays a role in falls and health care utilization in general. It may be more difficult for those with less financial means to make some of these lifestyle or environmental changes, and alternative interventions should be considered.

REFERENCES

1. Kakara R, Bergen G, Burns E, Stevens M. Nonfatal and fatal falls among adults aged ≥65 years – United States, 2020–2021. *MMWR Morb Mortal Wkly Rep.* 2023;72(35):938–943. doi:10.15585/mmwr.mm7235a1
2. Faulkner KA, Cauley JA, Studenski SA, et al. Lifestyle predicts falls independent of physical risk factors. *Osteoporos Int.* 2009;20(12):2025–2034. doi:10.1007/s00198-009-0909-y
3. Tiedemann A, Sturnieks DL, Burton E, et al. Exercise and Sports Science Australia updated position statement on exercise for preventing falls in older people living in the community. *J Sci Med Sport.* 2024;S1440–2440(24)00518-8. doi:10.1016/j.jsams.2024.09.003
4. Patti A, Zangla D, Sahin FN, et al. Physical exercise and prevention of falls: effects of a Pilates training method compared with a general physical activity program. *Medicine.* 2021;100(13):e25289. doi:10.1097/md.0000000000025289

5. Oliveira JS, Sherrington C, Lord S, et al. Yoga-based exercise to prevent falls in community-dwelling people aged 60 years and over: study protocol for the Successful AGEing (SAGE) yoga randomized controlled trial. *BMJ Open Sport Exerc Med.* 2020;6(1):e000878. doi:10.1136/bmjsem-2020-000878
6. Tang S, Liu M, Yang T, et al. Association between falls in elderly and the number of chronic diseases and health-related behaviors based on CHARLS 2018: health status as a mediating variable. *BMC Geriatr.* 2022;22(1). doi:10.1186/s12877-022-03055-x
7. Chen W, Li M, Li H, et al. Tai Chi for fall prevention and balance improvement in older adults: a systematic review and meta-analysis of randomized controlled trials. *Front Public Health.* 2023;11:1236050. doi:10.3389/fpubh.2023.1236050
8. Hamrick I, Norton D, Birstler J, et al. Association between dehydration and falls. *Mayo Clin Proc Innov Qual Outcomes.* 2020;4(3):259–265. doi:10.1016/j.mayocpiqo.2020.01.003
9. Eckert CD, Tarleton EK, Pellerin J, et al. Nutrition risk is associated with falls risk in an observational study of community-dwelling, rural, older adults. *J Aging Health.* 2022;34(6–8):1125–1134. doi:10.1177/08982643221096944
10. Essien SK, Feng CX, Sun W, et al. Sleep duration and sleep disturbances in association with falls among middle-aged and older adults in China: a population-based nationwide study. *BMC Geriatr.* 2018;18:196. doi:10.1186/s12877-018-0889-x
11. Zhu C, Sun J, Huang Y, Lian Z. Sleep and risk of hip fracture and falls among middle-aged and older Chinese. *Sci Rep.* 2024;14(1):23273. doi:10.1038/s41598-024-74581-4
12. Kolla BP, Lovely JK, Mansukhani MP, Morgenthaler TI. Zolpidem is independently associated with increased risk of inpatient falls. *J Hosp Med.* 2013;8(1):1–6. doi:10.1002/jhm.1985
13. Cho H, Myung J, Suh HS, Kang HY. Antihistamine use and the risk of injurious falls or fracture in elderly patients: a systematic review and meta-analysis. *Osteoporos Int.* 2018;29(10):2163–2170. doi:10.1007/s00198-018-4564-z
14. Rossman J. Cognitive-behavioral therapy for insomnia: an effective and underutilized treatment for insomnia. *Am J Lifestyle Med.* 2019;13(6):544–547. doi:10.1177/1559827619867677
15. Hallford DJ, Nicholson G, Sanders K, McCabe MP. The association between anxiety and falls: a meta-analysis. *J Gerontol B Psychol Sci Soc Sci.* 2017;72(5):729–741. doi:10.1093/geronb/gbv160
16. Jacob L, Kostev K, Shin JI, et al. Falls increase the risk for incident anxiety and depressive symptoms among adults aged ≥50 years: an analysis of the Irish longitudinal study on ageing. *Arch Gerontol Geriatr.* 2023;114:105098. doi:10.1016/j.archger.2023.105098
17. Asai T, Oshima K, Fukumoto Y, et al. The association between fear of falling and occurrence of falls: a one-year cohort study. *BMC Geriatr.* 2022;22:393. doi:10.1186/s12877-022-03018-2
18. Fink HA, Kuskowski MA, Marshall LM. Association of stressful life events with incident falls and fractures in older men: the Osteoporotic Fractures in Men (MrOS) Study. *Age Ageing.* 2014;43(1):103–108. doi:10.1093/ageing/aft117
19. Sun Y, Zhang B, Yao Q, et al. Association between usual alcohol consumption and risk of falls in middle-aged and older Chinese adults. *BMC Geriatr.* 2022;22(1):750. doi:10.1186/s12877-022-03429-1
20. Yuan K, Haddad Y, Law R, et al. Emergency department visits for alcohol-associated falls among older adults in the United States, 2011 to 2020. *Ann Emerg Med.* 2023;82(6):666–677. doi:10.1016/j.annemergmed.2023.04.013
21. Kojima G, Iliffe S, Walters K. Smoking as a predictor of frailty: a systematic review. *BMC Geriatr.* 2015;15:131. doi:10.1186/s12877-015-0134-9

22. Fried LP, Tangen CM, Walston J, et al. Frailty in older adults: evidence for a phenotype. *J Gerontol A Biol Sci Med Sci.* 2001;56(3):M146–M157. doi:10.1093/gerona/56.3.M146
23. Cheng MH, Chang SF. Frailty as a risk factor for falls among community-dwelling people: evidence from a meta-analysis. *J Nurs Scholarsh.* 2017;49(5):529–536. doi:10.1111/jnu.12322
24. Woolcott JC, Richardson KJ, Wiens MO, et al. Meta-analysis of the impact of 9 medication classes on falls in elderly persons. *Arch Intern Med.* 2009;169(21):1952–1960. doi:10.1001/archinternmed.2009.357
25. Petersen N, König HH, Hajek A. The link between falls, social isolation, and loneliness: a systematic review. *Arch Gerontol Geriatr.* 2020;88:104020. doi:10.1016/j.archger.2020.104020
26. Zeytinoglu M, Wroblewski KE, Vokes TJ, et al. Association of loneliness with falls: a study of older U.S. adults using the National Social Life, Health, and Aging Project. *Gerontol Geriatr Med.* 2021;7:2333721421989217. doi:10.1177/2333721421989217
27. Khalatbari-Soltani S, Stanaway F, Sherrington C, et al. The prospective association between socioeconomic status and falls among community-dwelling older men. *J Gerontol A Biol Sci Med Sci.* 2021;76(10):1821–1828. doi:10.1093/gerona/glab038
28. Clemson L, Stark S, Pighills AC, et al. Environmental interventions for preventing falls in older people living in the community. *Cochrane Database Syst Rev.* 2019;(2):CD013258. doi:10.1002/14651858.CD013258

24 Obesity in Older Adults
Lifestyle Medicine Perspective

Shenbagam Dewar and John A. Batsis

INTRODUCTION

The prevalence of obesity has been increasing steadily among older adults,[1] especially in older adults who are admitted to nursing homes.[2] Obesity is known to affect quality of life and can accelerate the aging process, and concomitantly the exaggerated loss of muscle mass and strength may lead to disability and impaired function. Although obesity is a complex multifactorial chronic disease, healthy lifestyle behaviors consisting of dietary and exercise interventions have a favorable effect on adipose tissue and can significantly decrease the risk of mortality among patients with obesity.[3]

Obesity is assessed in clinical settings using Body Mass Index (BMI) due to its ease as a practical measure compared to body composition, despite its impreciseness. BMI is calculated as weight in kilograms divided by height in square meters. Yet, as a proxy for adipose tissue, BMI has poor diagnostic accuracy in older individuals due to loss of height, and its limitation in identifying visceral adiposity and alterations in body composition, specifically an inability to distinguish between fat and fat-free mass.[4] The World Health Organization (WHO) has defined specific categories as follows: overweight as a BMI greater than 25 kg/m² but less than 30 kg/m², obesity as a BMI greater than 30 kg/m², Class I obesity as a BMI from 30 to 34.9 kg/m², Class II as a BMI from 35 to 39.9 kg/m² and Class III as a BMI of 40.0 kg/m² or greater. The surgical community classifies further into "super obesity" as a BMI greater than 50 kg/m² and a BMI greater than 60 kg/m² as super-super obesity.

Lifestyle behaviors learned, adopted and practiced over the lifecycle can influence the health and aging trajectory of older adults.[5] Lifestyle medicine is an evidence-based practice of medicine that helps individuals and families with the adoption of healthy behaviors, and has been proven to positively impact outcomes in geriatric medicine[5] by preventing or delaying the onset of comorbidities, delaying the decline in both physical function and cognitive function and delaying the onset of sarcopenia and frailty.[5] The six pillars of lifestyle medicine include: nutrition, physical activity, stress management, restorative sleep, avoidance of risky substances and social connections.[6] There exists further characterization of "risky substances" such

TABLE 24.1
BMI Classification: World Health Organization Body Mass Index Classification Criteria

BMI in kg/m²	BMI Class
Below 18.5	Underweight
18.5–24.9	Normal/Healthy weight
25–29.9	Overweight
30–34.9	Class I
35–39.9	Class II
40–49.9	Class III
50–59.9	"Super obesity"
Above 60	"Super-super obesity"

as smoking, opioid use and alcohol use as studied in the Million Veteran Program.[7] Lifestyle medicine approaches the disease by treating the underlying cause, leading to prevention, treatment and, potentially, reversal of diseases, thereby reducing health care expenditure on medications and surgical procedures.[8]

Healthy lifestyle habits have proven to help prevent 90% of cases of diabetes, 80% of coronary artery disease, 70% of cardiovascular and 50% of cancer-related mortality.[9–12] A recent study among veterans enrolled in the Million Veteran Program (2011–2019) has shown that lifestyle factors help lower the risk of premature mortality and help prolong life expectancy. With the rapid growth of the older population, including aging baby boomers who have onset of obesity and metabolic syndrome at an earlier age, health care providers are uniquely positioned to treat, as this cohort faced social changes in areas of lifestyle patterns, increased affluence, and psychological factors that happened in the last half of the 20th century.[13,14]

Regular physical activity also helps lower the risk of all-cause mortality, control comorbid medical conditions and improve quality of life. Despite the release of the Physical Activity Guidelines for Americans in 2008, the National Health and Nutrition Examination Survey (NHANES) study among adults with diabetes has shown that one in two remain sedentary.[15] Physical activity involves energy expenditure by any movement of skeletal muscle while exercise is a planned activity for health and fitness. Hence the Physical Activity Guidelines for Americans, 2nd Edition from the US Department of Health and Human Services emphasizes the need to reduce sedentary activity while promoting the goal "move more and sit less." Any nature of physical activity which helps to expend energy has been shown to influence survival in older adults.[16] A meta-analysis shows a positive association between obesity and physical inactivity and sedentary behavior with a high prevalence of sedentary behavior (35%) and physical inactivity (43%) in adults overall.[17] Sedentary behaviors are behaviors such as sitting or reclining that have low-energy expenditure and include activities such as television watching, computer use or other screen viewing.[18] With the advent of agriculture and recent urbanization and industrialization

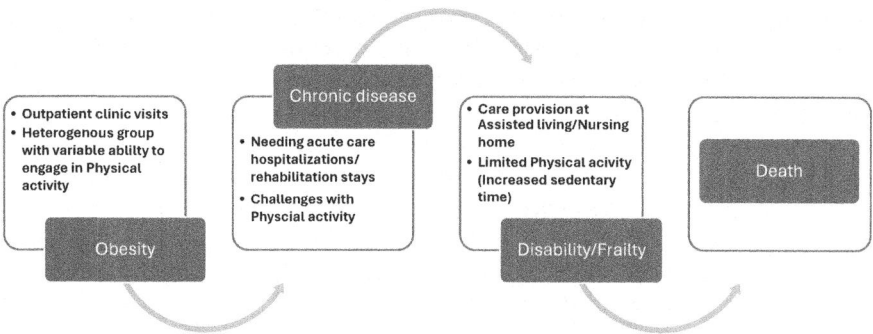

FIGURE 24.1 A schematic representation of various living and care environments of older adults with obesity.

leading to automation and motorized transportation, sedentary leisure time has increased, leading to physical inactivity and reduced energy expenditure. Sedentary behavior also increases with aging resulting in a high prevalence among older adults and leading to >8.5 hours a day spent sitting.[19] Sedentary lifestyle and the emergence of processed foods and high-calorie diets have contributed to the energy imbalance pendulum with a resultant obesity epidemic. Total sedentary time (ST) and long bouts of sedentary activity were associated with increased CVD risk in the Objective Physical Activity and Cardiovascular Health Study in women.[20]

Lifestyle interventions including diet and exercise are components of a comprehensive evidence-based treatment and can help adults attain 5–10% weight loss.[21] Further, among older Veterans with Post Traumatic Stress Disorder interventions targeting both diet quality and exercise activity have proven to avert the increased risk of obesity and cardiometabolic disease.[22] Older adults who were compliant with lifestyle intervention were able to achieve greater weight loss targets than young adults in the Diabetes Prevention Program, signaling that they are better candidates for lifestyle intervention.[23]

The type and intensity of physical activity and dietary recommendations need to be tailored to the varied residential settings and life stages of the older adult, as aging leads to potential transitions from community living to senior assisted living and nursing homes. The level of functional impairment, mobility limitation and cognitive capacity may limit the ability to engage in lifestyle programs.

PATHOPHYSIOLOGY AND RATIONALE FOR LIFESTYLE MEDICINE PILLARS

The understanding of the biology and pathophysiology of obesity continues to evolve. Obesity is a heterogeneous disease whose course is shaped by the complex interactions between the biological attributes of adiposity (including genetics and multi-omics biomarkers), social, behavioral and environmental factors.[24] Healthy lifestyle behaviors are the basic construct and foundation of the behavioral component in an obesogenic environment with an abundance of calorie-dense foods, food processing, a sedentary lifestyle and an unfavorably built environment resulting in dependence on motorized transportation and environmental obesogens.[25]

Evidence supporting lifestyle intervention including aerobic and resistance exercises in combination with weight loss improves physical function in older adults with obesity.[26] Together this intervention helps to improve metabolic dysregulation and physical impairments due to obesity-related adiposity.[27] Hence lifestyle-based medicine is foundational to weight management along with other modalities such as pharmacological and surgical intervention.

IMPACT OF LIFESTYLE PILLARS

NUTRITION

Hippocrates noted, "Let food be thy medicine and let thy medicine be food," which holds true in the current century as health care acknowledges the concept of food-is-medicine.[28] This has led to food prescriptions which have proven to be a promising health care intervention. There is supporting evidence linking a poor diet (a diet low in whole grains, fruit and vegetables and high in sodium, refined grains and sugar) to obesity, chronic diseases and mortality.[29] There is a growing body of evidence that "medically tailored meals" could help improve chronic diseases such as diabetes and result in cost savings.[30] Food is considered one of the three foundational pillars of health and survival in the aging continuum.[31] Maintaining a healthy weight across life stages by moderate calorie restriction in the current obesogenic environment is crucial for longevity and healthy aging.[32]

Healthy plant-based diets enriched in fruits, vegetables, whole grains, nuts and legumes have been proven to reduce the incidence of obesity in adults[33] and lower the risk of frailty in older adults.[34] Interestingly, the Health and Retirement Study compared silent generation birth cohorts with a baby boomer cohort and revealed that the latter lagged behind in the adoption of lifestyle changes.[35] There has been a growing concern that as the population ages, with the Baby Boomers reaching their older ages, there could be a shift in consumption of unhealthy food patterns leading to obesity and chronic diseases.[36] Interestingly, men in this generation are developing obesity and associated conditions such as diabetes, chronic cardiovascular disease and metabolic syndrome at younger ages and would benefit from a tailored approach to achieve weight loss, bearing in mind they may struggle with acceptance of an aging body, goal setting and finding strategies.[37] An often overlooked interventional strategy is to include their intermediaries or loved ones as possible "care partners" in the process.[37]

Among the various diets, the Mediterranean diet has proven to be the most effective diet to promote weight loss in older adults, while helping prevent age-related decline in muscle mass and bone density, preserving the immune system and sexual capacity and preventing cardiovascular disease and neurocognitive decline.[38] Supplemental calcium up to 1,200 mg/day and 800–1,000 IU of vitamin D are recommended to prevent weight loss–induced bone density reduction. It is recommended to maintain a protein intake of 1–1.2 g/kg/day, and up to 1.4 g/kg/day (20–30% of total calories) to preserve lean muscle mass and to maintain function during a weight loss intervention in older adults. Ensuring 20–30 g of protein with each meal along with a protein snack post-exercise can help cut down elevated needs during those times.[39] Time-restricted eating (8 to 10 hours) as a lifestyle change combined with modest caloric restriction, modest increase in protein consumption, and resistance exercises can help achieve weight loss with improved cardiometabolic health and functional capacity.[40] This could be a more practical approach to achieve weight loss and improve cardiometabolic health in older adults where adherence to strict caloric restriction is often impractical.

The gut microbiome plays a role in the energy metabolism and immune response resulting in systemic inflammation and insulin resistance. A diet rich in fiber, polyphenols and polyunsaturated fatty acids quality can diversify the microbiome composition influencing the metabolic capacity and enhancing the gut and systemic immune function.[41] There is emerging evidence that poor diet and obesity alter the gut microbiome and cause metabolic dysfunction, predisposing older adults to cognitive impairment due to systemic and central inflammation as well as a compromised blood–brain barrier.[42] Aging is associated with dietary changes, constipation and ingestion of multiple medications for disease management including antibiotics which cause perturbations of the gut microbiome leading to gut and systemic inflammation.[43] Furthermore, an older adult's living environment and socioeconomic status influence their diet, as meals in assisted living and nursing homes are often tailored to meet the nutritional needs of frail older adults with malnutrition and less geared towards caloric restriction and modified nutritional needs of residents who have or are at risk for obesity and sarcopenia.

Physical Activity

Physical activity is a key requirement and should be an integral part of any weight management intervention. Importantly, its effect on weight loss remains moderate, yet it still has significant health benefits.[44] A combination of aerobic and resistance exercise with caloric restriction is essential to reduce adiposity and improve physical and metabolic health.[45] The Physical Activity Guidelines for Americans recommends a multicomponent approach with aerobic, muscle-strengthening and balance exercises in older adults and this needs more emphasis in obese older adults due to the concern for postural imbalance with obesity. Robust studies recommended moderate- to high-intensity aerobic exercises to promote weight loss which is less achievable in older adults. The International Exercise Recommendations in Older Adults (ICFSR): Expert Consensus Guidelines suggest achieving this by alternate methods by intermittent intensity with resistance or interval training. Adherence to exercise in older adults with obesity is a challenge due to multiple limiting factors such as pain from osteoarthritis leading to unpleasant experiences, embarrassment of one's own appearance, rapid exhaustion due to functional limitation due to inactivity, safety concerns and lack of enjoyment with movement leading to lack of motivation.[46] Older adults may reside in various care settings apart from home, which influences the extent of the ST and physical inactivity, with higher rates of both in residential settings, aligning with higher obesity prevalence in those care settings. There exists a strong association between increased sedentary behavior and physical inactivity with obesity in older adults.[17] Older adults with obesity often perceive exercise as challenging and hence recommendations to improve light-intensity physical activity and therefore reducing ST can be beneficial to health. Aging is associated with changes in body composition with redistribution of fat mass to visceral adipose depots and reduction in bone and muscle mass and strength. In older adults with obesity, sarcopenia and hence sarcopenic obesity further impair physical function and inversely affect physical performance leading to frailty.[47]

STRESS MANAGEMENT

Stress, due to both physical (pain, inflammation, sleep deprivation and prescription glucocorticoids) and psychological stress is worse in older adults.[48] With aging there is a progression of chronic diseases, cognitive loss, psychological distress due to personal and financial losses, caregiving needs and roles and loss of independence[49] which adds to a cumulative stress burden. Stress is a risk factor which negatively influences eating patterns towards more energy-dense foods, energy homeostasis and physical inactivity.[50] Stress predisposes to the development and maintenance of obesity[51] and detrimental effects on physical and mental health in aging adults. Stress when further combined with smoking behavior leads to unfavorable changes in the composition of the gut microbiome resulting in gut microbiota dysbiosis leading to obesity.[52] Obesity increases multimorbidity, which is already prevalent in older adults, and can lead to a state of increased emotional distress.[53,54]

SLEEP

Insufficient sleep and circadian rhythm alterations in individuals predispose to metabolic stress and risk for obesity. Older adults with obesity suffer from sleep disorders with aging, further worsened by multimorbid chronic conditions, both of which activate the hypothalamic–pituitary axis, inducing a state of hypercortisolism leading to visceral obesity and metabolic syndrome.[55]

There exists a complex relationship between short duration of sleep and obesity and chronic diseases.[56,57] Epidemiological studies have shown an association of sleep loss with increased calorie intake.[58] There are studies linking negative energy balance during insufficient sleep and increased ghrelin and decreased leptin (appetite hormones) leading to increased hunger.[59,60] Low-calorie, high-protein diets have proven to influence sleep regulation promoting sleep quality, improving sleep-disordered breathing including sleep apnea and body composition in adults with obesity.[61] There is evidence that exposure to artificial light at night in older adults interferes with circadian rhythm and predisposes them to hypnotic drug use and obesity.[62,63] Prescription medications such as mirtazapine, often used to treat insomnia in older adults, coupled with a sedentary lifestyle, accelerate weight gain. Melatonin would be the recommended first-line medication for older adults with proven safety to help establish a circadian rhythm and it would be prudent to review the risk for weight gain and other side effects if other prescription hypnotics are considered,[64] as they often worsen sleep-related eating[65] promoting obesity and the risk of falls.

SOCIAL CONNECTION

Social connections are an important determinant of health and vary during the life course, and there is a dire need to understand the interaction in older adults.[66] Prevalence of social isolation and loneliness is high among older adults.[67] While earlier studies had indicated that obesity-related stigma was an underlying factor for social engagement among adults, later studies clarified that this concern exists only among young adults.[68] A recent systematic review showed an incomplete and inconclusive association with obesity.[69] The contribution of social connections to obesity differs in men and women; while marital status and social participation mattered in women, living arrangement and social participation played a role in the interaction of obesity and social connection in men.[70] The Canadian Longitudinal Study on Aging showed lower social participation among female participants with obesity than their male counterparts.[71] With the predicted rise in severe obesity, which is associated with higher rates of immobility, functional limitation and psychosocial dysfunction all of which can potentially worsen loneliness and social isolation, this would merit further study in this cohort with severe obesity.

AVOIDING TOXINS

Behavior and substance use disorders are on the rise among all adults. *Smoking* behavior, despite being lower than other age groups, still prevails (8.5%) among older adults but substance use disorders such as *opioid* use, and *alcohol* use have increased as a public health problem with population aging. All three toxins predispose older adults to unintended harm due to age-associated biological changes, social factors, increases in comorbidity and the use of medications that may interact with substances.

Older adults with obesity are at increased risk of lung diseases due to mechanical as well as metabolic alterations such as obstructive sleep apnea syndrome, obesity hypoventilation syndrome, asthma (asthma phenotype) and, likely, COPD (BMI association is still unclear). Smoking and higher BMI independently increase mortality risk and raise the index of disability-adjusted life years.[72] The above studies highlight the negative influence of smoking on the quality of life and mortality in older adults with obesity. Although older adults are less likely to quit, they are more successful when attempted.

The evidence linking obesity and increased alcohol consumption had been conflicting in earlier studies but recent literature is beginning to show associations with decision-making deficits.[73] A prospective cohort study on post-bariatric surgery patients identified an increased risk for alcohol use disorder (AUD) symptoms among Roux-en-Y gastric bypass (RYGB) highlighting the need for AUD screening, assessment, referral and treatment among this class of post-bariatric surgery patients.[74] High-risk individuals with poor lifestyle practices such as sedentary behavior, reduced physical activity, insufficient sleep and increased alcohol consumption have a higher predisposition to obesity and should be targeted for preventive therapies using lifestyle medicine pillars.

The prevalence of opioid use disorder has increased among adults with obesity due to the high burden of chronic pain due to osteoarthritis, low back pain, neuropathy, fibromyalgia and migraine among adults with obesity,[75-77] further worsened by aging. Although studies have reassured that pain is not undertreated in patients with obesity, further research is needed to ensure that they are not overtreated with pain medications[78] as it can increase their risk for respiratory failure, as seen in patients with obesity and heart failure with preserved ejection fraction (the most common form of heart failure in individuals with obesity) who have narrow ventilatory reserve.[79] Lifestyle interventions can be an effective intervention to promote weight loss and improve mobility and function in this growing segment of the population. This intervention could reduce the burden of prescription opioids which has partly led to the opioid epidemic and mortality in this high-risk population.

FUTURE OF THE LIFESTYLE MEDICINE ROLE IN CARING FOR OLDER ADULTS WITH OBESITY

New clinical models of obesity care will need to use a team-based multidisciplinary approach due to the multisystem involvement of the disease, complicated by aging and functional impairment, with an ongoing need for behavior change.[54,80] With the onset of disability due to the aforementioned factors, there exists an under-recognized need for assistance in navigating health care due to the multiple comorbid conditions. This results in a need for multiple health care provider visits, addressing competing health priorities, urgent need for ED visits and non-elective hospital admissions for acute medical and surgical conditions, as obesity severity increases. Currently, the Veterans Affairs health system adopts a population-based, behavioral modification program to offer a comprehensive, evidence-based, lifestyle modification intervention (CLMI) to veterans with overweight and obesity. In 2011, Centers for Medicare and Medicaid approved Intensive Behavioral Therapy for obesity counseling in adults. Both programs highlight the need for a behavioral approach to weight management with an emphasis on diet and physical activity. Yet, the uptake of these lifestyle modification standalone programs by multimorbid older adults with obesity and functional impairment remains a concern.[81] This could partly be explained by the heterogeneity of the older population in contrast to the middle-aged adults due to the cumulative burden of multimorbidity. Hence an obesity-focused and patient-centered medical home model involving a multidisciplinary team with a primary care provider, dietician, physical therapist (if pain and musculoskeletal impairments restrict self-directed exercise), behavioral therapist/programs, use of coach, social worker, exercise physiologist and multiple sub-specialists depending on the severity of the disease and system involvement will benefit the older adult with obesity. The primary care provider and a clinic care management program would serve as the anchor for the patient in the proposed patient- and obesity-centered model of care.

Future health care delivery models should involve community-based organizations and programs to help older adults with obesity as these programs have proven to be effective public health strategies among youth with both a preventive and curative approach. Current programs for older adults exist for diseases such as dementia and other chronic diseases focusing on self-management education for patients as well as caregivers. Since obesity prevalence is rising among older adults and is often the underlying driver of chronic cardiometabolic disorders, it is prudent to strategize a multipronged approach with goals of prevention and cure. This could involve education centered around healthy nutrition (access to food prescription programs) and incorporation of physical activity across settings with the intervention approach integrated with support services and partnerships with agencies which currently promote healthy aging.

Concurrently, changes at a societal level involving capacity building and macropolicy changes focusing on the built environment for older adults to access neighborhood parks and fitness centers, senior centers with education offerings and fitness equipment for varying levels of physical impairments, serving small portion sizes with quality serving (with a focus on whole grains, low caloric density, protein- and fiber-rich meals and reducing calorie dense snacks) and in residential care settings deserves focus and implementation. The current built obesogenic ecosystem needs to be modified to promote more active outdoor lifestyles which could involve urban planning, availability of public transportation and access to fresh produce.[82] Health care providers need to be mindful that older adults with obesity come from various residential settings and have varying degrees of resource availability, disability and caregiver support, limiting their ability to access resources. Above all, health care practitioners caring for older adults need to understand the challenges of enabling behavior change among this age group. They play a key role in helping patients engage in lifestyle medicine practices and provide education highlighting the linkage of increasing BMI with chronic diseases. All of this should be delivered without stigma, and should help improve self-efficacy, while providing ongoing support to achieve meaningful weight loss targets, with physical function and enhanced quality of life as overarching goals, along with weight loss maintenance.[83]

CLINICAL APPLICATIONS

- Older adults across all living environments are at increased risk for obesity and multiple obesity-related comorbid conditions which impact quality of life, increasing multimorbidity and mortality.
- Healthy plant-based diets with moderate caloric restriction, time-restricted eating, modest increase in protein consumption and resistance exercises can help achieve weight loss.
- Combined aerobic and resistance exercise with caloric restriction is essential for improving cardiometabolic health and functional capacity.

- A tailored approach is pivotal, taking into consideration patients' functional limitations, underlying stress, presence of sleep disorder, chronic pain and psychological conditions in the context and limitations of the living environment.
- A multidisciplinary team-based model of care with behavioral and coaching support to enable lifestyle change will help to improve adherence and successful weight loss in older adults.

ABBREVIATIONS

BMI: Body Mass Index
CLMI: Comprehensive, Evidence-Based, Lifestyle Modification Intervention
COPD: Chronic Obstructive Pulmonary Disease
CVD: Cardiovascular Disease
ICFSR: International Exercise Recommendations in Older Adults
IU: International Units
NHANES: National Health and Nutrition Examination Survey
ST: Sedentary time

Conflicts of Interest: There are no potential conflicts of interest to disclose.

REFERENCES

1. Hales CM, Fryar CD, Carroll MD, Freedman DS, Ogden CL. Trends in obesity and severe obesity prevalence in US youth and adults by sex and age. *JAMA.* 2018;319(16):1723–1725.
2. Felix HC, Bradway C, Chisholm L, Pradhan R, Weech-Maldonado R. Prevalence of moderate to severe obesity among U.S. nursing home residents, 2000–2010. *Res Gerontol Nurs.* 2015;8(4):173–178. doi:10.3928/19404921-20150223-01
3. Matheson EM, King DE, Everett CJ. Healthy lifestyle habits and mortality in overweight and obese individuals. *J Am Board Fam Med.* 2012;25(1):9–15. doi:10.3122/jabfm.2012.01.110164
4. Batsis JA, Mackenzie TA, Bartels SJ, Sahakyan KR, Somers VK, Lopez-Jimenez F. Diagnostic accuracy of body mass index to identify obesity in older adults: NHANES 1999–2004. *Int J Obes.* 2016;40(5):761–767. doi:10.1038/ijo.2015.243
5. Friedman SM. Lifestyle (medicine) and healthy aging. *Clin Geriatr Med.* 2020;36(4):645–653. doi:10.1016/j.cger.2020.06.007
6. American College of Lifestyle Medicine. Core competencies. Accessed January 7, 2024. https://lifestylemedicine.org/Core-Competencies/
7. Nguyen X-MT, Li Y, Wang DD, et al. Impact of 8 lifestyle factors on mortality and life expectancy among United States veterans: the Million Veteran Program. *Am J Clin Nutr.* 2023;119(1):127–135. doi:10.1016/j.ajcnut.2023.10.032
8. Vodovotz Y, Barnard N, Hu FB, et al. Prioritized research for the prevention, treatment, and reversal of chronic disease: recommendations from the Lifestyle Medicine Research Summit. *Front Med.* 2020;7:585744. doi:10.3389/fmed.2020.585744
9. Stampfer MJ, Hu FB, Manson JE, Rimm EB, Willett WC. Primary prevention of coronary heart disease in women through diet and lifestyle. *N Engl J Med.* 2000;343(11):1496–1498. doi:10.1056/nejm200007063430103

10. Hu FB, Manson JE, Stampfer MJ, et al. Diet, lifestyle, and the risk of type 2 diabetes mellitus in women. *N Engl J Med.* 2001;345(11):790–797. doi:10.1097/00006254-200203000-00018
11. Li Y, Schoufour J, Wang DD, et al. Healthy lifestyle and life expectancy free of cancer, cardiovascular disease, and type 2 diabetes: prospective cohort study. *BMJ.* 2020;368:l6669. doi:10.1136/bmj.l6669
12. Loef M, Walach H. The combined effects of healthy lifestyle behaviors on all-cause mortality: a systematic review and meta-analysis. *Prev Med.* 2012;55(3):163–170. doi:10.1016/j.ypmed.2012.06.017
13. The Older Population. 2020. Accessed December 12, 2023. https://www.census.gov/library/publications/2023/decennial/c2020br-07.html
14. Buckley J. Baby boomers, obesity, and social change. *Obes Res Clin Pract.* 2008;2(2):73–82. doi:10.1016/j.orcp.2008.04.002
15. Dai J, Dai W, Li WQ. Trends in physical activity and sedentary time among U.S. adults with diabetes: 2007–2020. *Diabetes Metab Syndr Clin Res Rev.* 2023;17(10):102874. doi:10.1016/j.dsx.2023.102874
16. Manini TM, Everhart JE, Patel KV, et al. Daily activity energy expenditure and mortality among older adults. *JAMA.* 2006;296(2):171–179. doi:10.1001/jama.296.2.171
17. Silveira EA, Mendonça CR, Delpino FM, et al. Sedentary behavior, physical inactivity, abdominal obesity and obesity in adults and older adults: a systematic review and meta-analysis. *Clin Nutr ESPEN.* 2022;50:63–73. doi:10.1016/j.clnesp.2022.06.001
18. U.S. Department of Health and Human Services, Physical Activity Guidelines Advisory Committee Scientific Report. U.S. Department of Health and Human Services; 2018. Accessed January 6, 2024. https://health.gov/our-work/nutrition-physical-activity/physical-activity-guidelines/current-guidelines/scientific-report
19. Harvey JA, Chastin SFM, Skelton DA. Prevalence of sedentary behavior in older adults: a systematic review. *Int J Environ Res Public Health.* 2013;10(12):6645–6661. doi:10.3390/ijerph10126645
20. Bellettiere J, Lamonte MJ, Evenson KR, et al. Sedentary behavior and cardiovascular disease in older women: the OPACH Study. *Circulation.* 2019;139(8):1036–1046. doi:10.1161/CIRCULATIONAHA.118.035312
21. Elmaleh-Sachs A, Schwartz JL, Bramante CT, Nicklas JM, Gudzune KA, Jay M. Obesity management in adults: a review. *JAMA.* 2023;330(20):2000–2015. doi:10.1001/jama.2023.19897
22. Browne J, Morey MC, Beckham JC, et al. Diet quality and exercise in older veterans with PTSD: a pilot study. *Transl Behav Med.* 2021;12(11):2116–2122.
23. Wing RR. Achieving weight and activity goals among diabetes prevention program lifestyle participants. *Obes Res.* 2004;12(9):1426–1434. doi:10.1038/oby.2004.179
24. Fall T, Mendelson M, Speliotes EK. Recent advances in human genetics and epigenetics of adiposity: pathway to precision medicine? *Gastroenterology.* 2017;152(7):1695–1706. doi:10.1053/j.gastro.2017.01.054
25. Garvey WT. Is obesity or adiposity-based chronic disease curable: the set point theory, the environment, and second-generation medications. *Endocr Pract.* 2022;28(2):214–222. doi:10.1016/j.eprac.2021.11.082
26. Starr KNP, Do SRM, Bales CW. Obesity and physical frailty in older adults: a scoping review of lifestyle intervention trials. *J Am Med Dir Assoc.* 2014;15(4):240–250. doi:10.1016/j.jamda.2013.11.008
27. Colleluori G, Villareal DT. Aging, obesity, sarcopenia, and the effect of diet and exercise intervention. *Exp Gerontol.* 2021;155:111561. doi:10.1016/j.exger.2021.111561
28. Volpp KG, Berkowitz SA, Sharma SV, et al. Food is medicine: a presidential advisory from the American Heart Association. *Circulation.* 2023;148(18):1417–1439. doi:10.1161/CIR.0000000000001182

29. Boeing H, Bechthold A, Bub A, et al. Critical review: vegetables and fruit in the prevention of chronic diseases. *Eur J Nutr.* 2012;51(6):637–663. doi:10.1007/s00394-012-0380-y
30. Chang AR, Bailey-Davis L. Food is medicine, but are produce prescriptions? *Diabetes Care.* 2023;46(6):1140–1142. doi:10.2337/dci23-0020
31. Rattan SIS. Biogerontology: research status, challenges and opportunities. *Acta Biomed.* 2018;89(2):291–301. doi:10.23750/abm.v89i2.7403
32. Hu FB. Diet strategies for promoting healthy aging and longevity: an epidemiological perspective. *J Intern Med.* 2023:1–24. doi:10.1111/joim.13728
33. Satija A, Malik V, Rimm EB, Sacks F, Willett W, Hu FB. Changes in intake of plant-based diets and weight change: results from 3 prospective cohort studies. *Am J Clin Nutr.* 2019;110(3):574–582. doi:10.1093/ajcn/nqz049
34. Sotos-Prieto M, Struijk EA, Teresa Fung T, et al. Association between the quality of plant-based diets and risk of frailty. *J Cachexia Sarcopenia Muscle.* 2022;13:2854–2862. doi:10.1002/jcsm.13077.
35. Shen A. Religious attendance, healthy lifestyles, and perceived health: a comparison of baby boomers with the silent generation. *J Relig Health.* 2019;58(4):1235–1245. doi:10.1007/s10943-018-0736-6
36. Buckley J. Baby boomers, obesity, and social change. *Obes Res Clin Pract.* 2008;2(2):73–82. doi:10.1016/j.orcp.2008.04.002
37. James DCS, Wirth CK, Harville C, Efunbumi O. Weight-loss strategies used by baby boomer men: a mixed methods approach. *J Hum Nutr Diet.* 2016;29(2):217–224. doi:10.1111/jhn.12305
38. Hanna AMR. Solving the obesity crisis in older adults with the Mediterranean diet: policy brief. *J Nutr Health Aging.* 2023;27(11):966–971. doi:10.1007/s12603-023-1995-9
39. Al-Nimr RI. Optimal protein intake during weight loss interventions in older adults with obesity. *J Nutr Gerontol Geriatr.* 2019;38(1):50–68. doi:10.1080/21551197.2018.1544533
40. Panda S, Maier G, Villareal DT. Targeting energy intake and circadian biology to engage mechanisms of aging in older adults with obesity: calorie restriction and time-restricted eating. *J Gerontol A Biol Sci Med Sci.* 2023;78:79–85. doi:10.1093/gerona/glad069
41. Strasser B, Wolters M, Weyh C, Krüger K, Ticinesi A. The effects of lifestyle and diet on gut microbiota composition, inflammation and muscle performance in our aging society. *Nutrients.* 2021;13(6). doi:10.3390/nu13062045
42. Leigh SJ, Morris MJ. Diet, inflammation and the gut microbiome: mechanisms for obesity-associated cognitive impairment. *Biochim Biophys Acta Mol Basis Dis.* 2020;1866(6):165767. doi:10.1016/j.bbadis.2020.165767
43. Lee CJ, Sears CL, Maruthur N. Gut microbiome and its role in obesity and insulin resistance. *Ann N Y Acad Sci.* 2020;1461(1):37–52. doi:10.1111/nyas.14107
44. Oppert JM, Ciangura C, Bellicha A. Physical activity and exercise for weight loss and maintenance in people living with obesity. *Rev Endocr Metab Disord.* 2023;24(5):937–949. doi:10.1007/s11154-023-09805-5
45. Waters DL, Aguirre L, Gurney B, et al. Effect of aerobic or resistance exercise, or both, on intermuscular and visceral fat and physical and metabolic function in older adults with obesity while dieting. *Journals Gerontol A Biol Sci Med Sci.* 2022;77(1):131–139. doi:10.1093/gerona/glab111
46. Collado-Mateo D, Lavín-Pérez AM, Peñacoba C, et al. Key factors associated with adherence to physical exercise in patients with chronic diseases and older adults: an umbrella review. *Int J Environ Res Public Health.* 2021;18(4):1–24. doi:10.3390/ijerph18042023

47. Rolland Y, Lauwers-Cances V, Cristini C, et al. Difficulties with physical function associated with obesity, sarcopenia, and sarcopenic-obesity in community-dwelling elderly women: the EPIDOS (EPIDemiologie de l'OSteoporose) study. *Am J Clin Nutr.* 2009;89(6):1895–1900. doi:10.3945/ajcn.2008.26950
48. Charles ST, Piazza JR, Mogle J, Sliwinski MJ, Almeida DM. The wear-and-tear of daily stressors on mental health. *Psychol Sci.* 2013;24(5):733–741. doi:10.1177/0956797612462222
49. Lavretsky H, Newhouse PA. Stress, inflammation, and aging. *Am J Geriatr Psychiatry.* 2012;20(9):729–733. doi:10.1097/JGP.0b013e31826573cf
50. Dye L, Boyle NB, Champ C, Lawton C. The relationship between obesity and cognitive health and decline. *Proc Nutr Soc.* 2017;76(4):443–454. doi:10.1017/S0029665117002014
51. van der Valk ES, Savas M, van Rossum EFC. Stress and obesity: are there more susceptible individuals? *Curr Obes Rep.* 2018;7(2):193–203. doi:10.1007/s13679-018-0306-y
52. Geng J, Ni Q, Sun W, Li L, Feng X. The links between gut microbiota and obesity and obesity related diseases. *Biomed Pharmacother.* 2022;147:112678. doi:10.1016/j.biopha.2022.112678
53. Marengoni A, Angleman S, Melis R, et al. Aging with multimorbidity: a systematic review of the literature. *Ageing Res Rev.* 2011;10(4):430–439. doi:10.1016/j.arr.2011.03.003
54. Lynch DH, Petersen CL, Fanous MM, et al. The relationship between multimorbidity, obesity and functional impairment in older adults. *J Am Geriatr Soc.* 2022;70(5):1442–1449. doi:10.1111/jgs.17683
55. Section PE. The role of stress and the hypothalamic-pituitary-adrenal axis in the pathogenesis of the metabolic syndrome: Neuro-endocrine and target tissue-related causes. *Int J Obes.* 2000;6(2):50–55. Available from: www.nature.com/ijo
56. Dashti HS, Scheer FAJL, Jacques PF, Lamon-Fava S, Ordovás JM. Short sleep duration and dietary intake: Epidemiologic evidence, mechanisms, and health implications. *Adv Nutr.* 2015;6(6):648–659. doi:10.3945/an.115.008623
57. Bayon V, Leger D, Gomez-Merino D, Vecchierini MF, Chennaoui M. Sleep debt and obesity. *Ann Med.* 2014;46(5):264–272. doi:10.3109/07853890.2014.931103
58. Patterson RE, Emond JA, Natarajan L, et al. Short sleep duration is associated with higher energy intake and expenditure among African-American and non-Hispanic white adults. *J Nutr.* 2014;144(4):461–466. doi:10.3945/jn.113.186890
59. Spiegel K, Leproult R, L'Hermite-Balériaux M, Copinschi G, Penev PD, Van Cauter E. Leptin levels are dependent on sleep duration: relationships with sympathovagal balance, carbohydrate regulation, cortisol, and thyrotropin. *J Clin Endocrinol Metab.* 2004;89(11):5762–5771. doi:10.1210/jc.2004-1003
60. Broussard JL, Kilkus JM, Delebecque F, et al. Elevated ghrelin predicts food intake during experimental sleep restriction. *Obesity.* 2016;24(1):132–138. doi:10.1002/oby.21321
61. Javaheri FSH, Ostadrahimi AR, Nematy M, Arabi SM, Amini M. The effects of low calorie, high protein diet on body composition, duration and sleep quality on obese adults: a randomized clinical trial. *Heal Sci Reports.* 2023;6(11). doi:10.1002/hsr2.1699
62. Touitou Y, Reinberg A, Touitou D. Association between light at night, melatonin secretion, sleep deprivation, and the internal clock: health impacts and mechanisms of circadian disruption. *Life Sci.* 2017;173:94–106. doi:10.1016/j.lfs.2017.02.008
63. Min JY, Min KB. Outdoor artificial nighttime light and use of hypnotic medications in older adults: a population-based cohort study. *J Clin Sleep Med.* 2018;14(11):1903–1910. doi:10.5664/jcsm.7490
64. Cardinali DP, Brown GM, Pandi-Perumal SR. Melatonin's benefits and risks as a therapy for sleep disturbances in the elderly: current insights. *Nat Sci Sleep.* 2022;14:1843–1855. doi:10.2147/NSS.S380465

65. Nzwalo H, Ferreira L, Peralta R, Bentes C. Sleep-related eating disorder secondary to zolpidem. *BMJ Case Rep.* 2013:10–13. doi:10.1136/bcr-2012-008003
66. Pachucki MC, Goodman E. Social relationships and obesity: benefits of incorporating a lifecourse perspective. *Curr Obes Rep.* 2015;4(2):217–223. doi:10.1007/s13679-015-0145-z
67. Freedman A, Nicolle J. Social isolation and loneliness: the new geriatric giants. *Can Fam Physician.* 2020;66:176–182. https://www.cfp.ca/content/cfp/66/3/176.full.pdf
68. Zettel-Watson L, Britton M. The impact of obesity on the social participation of older adults. *J Gen Psychol.* 2008;135(4):409–424. doi:10.3200/GENP.135.4.409-424
69. Hajek A, Kretzler B, König HH. The association between obesity and social isolation as well as loneliness in the adult population: a systematic review. *Diabetes Metab Syndr Obes.* 2021;14:2765–2773. doi:10.2147/DMSO.S313873
70. Hosseini Z, Veenstra G, Khan NA, Conklin AI. Associations between social connections, their interactions, and obesity differ by gender: a population-based, cross-sectional analysis of the Canadian Longitudinal Study on Aging. *PLoS One.* 2020;15(7):1–19. doi:10.1371/journal.pone.0235977
71. Rao DP, Patel P, Roberts KC, Thompson W. Obesity and healthy aging: social, functional, and mental well-being among older Canadians. *Heal Promot Chronic Dis Prev Canada.* 2018;38(12):437–444. doi:10.24095/hpcdp.38.12.01
72. Kyu HH, Abate D, Abate KH, et al. Global, regional, and national disability-adjusted life-years (DALYs) for 359 diseases and injuries and healthy life expectancy (HALE) for 195 countries and territories, 1990–2017: a systematic analysis for the Global Burden of Disease Study 2017. *Lancet.* 2018;392(10159):1859–1922. doi:10.1016/S0140-6736(18)32335-3
73. Agarwal K, Demiral SB, Manza P, Volkow ND, Joseph PV. Relationship between BMI and alcohol consumption levels in decision making. *Int J Obes.* 2021;45(11):2455–2463. doi:10.1038/s41366-021-00919-x
74. King WC, Chen JY, Courcoulas AP, et al. Alcohol and other substance use after bariatric surgery: prospective evidence from a U.S. multicenter cohort study. *Surg Obes Relat Dis.* 2017;13(8):1392–1402. doi:10.1016/j.soard.2017.03.021
75. Okifuji A, Hare BD. The association between chronic pain and obesity. *J Pain Res.* 2015;8:399–408. doi:10.2147/JPR.S55598
76. Kulkarni K, Karssiens T, Kumar V, Pandit H. Obesity and osteoarthritis. *Maturitas.* 2016;89:22–28. doi:10.1016/j.maturitas.2016.04.006
77. Shiri R, Karppinen J, Leino-Arjas P, Solovieva S, Viikari-Juntura E. The association between obesity and low back pain: a meta-analysis. *Am J Epidemiol.* 2010;171(2):135–154. doi:10.1093/aje/kwp356
78. Cho G, Chang VW. Obesity and the receipt of prescription pain medications in the US. *J Gen Intern Med.* 2021;36(9):2631–2638. doi:10.1007/s11606-020-06581-9
79. Babb TG, Balmain BN, Tomlinson AR, et al. Ventilatory limitations in patients with HFpEF and obesity. *Respir Physiol Neurobiol.* 2023;318:104167. doi:10.1016/j.resp.2023.104167
80. Masood B, Moorthy M. Causes of obesity: a review. *Clin Med J R Coll Physicians London.* 2023;23(4):284–291. doi:10.7861/clinmed.2023-0168
81. Dewar S, Bynum J, Batsis JA. Uptake of obesity intensive behavioral treatment codes in Medicare beneficiaries, 2012–2015. *J Gen Intern Med.* 2019;35(1):368–370. doi:10.1007/s11606-019-05437-1
82. Caballero B. Humans against obesity: who will win? *Adv Nutr.* 2019;10:S4–S9. doi:10.1093/advances/nmy055
83. Dicker D, Alfadda AA, Coutinho W, et al. Patient motivation to lose weight: importance of healthcare professional support, goals, and self-efficacy. *Eur J Intern Med.* 2021;91:10–16. doi:10.1016/j.ejim.2021.01.019

25 Osteoporosis and Bone Health

Jatupol Kositsawat, Faryal Mirza and Patrick P. Coll

INTRODUCTION

As life evolved on Earth from unicellular organisms to multi-cellular organisms, there came a point at which larger organisms became structurally more complex. For many, this structural complexity included a support system or skeleton. Some organisms, such as insects, developed an exoskeleton and others including those that eventually evolved to be homo sapiens developed an endoskeleton. In some animals, such as sharks, the endoskeleton is cartilage. However, most land-based animals, including humans, have an endoskeleton composed of bone.

There is a complex set of cellular and sub-cellular processes involved in bone formation. At a very basic level, osteoblasts build bone, and osteoclasts break down bone. This is a dynamic, lifelong process. In human embryos and young adults, there is more bone production than bone breakdown, but later in life, the reverse is true. Though a decrease in bone mass is a normal part of aging, there are many factors that can accelerate this decrease in bone mass.

Our bony skeleton allows us to do many things that would be otherwise impossible. Things we take for granted such as walking, jumping, using a computer keyboard and holding a baby. It also provides protection for vital parts of our body such as our brain and spinal cord. Because we exert mechanical stress on our bony skeleton it must be sufficiently strong to withstand those stresses and maintain its structural integrity. The weight of our body alone when standing results in significant mechanical stress, which is increased when we move or fall. When sufficient force is applied, even healthy bone can break. However, the bone that is weakened because of a decrease in bone mass is more likely to break from a force or forces that would not damage normal-density bone. A sudden mechanical force such as a fall can result in the painful fracture of a large bone such as the femur. Micro asymptomatic fractures are also more likely to occur in low-density bone. These are particularly common in the vertebral bodies of older adults and over time can contribute to a decrease in height and curvature of the spine.

Osteoporosis is defined as a systemic skeletal disease characterized by low bone mass and micro-architectural deterioration of bone tissue, with a consequent increase in bone fragility and susceptibility to fracture. Osteopenia is a decrease in bone mineral density below normal reference values, yet not low enough to meet the diagnostic criteria to be considered osteoporosis.

DOI: 10.1201/9781032638560-28

In the United States (US), an estimated 10 million people 50 years of age and older have osteoporosis. Most of these are women, but about 2 million are men. Just over 43 million more people, including 16 million men have low bone mass consistent with osteopenia, putting them at increased risk for osteoporosis.[1] Large bone fractures are painful, can lead to both temporary and permanent disability, may require surgical repair and can increase mortality.[2]

Lifestyle factors including most importantly nutrition and physical exercise play an important role in bone health for older adults. Smoking cigarettes and excessive alcohol consumption both have a toxic effect on bone density. Because of the strong connection between renal function and bone health, renal toxins such as organochlorine pesticides can indirectly cause osteoporosis. There are also many medications that can have a negative impact on bone density, most importantly glucocorticoids. Excessive thyroid hormone replacement can also result in a decrease in bone density. Though there is evidence that bisphosphonates can help preserve bone density in patients with osteoporosis, they can in some situations increase long-bone fragility. There is also a growing body of evidence that both air and water pollutants can contribute to low bone density.[3-5] Cadmium has been recognized as being toxic for bone and not only is cadmium an environmental pollutant, but it is also found in many tobacco products.

NUTRITION AND BONE HEALTH

Good nutrition is important for bone health. Older adults however are at risk for nutritional deficiency, including nutritional deficiencies that result in reduced bone density.[6] Contributing factors include reduced taste and smell, poor oral health and associated trouble with chewing, reduced absorption of certain nutrients, inadequate education regarding healthy food choices and for some, reduced access to healthy foods. In the United States, approximately one-third of older adults are deficient in one or more micronutrients. A high percentage of older adults consume less than the Recommended Dietary Allowance (RDA) of protein (13% of men and 21% of women aged >70 years of age).

Lifestyle interventions including good nutrition and exercise (discussed elsewhere in this chapter) are preferable to the use of medications to prevent and treat osteoporosis.[7] It is also worth noting that whereas the medications used to treat osteoporosis primarily impact bone, good nutrition and exercise have a positive impact on both bone and muscle which is particularly important since many patients with osteoporosis also have sarcopenia (osteosarcopenia).[8] Multifaceted nutritional interventions can ameliorate deteriorating bone health through three major mechanistic pathways including oxidative stress, inflammation and anabolic/anticatabolic pathways.[9] Correction of insufficient micro- and macronutrient intake[10] may slow down or improve musculoskeletal aging. Micronutrients include trace elements, minerals and vitamins, whereas macronutrients include protein and fatty acids. In addition to discussing specific micro- and macronutrients, the importance of an overall healthy diet to optimize bone health, including Mediterranean[11] and vegetarian/vegan[12] diets will be discussed.

Finally, it is also important to note that combining healthy lifestyle practices has a positive impact on bone health. Data from the Tromsø longitudinal population-based study in Norway that included men and women aged 24–84 years, showed that a combination of healthy lifestyle practices (increased physical activity, avoiding weight loss and not smoking) reduced bone loss and reduced the incidence of distal radial fractures.[13]

DIETARY NUTRIENTS

PROTEIN

Protein is essential for collagen synthesis, a major component of bone. Collagen makes up about 50% of bone volume and one-third of bone mass.[14] Protein also influences insulin-like growth factor-1 (IGF-1) production. IGF-1 promotes the growth of various cells including osteoblasts and stimulates intestinal absorption of calcium and the renal reabsorption of phosphate. The Framingham Osteoporosis Study showed that older men and women with less dietary protein intake experienced more bone loss.[15] The same study did not find any adverse effects from increased animal protein intake. Though there is a concern that excess protein intake may lead to a negative calcium balance due to high acid renal load and resulting urinary calcium loss, this is uncommon in older adults.

VITAMIN D

Vitamin D promotes calcium absorption in the gastrointestinal tract and helps maintain adequate serum calcium and phosphorus concentrations which facilitates normal bone mineralization. Vitamin D is an essential component of a healthy diet, but in distinction to other vitamins which need to be ingested, the body can produce vitamin D. Though it is possible to get sufficient vitamin D from nutritional sources (Table 25.1), for many older adults, supplementation may be necessary. There are different opinions regarding the optimal serum vitamin D level ranging from a low of 30 ng/mL to a high of 60 ng/mL, with most recommendations favoring a higher level in older adults. It is also worth noting that as a fat-soluble vitamin, one can take too much vitamin D which can result in significant health issues, including negative impacts on bone health.

According to the European Society of Clinical and Economical Aspects of Osteoporosis, Osteoarthritis and Musculoskeletal Diseases (ESCEO) working group, 1,000 units of vitamin D supplementation is recommended for those at high risk for vitamin D deficiency, which includes many older adults.[16] However as noted above if someone is mindful about eating foods rich in vitamin D, supplementation may not be necessary.

Even within the medical community, the need for vitamin D supplementation is controversial.[17] Currently the US Preventive Services Task Force (USPSTF) has recommended against vitamin D supplementation to prevent falls in community-dwelling adults ≥65 years of age. The USPSTF also recommends against both

TABLE 25.1
Dietary Sources of Calcium and Vitamin D

Dietary Sources	Ca (mg)	Vitamin D (IU)
Dairy Products and Plant Milk Alternatives		
Low-fat plain yogurt (8 ounces)	448	116
1% Low-fat milk (8 ounces)	305	117
Cheese, low, or fat free (1.5 ounces)	115–485	85
Soy milk (8 ounces)	301	119
Almond milk (1 cup)	442	107
Vegetables		
Mustard spinach (1 cup)	284	n/a
Collard greens (1 cup)	268	n/a
Spinach (1 cup)	245	n/a
Kale (1 cup)	177	n/a
Mushroom, raw (1 cup)	n/a	114–1,110
Protein Foods		
Tofu (1/2 cup)	434	n/a
Sardines, canned (3 ounces)	325	160
Salmon (3 ounces)	181	385–570
Rainbow trout (3 ounces)	n/a	645
Fruit		
Orange juice, fortified (1 cup)	349	100

vitamin D and calcium supplementation for the primary prevention of fractures in community-dwelling postmenopausal women.[18] The amount of vitamin D necessary to optimize bone health and the dose and frequency of vitamin D supplementation are unclear. In one randomized clinical trial in Canada, high-dose vitamin D supplementation (≥4,000 IU/d) for 3 years did not improve bone density among healthy adults (mean age 62.2 years).[19] Intermittent (monthly and annually) high-dose vitamin D supplementation has been shown to increase falls and fractures and should be avoided.[20–22]

CALCIUM AND PHOSPHORUS

Calcium is the most abundant mineral in the body. Together with phosphorus, they are the key components of inorganic bone matrix including calcium phosphate hydroxyapatite that contribute to bone rigidity. Dairy products are the most common and best dietary source of calcium. Dietary sources of calcium are summarized in Table 25.1. The RDA of calcium is 800–1,200 mg/day. Ensuring adequate calcium intake in the diet is preferred but for older adults who do not have adequate calcium from dietary sources, supplementation may be necessary. However, as noted above there continues to be uncertainty regarding the benefits of calcium supplementation on bone health. If supplementation is being considered, calcium carbonate is less expensive and contains more elemental calcium than calcium citrate. However, its absorption is less than calcium citrate for those who have decreased gastric acid secretion, which is more common in older adults and especially those who take gastric acid-reducing medications such as proton pump inhibitors. Potential side effects of calcium supplements include gastrointestinal symptoms including constipation and renal and urinary tract stone formation. There is no evidence of benefits for total intake to be above 1,500 mg/day.[23]

Phytoestrogens

Some foods, especially soybeans, contain phytoestrogens. They have structural similarities to 17-estradiol and have been shown to have a positive impact on bone health without the concerning side effects of estrogens. The effect of phytoestrogens on bone health may vary according to the dose, duration and age.[24] There are four phenolic compounds classified as phytoestrogens including isoflavones, stilbene, coumestan and lignan, with isoflavones being the most common. Phytoestrogen benefits on bone health are primarily related to decreased osteoclast-induced bone loss, though they may also increase calcium absorption. Though there remains uncertainty regarding the benefits of phytoestrogens, in a randomized clinical trial, a daily supplement of the phytoestrogen genistein for 24 months was shown to benefit BMD in osteopenic postmenopausal women.[25] However, data are lacking on the impact of phytoestrogens on fracture risk.[26] To date, most clinical trials involving phytoestrogens have not shown consistent benefits regarding the prevention of bone loss or fracture risk.[10]

Unsaturated Fatty Acids

Unsaturated fatty acids have anti-inflammatory effects and have also been shown to increase calcium absorption and decrease calcium excretion. Recent National Health and Nutrition Examination Survey (NHANES) data from 2011 to 2018 showed an association between increased fatty acid intakes (saturated, polyunsaturated and monounsaturated) and higher BMD in adults 20–59 years of age.[27] However, in another study looking at the impact of dietary omega-3 (ω-3) fatty acids which are polyunsaturated fatty acids, on fractures, no benefit was found.

Iron

Iron (Fe) is important for most basic cellular activities. It plays an essential role in collagen synthesis and vitamin D metabolism.[28] Fe deficiency is the most prevalent nutritional deficiency, especially in young children and premenopausal women. It is also common in older adults due to poorer absorption. Inappropriate long-term use of proton pump inhibitors can have a potential negative impact on critical nutrients' absorption, including Fe.[29] Fe deficiency has been shown to be associated with osteopenia or osteoporosis in animal models and in several clinical observations.

Dietary Fiber

There is evidence that dietary fiber may have a positive impact on bone density.[30] It is thought that fiber promotes an increase in gut microbiome production of short-chain fatty acids (SCFA), particularly butyrate, the primary metabolites of microbial fermentation in the gut.[31] SCFA are regulators of osteoclast metabolism and bone mass in vivo.[32]

Vitamin K

Vitamin K is essential for bone health.[33] It regulates many bone-related proteins, osteoblasts and bone resorption. Its level can also be affected by vitamin K antagonist anticoagulants. Low serum vitamin K1 may increase the risk of fracture and lower BMD. However, data on the amount of vitamin K needed for optimal bone health remain inconclusive.

DIETARY PATTERNS

As has been pointed out above, many nutrients have an impact on bone health. Therefore, rather than concentrating on a specific nutrient and specific dietary supplements, recommendations regarding someone's overall diet may be a more satisfactory approach to promoting good bone health.

Mediterranean Diet

Epidemiological studies have demonstrated that Mediterranean countries have a lower incidence of osteoporosis and osteoporotic fractures compared to northern European countries. It is felt that lifestyle factors and especially dietary differences are in large part responsible for these findings. The Mediterranean diet is based on olive oil (monounsaturated fatty acid), fruits, vegetables, legumes, dairy products (especially fermented dairy products), fish and poultry and minimal consumption of processed foods. Of all the dietary patterns reviewed, the Mediterranean diet shows the greatest benefits for bone health.[10] Data from the Women's Health Initiatives showed its association with lower risk for hip fracture in postmenopausal women.[34]

The Mediterranean diet includes many antioxidant nutrients including phytochemicals (carotenoids), polyphenols in olive oil, resveratrol in red wine and omega-3 polyunsaturated fatty acids, vitamin C, vitamin E, among others. Polyphenols from olives have both antioxidative and anti-inflammatory effects which favor the growth and differentiation of pro-osteoblasts and decrease osteoclasts which break down bone. Most fish contain high-quality protein, omega-3 fatty acids, vitamin A, vitamin D and minerals including calcium, zinc, selenium and iodine, which all promote good bone health. In addition, Mediterranean diets high in whole grains, and legumes provide B vitamins, calcium and phytochemicals.

Vegetarian and Vegan Diet

Plant-based diets are becoming increasingly more popular. Fruits and vegetables contain phytochemicals with antioxidant properties. Plant-based diets are also high in fiber. Fiber, a non-digestible food substrate, is a significant source of prebiotics. Prebiotics undergo fermentation within the large bowel causing a reduction in bowel pH and an increase in calcium absorption. In the Framingham Offspring Study, lower dietary fiber intake was associated with decreased bone density in the femoral neck. Vegetarian diets are also high in nutrients such as magnesium, potassium, vitamin K, vitamin C, vitamin E, carotenoids and anti-inflammatory phytonutrients that are beneficial for bone health. Despite these benefits, there are conflicting results regarding the impact of a plant-based diet on bone health and fracture risk. Those who follow a plant-based diet have to be thoughtful of their food choices so that they can ensure an adequate intake of important nutrients, and for some, enriching their diet either with fortified foods or supplements may be necessary.[35] Though a vegetarian diet may include dairy products including milk and eggs, a vegan diet is based solely on plant sources. Milk, milk products and eggs are rich in both calcium and vitamin D. Though with planning it is possible to get adequate calcium and vitamin D as a vegan, data does indicate that many vegans are at risk for both reduced BMD and a higher incidence of fracture.

EXERCISE AND BONE HEALTH

Effect of Exercise on Bone Density in Healthy Adults

The evidence supporting the role of physical activity for osteoporosis prevention in people aged 65 and older was reviewed in a recent meta-analysis evaluating 59 studies.[36] The data suggested that physical activity improved bone health and prevented osteoporosis in older adults with moderate certainty. Physical activity programs involving aerobic and resistance exercises were noted to be most effective. The duration, frequency and consistency of the exercise program also made a difference. Exercise programs that lasted 60 minutes or longer and occurred 2 to 3 times a week for at least 7 months or longer had the most significant impact on bone health. It was also noted that physical activity had a greater impact on lumbar spine bone density than on hip bone density, although bone density showed improvement at both sites. Higher levels of exercise intensity, longer periods of exercise and resistance exercises were noted to be most effective in improving bone health.

In another metanalysis evaluating 53 trials in healthy postmenopausal women aged 51–79 years of age, the effect of different types of exercise at various degrees of intensity was evaluated with respect to its impact on bone density in the lumbar spine, femoral neck and total hip.[37] Although exercise at each intensity level had positive effects on lumbar spine bone density, high intensity (exercises involving impact for ground reaction forces at 4 times the weight, e.g., body weight jumps with stiff leg at landing) and moderate intensity resistance exercises and impact training (rope skipping, aerobics, jumps with soft landings, heel drops and impact for ground reaction forces at two to four times the body weight) were found to be most effective compared to low-intensity exercises. Among low-intensity exercises (walking, jogging, cycling, aquatic interventions, Tai Chi, body weight exercises, resistance training using elastic bands and exercises with impact for ground reaction forces at greater than two times the body weight), resistance training was noted to be most effective.[37]

In another systematic review and meta-analysis, the effects of dynamic resistance exercise (exercises involving main muscle groups using machines and free weights) on bone mineral density were evaluated in mostly healthy postmenopausal women.[38] The effect of intervention length, type of dynamic resistance training, training frequency, exercise intensity and exercise volume were also evaluated in subgroup analysis. The authors reported that a lower training frequency (less than two sessions per week) was associated with greater bone density increase at lumbar spine and total hip compared to a higher training frequency, and that free weights fared better compared to dynamic resistance training devices for improving total hip bone density. Overall, they reported low to moderate effect of dynamic resistance exercise on bone mineral density changes in postmenopausal women. Subgroup analyses in this metanalysis did not reveal meaningful results to make specific recommendations for exercise. However, subgroup analysis in another larger metanalysis did show a significant positive effect of weight-bearing and dynamic resistance exercises when done separately or in combination on bone mineral density of the lumbar spine, femoral, neck and total hip, with an improvement in bone density at these sites.[39]

EFFECT OF EXERCISE ON BONE DENSITY IN ADULTS WITH OSTEOPENIA OR OSTEOPOROSIS

In a large meta-analysis spanning 97 studies in patients with osteopenia or osteoporosis, the effect of various forms of physical exercise was studied without limitation on the type of exercise, the intensity or the duration.[40] Interventions were divided up into either no exercise, aerobic exercise (walking/running/cycling), resistance exercise (using elastic bands or weight machines with the intent to increase muscle, strength and power), combined exercise (at least two types of exercise, such as aerobic/resistance/balance training), whole body vibration and mind–body exercise (Tai Chi, yoga and dance). Aerobic exercises, resistance exercises, combined exercises and mind–body exercises were all effective in improving lumbar spine bone density compared to no exercise. Whole-body vibration was not effective, while mind–body exercise was most effective in improving bone density in the lumbar spine.

The benefit of exercise was evaluated in postmenopausal women with osteopenia by the Lifting Intervention for Training Muscle and Osteoporosis Rehabilitation (LIFTMOR) trial. This was a prospective study in which postmenopausal women with osteopenia were randomized to 8 months of 30 minutes of supervised high-intensity resistance and impact training exercise program twice a week, or a home-based low-intensity exercise program, and bone density was followed.[41] High-intensity exercise was found to be superior to low-intensity exercise and resulted in greater improvements in the lumbar spine and femoral neck bone density, in addition to producing greater improvement in the functional performance scores for the study subjects. It also put to rest concerns that high-intensity resistance and impact training exercises may be harmful in postmenopausal women with osteopenia, as no increase in adverse outcomes was reported in this study.

OSTEOSARCOPENIA

It has become increasingly clear that there is a strong correlation between bone health and muscle health.[42] Decreasing bone density, reduced muscle mass and reduced muscle strength are common in older adults. Many of the lifestyle interventions, including physical exercise that promote good bone health, also promote healthy muscle.[43,44]

OTHER LIFESTYLE FACTORS THAT IMPACT BONE HEALTH

In addition to nutrition and exercise, there are several other lifestyle factors that have an impact on bone health that need to be addressed. Though excessive alcohol intake can result in a decrease in bone density and is a risk factor for osteoporosis, there are data which show that low and even moderate amounts of alcohol consumption can have a positive impact on bone density.[45,46] However because of the potential negative impacts of alcohol on overall health, health care professionals should not recommend alcohol consumption for bone health and those who do consume alcohol should be recommended to moderate their intake, in the realm of one alcoholic beverage per day.

Smoking tobacco is a risk factor for osteoporosis.[47,48] There are many other negative health impacts from smoking tobacco. It is important that children and young adults are educated regarding the health hazards of smoking, including negative impacts on bone health and those who currently smoke should be encouraged and assisted with smoking cessation.

PUBLIC POLICY SUPPORTING A BONE-HEALTHY LIFESTYLE

Though most lifestyle interventions that promote health in general and in this case, bone health are individual choices, public policy plays an important role. Public education regarding healthy food choices, the benefits of regular exercise, the dangers of smoking tobacco and the dangers of drinking excessive amounts of alcohol are all important. Ensuring access to healthy foods is a public health priority. Public policy that facilitates walkable neighborhoods and green spaces has been shown to reduce fracture risk.[49] There are several environmental toxins including selenium and cadmium that have been shown to have a negative impact on bone density.[3,50,51] Public policy that reduces environmental toxins has multiple positive impacts on overall health, including bone health. Bone health in adults is determined to a significant degree by bone development in childhood and adolescence. Healthy school meals and school exercise programs are also public health interventions that promote bone health.

CLINICAL APPLICATIONS

- All older adults should be educated regarding a bone healthy diet, including adequate amounts of protein, vitamin D and foods that are high in phytoestrogens such as soy.
- A Mediterranean diet, historically recognized for its cardiovascular benefits, also promotes good bone health.
- Older adults' access to bone healthy nutrition is often impacted by socioeconomic and cultural factors that may require the input of other clinicians including nutritionists and social workers.
- Aerobic, muscle strengthening and balance exercise, all promote optimal bone health.
- Though there are many reasons to avoid smoking tobacco products and drinking excessive amounts of alcohol, bone health is negatively impacted by both.

REFERENCES

1. Wright NC, Looker AC, Saag KG, et al. The recent prevalence of osteoporosis and low bone mass in the United States based on bone mineral density at the femoral neck or lumbar spine. *J Bone Miner Res.* 2014;29(11):2520–2526.
2. Bliuc D, Nguyen ND, Milch VE, Nguyen TV, Eisman JA, Center JR. Mortality risk associated with low-trauma osteoporotic fracture and subsequent fracture in men and women. *JAMA.* 2009;301(5):513–521.
3. Mousavibaygei SR, Bisadi A, ZareSakhvidi F. Outdoor air pollution exposure, bone mineral density, osteoporosis, and osteoporotic fractures: a systematic review and meta-analysis. *Sci Total Environ.* 2023;865:161117.
4. Snega Priya P, Pratiksha Nandhini P, Arockiaraj J. A comprehensive review on environmental pollutants and osteoporosis: insights into molecular pathways. *Environ Res.* 2023;237(Pt 2):117103.
5. Luo H, Gu R, Ouyang H, et al. Cadmium exposure induces osteoporosis through cellular senescence, associated with activation of NF-kappaB pathway and mitochondrial dysfunction. *Environ Pollut.* 2021;290:118043.
6. Roberts SB, Silver RE, Das SK, et al. Healthy aging-nutrition matters: start early and screen often. *Adv Nutr.* 2021;12(4):1438–1448.
7. Guo D, Zhao M, Xu W, He H, Li B, Hou T. Dietary interventions for better management of osteoporosis: an overview. *Crit Rev Food Sci Nutr.* 2023;63(1):125–144.
8. Sharma AR, Chatterjee S, Lee YH, Lee SS. Targeting crosstalk of signaling pathways among muscles-bone-adipose tissue: a promising therapeutic approach for sarcopenia. *Aging Dis.* 2024;15(4):1619–1645.
9. Kositsawat J, Duque G, Kirk B. Nutrients with anabolic/anticatabolic, antioxidant, and anti-inflammatory properties: targeting the biological mechanisms of aging to support musculoskeletal health. *Exp Gerontol.* 2021;154:111521.
10. Rizzoli R, Biver E, Brennan-Speranza TC. Nutritional intake and bone health. *Lancet Diabetes Endocrinol.* 2021;9(9):606–621.
11. Andreo-Lopez MC, Contreras-Bolivar V, Garcia-Fontana B, Garcia-Fontana C, Munoz-Torres M. The influence of the Mediterranean dietary pattern on osteoporosis and sarcopenia. *Nutrients.* 2023;15(14).

12. Galchenko A, Gapparova K, Sidorova E. The influence of vegetarian and vegan diets on the state of bone mineral density in humans. *Crit Rev Food Sci Nutr.* 2023;63(7):845–861.
13. Wilsgaard T, Emaus N, Ahmed LA, et al. Lifestyle impact on lifetime bone loss in women and men: the Tromso study. *Am J Epidemiol.* 2009;169(7):877–886.
14. Heaney RP, Layman DK. Amount and type of protein influences bone health. *Am J Clin Nutr.* 2008;87(5):1567S–1570S.
15. Hannan MT, Tucker KL, Dawson-Hughes B, Cupples LA, Felson DT, Kiel DP. Effect of dietary protein on bone loss in elderly men and women: the framingham osteoporosis study. *J Bone Miner Res.* 2000;15(12):2504–2512.
16. Chevalley T, Brandi ML, Cashman KD, et al. Role of vitamin D supplementation in the management of musculoskeletal diseases: update from an European Society of Clinical and Economical Aspects of Osteoporosis, Osteoarthritis and Musculoskeletal Diseases (ESCEO) working group. *Aging Clin Exp Res.* 2022;34(11):2603–2623.
17. Gallagher JC, Rosen CJ. Vitamin D: 100 years of discoveries, yet controversy continues. *Lancet Diabetes Endocrinol.* 2023;11(5):362–374.
18. Force USPST, Grossman DC, Curry SJ, et al. Vitamin D, calcium, or combined supplementation for the primary prevention of fractures in community-dwelling adults: US preventive services task force recommendation statement. *JAMA.* 2018;319(15):1592–1599.
19. Burt LA, Billington EO, Rose MS, Raymond DA, Hanley DA, Boyd SK. Effect of high-dose vitamin D supplementation on volumetric bone density and bone strength: a randomized clinical trial. *JAMA.* 2019;322(8):736–745.
20. Ataide FL, Carvalho Bastos LM, Vicente Matias MF, Skare TL, Freire de Carvalho J. Safety and effectiveness of vitamin D mega-dose: a systematic review. *Clin Nutr ESPEN.* 2021;46:115–120.
21. Sanders KM, Stuart AL, Williamson EJ, et al. Annual high-dose oral vitamin D and falls and fractures in older women: a randomized controlled trial. *JAMA.* 2010;303(18):1815–1822.
22. Waterhouse M, Ebeling PR, McLeod DSA, et al. The effect of monthly vitamin D supplementation on fractures: a tertiary outcome from the population-based, double-blind, randomised, placebo-controlled D-Health trial. *Lancet Diabetes Endocrinol.* 2023;11(5):324–332.
23. Tabatabai LS, Sellmeyer DE. Nutritional supplements and skeletal health. *Curr Osteoporos Rep.* 2021;19(1):23–33.
24. Patisaul HB, Jefferson W. The pros and cons of phytoestrogens. *Front Neuroendocrinol.* 2010;31(4):400–419.
25. Marini H, Minutoli L, Polito F, et al. Effects of the phytoestrogen genistein on bone metabolism in osteopenic postmenopausal women: a randomized trial. *Ann Intern Med.* 2007;146(12):839–847.
26. Cassidy A, Albertazzi P, Lise Nielsen I, et al. Critical review of health effects of soyabean phyto-oestrogens in post-menopausal women. *Proc Nutr Soc.* 2006;65(1):76–92.
27. Fang ZB, Wang GX, Cai GZ, et al. Association between fatty acids intake and bone mineral density in adults aged 20-59: NHANES 2011–2018. *Front Nutr.* 2023;10:1033195.
28. Yang J, Li Q, Feng Y, Zeng Y. Iron deficiency and iron deficiency anemia: potential risk factors in bone loss. *Int J Mol Sci.* 2023;24(8).
29. Heidelbaugh JJ. Proton pump inhibitors and risk of vitamin and mineral deficiency: evidence and clinical implications. *Ther Adv Drug Saf.* 2013;4(3):125–133.
30. Dai Z, Zhang Y, Lu N, Felson DT, Kiel DP, Sahni S. Association between dietary fiber intake and bone loss in the framingham offspring study. *J Bone Miner Res.* 2018;33(2):241–249.
31. Castaneda M, Smith KM, Nixon JC, Hernandez CJ, Rowan S. Alterations to the gut microbiome impair bone tissue strength in aged mice. *Bone Rep.* 2021;14:101065.

32. Lucas S, Omata Y, Hofmann J, et al. Short-chain fatty acids regulate systemic bone mass and protect from pathological bone loss. *Nat Commun.* 2018;9(1):55.
33. Rodriguez-Olleros Rodriguez C, Diaz Curiel M. Vitamin K and bone health: a review on the effects of vitamin K deficiency and supplementation and the effect of non-vitamin K antagonist oral anticoagulants on different bone parameters. *J Osteoporos.* 2019;2019:2069176.
34. Haring B, Crandall CJ, Wu C, et al. Dietary patterns and fractures in postmenopausal women: results from the women's health initiative. *JAMA Intern Med.* 2016;176(5):645–652.
35. Falchetti A, Cavati G, Valenti R, et al. The effects of vegetarian diets on bone health: a literature review. *Front Endocrinol (Lausanne).* 2022;13:899375.
36. Pinheiro MB, Oliveira J, Bauman A, Fairhall N, Kwok W, Sherrington C. Evidence on physical activity and osteoporosis prevention for people aged 65+ years: a systematic review to inform the WHO guidelines on physical activity and sedentary behaviour. *Int J Behav Nutr Phys Act.* 2020;17(1):150.
37. Kistler-Fischbacher M, Weeks BK, Beck BR. The effect of exercise intensity on bone in postmenopausal women (part 2): a meta-analysis. *Bone.* 2021;143:115697.
38. Shojaa M, von Stengel S, Kohl M, Schoene D, Kemmler W. Effects of dynamic resistance exercise on bone mineral density in postmenopausal women: a systematic review and meta-analysis with special emphasis on exercise parameters. *Osteoporos Int.* 2020;31(8):1427–1444.
39. Kemmler W, Shojaa M, Kohl M, von Stengel S. Effects of different types of exercise on bone mineral density in postmenopausal women: a systematic review and meta-analysis. *Calcif Tissue Int.* 2020;107(5):409–439.
40. Zhang S, Huang X, Zhao X, et al. Effect of exercise on bone mineral density among patients with osteoporosis and osteopenia: a systematic review and network meta-analysis. *J Clin Nurs.* 2022;31(15–16):2100–2111.
41. Watson SL, Weeks BK, Weis LJ, Harding AT, Horan SA, Beck BR. High-intensity resistance and impact training improves bone mineral density and physical function in postmenopausal women with osteopenia and osteoporosis: the LIFTMOR randomized controlled trial. *J Bone Miner Res.* 2018;33(2):211–220.
42. Zanker J, Duque G. Osteosarcopenia: the path beyond controversy. *Curr Osteoporos Rep.* 2020;18(2):81–84.
43. Shen Y, Shi Q, Nong K, et al. Exercise for sarcopenia in older people: a systematic review and network meta-analysis. *J Cachexia Sarcopenia Muscle.* 2023;14(3):1199–1211.
44. Wu PY, Huang KS, Chen KM, Chou CP, Tu YK. Exercise, nutrition, and combined exercise and nutrition in older adults with sarcopenia: a systematic review and network meta-analysis. *Maturitas.* 2021;145:38–48.
45. Berg KM, Kunins HV, Jackson JL, et al. Association between alcohol consumption and both osteoporotic fracture and bone density. *Am J Med.* 2008;121(5):406–418.
46. Feskanich D, Korrick SA, Greenspan SL, Rosen HN, Colditz GA. Moderate alcohol consumption and bone density among postmenopausal women. *J Womens Health.* 1999;8(1):65–73.
47. Cusano NE. Skeletal effects of smoking. *Curr Osteoporos Rep.* 2015;13(5):302–309.
48. Hou W, Chen S, Zhu C, Gu Y, Zhu L, Zhou Z. Associations between smoke exposure and osteoporosis or osteopenia in a US NHANES population of elderly individuals. *Front Endocrinol (Lausanne).* 2023;14:1074574.
49. Zhu Z, Yang Z, Xu L, et al. Exposure to neighborhood walkability and residential greenness and incident fracture. *JAMA Netw Open.* 2023;6(9):e2335154.
50. Galvez-Fernandez M, Grau-Perez M, Garcia-Barrera T, et al. Arsenic, cadmium, and selenium exposures and bone mineral density-related endpoints: the HORTEGA study. *Free Radic Biol Med.* 2021;162:392–400.
51. Chung SM. Long-term sex-specific effects of cadmium exposure on osteoporosis and bone density: a 10-year community-based cohort study. *J Clin Med.* 2022;11(10).

26 A Lifestyle Medicine Approach to Constipation

Aarti Oza Bedi, Susan Spell and Deborah Chielli

INTRODUCTION

Constipation is one of the most common gastrointestinal (GI) complaints and a frequent reason people seek primary care for which they are referred to GI specialists. Implications for older adults include negative impacts on physical and emotional health, decreased quality of life and financial burden. Constipation occurs across the lifespan and can be classified as acute or chronic, as well as primary (also called functional or idiopathic) or secondary. This chapter focuses primarily on chronic idiopathic constipation (CIC; or functional constipation) in adults >65 years of age, integrating both the conventional approach in combination with specific evidence and considerations as they relate to the six pillars of lifestyle medicine. Chronic constipation is a complex, multifactorial condition that poses clinical challenges to both diagnosis as well as effective long-term management. In older adults, these challenges are often compounded by age-related factors such as the presence of multiple chronic conditions and/or associated polypharmacy, physical inactivity with or without limited mobility, poor quality diet that may be a result of physical factors (poor dentition, dysphagia, etc.) and/or psychosocial or financial factors, lack of proper hydration and age-related changes of the enteric nervous system (ENS), to name a few.

We begin by exploring the epidemiology and common defining clinical features of the condition and then move into the pathophysiology of the disorder. After touching on the basic initial evaluation and assessment for red flags that should prompt referral to a specialist, we briefly review conventional management strategies and therapies. After this foundation is laid, we invite the reader to reframe their approach through the lens of the six pillars of lifestyle medicine to consider evidenced-based and evidence-informed interventions for chronic constipation. Randomized controlled trials using lifestyle medicine interventions for chronic constipation in older adults are sparse. As such, the authors also include evidence from adult data sets and clinical experience.

Within the United States, there are several societies and organizations related to gastroenterology and associated sub-specialties that clinicians should be aware of

TABLE 26.1
Gastroenterology Organizations

American College of Gastroenterology (ACG) *gi.org*	American Gastroenterological Association (AGA) *gastro.org*
American Society of Gastrointestinal Endoscopy	Society of Gastroenterology Nurses and Associates (SGNA) *sgna.org*
North American Society for Pediatric Gastroenterology, Hepatology, and Nutrition (NASPGHN) *naspghn.org*	Society of State–affiliated societies such as the Florida Gastroenterologic Society (FGS) *flgastro.org*
The Rome Foundation *theromefoundation.org*	International Foundation for Gastrointestinal Disorders *iffgd.org*

(see Table 26.1). Noteworthy is the fact that leading agencies that provide clinical practice guidelines and generate evidence-based information do not place as much emphasis on the impacts of diet, stress, sleep and other lifestyle factors that drive the development, or improvement, of constipation for many. This creates a tremendous opportunity for lifestyle medicine providers to serve their patients by bridging this gap.

EPIDEMIOLOGY

PREVALENCE

The exact prevalence of chronic constipation is difficult to ascertain given the lack of both a uniform definition and diagnostic criteria used.[1] Estimates typically fall around 15–17%, with increasing rates in those 65 years of age and older, continue to increase with advancing age and vary by setting.

According to statista.com, in 2023 over-the-counter (OTC) laxative revenue was around US$1.93 billion and the sales of OTC medications for this condition have increased by over 200% in the last 20 years.[2] This alone speaks to the pervasiveness of constipation.

RISK FACTORS

The increased risk for chronic constipation with age is significantly influenced by the variety of medical conditions that older adults face.[3] Risk factors for constipation in older adults are many and include poor diet (lack of diverse sources of fiber and resistant starches), lack of adequate hydration, sedentary lifestyle, female gender, increasing age and low socioeconomic status.[4] Older adults face additional risk factors such as changes in colonic motility with advancing age, sedentary lifestyle with or without mobility concerns, malnutrition or poor nutrition, muscle weakness (of the abdominal wall and/or pelvic floor muscles), chronic medical conditions with or without polypharmacy, rectal hyposensitivity with or without ignoring the call to defecate and changes in the microbiome. Common behavioral factors in older adults act to further compound these risks. For example, an elderly patient may avoid hydrating so as to minimize the need to use the bathroom, because of a fear of falling due to difficulties in ambulation.

In addition to risk factors contributing to constipation, constipation itself can precipitate or worsen GI (and non-GI) conditions such as abdominal pain and bloating, hemorrhoids, anal fissures, rectal bleeding and fecal impaction. Fecal impaction can lead to non-GI issues such as restlessness, negative impact on cognition, mood changes such as increased anxiety, urinary tract problems and even skin rashes. In severe and extreme cases of fecal impaction, there is a risk of bowel perforation – a life-threatening condition.[5]

PATHOPHYSIOLOGY AND DEFINITIONS

Constipation at any age can be complicated and multi-factorial, varies geographically and has a wide range of potential risk factors and drivers.[6] It is critical to understand the physiology and pathophysiology of the GI tract in order to recognize constipation as early as possible and adequately intervene with an individualized, effective therapeutic intervention based on the primary drivers of the condition, which differ from patient to patient.

Constipation is characterized by infrequent, inadequate or difficulty passing stool. Common symptoms of constipation include one or more of the following: firm stool, straining to pass stool, less than three bowel movements a week and a feeling of incomplete evacuation. Less commonly, constipation may be accompanied by overflow incontinence, abdominal pain, bloating, use of manual maneuvers to remove stool from the rectum and even upper GI symptoms such as gastroesophageal reflux, nausea and or decreased appetite. It is important to note those characteristics that are more common in older adults and they include:

- Overflow fecal incontinence.[7]
- Straining to have a bowel movement, but not less frequent bowel movements[8]
- Association with urinary tract issues or symptoms.[7]
- Increased risk of bowel obstruction and perforation.[9]

The diagnosis of constipation is made clinically based on patient symptoms. Rome IV criteria (see Table 26.2) include symptom onset at least 6 months prior and criteria fulfilled for the last 3 months. Patients with concerns for underlying pathology should be sent to a gastroenterologist for further evaluation. Such evaluation may include endoscopic examination, and symptom-specific testing such as anorectal manometry (ARM) or motility testing, etc. (Table 26.3).

TABLE 26.2
Rome IV Criteria for Diagnosing Primary Chronic Constipation

(1) Must include one of the following: • Straining in > 25% of defecations • Lumpy or hard stools in > 25% of defecations • Sensation of incomplete evacuation in > 25% of defecations • Sensation of anorectal obstruction/blockage in > 25% of defecations • Manual maneuvers to facilitate > 25% of defecations (i.e. digital evacuation and support of the pelvic floor)
(2) Loose stools are rarely present without the use of laxatives
(3) Insufficient criteria for the diagnosis of irritable bowel syndrome (IBS)

Source: From *Rome IV Diagnostic Criteria for Disorders of Gut-Brain Interaction (DGBI)* (2023).[41]

TABLE 26.3
Modification of Rome Criteria for Clinical Practice Diagnosis[42]

Clinical criteria should be based on previously validated Rome IV symptom descriptors	Bothersomeness must be considered when symptoms interfere with daily life.	Frequency of symptoms is an important factor to consider but should not be an obligatory criteria for all cases.	Physicians can shorten the duration criteria when all the other diagnoses can confidently be excluded.

It is important to recognize the specific terms used when discussing constipation, as they guide the steps in evaluation, diagnosis and treatment. First, determine if constipation is acute (symptoms present $\leq$ 3 months) or chronic (symptoms present > 3 months). Acute constipation is short-lived and may be related to travel, disrupted routine, a change in diet, an illness or even a scenario such as surgery or hospitalization. Chronic constipation is longer term, and accurate diagnosis is essential to crafting an individualized plan of care that maximizes effectiveness while minimizing side effects. Second, determine if chronic constipation is primary (idiopathic/functional) or secondary (due to organic pathology).

Primary chronic constipation is due to inherent dysfunction with the colorectal organ, whereas secondary chronic constipation is a result of a variety of conditions and contributing factors. A full exploration into secondary causes is beyond the scope of this chapter but will be considered in the following discussion. Lifestyle interventions may be appropriate for both acute and chronic constipation at any age.

Primary chronic constipation, aka "chronic idiopathic constipation," or CIC, is diagnosed when there is no organic pathology (i.e. no mucosal or structural problem in the colon). "Structural" relates to anything that obstructs the movement of stool and includes spasms, ulcers, tumors, rectal prolapse and other structures. Etiologies of primary chronic constipation include issues with colonic motility (i.e. delayed or slowed transit versus normal transit), visceral hypersensitivity/pain with constipation (constipation-predominant IBS) or issues related to uncoordinated defecation (dyssynergic defecation). CIC is further divided into three sub-types, including normal transit (most common, often called "functional"), slow transit or dyssynergic defecation. An individual can have symptoms overlapping the different subtypes. Pathophysiology-specific pharmacologic and physiotherapeutic treatments for the various subtypes of CIC are best managed by the specialist, but all patients with CIC would benefit from an assessment of secondary etiologies and recommendations of lifestyle-based therapies, which are foundational to any treatment regimen. Overall, the most common form of constipation is normal transit/functional constipation. However, changes in anorectal function contribute more to chronic constipation in older adults.[8] The review article, "Chronic Constipation in the Elderly Patient: Updates in Evaluation and Management" highlights the fact that older adults with constipation report the need for prolonged abdominal pressure while defecating. In addition, they more frequently have the sensation of outlet obstruction, and more reports of digitalization to relieve impacted stool.[5]

Secondary chronic constipation results from a variety of conditions and/or use of certain medications to treat those conditions (see Table 26.4). A lifestyle medicine provider, in primary care or specialty practice, can potentially provide the most impactful recommendations when assessing primary as well as secondary etiologies.

INITIAL EVALUATION AND CONSIDERATIONS

Using a stepwise approach when evaluating patients with a complaint of constipation is essential at any age. Start with a focused but thorough history and physical exam, with careful identification of any red flags or alarm signs that necessitate referral to a GI specialist or even emergency care (see Table 26.5).

A careful and thorough review of the patient's history will include onset, duration and progression of symptoms, any accompanying non-GI symptoms, changes in comorbid conditions or medication use, degree of mobility and ability to independently engage in activities of daily living (ADLs), overall lifestyle and attention to social determinants of health. GI-specific elements of the history should start at the mouth and work down to the anus, eliciting information about appetite, oral health and/or the presence of dry mouth, dentition, dysphagia, globus sensation, gastroesophageal reflux (overt or manifested as chronic cough), gas, bloating, abdominal pain, rectal pain or fissures or any history of bowel surgery. Bowel movements are assessed for frequency, consistency (often aided by the validated Bristol Stool Chart from The Rome Foundation), sensation of complete or incomplete evacuation, incontinence of bowel or bladder and impact of symptoms on daily life. Questionnaires such as the PAC-SYM and PAC-QOL may be helpful tools to elicit symptom severity and their impact on quality of life.[10] The Bristol Stool Scale is a validated visual guide that is easily incorporated into clinical care. Stool consistency correlates with

TABLE 26.4
Examples of Medical Conditions and Corresponding Medications Associated with Chronic Constipation (Alone or in Combination)[5,43]

Chronic Pain	• Rheumatoid arthritis • Cancer-related pain • Fibromyalgia	• Opioids • Nonsteroidal anti-inflammatories
Psychiatric	• Anxiety • Depression • Eating disorders	• Tricyclic antidepressants • Monoamine oxidase inhibitors • Antipsychotics • Hypnotics • Lithium • Neuroleptics with antimuscarinic properties (e.g., chlorpromazine, trifluoperazine)
Cardiovascular	• Hypertension • Dysrhythmias • Chronic kidney disease	• Calcium channel blockers • Diuretics • Centrally acting antihypertensive drugs • Antiarrhythmics • Beta-adrenoreceptor antagonist
Gastrointestinal	• IBS • Pelvic floor dysfunction • Rectoceles • Crohn's and ulcerative colitis	• Antacids (aluminum or calcium-containing) • Bile acid sequestrants • Bismuth • 5-hydroxytryptamine 3 receptor antagonists
Neurologic	• Parkinson's disease • Multiple sclerosis • Spinal cord lesions • Seizures	• Anti-Parkinson's medication • Anticonvulsants
Genitourinary	• Overactive bladder • Prostate enlargement	• Anticholinergics (e.g., oxybutynin, tolterodine, trospium chloride) • Antispasmodics (e.g., hyoscine, dicyclomine, propantheline)
Endocrine	• Diabetes • Thyroid disease • Hormone changes • Hyperparathyroidism	• GLP-1 agonists • SGLT-2 inhibitors
Other	• Vitamin and mineral deficiencies • Osteoporosis • Allergies	• Antihistamines with antimuscarinic properties (diphenhydramine, chlorpheniramine) • Calcium supplements • Oral iron • Bisphosphonates • Vinca alkaloids • Sympathomimetics • Alkylating agents

TABLE 26.5
Alarm Signs ("Red Flags" That Necessitate Consideration and Evaluation for Organic Pathology)[5,44]

New onset ≥ 50 years old
Hematochezia (blood in stool, gross or occult)
Iron deficiency anemia
Fever
Unintended weight loss (> 5% of body weight in the previous 6–12 months)
Loss of appetite
Abdominal or rectal mass
Rectal prolapse
Anal fissures or ulcerations
Family or personal history of GI cancer
Family or personal history of Crohn's or ulcerative colitis
Severe, persistent and or treatment-refractory constipation

transit time, but bowel movement frequency may not.[4] It is important to be mindful that a patient can report daily bowel movements and still be constipated, which is why a tool such as the Bristol Stool Scale is helpful.

A careful physical exam includes assessment for the presence of cachexia, general mobility, cognition and oral health including the fit of any dental prostheses, any difficulty clearing the throat or choking on saliva and an abdominal exam noting bowel sounds and any masses.[11] A basic digital rectal exam should be performed to assess for rectal tone, old or fresh hematin material in the rectal vault, hard impacted stool in the rectum or contrarily the presence of liquid stool or the presence or absence of any of the following: rectal masses, compression from prostate or vaginal pathology and signs of trauma from retention or passage of stool such as fissures, ulcerations and hemorrhoids.

Initial evaluation may include basic laboratory tests (complete blood count, comprehensive metabolic profile, thyroid studies, hemoglobin A1C) and abdominal imaging (abdominal flat plate/KUB). Basic abdominal imaging is useful in determining the degree of fecal loading, particularly in those with altered mentation or expressive faculties.[11]

Once it is determined that referral to a specialist is not necessary (or is complete), attention can be turned to developing an individualized therapeutic plan. Again, a stepwise approach is necessary, guided by the patient's underlying drivers of chronic constipation and starting with the least risk of adverse effects. For mild to moderate symptoms, incorporating the six pillars of lifestyle medicine (or a carefully selected few) may be all that is needed. Unfortunately, these are often overlooked by primary care clinicians and specialists alike once organic pathology has been ruled out.[9] Lifestyle medicine clinicians are perfectly positioned to profoundly improve quality of life and reduce serious complications for older adults with chronic constipation.

CONVENTIONAL APPROACHES AND THERAPIES

Management of chronic constipation in older adults requires a multifactorial approach. Using a stepwise approach of lifestyle interventions in combination with pharmacologic methods is often needed, allowing an adequate trial period (4 to 8 weeks) for each step before escalation of therapy. Leveraging the pillars of lifestyle medicine in combination with pharmacologic therapy will foster synergy and likely reduce dependence on pharmacologic therapies. This should reduce the risk of side effects, adverse effects and the financial and psychological burden of polypharmacy. The goal of management is the improvement of the patient's clinical symptoms, often defined as passing stool without significant straining or pain, three times a week to three times a day.[12]

The first step in addressing chronic constipation is to prescribe lifestyle and dietary modifications. This involves increasing fiber intake (with a whole food first approach with or without fiber supplementation), adequate hydration and increased physical activity. Congruent with a fundamental underpinning of lifestyle medicine, the patient (and caregivers, if necessary) should be an active participant in their care and arming the patient with evidenced-based knowledge is critical in securing that participation. In 2014, Nour-Elden et al. conducted a study in a long-term care facility in Egypt with the aim of improving the quality of life in older adult residents. They showed that an education program using lifestyle modification for residents with functional constipation improved healthy lifestyle behaviors, constipation severity and quality of life related to constipation. Behavioral improvements included consumption of regular meals, increased fiber-rich foods, exercise and fluid consumption.[13]

One consideration to keep in mind is that often patients have already been placed on higher steps without exhausting options at lower ones. Thus, the therapeutic intervention may include delicately re-balancing therapies related to lifestyle and dietary modifications, while simultaneously making efforts to de-escalate pharmacologic therapies. The second step in addressing constipation, particularly for patients who do not respond to lifestyle and dietary modifications, is to incorporate pharmaceuticals and/or nutritional supplements. Osmotic laxatives are the initial pharmacologic therapy recommended. This is followed by stimulant laxatives, addressing pelvic floor dysfunction with therapy (if indicated) and then consideration for the use of secretagogues or prokinetics. The 2023 AGA/ACG clinical practice guideline and clinical decision support tool for CIC are helpful at this stage. The decision algorithm is nicely illustrated within the guideline. It is intended to provide a framework for clinical decision-making in the use of over-the-counter and pharmaceutical medications for CIC and is appropriate for use in primary care as well as specialty settings.[14]

A Note about Fiber!

Whole plant foods in a diverse array of colors provide more than just fiber. They also contain many phenols (and polyphenols), minerals, vitamins and other micronutrients that contribute to thousands of processes within the body along with providing nourishment for all the health-promoting microbiota that live in the human GI tract.

Lifestyle Medicine Approach to Constipation

Fiber is a carbohydrate in plant sources that is not affected by gastrointestinal processes. As fiber does not get broken down, it passes through the body undigested. There are two types of dietary fiber to consider, insoluble and soluble. Soluble fiber, also described as viscous fiber, dissolves in water and insoluble fiber does not. Thus, one can think of soluble fiber as retaining water, slowing down digestion and thus lowering blood glucose levels and cholesterol. Good sources of soluble fiber come from chia seeds, oats, lentils, beans, nuts, apples and berries. Insoluble fiber can be thought of as a "bristle brush" that helps move products through the intestines and prevent constipation. As this type of fiber works on moving things through the intestine, it is important that the patient's hydration is maintained and optimized. Natural sources of insoluble fiber are wheat bran and wheat products, artichokes, quinoa, leafy greens, legumes and brown rice. Fiber can further be described as "fermentable" or not depending on whether colonic bacteria can break down the fiber into short-chain fatty acids (SCFA), the exclusive intestinal nutrition source, by anaerobic intestinal microbiota. The Nutrition Source site of the Harvard School of Public Health has an excellent overview of fiber.[15] McRorie & McKeown (2017) present a comprehensive review of fiber in their publication, "Understanding the Physics of Functional Fibers in the Gastrointestinal Tract: An Evidence-Based Approach to Resolving Enduring Misconceptions about Insoluble and Soluble Fiber" in the *Journal of the Academy of Nutrition and Dietetics* that is an excellent resource.[16] Widely accepted recommendations for fiber consumption are around 25–35 grams/day with the focus not being on types of fiber and counting grams consumed, but rather on eating a variety of whole food and plant-based foods on a daily basis. See Table 26.6 for the nuances of fiber used for chronic constipation. These agents are generally very well tolerated, have very few to no adverse effects or drug interactions and do not create any dependency. They can be used in conjunction with dietary fiber, or alone. Common agents in this category include psyllium husk (e.g., Metamucil), methylcellulose (e.g., Citrucel), calcium polycarbophil (e.g., FiberCon) and wheat dextrin (e.g., Benefiber). To note, the joint AGA/ACG practice guideline recommends only psyllium in the fiber category, noting that flatulence is a common effect of increasing fiber and that caution should be exercised in patients with strictures or obstructive processes.[14]

The next step for patients who do not respond adequately to lifestyle interventions and fiber is a trial of osmotic laxatives. Osmotic laxatives draw water into the lumen of the large intestine via osmosis thus increasing fecal mass and softening stool consistency, which results in a laxative effect and improved frequency of bowel movements. Common agents, in order of strongest to weakest in the AGA/ACG practice guideline, include polyethylene glycol (PEG or Miralax – strong recommendation), magnesium oxide and lactulose (both conditionally recommended).[14] In clinical practice, the authors have also utilized other forms of magnesium (citrate, sulfate) and sorbitol. Adverse effects of osmotic laxatives include bloating, cramping, fecal urgency and renal toxicity (with the magnesium compounds). Sorbitol tends to be better tolerated than lactulose with less bloating and flatulence.

If treatment with lifestyle interventions, fiber and osmotic laxatives are ineffective (or sub-optimal) after an adequate trial, stimulant laxatives can be added for rescue

TABLE 26.6
Nutritional Interventions for Chronic Constipation

Nutritional Intervention	Examples
Food first approach	Eat at least 30 different whole plant foods daily for optimal gut health (the Gut Microbiome Project)[18]
Fiber	Tips for adding fiber as we age:[45] • Eat seeds generously (chia, hemp, ground flax) – sprinkle on granola, salad, yogurt, hummus, etc. • Use alternative types of pasta such as chickpea or lentil pasta • Experiment with bean dips and hummus • Add quinoa, bulgur wheat or pearled barley to salads • Incorporate a small amount of dark chocolate (85% cocoa) after dinner (ex: Lily's makes great tasting sugar free chocolate bars) • Add avocado slices to salads and sandwiches, make fresh guacamole or spread onto whole grain toast • Intentionally add citrus fruits such as kiwi, dragon fruit and passion fruit Fiber supplementation: • Psyllium (high viscosity, low fermentation fiber – great for constipation as well as diarrhea) • Guar gum • B-glucans Half a cup of prune juice daily was found to both soften stool (after 4 weeks) and increase bowel movements (after 7 weeks) in a double-blind RCT.[46]
Magnesium	Magnesium-rich foods (should be consumed daily; average RDA is 300–400 mg/day): • Whole grains – brown rice, oatmeal, quinoa • Vegetables – spinach, avocado, kale, lima beans • Legumes – lima, black and kidney beans, edamame, tofu • Nuts and seeds – squash and pumpkin seeds, almonds • Miscellaneous – dark chocolate (85% cocoa), non-fat yogurt Supplements: Unabsorbed magnesium creates a laxative effect, so using forms with a higher dose and lower bioavailability will be the best for constipation. For example, magnesium oxide contains 60% magnesium (the most of any form), but has the lowest absorption and most targeted effect for constipation. Alternatives to magnesium oxide: • Magnesium hydroxide (milk of magnesia) • Magnesium sulfate (epsom salt), one to two cups added to a warm evening bath, which also promotes sleep Drug-induced depletion of magnesium with: acid reducers (PPIs and H2 blockers), diuretics, corticosteroids, oral contraceptives, macrolide antibiotics and nephrotoxic medications. Caution applied for patients with kidney disease.[47,48]

(Continued)

TABLE 26.6 (Continued)

Nutritional Intervention	Examples
Hydration	Individual needs vary – eight 8 oz glasses of water has no real scientific evidence to support this recommendation. Consider overall health, comorbidities, medications, mobility, etc., with care to avoid dehydration. The AHA suggests that if urine is pale you are well hydrated. If urine is dark yellow or amber, you are dehydrated. Note: Vegetables and fruits have high water and fiber content, and can be accounted for regarding hydration. Tips to stay well hydrated for older adults: • Keep water with you (ideally a refillable stainless steel or glass bottle, avoiding plastic when possible – consider keeping one near the favorite chair, in the bedroom, or anywhere the individual spends time) • Eat water-rich foods (e.g., watermelon, cucumber, lettuce, celery, tomatoes) • Soups and stews are excellent choices (favor vegetable-rich versions) • Incorporate green smoothies • Jazz up plain water with fruit, vegetables or herbs (e.g., add a few frozen berries to a glass of water) • Limit food and fluids with diuretic effects (e.g., alcohol, caffeine, parsley)

Note: Many older adults avoid drinking due to the need to urinate frequently. This must be part of the individualized assessment and additional evaluation undertaken as indicated.[49,50]

or as a short-term adjunct. The AGA/ACG guidelines recommend their use in conjunction with lower-level therapies rather than as single agents, favoring bisacodyl or sodium picosulphate.[14] Senna is a less favored alternative. Common side effects include abdominal pain, cramping and diarrhea, so the recommendation to start at a low dose and increase if needed should be followed. Stimulants enhance colonic transport and motility by altering electrolyte transport across the intestinal mucosa and are certainly effective, but long-term safety is not known.[14]

Suppositories are not very effective for chronic constipation given the localized effect of this delivery method. Accordingly, suppositories (glycerin or bisacodyl) and enemas (tap water or soapsuds) only have a role in the treatment of fecal impaction. Sodium phosphate enemas should be used with caution in older patients given reports of hypotension, dehydration, several electrolyte imbalances and resultant acid/base disturbances, renal toxicity and EKG changes.

Following a combination of lifestyle interventions, increased fiber, osmotic laxatives, stimulants for rescue and or pelvic floor therapy (if indicated), options include a change to or addition of secretagogues or a prokinetic. Colon secretagogues (lubiprostone, linaclotide and plecanatide) act on receptors which increase fluid secretion into the intestinal lumen, whereas prokinetics such as prucalopride (5HT-4 receptor agonists) increase colonic motility.

For patients on chronic opioid therapy, opioid antagonists can be helpful to mitigate secondary chronic constipation as they act on peripheral mu-opioid receptors. They do not cross the blood–brain barrier, so they do not impair the analgesic effects of opioids. In patients with dyssynergic defecation, referral to a specialist for biofeedback therapy is utilized.

LIFESTYLE MEDICINE PILLARS AND CONSTIPATION

NUTRITION

Nutrition is one of the most important lifestyle medicine pillars when it comes to constipation at any age, but especially for older adults. Overall dietary pattern and hydration, alone or in combination with physical activity, may be all that is needed for mild or even moderate constipation. It's also foundational for moderate to severe constipation, even when other therapeutic interventions are needed. See Table 26.6 for a compilation of nutritional interventions.

A thorough assessment is needed to create a personalized, effective plan of care. Engage a registered dietitian to help personalize and optimize management. For the older adult, adequate attention to dentition, mastication, swallowing, appetite, satiety, financial constraints, ability to engage in activities of daily living (such as meal preparation) and other factors are important elements of the initial assessment. In general, a dietary pattern that is rich in the amount and diversity of whole plant foods, in combination with adequate hydration, helps optimize GI function including the normalization of bowel movements and reduces the risk of constipation. See the section "Conventional Approaches and Therapies" above for details regarding fiber.

Nutritional interventions to prevent or improve constipation include the following:

- Avoidance of constipating foods such as cheese and other dairy products, high fat meats, eggs, and processed foods.[17]
- Consumption of a diverse array of fiber-rich foods, which are only found in plant-based foods (ideally, 30 different whole plant foods weekly – vegetables, fruits, whole grains, legumes, nuts, seeds and spices).[18] Mechanisms of action of fiber-rich food, and fruit in particular, are presumed to have positive effects on gut microbiota as well as gut motility, both of which improve constipation.[19]
- Fruits rich in polyphenols and fiber including kiwifruit (gold and green), grapes, raisins, prunes and others.
- Maintenance of adequate hydration (with water or herbal tea).
- Targeted fiber supplementation, predominantly with high-viscosity fibers including psyllium, raw guar gum and gel-forming b-glucans.
- Targeted supplementation with magnesium – oxide, hydroxide and possibly magnesium sulfate-rich mineral water.[20]
- Elimination of medication(s) that negatively impact thirst, appetite, absorption of nutrients, gut motility or microbiome (see "Risky Substances: Medications" section of this chapter).

STRESS

The concept of the gut–brain axis continues to gain popularity and research support. There has been exponential growth in the evidence base related to the gut–brain connection and our understanding is evolving quickly. Psychological stress is known to negatively influence the GI tract.

Stressors change throughout the lifespan and perception of those stressors is incredibly individual. Aging adults may have additional stressors such as health concerns (for themselves or loved ones), isolation and loneliness, financial concerns, functional and/or cognitive decline, worry about being a burden to others, change in lifestyle or living situation and physiologic stressors such as loss of appetite, dysphagia and even poor dentition that contributes to difficulty chewing.

There are many tactics to reduce stress and clinicians will need to take into account the individual's health status, comorbidities, likes and desires, safety and willingness to try practices they are not used to. The most robust literature around stress management and constipation comes from the sub-group of irritable bowel syndrome (IBS). Mindfulness-Based Stress Reduction (MBSR) and yoga are two examples of effective stress reduction techniques that improve bowel function.[21,22] Table 26.7 summarizes interventions to mitigate stress and Table 26.9 presents a

TABLE 26.7
Stress Reduction Techniques That May Help Relieve Constipation

Category	Examples
Mind–body therapies	• Meditation • Mindfulness-based stress reduction • Mindful eating • Progressive relaxation • Guided imagery • Yoga • Prayer • Art, music, dance therapies • Psychotherapy or support groups • Journaling • Breathwork (e.g., heart math)
Biologically based therapies	• Diet and nutrition • Supplements • Probiotics
Energy therapies	• Vagus nerve stimulation • Healing touch • Acupuncture
Manual and body-based practices	• Physical therapy • Massage • Abdominal massage[51] • Chiropractic care

variety of interventions that leverage multiple LM pillars simultaneously, which may in turn improve constipation.

SLEEP

Evidence exists linking sleep and constipation, but it is limited in the older adult population. A 2023 study identified poor sleep quality as a new and independent risk factor for constipation among community-dwelling older adults.[23] This study also found that sleep quality and constipation are associated in a dose-response manner. Drawing from adult data, Yun, et. al. (2021) identified a strong correlation between insomnia and constipation among shift workers[22] and Liu et. al. (2022) identified an association between sleep deficiency with worse constipation, as well as altered anorectal and autonomic functions in people with CIC.[24,25] It seems that sleep disturbance negatively affects bowel function and can lead to constipation.

Sleep quality and quantity have profound impacts on mental, emotional and physical well-being throughout the lifecycle. Restorative sleep and alignment of circadian rhythms more generally, are foundational to the functioning of every other body system, including the GI tract. There are a number of promising interventions to consider for older adults to optimize sleep (see Table 26.8).

Again, an individualized approach will be the most effective and considerations include, but are not limited to:

1. Address medical conditions that may interrupt sleep, such as prostate enlargement, sleep apnea, restless legs syndrome and gastroesophageal reflux.
2. Address medications (see the "Risky Substances" section for additional information) that can interfere with restful sleep, such as opioids, antidepressants, antihypertensives and medications for dementia.
    a. Opioids may cause daytime drowsiness and napping, which impacts both quality and quantity of sleep at night.
    b. Antidepressants can cause arousal, somnolence, bothersome dreams and/or changes in bowel movements that may affect sleep.
    c. Antihypertensives can cause frequent cough (ACE inhibitors), reduce endogenous melatonin production or cause nightmares (beta-blockers).[26]
    d. Medications for dementia may promote wakefulness, further worsening disrupted sleep–wake cycles for those suffering from dementia.
3. Address behavioral factors, such as the use of alcohol, caffeine and nicotine, and promote sleep hygiene.
4. Obtain an evaluation by a sleep specialist if a new sleep disorder is suspected.

EXERCISE/PHYSICAL ACTIVITY

Physical inactivity and living a sedentary lifestyle, particularly for older adults, are known risk factors for the development of constipation. It is unclear whether physical activity alone is an effective therapeutic lifestyle intervention specifically for

TABLE 26.8
Improving Sleep

Daytime	Nighttime
Same wake time every day: • Ideal is within 1 hour of sunrise	Same bedtime every day: • Ideal is within 2 hours of sunset
Exposure to natural sunlight outside (not through a window) within 30–60 minutes of waking for 10–20 minutes, without sunglasses, even if it is cloudy: • Pair this with walking for physical activity • Pair this with time in nature for overall restorative benefits • Pair this with grounding	Bedroom for sleep and sex only
If napping during the day: • Limit naps to 20–30 minutes • Limit naps after 2–3 pm	Avoid electronics/screens and bright lights for 1 to 2 hours before bed • If unable to disconnect, use blue light–blocking glasses or screen dimming • Dim the lights
If using caffeine, limit use to 2 cups a day and none after 2–3 pm	Develop an evening wind-down routine: • Wash face, brush teeth, urinate, etc. • If able, take a warm bath before bed
Ensure physical activity during the day, preferably earlier in the day (i.e., not within the 3 hours before bedtime)	Dark bedroom (only red light numbers on an alarm clock, if needed)
Meal timing and volume: • Largest meal should be lunch • Smallest meal should be dinner • No eating within 2 hours of bedtime, ideally not after 7–8 pm	Cool temperature in the bedroom (65–67°F)

constipation in older adults and conflicting evidence exists. Physical activity, adequate hydration, optimal fiber consumption, stress mitigation, restorative sleep and other behaviorally based interventions, can alleviate both acute and chronic constipation at any age. This approach can be very effective for mild constipation but may not be fully effective in moderate to severe cases.

The recommendation for 150 minutes of moderate-intensity physical activity seems to be the most beneficial for functional constipation in any age group including those over age 65. Movement paradigms that upregulate parasympathetic nervous system activity and have multiple other benefits, such as Tai Chi and yoga, are reasonable additions to any physical activity plan of care across the lifespan when treating constipation. A thorough assessment of baseline physical fitness, with consideration of any comorbidities and mobility limitations, is essential to craft an individualized activity plan. Collaborate with local pelvic floor physical therapists, occupational therapists, exercise physiologists or other qualified professionals that focus on safely working with the elderly population to slowly improve physical fitness levels without injury.

At the time of this writing, no clear-cut evidence exists regarding the best type and dose of exercise to alleviate constipation in older adults. Core strengthening exercises were not found to provide any benefit for constipation, and high-intensity cardiovascular exercise may be detrimental. Many researchers and commentators note the detrimental effects of high-intensity exercise, especially diarrhea, with a proposed mechanism of ischemia due to blood being shunted to other organs and tissues during vigorous exercise. Commonalities across studies and meta-analyses indicate that mild to moderate-intensity cardiovascular exercise is an ideal adjunct for the treatment of constipation, including for older adults and those in long-term care facilities. The best effect is when exercise is combined with increased fiber and water intake.

Yoga is a promising form of physical activity with many benefits and multiple suspected mechanisms of action. One recent randomized controlled trial (RCT) from India identifies possible mechanisms including regulation of the nervous system (increased parasympathetic activity), mechanical pressure and movement on the abdominal organs and an indirect gastrointestinal benefit due to improved quality and quantity of sleep.[21] Other potential mechanisms of action related to exercise and improved constipation include improved colon motility, improved GI tract musculature, improved circulation to the GI tract and improved quality of life overall resulting in stress mitigation. For dyssynergic defecation, pelvic floor therapy and pelvic floor exercises aimed at strengthening those muscles can be particularly helpful.

Tai Chi has many physical and psychological benefits. A study is in progress at Chengdu University of Traditional Chinese Medicine comparing Tai Chi (Taiji) and aerobic exercise for functional constipation. The investigators hope to identify correlations among variables and elucidate specific therapeutic effects of Tai Chi, particularly for those with functional constipation.[25]

In 2012, a single-blinded, randomized controlled trial was conducted in Taiwan that evaluated whole-body vibration for functional constipation. External mechanical vibration was applied to the abdomen of individuals with severe constipation. This non-invasive, low-intensity therapy was found to be safe and beneficial, lowering constipation severity as well as the obstructive defecation score of study participants. This is similar to TENS therapy used by many physical therapists and can even be done at home.[26] See Table 26.9 for a variety of ideas to leverage multiple LM pillars simultaneously.

Social Connection

There is much to be elucidated about how social connectedness influences functional GI disorders and research in this area is in its infancy, but clinicians must assess a patient's social connections, as they are instrumental in overall well-being. The detrimental effects of loneliness and isolation may impact the GI tract, possibly via stress and activation of the sympathetic nervous system and through the impact on behaviors such as poor diet, sedentary lifestyle, lack of exercise or even use of risky

TABLE 26.9
Ideas That May Increase Social Connection and Physical Activity, Mitigate Stress and Improve Sleep in Older Adults

Group mindfulness activities such as Tai Chi and yoga	Communal dining or dining with friends and family	Gardening, art or other community clubs	Volunteering
Shared interest/hobby groups (gardening, knitting, book clubs, etc.)	Exercise groups, such as Silver Sneakers or Walk With A Doc or community pickleball	Playing games at community centers for older adults	Pet companionship or visits from local pets
Faith community and related activities	"Befriending" and peer visiting services	Spend 120 minutes per week in nature (green spaces and forests in particular)[29]	Traveling with friends and family
National organizations that offer resources for loneliness in older adults[52]			
• AARP • National Council on Aging • National Institute on Aging • Eldercare Locator • Area Agencies on Aging			

substances. There is no published evidence that directly links social connectedness with constipation in the elderly. However, scientific research related to the bidirectionality of the gut–brain connection via the microbiome and the vagus nerve is rapidly emerging, with promising insights into the powerful connection between the gut and overall health. Social connectedness with one another and connection with our natural world have physical and psychological benefits, which may positively impact functional constipation. Spending time in nature has healing properties via various mechanisms that result in a more diverse and resilient gut microbiome. In a 2019 study, more diverse yard vegetation correlated with a healthier gut microbiome of 48 older individuals in Finland.[27] That same year, White et al. published the best dose for time in nature to be 120 minutes a week, spread out across the week or in weekend warrior style (accumulating all 120 minutes in 1–2 days), as the effects last at least 7 days.[28] Many fun and engaging outdoor activities should be considered for older adults with functional constipation including gardening, walks in nature and outdoor exercise. See Table 26.9 for specific ways to increase social connectedness for the elderly population.

RISKY SUBSTANCES

Traditionally, alcohol and tobacco are the substances addressed in this pillar of lifestyle medicine. Both of these substances have an association with intestinal health and motility. As polypharmacy is common in this population, we have also included the major groups of culprit medications with known effects on intestinal motility and function which predisposes patients to constipation. We would not characterize these medications, many of which are medically necessary, as "risky substances," however, including them in the discussion within this pillar does remind practitioners to not overlook the effect of prescribed medications on the presenting complaints, and not forego the opportunity to de-escalate or de-prescribe medications.

The effect of alcohol abuse on constipation is multifactorial. There is strong evidence showing a negative effect on consumption of dietary caloric intake in patients abusing alcohol.[29–31] There is also a documented associated increase in gastric emptying times and in mouth-to-cecum transit times, all of which can be grouped under impaired gastrointestinal motility.[32,33] There is an alteration in gut permeability and jejunal microbiota noted in those abusing alcohol as well as a reduction in sodium and water absorption in the small intestine.[34,35] This alone would predispose one to diarrhea; however, when combined with deficient caloric intake, decreased water intake, nausea and vomiting, one can find dehydration to be a problem which can then contribute to constipation. The higher risk for inactivity, as well as the increased risk of concomitant depression and social isolation in those abusing alcohol, also contributes to constipation in these patients; thus, one can see how this one substance has such a profound impact on so many pillars.

Marijuana usage has been increasing over the last few years. Due to recent legalization in many parts of the United States and globally, cannabis has increasingly become a controlled substance used to treat various disorders, within and beyond gastroenterology. Cannabis is comprised of more than 60 aromatic hydrocarbon compounds, with the two best known being THC (Delta-9-tetra-hydrocannabinoil) and CBD (cannabidiol). THC is implicated in the psychotropic effects and CBD in pathways regulating inflammation, pain and motility. These compounds interact with CB1 and CB2 receptors both centrally and peripherally. There is a very high concentration of CB1 receptors in the colonic epithelium. Cannabis is felt to reduce GI motility via agonistic activation of CB1 receptors of the myenteric plexus which results in decreased peristalsis and contractility by reduced acetylcholine and substance P. These two neurotransmitters are traditionally excitatory. With respect to the effect of cannabis on gastrointestinal motility, the jury is still out. Data is limited and conflicting and we hope to see more investigation in this space.

Tobacco is a stimulant that actually facilitates gastric and intestinal emptying. It also is an appetite suppressant via suppression of ghrelin and cortisol.[36,38] However, the overall detrimental effects of tobacco usage far outweigh any benefits; thus, there is consensus in the medical community that its use should be discouraged. We want to highlight that smoking cessation can actually lead to constipation in patients and has been reported in numbers as high as 17% of individuals undergoing smoking cessation as well as a noteworthy impact on 9% of those who have quit. These effects are usually short-lived, lasting from 2 to 4 weeks.[38] It is critical the providers support the patient with hydration, nutritional support with attention to fiber intake, physical activity, and stress relief methods throughout this time.

Medications often contribute to the presence and evaluation of constipation, particularly in older adults who have larger medication lists. Some of this may be due to multiple medical comorbidities and necessity; however, avoiding "benign neglect" of medications should be emphasized. The mechanism of action of the various medications is beyond the scope of this chapter, but direct alterations in motility and function are among the etiologies. Opioid-induced constipation is the most prevalent with estimates as high as 81% in patients receiving these medications.[39] This is due to the direct effect on their receptors in the gastrointestinal tract. We mention this because the available peripherally acting Mu-opioid receptor antagonists used to manage opioid-induced constipation selectively act on peripheral receptors. One such agent, methylnaltrexone (Relistor), does not cross the blood–brain barrier; thus, its use will not affect the analgesic effect of the medication or induce symptoms of opioid withdrawal.[40] Patients should be referred to a gastroenterologist to discuss whether this medication would be appropriate in the patient's care.

CONCLUSIONS

In conclusion, constipation is a complex, multifactorial condition that is widely present in patients of all ages. In older adults, the challenges surrounding diagnosis and management are often compounded by age-related factors such as the presence of multiple chronic conditions, polypharmacy, physical inactivity with or without mobility issues, poor quality diet, etc. Approaching patients mindfully, while framing assessment and management using the six pillars of lifestyle medicine, allows the practitioner to provide a logical, comprehensive and evidence-based treatment plan from which to start. It is also crucial to identify and acknowledge that these pillars are very interconnected. In older patients, the impact of changes in behavior in one pillar needs to be weighed against their effects on the other pillars before making generalized recommendations. For example, increasing hydration in a patient on a diuretic, who already has mobility concerns and poor sleep will not be a positive or productive recommendation.

Nutrition considerations aimed at increasing hydration, and the amount of fiber-rich, whole food plant-based items are crucial. Items such as kiwi can be easily incorporated into the diet, with impactful results. It is equally important to assess dentition, mobility and financial considerations in this population when making recommendations.

Psychological stress is known to negatively influence the GI tract through a few different mechanisms that may contribute to the development of constipation. It is thought that the parasympathetic/sympathetic nervous systems are one of the pathways for this. Stressors do not disappear, but rather change throughout life. Approaches to learning coping strategies should be sought regardless of age.

Sleep hygiene and avoidance of habits and substances that impact it should be assessed. Restorative sleep is important for not just gastrointestinal health, but overall health as well.

Physical inactivity and living a sedentary lifestyle, particularly for older adults, are known risk factors for the development of constipation.

Scientific research related to social connectedness and the bidirectionality of the gut–brain connection via the microbiome and the vagus nerve is rapidly emerging, with promising insights into the powerful connection between the gut and overall health.

The medication list should be viewed in the light of "Risky Substances" in the older patient population. Assessment of prescribed medications and their potential contribution to constipation should be assessed routinely. One should attempt to reduce the medication burden and avoid "benign neglect" of a patient's prescribed medications at all times.

CLINICAL APPLICATIONS

- Nutrition considerations aimed at increasing hydration, and the amount of fiber-rich, whole food plant-based items is crucial. Items such as kiwi can be easily incorporated into the diet, with impactful results.
- Psychological stress is known to negatively influence the GI tract through a few different mechanisms that may contribute to the development of constipation. Stressors do not disappear, but rather change throughout life. Approaches to learning coping strategies should be sought regardless of age.
- Sleep hygiene, and avoidance of habits and substances that impact it, should be assessed.
- Physical inactivity and living a sedentary lifestyle, particularly for older adults, are known risk factors for the development of constipation.
- There is no published evidence that directly links social connectedness with constipation in older adults. However, scientific research related to the bidirectionality of the gut–brain connection via the microbiome and the vagus nerve is rapidly emerging, with promising insights into the powerful connection between the gut and overall health.
- Assessment of prescribed medications and their potential contribution to constipation should be assessed routinely. One should attempt to reduce the medication burden and avoid "benign neglect" of a patient's prescribed medications at all times.

REFERENCES

1. Salari N, Ghasemianrad M, Ammari-Allahyari M, Rasoulpoor S, Shohaimi S, Mohammadi M. Global prevalence of constipation in older adults: a systematic review and meta-analysis. *Wien Klin Wochenschr.* 2023;135(15–16):389–398. doi:10.1007/s00508-023-02156-w
2. Laxatives OTC revenue in U.s. 2017–2023. Statista. Accessed February 15, 2024. https://www.statista.com/statistics/506583/otc-revenue-of-laxatives-in-the-us/
3. Staller K, Cash BD. Myths and misconceptions about constipation: a new view for the 2020s. *Am J Gastroenterol.* 2020;115(11):1741–1745. doi:10.14309/ajg.0000000000000947

4. Black CJ, Ford AC. Chronic idiopathic constipation in adults: epidemiology, pathophysiology, diagnosis and clinical management. *Med J Aust.* 2018;209(2):86–91. doi:10.5694/mja18.00241
5. Mari A, Mahamid M, Amara H, Baker FA, Yaccob A. Chronic constipation in the elderly patient: updates in evaluation and management. *Korean J Fam Med.* 2020;41(3):139–145. doi:10.4082/kjfm.18.0182
6. Forootan M, Bagheri N, Darvishi M. Chronic constipation: a review of literature. *Medicine (Baltimore).* 2018;97(20):e10631. doi:10.1097/md.0000000000010631
7. McCrea GL, Miaskowski C, Stotts NA, Macera L, Varma MG. Pathophysiology of constipation in the older adult. *World J Gastroenterol.* 2008;14(17):2631–2638. doi:10.3748/wjg.14.2631
8. Dumic I, Nordin T, Jecmenica M, Stojkovic Lalosevic M, Milosavljevic T, Milovanovic T. Gastrointestinal tract disorders in older age. *Can J Gastroenterol Hepatol.* 2019;2019:1–19. doi:10.1155/2019/6757524
9. De Giorgio R, Ruggeri E, Stanghellini V, Eusebi LH, Bazzoli F, Chiarioni G. Chronic constipation in the elderly: a primer for the gastroenterologist. *BMC Gastroenterol.* 2015;15(1). doi:10.1186/s12876-015-0366-3
10. Miller LE, Ibarra A, Ouwehand AC. Normative values for colonic transit time and Patient Assessment of constipation in adults with functional constipation: systematic review with meta-analysis. *Clin Med Insights Gastroenterol.* 2017;10:117955221772934. doi:10.1177/1179552217729343
11. Aziz I, Whitehead WE, Palsson OS, Törnblom H, Simrén M. An approach to the diagnosis and management of Rome IV functional disorders of chronic constipation. *Expert Rev Gastroenterol Hepatol.* 2020;14(1):39–46. doi:10.1080/17474124.2020.170871
12. Sood R, Ford AC. Rome IV criteria for FGIDs — an improvement or more of the same? *Nat Rev Gastroenterol Hepatol.* 2016;13(9):501–502. doi:10.1038/nrgastro.2016.110
13. Nour-Eldein H, Salama H, Abdulmajeed A, Heissam K. The effect of lifestyle modification on severity of constipation and quality of life of elders in nursing homes at Ismailia city, Egypt. *J Family Community Med.* 2014;21(2):100. doi:10.4103/2230-8229.134766
14. Chang L, Chey WD, Imdad A, et al. American Gastroenterological Association–American College of Gastroenterology clinical practice guideline: pharmacological management of chronic idiopathic constipation. *Gastroenterology.* 2023;164(7):1086–1106. doi:10.1053/j.gastro.2023.03.214
15. Fiber. The nutrition source. September 18, 2012. Accessed February 10, 2024. https://nutritionsource.hsph.harvard.edu/carbohydrates/fiber/
16. McRorie JW Jr, McKeown NM. Understanding the physics of functional fibers in the gastrointestinal tract: an evidence-based approach to resolving enduring misconceptions about insoluble and soluble fiber. *J Acad Nutr Diet.* 2017;117(2):251–264. doi:10.1016/j.jand.2016.09.021
17. Concerned about constipation? NIH National Institute on Aging. October 22, 2022. Accessed January 8, 2024. https://www.nia.nih.gov/health/constipation/concerned-about-constipation
18. McDonald D, Hyde E, Debelius JW, et al. American gut: an open platform for citizen science microbiome research. *mSystems.* 2018;3(3). doi:10.1128/msystems.00031-18
19. Katsirma Z, Dimidi E, Rodriguez-Mateos A, Whelan K. Fruits and their impact on the gut microbiota, gut motility and constipation. *Food Funct.* 2021;12(19):8850–8866. doi:10.1039/d1fo01125a
20. Dupont C, Hébert G. Magnesium sulfate-rich natural mineral waters in the treatment of functional constipation–A review. *Nutrients.* 2020;12(7):2052. doi:10.3390/nu12072052
21. Shree Ganesh HR, Subramanya P, Rao M R, Udupa V. Role of yoga therapy in improving digestive health and quality of sleep in an elderly population: a randomized controlled trial. *J Bodyw Mov Ther.* 2021;27:692–697. doi:10.1016/j.jbmt.2021.04.012

22. Naragatti S, Yoga Therapist, Central Council for Research in Yoga and Naturopathy, New Delhi, India. Management of constipation through yogic therapy. *J Adv Res Ayurveda Yoga Unani Sidhha Homeopathy*. 2021;08(1 & 2):18–23. doi:10.24321/2394.6547.202104
23. Nakagawa H, Takeshima T, Ozaka A, et al. Poor sleep quality as a risk factor for constipation among community-dwelling older adults in Japan. *Cureus*. Published online 2023. doi:10.7759/cureus.46175
24. Yun BY, Sim J, Yoon JH, Kim SK. Association between insomnia and constipation: a multicenter three-year cross-sectional study using shift workers' health check-up data. *Saf Health Work*. 2022;13(2):240–247. doi:10.1016/j.shaw.2022.01.001
25. Liu J, Wang W, Tian J, et al. Sleep deficiency is associated with exacerbation of symptoms and impairment of anorectal and autonomic functions in patients with functional constipation. *Front Neurosci*. 2022;16. doi:10.3389/fnins.2022.912442
26. Garling A. 10 Common medications that can affect sleep. www.aarp.org. April 8, 2013. Accessed January 10, 2024.
27. Wu TJ, Wei TS, Chou YH, et al. Whole-body vibration for functional constipation: a single-centre, single-blinded, randomized controlled trial. *Colorectal Dis*. 2012;14(11). doi:10.1111/codi.12021
28. Parajuli A, Hui N, Puhakka R, et al. Yard vegetation is associated with gut microbiota composition. *Sci Total Environ*. 2020;713(136707):136707. doi:10.1016/j.scitotenv.2020.136707
29. White MP, Alcock I, Grellier J, et al. Spending at least 120 minutes a week in nature is associated with good health and wellbeing. *Sci Rep*. 2019;9(1):1–11. doi:10.1038/s41598-019-44097-3
30. Lieber CS. ALCOHOL: its metabolism and interaction with nutrients. *Annu Rev Nutr*. 2000;20(1):395–430. doi:10.1146/annurev.nutr.20.1.395
31. Kimball SR, Lang CH. Mechanisms underlying muscle protein imbalance induced by alcohol. *Annu Rev Nutr*. 2018;38(1):197–217. doi:10.1146/annurev-nutr-071816-064642
32. Bode JC. Alcohol and the gastrointestinal tract. *Ergeb Inn Med Kinderheilkd*. 1980;45:1–75. doi:10.1007/978-3-642-67632-1_1
33. Wegener M, Schaffstein J, Dilger U, Coenen C, Wedmann B, Schmidt G. Gastrointestinal transit of solid-liquid meal in chronic alcoholics. *Dig Dis Sci*. 1991;36(7):917–923. doi:10.1007/bf01297141
34. Bode JC, Bode C, Heidelbach R, Dürr HK, Martini GA. Jejunal microflora in patients with chronic alcohol abuse. *Hepatogastroenterology*. 1984;31(1). Accessed April 8, 2024. https://pubmed.ncbi.nlm.nih.gov/6698486/
35. Bode C, Bode JC. Effect of alcohol consumption on the gut. *Best Pract Res Clin Gastroenterol*. 2003;17(4):575–592. doi:10.1016/s1521-6918(03)00034-9
36. Gnanadesigan N, Fung CH. Quality indicators for screening and prevention in vulnerable elders. *J Am Geriatr Soc*. 2007;55(s2). doi:10.1111/j.1532-5415.2007.01350.x
37. Lehrer S, Rheinstein PH. Constipation and cigarette smoking are independent influences for Parkinson's disease. *Cureus*. Published online 2022. doi:10.7759/cureus.21689
38. Mahyoub MA, Al-Qurmoti S, Rai AA, et al. Adverse physiological effects of smoking cessation on the gastrointestinal tract: a review. *Medicine (Baltimore)*. 2023;102(38):e35124. doi:10.1097/MD.0000000000035124
39. Ueki T, Nakashima M. Relationship between constipation and medication. *J UOEH*. 2019;41(2):145–151. doi:10.7888/juoeh.41.145
40. Naloxegol (Movantik) for Opioid-induced constipation. *JAMA*. 2016;315(2):194. doi:10.1001/jama.2015.17459
41. ROME IV Criteria Booklet. Rome Foundation. March 6, 2023. Accessed February 16, 2024. https://theromefoundation.org/resources/rome-iv-criteria-booklet/

42. Drossman DA, Tack J. Rome Foundation clinical diagnostic criteria for disorders of gut-brain interaction. *Gastroenterology.* 2022;162(3):675–679. doi:10.1053/j.gastro.2021.11.019
43. Schuster BG, Kosar L, Kamrul R. Constipation in older adults: stepwise approach to keep things moving. *Can Fam Physician.* 2015;61(2):152–158.
44. Heidelbaugh J, Martinez de Andino N, Pineles D, Poppers DM. Diagnosing constipation spectrum disorders in a primary care setting. *J Clin Med.* 2021;10(5). doi:10.3390/jcm10051092
45. Bale R. 8 easy ways to get more fiber. AARP. November 21, 2023. Accessed April 8, 2024. https://www.aarp.org/health/healthy-living/info-2023/ways-to-eat-more-fiber.html
46. Koyama T, Nagata N, Nishiura K, Miura N, Kawai T, Yamamoto H. Prune juice containing sorbitol, pectin, and polyphenol ameliorates subjective complaints and hard feces while normalizing stool in chronic constipation: a randomized placebo-controlled trial. *Am J Gastroenterol.* 2022;117(10):1714–1717. doi:10.14309/ajg.0000000000001931
47. Whitbread D. Top 10 foods highest in magnesium. *My Food Data.* July 15, 2009. Accessed April 8, 2024. https://www.myfooddata.com/articles/foods-high-in-magnesium.php
48. Guilliams TG. *Supplementing Dietary Nutrients, A Guide for Healthcare Professionals*, 2nd edn. The Point Institute; 2020. Accessed January 8, 2024. https://www.pointinstitute.org/product/supplementing-dietary-nutrients-second-edition
49. McPherson G. The 6 best natural diuretic foods and drinks, according to a dietitian. *EatingWell.* July 7, 2023. Accessed April 8, 2024. https://www.eatingwell.com/article/8056023/best-natural-diuretic-foods/
50. National Council On Aging. Hydration for older adults – how to stay hydrated for better health. *Ncoa.org.* March 18, 2024. Accessed March 29, 2024. https://www.ncoa.org/article/how-to-stay-hydrated-for-better-health
51. Doğan İG, Gürşen C, Akbayrak T, et al. Abdominal massage in functional chronic constipation: a randomized placebo-controlled trial. *Phys Ther.* 2022;102(7). doi:10.1093/ptj/pzac058
52. Demographic Change. Social isolation and loneliness among older people: advocacy brief. *Who.int.* July 29, 2021. Accessed February 10, 2024. https://www.who.int/publications/i/item/9789240030749

Index

Activities of daily living (ADLs), 7, 18, 106, 168, 185, 209, 220, 264, 304, 328, 329, 383, 390
Adrenergic receptors, 265
Advance care planning (ACP), 7, 303–304, 316
Adverse childhood experiences (ACEs), 18, 19
Adverse drug events (ADEs), 320
Aerobic exercises, 254, 357, 374
Ageism
  with language
    age-based language, 46
    ageist communication patterns, 46, 47
    combat ageism campaign, 48
    disease-centered language, 47
    in health care, 45–46
    hidden curriculum, 48
    stigma around aging, 47
    stigmatizing age-based language, 46
  with lifestyle medicine, 48–49
Alcohol, 19, 20, 25, 27, 36, 122, 127, 156, 159, 160, 165, 167, 178, 191–196, 199–202, 212, 230, 238–241, 251, 258, 271, 274, 277, 284, 292, 295, 307, 309, 324, 325, 346, 347, 350, 354, 359, 360, 368, 375, 376, 392, 395, 396
Alcohol use disorder (AUD), 140, 144, 154, 192, 216, 315, 359
Alpha-blockers, 267
Alzheimer's disease (AD), 24–26, 236, 284
American Cancer Society (ACS), 315
American College of Lifestyle Medicine (ACLM), 3, 21, 81, 118
American Geriatric Society (AGS), 3, 17, 37, 52, 111, 142, 217, 320
American Heart Association (AHA), 307
Angiotensin-converting enzyme (ACE) inhibitors, 268
Angiotensin receptor blockers (ARBs), 268
Anorectal manometry (ARM), 381
Anorexia, 134, 137
Antidepressants, 267, 392
Antihistamines, 97, 271
Antihypertensives, 268, 392
Antipsychotics, 267
Apolipoprotein E (APOE), 305
Atheromas formation, 22
Atherosclerosis, 22, 23

Biomarkers, 284–285, 291

Blue Zones, 118, 348
Body Mass Index (BMI), 27, 134, 143, 296, 353, 354, 359, 361
Brain-derived neurotrophic factor (BDNF), 92, 252–253
Brief Resilient Coping Scale (BRCS), 289, 297
Bristol Stool Scale, 383, 385

Cachexia, 217
Cannabidiol (CBD), 199, 396
Cannabis, 199–202
Cardiovascular disease (CVD), 21–23, 89, 91, 93, 107, 120, 123, 138, 152, 153, 156, 167, 168, 178, 179, 194, 196, 199, 214, 222, 238, 268, 295, 306, 307, 311, 313–315, 321–324, 356
Caregivers
  clinical applications, 337–338
  epidemiology, 328
  health and well-being, 329–330
    engagement, 332, 335
    lifestyle medicine, 331–332
    pathophysiology, 330–331
    physical activity, 334–335
    sleep, 335
    social connectedness, 335–336
    stress management, 336–337
    Zarit Burden Interview, 333
  proactive approach, 337
Centers for Disease Control and Prevention (CDC), 36, 89, 104
Chronic idiopathic constipation (CIC), 382–383
Chronic obstructive pulmonary disease (COPD), 305–306
Chronic sleep deprivation, 323
Chronic urinary retention, 266
Climate change
  environmental degradation, 52
  geriatric medicine, 54–56
  greenhouse gas emissions, 52
  health care system, 52–53
  lifestyle medicine, 56
    avoiding risky substances, 58
    interventions, 57
    nutrition, 57–58
    physical activity, 57
    sleep, 59
    social connection, 60–61
    stress management, 59–60

403

Cognitive behavioral therapy (CBT), 311, 345
Cognitive behavioral therapy for insomnia (CBT-I), 155–158, 255
Cognitive health
    chronic stress and, 234–236
    effect of diet on cognitive health, 229–232
    exercise and, 232–234
    geriatric substance, 237–244
    neurocognitive well-being, 234–235
Cognitive Reserve Unit Scale (CRUS), 284
Comprehensive geriatric assessment (CGA), 6–8, 154, 180
Connor–Davidson Resilience Scale, 287, 289
Constipation
    challenges, 397–398
    clinical applications, 398
    conventional therapies, 386
        fiber, 386–390
    epidemiology, 380–381
    initial evaluation, 383–385
    lifestyle medicine pillars
        nutrition, 390
        risky substances, 395–397
        sleep, 392
        social connection, 394–395
        stress, 391–392
    pathophysiology, 381–383
Cornell Scale for Depression in Dementia (CSDD), 185
Coronary artery disease, 22–24, 152, 321, 354
COVID-19, 56, 80, 162, 282

Definition of Aging, 33–34
    Geriatric 5Ms framework *see* Geriatric 5Ms framework
    pillars of lifestyle medicine, 89–208
        nutrition, 39
        sleep, 39–40
        socialization, 38
Dementia, 25, 47, 138, 143, 184, 185, 229, 230, 232–234, 304
Depression
    clinical considerations, 258–259
    epidemiology of, 248–250
    lifestyle pillars impact of, 253–258
    pathogenesis of, 250–253
Detrusor muscle, 265, 267
Diabetes Prevention Program (DPP), 355
Dietary Approaches to Stop Hypertension (DASH), 230, 231, 293
Diphenhydramine, 152, 345
Diuretics, 268, 347
Do Not Hospitalize (DNH), 303
Do Not Intubate (DNI), 303
Do Not Resuscitate (DNR) orders, 303
Dysphagia, 138, 143

Dyspnea, 306, 309

Endurance training, 343, 344
Enteric nervous system (ENS), 379
Excessive Daytime Sleepiness (EDS), 153
Exercise
    benefits, 90
        cardiovascular systems, 91–92
        endocrine, 93
        falls, 94
        immunological, 92
        metabolism, 93
        musculoskeletal, 92–93
        neurological, 92
        psychological, 93–94
        pulmonary systems, 91–92
Expected recovery differential (ERD), 286, 287

Fall risk-increasing drugs (FRIDs), 320
Falls, 342
    avoidance of harmful substances, 346–348
    clinical applications, 349–350
    environmental hazards, 348
    exercise, 343–344
    nutrition, 344–345
    overview of, 349
    sleep, 345
    social connection, 348
    socioeconomic disparities, 349
    stress management, 346
Fibronectin Type III Domain-Containing Protein 5 (FNDC5), 233
Flexibility training, 343
Food Frequency Questionnaire (FFQ), 322
Frailty, 34, 98, 111–112, 217, 347
Functional incontinence, 266

Gait speed, 37, 219, 220
Generating Engagement in Network Support (GENIE), 314
Genome-Wide Association Studies (GWAS), 285
Geriatric 5Ms framework
    matters most, 7, 11, 28, 35, 38, 296, 298, 303
    medications, 7, 11, 35, 37, 56, 296
    mind, 7, 11, 35–36
    mobility, 7, 12, 36–37, 56, 296, 298
    multicomplexity, 7, 11, 35, 37–38
Geriatric Anxiety Scale, 180
Geriatric primary care
    5Ms model, 73–75
    comprehensive geriatric assessment, 73–75
    integrating lifestyle medicine tools
        community resources, 80
        follow-ups, 80–81
        interdisciplinary team members, 79
        lifestyle prescriptions, 80

metrics review, 81
potential barriers, 81–82
registry, 81
reimbursement, 81
resources, 80
team huddles, 79
lifestyle pillars assessment, 75
lifestyle vital signs, 75–77
shared decision-making, 78
stages of change, 78
physical activity
  barriers, 98–99
  chronic disease, 97–98
  common injuries, 94
  frailty, 98
  injury prevention, 94–96
  medication management, 96–97
  motivations, 98–99
  primary care team, 71–73
Geriatric syndromes, 5, 12, 81, 133
Glucocorticoids, 368
Goals of care (GOC), 9, 63, 143, 303–305, 307, 316
Greenhouse gas emissions, 52–54
Greenhouse Gas Protocol, 53
Gut–brain axis, 293, 391
Gut microbiome, 221, 357, 358

Healthy aging across the lifecycle
  chronic diseases, 18
    Alzheimer's disease, 24–26
    coronary artery disease, 22–24
    hip fractures, 26–28
    osteoporosis, 26–28
  definition of, 17
  glidepaths, 8–9
  lifestyle changes, 19–20
    to address chronic diseases, 21–22
  morbidity compression, 8–9
  motivation, 20–21
  promoting among older adults, 28
  social determinants, 18–19
  successful aging, 8
  three-component model, 17
Healthy People 2030 initiative, 19
Heart failure (HF), 40, 91, 305
Hip fractures, 26–28
HITECH Act of 2009, 80
Homeostasis, 4, 111, 134, 293
Homeostenosis, 4, 34
Hyperglycemia, 215
Hypothalamic–pituitary–adrenal (HPA), 252, 291

Indian Health Services (IHS), 303
Insomnia, 155–158, 255, 309, 311, 345
Insulin-like growth factor-1 (IGF-1), 369

International Exercise Recommendations in Older Adults (ICFSR), 357
Irritable bowel syndrome (IBS), 391

Lancet Commission on Dementia Prevention, Intervention and Care, 24–26
Levatorani, 265, 268
Life expectancy, 6, 8, 9, 40
Lifestyle Medicine Research Summit, 21
Lifestyle vital signs, 75–77

Malnutrition
  causes of, 136–140
  epidemiology of, 134–136
  evaluation of, 140–145
  lifestyle medicine approaches, 133–134
  management of, 140–145
  predictors of, 135
Malnutrition Quality Improvement Initiative (MQII), 141
Medical Orders for Life-Sustaining Treatment (MOLST), 303
Mediterranean–DASH Interventions for Neurocognitive Delay (MIND), 293
Mind–body exercises, 374
Mindfulness-based stress reduction (MBSR), 273, 274, 295, 391
Mini Nutritional Assessment (MNA), 39, 141
Mobility and Vitality Lifestyle Program (MOVE UP), 334
Monoamine neurotransmitters, 250
Multimorbidity, 217, 296
Muscarinic receptors, 265

National Institutes of Health (NIH), 294
Neuroimaging diagnostic tools, 285
Nutrition care
  Blue Zones, 118
  dietary guidelines, 117–118
  dietary supplements, 127–128
  nutrient recommendations and requirements, 118, 120
    alcohol, 122, 127
    antioxidants, 123–124
    carbohydrates, 120
    fats, 120–121
    fiber, 120
    fluids, 121
    folate, 122
    magnesium, 124
    micronutrients, 122
    protein, 121
    sodium, 123
    total energy, 120
    vitamin B6, 122

vitamin B12, 122
vitamin D, 123
zinc, 124
promoting healthy lifestyles, 128–129
promoting nutrition, 128–129
Nutrition-focused physical exam (NFPE), 140

Obesity
  clinical applications, 361–362
  impact of
    avoidance of toxins, 359–360
    lifestyle medicine role, 360–361
    nutrition, 356–357
    physical activity, 357–358
    sleep, 358–359
    social connection, 359
  pathophysiology, 355–356
  rationale, 355–356
Obstructive sleep apnea (OSA), 152, 159, 272
Opioids, 271, 392
Osteoporosis and bone health
  clinical applications, 376
  dietary nutrients
    calcium, 370–371
    fiber, 372
    iron, 371
    phosphorus, 370–371
    protein, 369
    vitamin D, 369–370
    vitamin K, 372
  dietary patterns, 372
    Mediterranean diet, 372
    vegetarian diets, 373
  exercise and bone health
    in healthy adults, 373–374
    lifestyle factors, 375
    with osteopenia/osteoporosis, 374–375
    osteosarcopenia, 375
    public policy, 375
  nutrition, 368–369
  phytoestrogens, 371
  unsaturated fatty acids, 371
Osteoporotic fractures, 152
Osteosarcopenia, 375
Overactive bladder disease (OAB), *see* Urge urinary incontinence
Overflow incontinence, 266
Over-the-counter (OTC), 380
Oxidative stress, 251–252

Palliative care
  advance care planning, 303–304
  cardiac disorders, 305
  chronic health conditions, 304–305
  clinical applications, 316
  epidemiology, 303
  goals of care, 303–304
  lifestyle medicine approaches, 306
    avoidance of risky substances, 314–315
    nutrition, 306–308
    physical activity, 308–309
    sleep, 309, 311
    social connection, 313–314
    stress management, 311–312
  outcomes, 315–316
  performance scale descriptors, 310
  pulmonary disorders, 305–306
Palliative Performance Scale (PPS), 308–309
Pelvic floor muscle training (PFMT), 274–276
Perceived Stress Scale, 179
Periodic Limb Movement Disorder (PLMD), 152, 153
Periodic Limb Movements of Sleep (PLMS), 153
Physical activity and exercise
  in daily life, 106
  and disability, 112
  exercise guidelines, 104–106
  in fall prevention, 109–111
  and frailty, 111–112
  health coaches, 107
  monitors, 108
  nutrition requirements, 108–109
  as part of life, 112
  prescription for older adults, 106
  providers role, 106–107
  social connections, 112
  special considerations, 109
Physical resilience, 285–286
Physical Resilience Instrument for Older Adults (PRIFOR), 286
Physical Resilience Scale (PRS), 286
Physician Orders for Life-Sustaining Treatment (POLST), 303
Plant-based diets, 58, 60, 65, 230, 356, 361, 373
Polypharmacy
  clinical applications, 325
  lifestyle medicine pillars, 321
    avoidance of risky substances, 324–325
    physical activity, 321–322
    sleep, 323
    social connection, 324
    stress management, 323
    whole food plant-based nutrition, 322
  in older adults, 320–321
Polyphenols, 372
Potentially inappropriate medications (PIMs), 320, 322
Potentially inappropriate prescriptions (PIPs), 322
Problem Adaptation Therapy (PATH), 185

Index

Protein-calorie malnutrition, 38–39
Pseudoephedrine, 271

Quality of life (QOL), 302

Racial differences in stress exposure, 177, 178
Randomized controlled trials (RCTs), 253, 254, 308, 394
Rationale for lifestyle medicine in geriatrics
  aging physiological changes, 4
  climate change, 61–64
  comprehensive geriatric assessment (CGA), 6–8
  geriatrics trends, 5–6
  geriatric syndromes, 6
  healthy aging, 8–9
  history of, 3–4
  inter-relationship of, 10–11
  pillars of lifestyle, 11–12
  principles of geriatrics, 12–13
Recommended dietary allowance (RDA), 368
Recovery phenotype, 286, 287
Registered Dietitian Nutritionist (RDN), 118, 121, 128, 129, 140
Resilience
  and aging, 282–283
  characteristics of, 288
  clinical applications, 298
  cognitive, 283–284
    biomarkers, 284–285
    genetic factors, 285
  interventions
    avoidance of risky substances, 295
    exercise, 293–294
    nutrition, 292–293
    physical activity, 293–294
    positive psychology, 295–296
    sleep, 294
    stress management, 295
  optimization of, 296–298
  physical, 285–286
    measurement of, 286–287
  psychological, 289
    biomarkers, 291
    measurement scales, 289–291
    stress-related diseases, 291–292
Resilience Scale™ (RS™), 289
Resistance exercises, 374
Restless Legs Syndrome (RLS), 152
Roux-en-Y gastric bypass (RYGB), 359

SARC-F, 218
Sarcopenia, 37
  coexisting medical, 217
  definition, 209–210
  diagnosis, 217–220
  management, 220–223
  molecular changes, 216
  prevalence of, 210–212
  risk factors, 212–216
Screening Tool of Older Persons' Prescriptions (STOPP), 320
Sedative hypnotics, 268
Sedentary behavior, 89
  physiological effects, 90
Sedentary behaviors, 5, 213, 354
Self-determination theory, 21
Senna, 389
Sensory impairment, 38, 166, 184, 249
Short-chain fatty acids (SCFAs), 230, 372, 387
Sleep-disordered breathing (SDB), 309
Sleep disturbance
  age-related changes in, 150–152
  cognitive behavioral therapy for insomnia (CBT-I), 155–158
  common disorders, 152–153
  comorbid diseases, 159–160
  evaluation of, 153–155
  medications and, 158–159
  older adults, 149–150
  treatment of, 153–155
Sleep latency, 151
SMART goals, 80, 82, 112, 258, 315
Social connection
  barriers to connection, 166–167
  emotional consequences, 167–168
  epidemiology, 163–166
  evaluation, 168–169
  functional consequences, 167–168
  interventions, 169–172
  loneliness, 163
  medical consequences, 167–168
  and social isolation, 163
Social engagement, 335
Social isolation, 5, 18, 25, 26, 36, 38, 110, 121, 139, 144, 154, 162–172, 239, 240, 242, 243, 250, 252, 256, 257, 272, 273, 276, 277, 295, 313, 314, 324, 330, 342, 348, 350, 359, 396
Sorbitol, 387
Stimulus Control Therapy (SCT), 157
Strength training, 343
Stress management
  age-related considerations, 184–187
  approaches to assessment, 179–182
  focus on epidemiology, 177–179
  lifestyle medicine, 183–184
  screening for, 182–183
Stress urinary incontinence (SUI), 266
Substance Abuse and Mental Health Services Administration (SAMHSA), 324
Successful Ageing Evaluation (SAGE), 295, 343

Suppositories, 389
Suprachiasmatic Nucleus (SCN), 152

Tai Chi, 293, 294, 343, 344, 394
Tannins, 274
Telomere length, 4
Tetrahydrocannabinol (THC), 199
Tobacco, 196–199, 347, 396
Toxins
    alcohol, 191–196
    cannabis, 199–202
    tobacco, 196–199

Unsaturated fatty acids, 371
Urge urinary incontinence (UUI), 266
Urinary incontinence (UI)
    clinical applications, 277
    epidemiology, 264
    lifestyle medicine pillars, 271
        avoidance of risky substances, 274
        behavioral approaches, 274–276
        fluid intake, 272
        nutrition, 271
        physical activity, 273
        sleep, 272
        social connectedness, 272–273
        stress management, 273
    mixed incontinence, 266
    pathophysiology, 264–265
    prescribed medications, 267–271
    treatment of, 276–277
    types of, 265–266
US Preventive Services Task Force (USPSTF), 182–183, 369

Vaginal cones, 276
Vaginal estrogen, 268
Veterans Administration (VA), 303

Weight-bearing exercise, 27
Whole food plant-based (WFPB) diets, 305
Whole food plant-predominant diet (WFPPD), 118
World Health Organization (WHO), 33, 40, 133, 302, 353

Yoga, 343, 394

Zarit Burden Interview, 332
Z-hypnotics, 240

Made in the USA
Monee, IL
03 May 2026

49437846R00234